The Measurement of Association

Kenneth J. Berry • Janis E. Johnston •
Paul W. Mielke, Jr.

The Measurement of Association

A Permutation Statistical Approach

Springer

Kenneth J. Berry
Department of Sociology
Colorado State University
Fort Collins
Colorado, USA

Janis E. Johnston
Alexandria
Virginia, USA

Paul W. Mielke, Jr.
Department of Statistics
Colorado State University
Fort Collins
Colorado, USA

ISBN 978-3-319-98925-9 ISBN 978-3-319-98926-6 (eBook)
https://doi.org/10.1007/978-3-319-98926-6

Library of Congress Control Number: 2018954500

Mathematics Subject Classification (2010): 62gxx, 62-07, 62-03, 62axx

This Springer imprint is published by the registered company Springer Nature Switzerland AG
The registered company address is: Gewerbestrasse 11, 6330 Cham, Switzerland

For our families: Nancy T. Berry, Ellen E. Berry, and Laura B. Berry; Lindsay A. Johnston, James B. Johnston, Tayla, Malia, Ollie, Cami, and Brian; and Roberta R. Mielke, William W. Mielke, Emily (Mielke) Spear, and Lynn (Mielke) Basila.

Preface

The Measurement of Association: A Permutation Statistical Approach utilizes exact and Monte Carlo resampling permutation statistical procedures to generate probability values for a variety of measures of association. Association is broadly defined to include measures of correlation for two interval-level variables; association for two nominal-level; two ordinal-level, or two interval-level variables, and agreement for two nominal-level or two ordinal-level variables. Measures of association have historically been constructed for three levels of measurement, i.e., nominal, ordinal, and interval. Additionally, measures of association for mixtures of the three levels of measurement have been considered, i.e., nominal–ordinal, nominal–interval, and ordinal–interval. The book is structured according to the three levels of measurement.

S.S. Stevens promoted the typology of scales containing four levels of measurement: nominal, ordinal, interval, and ratio, but it should be noted that a number of writers have taken exception to the organization of statistical tests and measures by levels of measurement, arguing that there is no relationship between levels of measurement and statistical techniques used, while others have suggested different typologies. Stevens also recognized that a too rigid adoption of his suggested typology could be counterproductive. In this book, the interval and ratio scales are considered together as simply "interval" and the nominal, ordinal, and interval typology is utilized strictly as a pragmatic organizational framework. The 10 chapters of the book provide:

Chapter 1: An introduction to, and the criteria necessary for, creating valid measures of association.

Chapter 2: A description and comparison of two models of statistical inference: the population model and the permutation model. Permutation methods, which are used almost exclusively in this book, are further detailed and illustrated, including exact, moment-approximation, and Monte Carlo resampling permutation methods.

Chapter 3: Presentation, discussion, and examples of measures of association for two nominal-level variables that are based on Pearson's chi-squared test statistic.

Chapter 4: Presentation, discussion, and examples of measures of association for two nominal-level variables that are based on criteria other than Pearson's chi-squared test statistic.
Chapter 5: Presentation, discussion, and examples of measures of association for two ordinal-level variables that are based on pairwise comparisons between rank scores.
Chapter 6: Presentation, discussion, and examples of measures of association for two ordinal-level variables that are based on criteria other than pairwise comparisons between rank scores.
Chapter 7: Presentation, discussion, and examples of measures of association for two interval-level variables.
Chapter 8: Presentation, discussion, and examples of measures of association for two variables at different levels of measurement: nominal–ordinal, nominal–interval, and ordinal–interval.
Chapter 9: Presentation, discussion, and examples of fourfold contingency tables as a special application of measures of association.
Chapter 10: Presentation, discussion, and examples of measures of association applied to symmetrical fourfold contingency tables.

The Measurement of Association adopts a permutation approach for generating exact and resampling probability values for various measures of association. Permutation statistical measures possess several advantages over classical statistical methods in that they are optimal for small samples, can be utilized to analyze nonrandom samples, are completely data dependent, are free of distributional assumptions, and yield exact probability values. Today, permutation statistical tests are considered by many to be a gold standard against which conventional statistical tests should be evaluated and validated. An obvious drawback to permutation statistical methods is the amount of computation required. While it took the advent of high-speed computing to make permutation methods feasible for many problems, today powerful computational algorithms and modern computers make permutation analyses practical for many research applications.

A comparison of two models of statistical inference begins the book: the conventional population model and the permutation statistical model. The population model assumes random sampling from one or more specified populations. Under the population model, the level of statistical significance that results from applying a statistical test to the results of an experiment or survey corresponds to the frequency with which the null hypothesis would be rejected in repeated random samplings from a specified population. Because repeated sampling of the specified population is impractical, it is assumed that the sampling distribution of test statistics generated under repeated random sampling conforms to an approximating theoretical distribution, such as the normal distribution. The size of a statistical test is the probability under the null hypothesis that repeated outcomes based on random samples of the same size are equal to or more extreme than the observed outcome.

In contrast, the permutation model does not assume, nor require, random sampling from a specified population. For the exact permutation model, a test statistic is computed for the observed data. The observations are then permuted over all possible arrangements of the observed data, and the selected test statistic is computed for each of the possible arrangements. The proportion of arrangements with test statistic values equal to or more extreme than the observed test statistic yields the exact probability of the observed test statistic value. When the number of possible arrangements of the observed data is very large, exact permutation methods are impractical and Monte Carlo resampling permutation methods become necessary. Resampling methods generate a random sample of all possible arrangements of the observed data, and the resampling probability value is the proportion of arrangements with test statistic values equal to or more extreme than the value of the observed test statistic.

As described, *vide supra*, this book provides permutation statistical methods for different measures of association for nominal-, ordinal-, and interval-level variables and is organized into 10 chapters.

Chapter 1 defines association in general terms and examines four dimensions of association: symmetry and asymmetry; one- and two-way association; models of association including maximum-corrected, chance-corrected, and proportional-reduction-in-error measures; and measures of correlation, association, and agreement. Chapter 1 concludes with sections on choosing criteria for creating useful measures of association, assessing the strength of association, and selecting an appropriate measure of association.

Chapter 2 compares and contrasts two models of statistical inference: the population model and the permutation model. Under the permutation model, three types of permutation tests are described: exact, Monte Carlo resampling-approximation, and moment-approximation statistical tests. Permutation and parametric statistical tests are compared and contrasted in terms of sample size, data dependency, and the assumptions of random sampling and normality.

Chapter 3 introduces permutation statistical methods for measures of association designed for two nominal-level (categorical) variables. Included in Chap. 3 are the usual chi-squared-based measures, Pearson's ϕ^2, Tschuprov's T^2, Cramér's V^2, and Pearson's contingency coefficient, C. The discussion of the four chi-squared-based measures of association is followed by an analysis of permutation-based goodness-of-fit tests. Chapter 3 concludes with an examination of the relationship between chi-squared and Pearson's product-moment correlation coefficient.

Chapter 4 introduces permutation statistical methods for measures of association designed for two nominal-level variables that are based on criteria other than Pearson's chi-squared test statistic. Included in Chap. 4 are discussions of Goodman and Kruskal's two asymmetric measures of nominal-level association, λ and τ, McNemar's Q and Cochran's Q tests for change, Cohen's unweighted κ measure of inter-rater chance-corrected agreement, the Mantel–Haenszel test of independence for combined 2×2 contingency tables, and Fisher's exact probability test applied to a variety of $r\times c$ contingency tables.

Chapter 5 introduces permutation statistical methods for measures of association designed for ordinal-level variables based on pairwise comparisons between rank scores. Included in Chap. 5 are Kendall's τ_a and τ_b measures, Stuart's τ_c measure,

Goodman and Kruskal's γ measure, Somers' d_{yx} and d_{xy} measures, Kim's $d_{y \cdot x}$ and $d_{x \cdot y}$ measures, Wilson's e measure, Whitfield's S measure of ordinal association between an ordinal-level variable and a binary variable, and Cureton's rank-biserial correlation coefficient.

Chapter 6 introduces permutation statistical methods for measures of association designed for two ordinal-level variables that are based on criteria other than pairwise comparisons between rank scores. Included in Chap. 6 are Spearman's rank-order correlation coefficient, Spearman's footrule measure of inter-rater agreement, Kendall's coefficient of concordance, Kendall's u measure of agreement, Cohen's weighted kappa measure of agreement with both linear and quadratic weighting, and Bross's ridit analysis.

Chapter 7 introduces permutation statistical methods for measures of association designed for interval-level variables. Included in Chap. 7 are simple and multiple ordinary least squares (OLS) and least absolute deviation (LAD) regression using permutation statistical methodology. Fisher's r_{xy} to z transform is described and evaluated as to its utility in transforming skewed distributions for both hypothesis testing and confidence intervals. Point-biserial and biserial correlation are described and tested with exact and Monte Carlo resampling permutation methods. Chapter 7 concludes with a discussion of the intraclass correlation.

Chapter 8 introduces permutation statistical methods for measures of association designed for mixed variables: nominal–ordinal, nominal–interval, and ordinal–interval. Included in Chap. 8 are Freeman's θ, Agresti's $\hat{\delta}$, Piccarreta's $\hat{\tau}$, and Berry and Mielke's $\Re$ for the measurement of nominal–ordinal association. Also, Whitfield's S measure and Cureton's rank-biserial measure for a dichotomous nominal-level variable and an ordinal-level variable are described. For nominal–interval association: Pearson's η^2, Kelley's ϵ^2, and Hays' $\hat{\omega}^2$ are presented. Chapter 8 concludes with a discussion of permutation statistical methods for Jaspen's multiserial correlation coefficient for an ordinal-level variable and an interval-level variable.

Chapter 9 introduces permutation statistical methods for measures of association usually reserved for 2×2 contingency tables. Included in Chap. 9 are discussions of Yule's Q and Yule's Y measures of nominal-level association, Pearson's ϕ^2 measure, simple percentage differences, Goodman and Kruskal's t_a and t_b measures, Somers' d_{yx} and d_{xy} measures, the Mantel–Haenszel test, Fisher's exact probability test, tetrachoric correlation, and the odds ratio.

Chapter 10 continues the discussion of 2×2 contingency tables initiated in Chap. 9 with consideration of symmetrical 2×2 contingency tables. Included in Chap. 10 are permutation statistical methods applied to Pearson's ϕ^2, Tschuprov's T^2, Cramér's V^2, Pearson's product-moment correlation coefficient, Leik and Gove's d_N^c measure, Goodman and Kruskal's t_a and t_b asymmetric measures, Kendall's τ_b and Stuart's τ_c measures, Somers' d_{yx} and d_{xy} asymmetric measures, simple percentage differences, Yule's Y measure of nominal association, and Cohen's unweighted and weighted κ measures of inter-rater chance-corrected agreement.

Acknowledgments. The authors wish to thank the editors and staff at Springer-Verlag. Very special thanks to Dr. Eva Hiripi, Statistics Editor, Springer, who guided the project from beginning to end. We are grateful to Roberta Mielke who read the entire manuscript. Finally, we wish to thank Steve and Linda Jones, proprietors of the Rainbow Restaurant, 212 West Laurel Street, Fort Collins, Colorado, for their gracious hospitality. Like our previous books, much of this book was written at Table 22 in their restaurant adjacent to the Colorado State University campus.

Fort Collins, CO, USA — Kenneth J. Berry
Alexandria, VA, USA — Janis E. Johnston
Fort Collins, CO, USA — Paul W. Mielke, Jr.
August 2017

Contents

Chapter 1
Introduction

The focus of this research monograph on *The Measurement of Association* is a permutation approach to the measurement of statistical association, broadly defined to include measures of correlation, association, and agreement. As sociologist Herbert Costner wrote in 1965:

> We suffer an embarrassment of riches with regard to measures of association. Ranging from product-moment correlation to a simple percentage difference in a fourfold table, so many measures have been designed to represent the degree of association between two variables that few [researchers] would pretend detailed knowledge of them all.... It is frequently difficult to decide which specific measure is suited to one's needs, and even more difficult to interpret certain measures that do appear appropriate [7, p. 341].

While a plethora of methods exist for measuring the magnitude of association between two variables, there is considerable difficulty in interpreting and comparing the various measures, as they often differ in structure, logic, and interpretation. Moreover, how can a responsible researcher choose, for example, from among Pearson's[1] coefficient of mean-square contingency ϕ^2, Yule's Q, Yule's coefficient of colligation Y, Pearson's tetrachoric r, McNemar's Q test, or a simple percentage difference for a 2×2 contingency table; among Pearson's coefficient of contingency C, Tschuprov's T^2, Cramér's V^2, Goodman and Kruskal's t_a and t_b, or Goodman and Kruskal's λ_a and λ_b for larger categorical contingency tables; Goodman and Kruskal's γ, Somers' d_{yx} and d_{xy}, or Spearman's rank-order correlation coefficient ρ for rank scores; Pearson's product-moment r_{xy}, biserial r_b, point-biserial r_{pb}, or Cureton's rank-biserial r_{rb} for measuring correlation; or Scott's π, Robinson's A, Spearman's footrule, Kendall's u coefficient, Cohen's unweighted kappa, Cohen's weighted kappa with linear weighting, or Cohen's weighted kappa with quadratic weighting for the measurement of inter-rater agreement?

[1]There are two prominent statisticians with the surname Pearson: Karl Pearson, the father, and Egon S. Pearson, the son. Unless specified otherwise, in this book "Pearson" refers to Karl Pearson (1857–1936).

K. J. Berry et al., *The Measurement of Association*,
https://doi.org/10.1007/978-3-319-98926-6_1

The organization of *The Measurement of Association* is based on three levels of measurement: nominal, ordinal, and interval/ratio. A number of writers have taken exception to the organization of statistical tests and measures by levels of measurement. Gaito, for example, argued that there is no relationship between levels of measurement and which statistical techniques are used [11, p. 564]. Mosteller and Tukey suggested that a sixfold typology based on grades, ranks, counted fractions, counts, amounts, and balances would be more useful [22]. See also discussions by Borgatta and Bornstedt [5], Lord [18], Luce, Krantz, Suppes, and Tversky [19], and Vellman and Wilkinson [27]. S.S. Stevens, who originated the typology of scales containing four levels of measurement in 1946, recognized that an inflexible invocation of that typology would be counterproductive [25, p. 26]. In this book, the nominal, ordinal, interval/ratio typology is utilized simply as a pragmatic organizational framework.

As Leik and Gove noted many years ago, when data progress from nominal to ordinal to interval levels of measurement, measures of association should ideally incorporate the added properties of the level of measurement into the logic utilized at the previous level [16, p. 279]. Unfortunately, such is not the case with the numerous and diverse measures of association currently in use. Thus, the various measures of association developed over the years constitute a hodgepodge of approaches, logic, structure, and interpretation. It is convenient to categorize the various measures of association by the level of measurement for which they were originally designed and for which they are most appropriate, recognizing that some measures are suitable for more than one level of measurement, especially the many measures originally designed for the analysis of 2×2 contingency tables where the level of measurement is often irrelevant.

Besides consideration of structure, logic, and interpretation, a major drawback to measures of association is the determination of the probability of the obtained measure under the null hypothesis. There are two major approaches to determining probability values for measures of association: the Neyman–Pearson population model and the Fisher–Pitman permutation model [4, pp. 2–3].[2] The population model is rife with assumptions that are seldom satisfied in practice and are often inappropriate for the lower levels of measurement, e.g., independence, random sampling from a parent population, an underlying Gaussian distribution for the target variable in the population, and homogeneity of variance (and covariance, when appropriate). In this book, the permutation model is used almost exclusively as it is free of any distributional assumptions, does not require random sampling, is completely data-dependent, provides exact probability values, and is ideally suited for the analysis of small samples.

[2]The Neyman–Pearson population model is named for Jerzy Neyman (1894–1981) and Egon Pearson (1895–1980) and the Fisher–Pitman permutation model is named for Ronald Aylmer Fisher (1890–1962) and Edward James George Pitman (1897–1993).

1.1 Definition of Measurement

Given that the title of the book is *The Measurement of Association*, it bodes well to define "measurement" and "association." George Bornstedt put it simply: "Measurement is a *sine qua non* of any science" [6, p. 69]. Praveen Fernandes argued: "If something is not counted, it is neither seen nor understood. For all intents and purposes, it does not exist" [10, p. A25]. In the late 19th century, the eminent Scottish mathematician and physicist William Thomson, Lord Kelvin of Largs, delivered a lecture at the Institution of Civil Engineers on 3 May 1883, later published in *Popular Lectures and Addresses*, in which he wrote:

> I often say that when you can measure what you are speaking about, and express it in numbers, you know something about it; but when you cannot measure it, when you cannot express it in numbers, your knowledge is of a meagre and unsatisfactory kind: it may be the beginning of knowledge, but you have scarcely, in your thoughts, advanced to the stage of science whatever the matter might be [26, pp. 73–74].

Ian Mortimer, writing on the Restoration period in England (1660–1700), noted:

> Perhaps the most significant shift of thinking connected with all this scientific work is the belief that everything can be subject to quantification. Newton can mathematically determine the depth of a film of air between a lens and a flat sheet of glass to the accuracy of 1/100,000 of an inch; Robert Boyle can calculate the relationship between the volume and pressure of a gas; Flamsteed the progress of comets; Halley the life expectancy of the population; and so on. ... You don't need to be a scientist to see how much the modern world owes to the rise of statistical thinking in the Restoration period: it underpins all the technological and social progress on which we depend [21, pp. 138–139].

As the discipline of statistics has progressed from its earliest days, the discipline has become increasingly concerned with quantification as a means of describing events. Florence Nightingale once observed:

> To understand God's thoughts we must study statistics, for these are the measure of His purpose.

(quoted in Everitt, *Chance Rules: An Informal Guide to Probability, Risk, and Statistics* [9, p. 135]).

Precise descriptions of events and the relationships among them are best achieved by measurement. Measurement has been a fundamental feature of human civilization from its very beginnings. Thus, measurement is the application of mathematics to events—the use of numbers to designate objects and events and the relationships that obtain among them [8, p. 39]. More formally, measurement is the process of mapping empirical phenomena onto a system of numbers.

As noted, *vide supra*, in 1946 S.S. Stevens distinguished four levels or scales of measurement: nominal, ordinal, interval, and ratio [24].[3] The *nominal* level of measurement does not measure quantities; it simply classifies events into a number of unordered categories and those events with characteristics in common are grouped together. Examples of nominal classifications are Gender (Female, Male), Blood Type (A, B, AB, O), Political Affiliation (Democrat, Republican, Libertarian, Green, Independent), and Marital Status (Single, Married, Widowed, Divorced, Separated).

The essence of the *ordinal* level of measurement is that it employs the characteristics of "greater than" (>) or "less than" (<). The relations (>) and (<) are irreflexive, asymmetrical, and transitive. Irreflexivity is the logical property that for any a, it is not true that $a > a$. Asymmetry simply means that if $a > b$, then $b \not> a$. Transitivity means that if $a > b$ and $b > c$, then $a > c$. Examples of ordinal scales are Birth Order (1st, 2nd, 3rd, ...), Academic Rank (Instructor, Assistant Professor, Associate Professor, Professor), and Likert Scales (Strongly Agree, Agree, Neutral, Disagree, Strongly Disagree). Steven's measurement typology of nominal, ordinal, interval, and ratio levels is itself an ordinal scale.

Interval-level scales introduce another dimension to the measurement process and order the events on equally appearing intervals. In interval scales, there is no absolute zero point—if there is a value of zero, then zero is arbitrarily defined. Temperatures measured as degrees Fahrenheit or Centigrade are traditional examples of interval measurement. When, in 1714, the German physicist Daniel Gabriel Fahrenheit observed that equal amounts (by weight) of pure table salt and distilled water froze at sea level, he marked it zero, and thirty-eight years later when Anders Celsius, the Swedish astronomer, observed that distilled water froze at sea level, he marked it zero. Thus, 0°F and 0°C are arbitrarily defined. Because there is no absolute zero value, proper ratios cannot be formed; thus, 20°C cannot be said to be twice as warm as 10°C.

Ratio-level scales are scales that not only incorporate all the characteristics of an interval scale, but have absolute zero points, allowing for the construction of meaningful ratios. Examples of interval scales are time, age, years of education, and height. Thus, a person who is six feet tall is twice as tall as a person who is three feet tall, and a person who is twenty years old is twice as old as a person who is ten years old. In terms of temperature, 200 Kelvins is twice as warm as 100 Kelvins because 0 Kelvins is absolute zero (−273.15°C or −459.67°F), defined as the absence of molecular motion.[4] Statistically, interval- and ratio-level measurements are usually treated together and, in general, simply referred to as interval-level measurements.

[3]Other typologies of scales of measurement exist. See, for example, those by Anderson, Balilevsky, and Hum [2], Mosteller and Tukey [22], and Pfanzagl [23].

[4]Kelvins are named for Scottish physicist William Thomson, Lord Kelvin of Largs (1866–1892).

1.2 Definition of Association

While there are many ways of defining association, perhaps the simplest and most useful definition is:

> Two variables are associated when the distribution of values of one variable differs for different values of the other variable.

Moreover, if a change in the distribution of values of one variable does not result in a change in the distribution of values in the other variable, the variables are said to be *independent* of each other. It should be noted that nearly every discussion of association implies a comparison of subgroups. So, alternatively, independence holds when subgroups of variables do not differ, and when subgroups do differ, association holds. Tables 1.1 and 1.2 illustrate independence and association, respectively, for two ordinal-level variables: Occupation Level and Job Satisfaction. For example, the cell frequencies in Table 1.1 are those expected under randomness and a measure of association such as Goodman and Kruskal's gamma measure of ordinal association is $\gamma = 0.00$. In contrast, the cell frequencies in Table 1.2 differ from those expected under randomness and for the data given in Table 1.2, $\gamma = +0.1921$.

Table 1.1 Job satisfaction within middle-class occupations, illustrating statistical independence

	Satisfied		Dissatisfied		Total	
Occupation	Number	Percent	Number	Percent	Number	Percent
Professionals	21	78	6	22	27	100
Managers	21	78	6	22	27	100
Salesmen	14	78	4	22	18	100
Total	56	78	16	22	72	100

Table 1.2 Job satisfaction within middle-class occupations, illustrating statistical association

	Satisfied		Dissatisfied		Total	
Occupation	Number	Percent	Number	Percent	Number	Percent
Professionals	24	90	3	10	27	100
Managers	17	63	10	37	27	100
Salesmen	15	83	3	17	18	100
Total	56	78	16	22	72	100

1.3 Dimensions of Association

There are several dimensions to be considered when measuring association. First and foremost, measures of association have historically been constructed for different levels of measurement: nominal-level (categorical), ordinal-level (ranked), and interval-level variables [17, p. 86]. Also, in a few cases, mixtures of the three levels of measurement are considered: nominal- and ordinal-level, nominal- and interval-level, and ordinal- and interval-level variables.

Examples of nominal-level measures of association include, but are not limited to, the symmetric chi-squared-based measures such as Pearson's ϕ^2, Tschuprov's (Čhuprov's) T^2, Cramér's V^2, and Pearson's C, as well as Goodman and Kruskal's asymmetric t_a and t_b measures and Cohen's unweighted kappa (κ) coefficient of agreement. Examples of ordinal-level measures of association include Cohen's weighted kappa (κ_w) measure of agreement, Goodman and Kruskal's gamma (γ) measure of weakly monotonic ordinal association, Spearman's rank-order correlation coefficient (ρ), Kendall's asymmetric (τ_a and τ_b) measures of ordinal association, and Somers' d_{yx} and d_{xy} asymmetric measures of ordinal association. Examples of interval-level measures of association include Pearson's product-moment (interclass) correlation coefficient (r_{xy} or r_{xy}^2) and Pearson's intraclass correlation coefficient (r_I or r_I^2). Examples of mixed-level measures include Freeman's θ for one nominal-level variable and one ordinal-level variable, Cureton's rank-biserial measure for one binary variable and one ordinal-level variable, Jaspen's multiserial correlation coefficient for one ordinal-level variable and one interval-level variable, and Pearson's η^2 for one nominal-level variable and one interval-level variable.[5]

1.3.1 Symmetry and Asymmetry

Second, a measure of association may be asymmetric, with well-defined independent and dependent variables, yielding two indices of the strength of association depending on which variable is considered to be the dependent variable. Or a measure of association may be symmetric, without a specified independent or dependent variable, yielding a single index of the strength of association. Examples of asymmetric measures of association include simple percentage differences, Goodman and Kruskal's t_a and t_b measures of nominal association, Kendall's τ_a and τ_b measures of ordinal association, and Somers' d_{yx} and d_{xy} measures of ordinal association. Examples of symmetric measures of association include the chi-squared-based measures for nominal-level variables such as Pearson's ϕ^2,

[5]The correlation ratio, η^2, was first described by Karl Pearson in 1911 and 1923 and later by R.A. Fisher in 1925.

Tschuprov's T^2, Cramér's V^2, and Pearson's C; measures of ordinal association such as Goodman and Kruskal's gamma and Spearman's rank-order correlation; and measures of correlation between two interval-level variables such as Pearson's product-moment correlation coefficient.

1.3.2 *One-Way and Two-Way Association*

Third, measures of association may quantify one-way association between variables based on the extent to which one variable implies the other, but not vice versa. On the other hand, two-way or mutual association refers to the extent to which the two variables imply each other. All asymmetric measures are measures of one-way association, and some symmetric measures are measures of one-way association. An example of one-way association is the simple percentage difference. Examples of mutual association include the standard chi-squared-based measures: Pearson's ϕ^2, Tschuprov's T^2, Cramér's V^2, and Pearson's C.

1.3.3 *Models of Interpretation*

Fourth, measures of association are variously based on different models, including maximum-corrected (MC), chance-corrected (CC), and proportional-reduction-in-error (PRE) models. While these models are neither exhaustive nor mutually exclusive, the taxonomy provides an important classification scheme. Examples of maximum-corrected measures of association include Pearson's ϕ^2, Tschuprov's T^2, Cramér's V^2, and Pearson's C.[6] Examples of chance-corrected measures of association include Scott's π measure of agreement, Robinson's A measure, Spearman's footrule measure, Kendall's u coefficient, and Cohen's unweighted and weighted kappa coefficients, κ and κ_w. Examples of proportional-reduction-in-error measures of association include Goodman and Kruskal's λ_a and λ_b measures of nominal association and Goodman and Kruskal's γ measure of ordinal association.

1.3.4 *Cross-Classification*

Fifth, measures of association have historically been constructed for data cross-classified into contingency tables or, alternatively, simple bivariate lists of response measurements. In addition, some measures are typically calculated both ways.

[6] Technically, Pearson's ϕ^2, Tschuprov's T^2, Cramér's V^2, and Pearson's C are maximum-corrected measures of association under only certain highly restrictive conditions.

Examples of measures of association for data organized into contingency tables include Cohen's unweighted and weighted kappa coefficients, κ and κ_w, and the usual chi-squared-based measures, including Pearson's ϕ^2, Tschuprov's T^2, Cramér's V^2, and Pearson's C. Examples of measures of association for data not organized into a contingency table include Kendall τ_a measure of ordinal-level association, Cochran's Q test for change, Spearman's rank-order correlation coefficient, and Pearson's product-moment correlation coefficient. Examples of measures of association that are often calculated both ways include Kendall's τ_a and τ_b measures of ordinal association, Whitfield's S measure for one binary and one ordinal-level variable, and Goodman and Kruskal's γ measure of ordinal association.

1.3.5 Correlation, Association, and Agreement

Sixth, measures of association may variously measure correlation, association, or agreement. Many writers have tried to distinguish between the concepts of correlation and association. There are two domains corresponding to the term "association." The wider domain includes all types of measures of association between two variables at all levels of measurement. The narrower domain is reserved for those measures specifically designed to measure the degree of relationship between two variables at the nominal and ordinal levels of measurement. Thus, association is used in two ways in this book. First, as an over-arching concept including measures of correlation, association, and agreement. Second, association is used more specifically as a measure of relationship between two nominal-level variables, two ordinal-level variables, or some combination of the two. Measures of association often label the two variables as A and B or a and b. Examples of measures of association include Goodman and Kruskal's λ_a and λ_b measures of nominal association, Kendall's τ_a and τ_b measures of ordinal association, and various chi-squared-based measures such as Pearson's ϕ^2, Tschuprov's T^2, Cramér's V^2, and Pearson's C.

In general, correlation usually refers to the class of measures of covariation derived from regression equations based on the method of ordinary least squares (OLS). An obvious exception is least-absolute-deviation (LAD) regression, which is based on ordinary Euclidean differences between measurements. Often, but not always, simple correlation measures the relationship between two variables at the interval level of measurement, where the two variables are typically labeled as X and Y or x and y. Exceptions are Spearman's rank-order correlation coefficient for two ordinal-level variables, Pearson's ϕ^2 for two binary variables, biserial and point-biserial correlation for one binary variable and one interval-level variable, Pearson's tetrachoric correlation for two binary variables, Cureton's rank-biserial correlation for one binary variable and one ordinal-level variable, and Jaspen's multiserial correlation for one ordinal-level variable and one interval-level variable.

Measures of agreement attempt to ascertain the identity of two variables at any level of measurement, i.e., $X_i = Y_i$ or $A_i = B_i$ for all i. Examples of measures of agreement include Scott's π measure of agreement, Robinson's A measure, Spearman's footrule measure, and Cohen's unweighted and weighted kappa coefficients. It is common that agreement and correlation are confused. Suppose that a researcher wishes to establish the relationship between observed and regression-predicted values, y and $\hat{y}$, respectively. Agreement implies that the functional relationship between y and $\hat{y}$ can be described by a straight line that passes through the origin with a slope of 45°, as depicted in Fig. 1.1 with $N = 5$ bivariate $(y, \hat{y})$ values: $(2, 2)$, $(4, 4)$, $(6, 6)$, $(8, 8)$, and $(10, 10)$. For the $N = 5$ data points depicted in Fig. 1.1, the intercept is $\hat{\beta}_0 = 0.00$, the unstandardized slope is $\hat{\beta}_1 = +1.00$, the squared Pearson product-moment correlation coefficient is $r^2_{y\hat{y}} = +1.00$, and the agreement percentage is 100 %, i.e., all five of the y and $\hat{y}$ paired values are in agreement.

In this context, the squared Pearson product-moment correlation coefficient, $r^2_{y\hat{y}}$, has also been used as a measure of agreement. However, $r^2_{y\hat{y}} = +1.00$ implies a linear relationship between y and $\hat{y}$, where both the intercept and slope are arbitrary. Thus, while perfect agreement is described by a value of +1.00, it is also true that $r^2_{y\hat{y}} = +1.00$ describes a linear relationship that may or may not reflect perfect agreement as depicted in Fig. 1.2 with $N = 5$ $(y, \hat{y})$ values: $(2, 4)$, $(4, 5)$, $(6, 6)$, $(8, 7)$, and $(10, 8)$. For the $N = 5$ bivariate data points depicted in Fig. 1.2, the intercept is $\hat{\beta}_0 = +3.00$, the unstandardized slope is $\hat{\beta}_1 = +0.50$, the squared Pearson product-moment correlation coefficient is $r^2_{y\hat{y}} = +1.00$, and the agreement percentage is 20 %, i.e., only one $(6, 6)$ of the $N = 5$ y and $\hat{y}$ paired values agree.

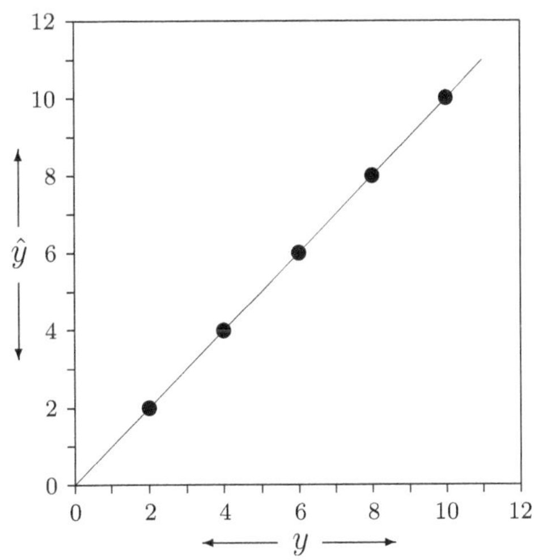

Fig. 1.1 Graphic depicting a regression line with perfect agreement between y and $\hat{y}$ with intercept equal to 0.00 and slope equal to +1.00

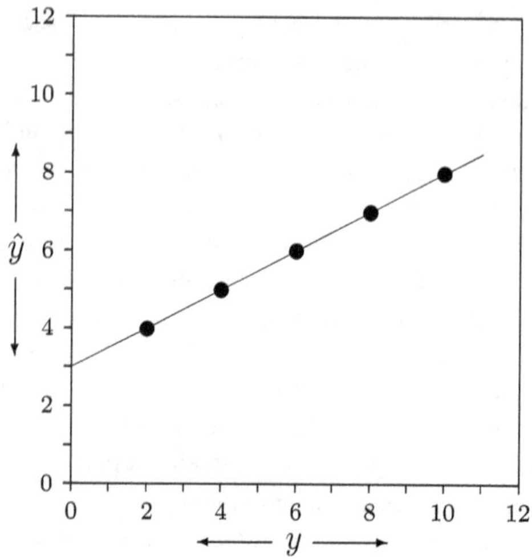

Fig. 1.2 Graphic depicting a regression line with perfect correlation between y and $\hat{y}$ with intercept equal to +3.00 and slope equal to +0.50

1.4 Criteria for Measures of Association

A number of researchers have written on important criteria for measures of association, most notably Costner [7] and Goodman and Kruskal [12, 13, 14, 15]. However, this section relies primarily on a discussion by Weiss [28, pp. 179–180]. Important criteria for measures of association include proper norming, interpretation, independence from marginal frequencies, and magnitude (degree or strength) of association.

Norming Ideally, the values of a measure of association should cover the same range as probability values, i.e., 0 to 1. Moreover, the measure of association should be zero when the variables are independent and one when there is perfect association. When it is appropriate to consider inverse association, then minus one should represent perfect negative association. The measures of association based on chi-squared—Pearson's ϕ^2, Tschuprov's T^2, Cramér's V^2, and Pearson's C—often do not have one as an upper bound, and the odds ratio has an upper bound of infinity. In addition, some proportional-reduction-in-error measures of association, such as Goodman and Kruskal's λ_a and λ_b, can be zero even when the two variables under consideration are not independent of each other.

Interpretation A measure of association should have a meaningful interpretation, such as proportional reduction in probable error, proportion of variance explained, or proportion above what would be expected by chance. Many measures of association are notably lacking in this regard. Indeed, many measures permit no interpretation except that a higher value indicates more association than a lower value, and even that is often questionable. The traditional measures based on chi-squared—Pearson's ϕ^2, Tschuprov's T^2, Cramér's V^2, and Pearson's C—are notably lacking in meaningful interpretation, except for the terminal values 0 and 1.

Independence from Marginal Frequencies Ideally, a measure of association should not change with an increase (decrease) in row or column frequency totals; that is, the measure of association should be independent of the marginal frequency totals. Some measures of association have this property, such as percentage differences and the odds ratio, but many others do not.

Degree of Association The values of a measure of association should increase (decrease) with increasing (decreasing) degrees of association. Thus, when the cell frequencies of a contingency table indicate changes in association, the measure of association should change concomitantly. Although proportionate-reduction-in-error measures of association, such as Goodman and Kruskal's γ measure of ordinal association and Somers' d_{yx} and d_{xy} asymmetric measures of ordinal association, are widely popular, they are somewhat dubious in this respect [28, p. 179]. In this regard, see also a 1971 article by Thomas Wilson in *Social Forces* on "Critique of ordinal variables" [29, pp. 438–439].

1.5 Degree of Association

Different measures of association assess the degree of association in a variety of ways. Among the various ways of measuring the strength of association are departure from independence, magnitude of subgroup differences, pairwise comparisons, incremental correspondence, and agreement.

Departure from Independence Measures of association that are based on departure from independence posit what the data would look like if the two variables were independent, i.e., there was no association, then measure the extent to which the observed data depart from independence. Examples of measures of association based on departure from independence include the chi-squared-based measures such as Pearson's ϕ^2, Tschuprov's T^2, Cramér's V^2, and Pearson's C, as well as others, not based on chi-squared, such as Goodman and Kruskal's λ_a, λ_b, t_a, and t_b measures of nominal association.

Magnitude of Subgroup Differences Given that some association exists, the degree of association may be measured by comparing subgroup proportions. Examples of measures of association based on subgroup differences are simple percentage differences, as well as a number of other measures designed for 2×2 contingency tables, including Yule's Q and Y measures of association and the odds ratio.

Pairwise Comparisons Some measures of association are based on pairwise comparisons where differences between response measurements are calculated between all possible pairs of measurements and divided into concordant and discordant pairs. A concordant pair is one in which the direction of a paired difference in one variable agrees with the direction of a paired difference in the second variable. A discordant pair is one in which the direction of a paired difference in one variable disagrees with the direction of a paired difference in the second variable. The degree of association is measured by the preponderance of one type of pair over the other. Examples of pairwise measures of ordinal association include Kendall's τ_a and τ_b measures, Stuart's τ_c measure, Goodman and Kruskal's γ measure of ordinal association, and Somers' d_{yx} and d_{xy} asymmetric measures of ordinal association.

Incremental Correspondence The degree of association is based on the extent to which an incremental increase (decrease) in one variable is accompanied by an increase (decrease) in the other variable. This approach is conventionally termed "correlation" rather than "association." A prime example is Pearson's product-moment correlation coefficient.

Agreement Between Variables The degree of association is measured by the extent to which the values in one variable disagree with the values in the other variable, above that expected by chance alone. Examples of measures of association based on agreement include Scott's π measure of agreement, Robinson's A measure, Spearman's footrule measure, Kendall's u coefficient, and Cohen's unweighted and weighted kappa measures, κ and κ_w.

1.6 The Choice of a Measure of Association

When selecting an appropriate measure of association, several criteria should be considered. In order to choose the correct measure of association, a researcher must first determine if the data are nominal, ordinal, or interval, which is the primary organizing theme of this book.[7] Second, a researcher should consider the purpose for the measure of association: prediction, agreement, association, or correlation. Liebetrau provides some guidelines for selecting an appropriate measure [17, pp. 86–88].

First, are the variables nominal, ordinal, interval, or some combination of the three? A measure of association for nominal-level (categorical) variables should not depend on ordered categories. On the other hand, a measure of association for ordinal-level (ranked) variables should depend on ordered categories. If the order of the categories is ignored, then information is lost. Moreover, squaring of differences between ordered categories or ranks is still controversial and should be avoided. A measure of association (correlation) for interval-level variables should ideally make use of all the information contained in the data. The choice between ordinary least squared (OLS) and least absolute deviation (LAD) regression and correlation may depend on, among other considerations, the presence of extreme values.

Second, is the measure designed to measure correlation, association, or agreement? In general, asymmetric measures are appropriate for prediction, while symmetric measures are appropriate for association or correlation, depending on the

[7] For a somewhat different organization using nominal, ordinal, and interval scales, see a 1983 book by A.M. Liebetrau on non-permutation *Measures of Association*.

level of measurement. If agreement is the intended objective where the variables are evaluated on their identity rather than some function among them, an appropriate measure of inter-rater agreement should be adopted. Commonly used measures of correlation include Pearson's product-moment correlation coefficient, Pearson's intraclass correlation coefficient, Spearman's rank-order correlation coefficient, Pearson's tetrachoric correlation coefficient, and Jaspen's multiserial correlation coefficient. Measures of association include the chi-squared-based measures such as Pearson's ϕ^2, Tschuprov's T^2, and Cramér's V^2 for nominal-level variables and Kendall's τ_a and τ_b measures for ordinal-level variables. Measures of agreement include Scott's π, Robinson's A, Spearman's footrule, Cohen's κ, and Kendall's u measures of inter-rater agreement.

Third, is the measure of association going to be used to make inferences, i.e., a probability value? Under the Neyman–Pearson population model, this requires knowledge of the standard error of the estimator and often requires making assumptions about the nature of the population as well as random sampling. Under the Fisher–Pitman permutation model, no knowledge of the standard error is required, random sampling is not necessary, distributional assumptions are irrelevant, and permutation tests are completely data-dependent. Permutation-based probability values may be exact, based on the entire reference set of all possible permutations of the observed data, or approximate, based on a large Monte Carlo random sample drawn from the reference set. Modern computing, even on a small desktop or a laptop computer, can easily generate a complete reference set of 100,000,000 values in just a few minutes, making exact permutation statistical methods increasingly popular.

Fourth, is the measure of association sensitive to marginal frequency totals? If the measure of association is unaltered by multiplying or dividing either or both the columns or rows of the contingency table by any arbitrary factor, then this is a very important property of the measure, as noted by Yule in 1912 [30, p. 587]. In general, values of a measure of association computed on two different samples cannot be compared if the measure depends on the marginal frequency totals [17, p. 88]. Nearly, all measures of association for nominal-level and ordinal-level variables are sensitive to changes in marginal frequency totals. Some notable exceptions are the odds ratio, percentage differences, and Yule's Q measure of association.

Fifth, is the measure of association stable under changes in the number of categories? A stable measure of association is one in which the value does not change when, for example, the number of categories is changed from five to four. Goodman and Kruskal's gamma measure of ordinal association is particularly unstable while Kendall's τ_b measure of ordinal association is relatively stable. Another form of stability is when a measure computed on a number of disjoint, ordered categories is similar to the value computed on the underlying continuous variable before it was divided into ordered categories, as noted by Agresti [1, p. 49].

Sixth, is the value of the measure of association easily interpretable? Some measures of association have clear and meaningful interpretations, such as proportional-reduction-in-error measures and chance-corrected measures. Other measures have no meaningful interpretation except when they possess the terminal values of 0, +1, or -1. For example, Goodman and Kruskal's gamma symmetric measure of ordinal association and Somers' d_{yx} and d_{xy} asymmetric measures of ordinal association possess proportional-reduction-in-error interpretations, where positive values indicate proportional improvement over guessing prediction errors with knowledge of both variables, compared with guessing prediction errors with knowledge of one variable only. Cohen's unweighted kappa and weighted kappa measures of inter-rater agreement and Spearman's footrule possess chance-corrected interpretations, where positive values indicate agreement above what is expected by chance, zero indicates chance agreement, and negative values indicate agreement below what is expected by chance. In general, measures of association based on Pearson's chi-squared test statistic have meaningful interpretations only when they possess values of 0 or 1.

Seventh, does the measure of association accommodate tied values? Some measures of association require complicated adjustments in order to accommodate tied values, while others incorporate tied values with no adjustment. For example, Spearman's rank-order correlation coefficient, as originally developed in 1904, required complex adjustments for tied values. Today, researchers are knowledgeable enough to simply calculate Pearson's product-moment correlation coefficient on the observed ranks, which automatically adjusts for any tied values. However, there are numerous other measures of association that require convoluted adjustments for tied values, some of which are highly questionable.

Eighth, will the measure of association easily generalize to multivariate data structures? Multivariate analysis has become increasingly important in contemporary research, so measures of association that will accommodate multivariate data are extremely useful. Some measures are easily generalized to multivariate structures, others are more difficult to generalize, and some are impossible. For years, researchers attempted to generalize Cohen's kappa measure of inter-rater agreement to more than two raters. Each time the generalization was found to have problems. Finally, in 2008 a solution was found and Cohen's kappa can now handle any number of judges with any type of weighting function [20]. Another example is Spearman's footrule measure of ordinal association. Developed in 1906 for two sets of rankings, a generalization to multiple rankings was finally established 92 years later in 1998 [3].

Ninth, for what type of association does the measure of association assume its extreme value? Some measures of association assume their extreme values, e.g., $+1$ in cases of weak association. For example, Goodman and Kruskal's gamma statistic is a measure of weakly monotonic association, reaching $+1$ under a variety of cell frequency configurations. Other measures of association assume their extreme values only in the case of strict perfect association. For example, Kendall's τ_b measure of ordinal association assumes a value of $+1$ only when strongly monotonic association is present, e.g., when all cell frequencies fall on the principal diagonal.

Tenth, is the measure of association easy to calculate? Some measures of association are notoriously difficult to calculate. One of the most difficult is Pearson's tetrachoric correlation measure for $2{\times}2$ contingency tables. Another is Leik and Gove's d_N^c measure of nominal association. Any measure employing a "sharper bounds" procedure requires complex algorithms and considerable computer time.

On the other hand, Spearman's footrule measure was specifically designed for ease of calculation and most measures of association based on chi-squared require very little effort to calculate.

1.7 Overview of Chaps. 2 Through 10

Chapter 2 describes and compares two models of statistical inference: the population model and the permutation model. Permutation methods are further detailed and illustrated, including exact, moment-approximation, and Monte Carlo resampling-approximation approaches. A number of limitations of the population statistical model are described, including the requirements of random sampling and the assumption of normality, as well as difficulties with the analysis of small sample sizes. The permutation statistical model is shown to require neither random sampling nor normality and is demonstrated to be ideal for small sample sizes.

Chapter 3 applies permutation statistical methods to measures of association for two nominal-level (categorical) variables that are based on Pearson's chi-squared test statistic. Included in Chap. 3 are exact and Monte Carlo resampling permutation statistical methods for the commonly used chi-squared-based measures: Pearson's ϕ^2, Tschuprov's T^2, Cramér's V^2, and Pearson's contingency coefficient, C. Also included in Chap. 3 is a discussion of the relationship between chi-squared and Pearson's product-moment correlation coefficient.

Chapter 4 continues the discussion initiated in Chap. 3 with permutation statistical methods applied to measures of association for two nominal-level variables that are based on criteria other than Pearson's chi-squared test statistic. Included in Chap. 4 are exact and Monte Carlo resampling permutation statistical methods for Goodman and Kruskal's asymmetric measures of nominal-level association, λ_a, λ_b, t_a, and t_b, McNemar's Q and Cochran's Q tests for change, Cohen's unweighted κ measure of agreement, the Mantel–Haenszel test of independence for combined $2{\times}2$ contingency tables, and Fisher's exact probability test for a variety of $r{\times}c$ contingency tables.

Chapter 5 applies permutation statistical methods to measures of association for two ordinal-level (ranked) variables that are based on pairwise comparisons of differences between rank scores. Included in Chap. 5 are exact and Monte Carlo resampling permutation statistical methods for Kendall's τ_a and τ_b measures, Stuart's τ_c measure, Goodman and Kruskal's γ measure, Somers' d_{yx} and d_{xy} measures, Kim's $d_{y \cdot x}$ and $d_{x \cdot y}$ measures, Wilson's e measure, Whitfield's S measure of ordinal association between one ordinal-level variable and one binary variable, and Cureton's rank-biserial correlation coefficient.

Chapter 6 continues the discussion in Chap. 5 with permutation statistical methods applied to measures of association for two ordinal-level variables that are based on criteria other than pairwise comparisons between rank scores. Included in Chap. 6 are exact and Monte Carlo resampling permutation statistical methods for Spearman's rank-order correlation coefficient, Spearman's footrule measure of agreement, Kendall's coefficient of concordance, Kendall's u measure of inter-rater agreement, Cohen's weighted kappa measure of agreement, and Bross's ridit analysis.

Chapter 7 applies permutation statistical methods to measures of association for two interval-level variables. Included in Chap. 7 are exact and Monte Carlo resampling permutation statistical methods for Pearson's product-moment (inter-class) correlation coefficient, Pearson's intraclass correlation coefficient, ordinary least squares (OLS) regression, least absolute deviation (LAD) regression, point-biserial correlation, biserial correlation, and a discussion of Fisher's normalizing transformation for Pearson's product-moment correlation coefficient.

Chapter 8 applies permutation statistical methods to measures of association for two mixed variables: nominal–ordinal, nominal–interval, and ordinal–interval. Included in Chap. 8 are exact and Monte Carlo resampling permutation statistical methods for Freeman's θ, Agresti's $\hat{\delta}$, and Piccarreta's $\hat{\tau}$ measures for a nominal-level independent variable and an ordinal-level dependent variable; Pearson's correlation ratio, η^2, Kelley's ϵ^2, and Hays' $\hat{\omega}^2$ for a nominal-level independent variable and an interval-level dependent variable; and Jaspen's coefficient of multiserial correlation for an ordinal-level variable and an interval-level variable.

Chapter 9 applies permutation statistical methods to measures of association usually reserved for 2×2 contingency tables. Because 2×2 tables are so prevalent in statistical analysis, and so controversial, special attention is devoted to 2×2 contingency tables in Chap. 9. Included in Chap. 9 are exact and Monte Carlo permutation statistical methods for Yule's Q and Yule's Y measures of nominal-level association, Pearson's ϕ^2 measure, simple percentage differences, Goodman and Kruskal's t_a and t_b measures, Somers' d_{yx} and d_{xy} measures, the Mantel–Haenszel test, Fisher's exact test for 2×2 tables, Pearson's tetrachoric correlation, and the odds ratio.

Chapter 10 continues the discussion of 2×2 contingency tables initiated in Chap. 9 with consideration of symmetrical 2×2 contingency tables. Included in Chap. 10 are permutation statistical methods applied to Pearson's ϕ^2, Tschuprov's T^2, Cramér's V^2, Pearson's product-moment correlation coefficient, Leik and Gove's d_N^c measure, Goodman and Kruskal's t_a and t_b asymmetric measures, Kendall's τ_b and Stuart's τ_c measures, Somers' d_{yx} and d_{xy} asymmetric measures, simple percentage differences, Yule's Y measure of nominal association, and Cohen's unweighted and weighted κ measures of inter-rater agreement. A discussion of extensions to multi-way contingency tables concludes the chapter.

1.8 Coda

Chapter 1 provided a broad overview of measures of association for various levels of measurement, a brief introduction to permutation statistical methods, and descriptions of the next nine chapters. Chapter 2 describes two models of statistical inference: the Neyman–Pearson population model and the Fisher–Pitman permutation model. Three types of permutation tests are detailed: exact, Monte Carlo resampling, and moment-approximation permutation procedures. Finally, common research problems involving random sampling, small sample sizes, and underlying assumptions are discussed.

References

1. Agresti, A.: The effect of category choice on some ordinal measures of association. J. Am. Stat. Assoc. **71**, 49–55 (1976)
2. Anderson, A.B., Balilevsky, A., Hum, D.P.J.: Missing data. In: Rossi, P.H., Wright, J.D., Anderson, A.B. (eds.) Handbook of Survey Research, chap. 12, pp. 415–479. Academic Press, New York (1983)
3. Berry, K.J., Mielke, P.W.: Extension of Spearman's footrule to multiple rankings. Psychol. Rep. **82**, 376–378 (1998)
4. Berry, K.J., Mielke, P.W., Johnston, J.E.: Permutation Statistical Methods: An Integrated Approach. Springer-Verlag, Cham, CH (2016)
5. Borgatta, E.F., Bornstedt, G.W.: Level of measurement—once over again. Sociol. Method Res. **9**, 147–160 (1980)
6. Bornstedt, G.W.: Measurement. In: Rossi, P.H., Wright, J.D., Anderson, A.B. (eds.) Handbook of Survey Research, chap. 3, pp. 69–121. Academic Press, New York (1983)
7. Costner, H.L.: Criteria for measures of association. Am. Sociol. Rev. **30**, 341–353 (1965)
8. Cowles, M.: Statistics in Psychology: An Historical Perspective, 2nd edn. Lawrence Erlbaum, Mahwah, NJ (2001)
9. Everitt, B.: Chance Rules: An Informal Guide to Probability, Risk, and Statistics, 2nd edn. Springer–Verlag, New York (2008)
10. Fernandes, P.: Don't send us back to the closet. NY Times **166**, A25 (11 May 2017)
11. Gaito, J.: Measurement scales and statistics: Resurgence of an old misconception. Psychol. Bull. **87**, 564–567 (1980)
12. Goodman, L.A., Kruskal, W.H.: Measures of association for cross classifications. J. Am. Stat. Assoc. **49**, 732–764 (1954)
13. Goodman, L.A., Kruskal, W.H.: Measures of association for cross classifications, II: Further discussion and references. J. Am. Stat. Assoc. **54**, 123–163 (1959)
14. Goodman, L.A., Kruskal, W.H.: Measures of association for cross classifications, III: Approximate sampling theory. J. Am. Stat. Assoc. **58**, 310–364 (1963)
15. Goodman, L.A., Kruskal, W.H.: Measures of association for cross classifications, IV: Simplification of asymptotic variances. J. Am. Stat. Assoc. **67**, 415–421 (1972)
16. Leik, R.K., Gove, W.R.: Integrated approach to measuring association. In: Costner, H.L. (ed.) Sociological Methodology, pp. 279–301. Jossey Bass, San Francisco, CA (1971)
17. Liebetrau, A.M.: Measures of Association. Sage, Beverly Hills, CA (1983)
18. Lord, F.: On the statistical treatment of football numbers. Am. Psychol. **8**, 750–751 (1953)
19. Luce, R.D., Krantz, D.H., Suppes, P., Tversky, A.: Foundations of Measurement, vol. 3. Academic Press, New York (1990)
20. Mielke, P.W., Berry, K.J., Johnston, J.E.: Resampling probability values for weighted kappa with multiple raters. Psychol. Rep. **102**, 606–613 (2008)
21. Mortimer, I.: The Time Traveler's Guide to Restoration Britain. Pegasus, New York (2017)
22. Mosteller, M., Tukey, J.W.: Data Analysis and Regression: A Second Course in Statistics. Addison–Wesley, Reading, MA (1977)
23. Pfanzagl, J.: Theory of Measurement. Wiley, New York (1968)
24. Stevens, S.S.: On the theory of scales and measurement. Science **103**, 667–680 (1946)

25. Stevens, S.S.: Mathematics, measurement, and psychophysics. In: Stevens, S.S. (ed.) Handbook of Experimental Psychology, chap. 1, pp. 1–49. Wiley, New York (1951)
26. Thomson, W.: Popular Lectures and Addresses. MacMillan, London (1889)
27. Vellman, P.F., Wilkinson, L.: Nominal, ordinal, interval and ratio typologies are misleading. Am. Stat. **47**, 65–72 (1993)
28. Weiss, R.S.: Statistics in Social Research: An Introduction. Wiley, New York (1968)
29. Wilson, T.P.: Critique of ordinal variables. Social Forces **49**, 432–444 (1971)
30. Yule, G.U.: On the methods of measuring association between two attributes. J. R. Stat. Soc. **75**, 579–652 (1912). [Originally a paper read before the Royal Statistical Society on 23 April 1912]

Chapter 2
Permutation Statistical Methods

In this second chapter of *The Measurement of Association*, two entirely different models of statistical inference are described: the population model and the permutation model. The permutation model includes three types of permutation statistical tests: exact, Monte Carlo resampling, and moment-approximation, each of which is detailed and illustrated. Several limitations of the population model, in contrast with the permutation model are discussed, including the requirements of random sampling and the assumption of normality, as well as difficulties with the analysis of small sample sizes, none of which is problematic for the permutation statistical model.

Permutation statistical methods were initially developed by R.A. Fisher, R.C. Geary, T. Eden, F. Yates, E.J.G. Pitman, and other mathematicians and scientists in the 1920s and 1930s for validating the normality and homogeneity assumptions of classical statistical methods, a point made repeatedly by Fisher in *The Design of Experiments* [43, Chaps. 20 and 21].[1] Subsequently, permutation statistical methods have emerged as an approach to data analysis in their own right [10].

Permutation statistical methods possess several advantages over classical statistical methods. First, permutation tests are entirely data-dependent in that all the information required for analysis is contained within the observed data. Second, permutation tests are appropriate for non-random samples, such as are common in many fields of research. Third, permutation tests are distribution-free in that they do not depend on the assumptions associated with traditional parametric tests. Fourth, permutation tests provide exact probability values based on the discrete permutation distribution of equally-likely test statistic values. Fifth, permutation tests are ideal for small data sets.

[1]For a brief overview of the development of permutation statistical methods, see a 2011 article in *Wiley Indisciplinary Reviews: Computational Statistics* by Berry, Johnston, and Mielke [9]. For a comprehensive history of the development of permutation statistical methods, see Berry, Johnston, and Mielke *A Chronicle of Permutation Statistical Methods: 1920–2000, and Beyond* [10].

K. J. Berry et al., *The Measurement of Association*,
https://doi.org/10.1007/978-3-319-98926-6_2

2.1 Two Models of Statistical Inference

Essentially, two models of statistical inference coexist: the population model and the permutation model; see, for example, extensive discussions by Curran-Everett [27], Hubbard [69], Kempthorne [75], Kennedy [76], Lachin [77], Ludbrook [85, 86], Ludbrook and Dudley [89], and May and Hunter [103]. The population model, formally proposed by Jerzy Neyman and Egon Pearson in a seminal two-part article on statistical inference in *Biometrika* in 1928, assumes random sampling from one or more specified populations [117, 118]. Under the Neyman–Pearson population model, the level of statistical significance that results from applying a statistical test to the results of an experiment or survey corresponds to the frequency with which the null hypothesis would be rejected in repeated random samplings from the same specified population(s). Because repeated sampling of the specified population(s) is usually impractical, it is assumed that the sampling distribution of the test statistics generated under repeated random sampling conforms to an approximating theoretical distribution, such as the normal distribution. The size of the statistical test, e.g., 0.05, is the probability under a specified null hypothesis that repeated outcomes based on random samples of the same size are equal to or more extreme than the observed outcome.

While the Neyman–Pearson population model of statistical inference is familiar to most, if not all, researchers, the permutation model may be less familiar, or even unfamiliar, to many researchers. The permutation model was introduced by R.A. Fisher in 1925 [42], further developed by R.C. Geary in 1927 [49] and T. Eden and F. Yates in 1933 [31], and made explicit in three seminal articles by E.J.G. Pitman in 1937 and 1938 [121, 122, 123]. These early publications were a harbinger of a multitude of articles and books on permutation statistical methods in subsequent years [10]. Under the Fisher–Pitman permutation model the only assumption is that experimental variability has caused the observed result. That assumption, or null hypothesis, is then tested as follows. A test statistic is computed for the observed data, then the observations are permuted over all possible arrangements of the data and the specified test statistic is computed for each possible, equally-likely arrangement of the observed data. The proportion of arrangements in the reference set of all possible arrangements possessing test statistic values equal to or more extreme than the observed test statistic yields the exact probability of the observed test statistic value.

2.2 Permutation Statistical Tests

Many statisticians have long felt that there should be something that statistics could say about those cases where few if any assumptions could be made about the properties of the population from which the sample was drawn [64, p. vii]. Because permutation methods under the Fisher–Pitman model make no assumptions about a parent population, permutation statistical tests are considered by many to be a gold standard against which conventional statistical tests should be evaluated and validated. In 1940 Friedman, comparing tests of significance for multiple rankings, referred to an exact permutation test as "the correct one" [47, p. 88]. In 1973 Feinstein remarked that conventional statistical tests "yield reasonably reliable approximations of the more exact results provided by permutation procedures" [39, p. 912]. In 1992 Good noted that Fisher regarded randomization as a technique for validating tests of significance, i.e., ensuring that conventional probability values were accurate [52, p. 263]. Bakeman, Robinson, and Quera remarked in 1996 that "like Read and Cressie…we think permutation tests represent the standard against which asymptotic tests must be judged" [2, p. 6]. And in 2007 Edgington and Onghena observed that "randomization tests…have come to be recognized by many…as the 'gold standard' of statistical tests for randomized experiments" [37, p. 9].[2]

The value of permutation statistical methods was recognized by early statisticians, even during periods in which the computationally intensive nature of permutation methods made them impractical. In 1955 Kempthorne wrote that "tests of significance in the randomized experiment have frequently been presented by way of normal law theory, whereas their validity stems from randomization theory" [73, p. 947] and "there seems little point in the present state of knowledge in using [a] method of inference other than randomization analysis" [73, p. 966]. Similarly, in 1959 Scheffé stated that the conventional analysis of variance F-ratio "can often be regarded as a good approximation to a permutation test, which is an exact test under a less restrictive model" [129, p. 313]. In 1966, Kempthorne re-emphasized that "the proper way to make tests of significance in the simple randomized experiments [sic] is by way of the randomization (or permutation) test" [74, p. 20] and "in the randomized experiment one should, logically, make tests of significance by way of the randomization test" [74, p. 21]. Later, in 1968, Bradley observed that "eminent statisticians have stated that the randomization test is the truly correct one and that the corresponding parametric test is valid only to the extent that it results in the same statistical decision" [18, p. 85]. In 2000 Howell, in discussing permutation statistical methods, noted:

> These can be very powerful techniques that do not require unreasonable assumptions about the populations from which you have sampled. I suspect that resampling statistics and related procedures will be in the mainstream of statistical analysis in the not-too-distant future [68, p. 204].

Because permutation statistical methods are inherently computationally intensive, it took the development of high-speed computing for permutation methods to achieve their potential. Today, a small laptop computer outperforms even the largest mainframe computers of previous decades [14, p. 4]. Consequently, in the 21st century permutation statistical methods have become both feasible

[2] In the literature, the terms "permutation" and "randomization" are often used interchangeably [39, p. 910].

and practical and have found applications in diverse fields of research ranging from agronomy to zoology. Research areas that often examine small non-random samples, such as atmospheric science, clinical psychology, early childhood development, ecology, biology, family studies, and clinical trials, have been especially receptive to permutation statistical methods where the objective is to examine differences among two or more groups or treatments and not to make inferences to a population or populations [39]. This is due in part to strong advocates of permutation statistical methods in these fields, including Hugh Dudley [89, 90, 91, 92], Eugene Edgington [32, 33, 34, 35, 36, 37], Alvan Feinstein [39, 40], Phillip Good [53, 54, 55, 56], Michael Hunter [70], Oscar Kempthorne [72, 73, 74, 75], John Ludbrook [85, 86, 87, 88], Bryan Manly [94, 95, 96, 97], Richard May [103], and John Tukey [20, 137, 138, 139].

Three types of permutation tests are common in the statistical literature: exact, Monte Carlo resampling, and moment-approximation permutation tests. Although the three types of permutation statistical tests are methodologically quite different, all three types are based on the same specified null hypothesis: each of M possible permutations of the observed data is equally likely, i.e, the probability of any permutation of the observed data is $1/M$.

2.2.1 Exact Permutation Tests

In an exact permutation statistical test, the first step is to calculate a test statistic value on the observed data. Second, all possible, equally-likely arrangements of the observed data are generated. Third, the desired test statistic is calculated for each arrangement of the observed data.[3] The probability of obtaining the observed value of the test statistic, or one more extreme, is the proportion of the enumerated test statistics with values equal to or more extreme than the value of the observed test statistic. For large samples the total number of possible arrangements can be considerable and exact permutation methods are quickly rendered impractical. For example, permuting two small samples of sizes $n_1 = n_2 = 30$ yields

$$M = \frac{(n_1 + n_2)!}{n_1!\, n_2!} = \frac{(30 + 30)!}{30!\; 30!} = 118{,}264{,}581{,}564{,}861{,}424$$

arrangements of the observed data; or in words, 118 million billion different arrangements of the observed data set—far too many statistical values to compute in a reasonable amount of time.

[3]The Mehta–Patel network enumeration algorithm cleverly circumvents the need to completely enumerate all possible arrangements of the data, yet still provides an exact probability value [105, 106].

An Exact Permutation Analysis Example

On 18 December 1934, R.A. Fisher presented an invited paper describing the logic of permutation statistical tests to the Royal Statistical Society, a paper that was subsequently published in *Journal of the Royal Statistical Society* [44]. Fisher described data on 30 criminal same-sex twins from a study originally conducted by Dr. Johannes Lange, Chief Physician at the Munich-Schwabing Hospital in Schwabing, a northern suburb of Munich.

The Lange data analyzed by Fisher consisted of 13 pairs of monozygotic (identical) twins and 17 pairs of dizygotic (fraternal) twins [79]. For each of the 30 pairs of twins, one twin was known to be a convict. The study considered whether the twin brother of the known convict was himself "convicted" or "not convicted," thus forming a 2×2 contingency table with 12 "convicted" and 18 "not convicted" twins cross-classified by the 13 "monozygotic" and 17 "dizygotic" twins. The 2×2 contingency table is presented in Table 2.1.

Fisher determined the reference set of all possible arrangements of the four cell frequencies, given the observed marginal frequency totals; in this case, $M = 13$ different arrangements of cell frequencies. For a 2×2 contingency table, it is relatively easy to determine the total number of possible tables, given fixed marginal frequency totals. Consider the 2×2 contingency table in Table 2.2. Denote by a dot $(\cdot)$ the partial sum of all rows or all columns, depending on the position of the $(\cdot)$ in the subscript list. If the $(\cdot)$ is in the first subscript position, the sum is over all rows and if the $(\cdot)$ is in the second subscript position, the sum is over all columns. Thus, $n_{i.}$ denotes the marginal frequency total of the ith row, $i = 1, \ldots, r$, summed over all columns, and $n_{.j}$ denotes the marginal frequency total of the jth column, $j = 1, \ldots, c$, summed over all rows. Therefore, $n_{1.}$ and $n_{2.}$ denote the marginal frequency totals for rows 1 and 2, $n_{.1}$ and $n_{.2}$ denote the marginal frequency totals for columns 1 and 2, n_{ij} denotes the cell frequencies for $i, j = 1, 2$, and $N = n_{11} + n_{12} + n_{21} + n_{22}$. Then the total number of possible values for any cell frequency, say, n_{11}, is given by

$$M = \min(n_{1.}, n_{.1}) - \max(0, n_{11} - n_{22}) + 1 .$$

Table 2.1 Convictions of like-sex criminal twins

Twin type	Convicted	Not convicted	Total
Monozygotic	10	3	13
Dizygotic	2	15	17
Total	12	18	30

Table 2.2 Conventional notation for a 2×2 contingency table

	Category		
Category	1	2	Total
1	n_{11}	n_{12}	$n_{1.}$
2	n_{21}	n_{22}	$n_{2.}$
Total	$n_{.1}$	$n_{.2}$	N

Thus, for the frequency data given in Table 2.1, there are

$$M = \min(13, 12) - \max(0, 10 - 15) + 1 = 12 - 0 + 1 = 13$$

possible arrangements of cell frequencies, given the observed row and column marginal frequency distributions, {13, 17} and {12, 18}, respectively.

Fisher then calculated the hypergeometric point probability value for each of the $M = 13$ cell arrangements, summing the probability values that were equal to or less than the hypergeometric point probability value of the observed cell frequency arrangement. Fisher concluded, "The test of significance is therefore direct, and exact for small samples. No process of estimation is involved" [44, p. 50]. The $M = 13$ arrangements of cell frequencies and the associated hypergeometric point probability values are listed in Table 2.3. Fisher observed, given that any 2×2 contingency table has only one degree of freedom, it is only necessary to compute the probability of one of the four cells; he chose the convicted dizygotic twins, the lower-left cell of the 2×2 contingency table in Table 2.1 with an observed cell frequency of $n_{21} = 2$.

Table 2.3 Listing of the 13 possible 2×2 contingency tables from Table 2.1 with associated exact hypergeometric point probability values

Table 1		Probability	Table 2		Probability
0	13	7.1543×10^{-5}	1	12	1.8601×10^{-3}
12	5		11	6	
Table 3		Probability	Table 4		Probability
2	11	1.7538×10^{-2}	3	10	8.0384×10^{-2}
10	7		9	8	
Table 5		Probability	Table 6		Probability
4	9	2.0096×10^{-1}	5	8	2.8938×10^{-1}
8	9		7	10	
Table 7		Probability	Table 8		Probability
6	7	2.4554×10^{-1}	7	6	1.2277×10^{-1}
6	11		5	12	
Table 9		Probability	Table 10		Probability
8	5	3.5414×10^{-2}	9	4	5.6212×10^{-3}
4	13		3	14	
Table 11		Probability	Table 12		Probability
10	3	4.4970×10^{-4}	11	2	1.5331×10^{-5}
2	15		1	16	
Table 13		Probability			
12	1	1.5030×10^{-7}			
0	17				

For a 2×2 contingency table, such as depicted in Table 2.2, the hypergeometric point probability of any specified cell, say, cell (2, 1), is given by

$$P(n_{21}|n_{2.}, n_{.1}, N) = \binom{n_{.1}}{n_{11}}\binom{n_{.2}}{n_{12}}\binom{N}{n_{1.}}^{-1} = \frac{n_{1.}!\, n_{2.}!\, n_{.1}!\, n_{.2}!}{N!\, n_{11}!\, n_{12}!\, n_{21}!\, n_{22}!} \ .$$

Computing the discrepancies from proportionality equal to or greater than the observed cell frequency configuration in Table 2.1, Fisher computed a one-tailed hypergeometric probability value for 2, 1, and 0 convicted dizygotic twins of

$$\begin{aligned} &P\{2|17, 12, 30\} + P\{1|17, 12, 30\} + P\{0|17, 12, 30\} \\ &\quad = \frac{13!\, 17!\, 12!\, 18!}{30!\, 10!\, 3!\, 2!\, 15!} + \frac{13!\, 17!\, 12!\, 18!}{30!\, 11!\, 2!\, 1!\, 16!} + \frac{13!\, 17!\, 12!\, 18!}{30!\, 12!\, 1!\, 0!\, 17!} \\ &\quad = 4.4970\times 10^{-4} + 1.5331\times 10^{-5} + 1.5030\times 10^{-7} \\ &\quad = 4.6518\times 10^{-4} \ . \end{aligned}$$

For the frequency data given in Table 2.1, a two-tailed hypergeometric probability value includes all hypergeometric point probability values equal to or less than the point probability value of the observed contingency table, i.e., $P = 4.4970\times 10^{-4}$. In this case, the additional probability value associated with Table 1 within Table 2.3 with 12 dizygotic convicts, i.e., $P = 7.1543\times 10^{-5}$. Thus, the two-tailed hypergeometric probability value is calculated as

$$\begin{aligned} &P\{2|17, 12, 30\} + P\{1|17, 12, 30\} + P\{0|17, 12, 30\} + P\{12|17, 12, 30\} \\ &\quad = \frac{13!\, 17!\, 12!\, 18!}{30!\, 10!\, 3!\, 2!\, 15!} + \frac{13!\, 17!\, 12!\, 18!}{30!\, 11!\, 2!\, 1!\, 16!} + \frac{13!\, 17!\, 12!\, 18!}{30!\, 12!\, 1!\, 0!\, 17!} + \frac{13!\, 17!\, 12!\, 18!}{30!\, 0!\, 13!\, 12!\, 5!} \\ &\quad = 4.4970\times 10^{-4} + 1.5331\times 10^{-5} + 1.5030\times 10^{-7} + 7.1543\times 10^{-5} \\ &\quad = 5.3672\times 10^{-4} \ . \end{aligned}$$

The point of the twin analysis—that exact tests are possible for small samples, eliminating the need for estimation—indicates an early understanding of the superiority of exact probability values computed from discrete permutation distributions, over approximations of probability values based on assumed theoretical distributions, i.e., abstractions based on a mathematical rule, that are presumed to match, or approximate, distributions of events in the real world [26, p. 68].

A Second Exact Permutation Analysis Example

Permutation statistical methods are applicable to analyses beyond simply measuring association. For a second example of an exact permutation analysis, consider a test

Table 2.4 Average per capita relief expenditures for Southampton and Suffolk counties in shillings: 1831

Southampton		Suffolk	
Parish	Relief	Parish	Relief
1	6.731808	6	26.383673
6	16.156615	10	16.727664
7	14.760218	11	27.628032
8	15.057353	13	19.914255
12	11.001482	19	13.833671
15	29.089955	24	33.827534
18	11.818136	28	19.050737
25	16.002180		
27	18.761256		
29	32.443278		
31	15.447992		
36	15.756267		
38	4.257547		
39	8.611310		
40	15.361136		

of differences between means instead of Fisher's exact probability test.[4] Table 2.4 contains the per capita relief expenditures in 1831, in shillings, for $N = 22$ parishes (identified only by number) in two counties in Great Britain: Southampton and Suffolk. In 1831, Southampton county consisted of $n_1 = 15$ parishes with a mean relief expenditure of $\bar{x}_1 = 15.4171$ shillings and a sample standard deviation of $s_1 = 7.4081$ shillings, and Suffolk county consisted of $n_2 = 7$ parishes with a mean relief expenditure of $\bar{x}_2 = 22.4808$ shillings and a sample standard deviation of $s_2 = 7.0321$ shillings.[5]

For the Southampton and Suffolk county relief data given in Table 2.4, a conventional Student's two-sample t test yields $t = -2.1147$ and with

$$n_1 + n_2 - 2 = 15 + 7 - 2 = 20$$

degrees of freedom, the two-sided probability value under the null hypothesis is $P = 0.0472$. There are only

$$M = \frac{(n_1 + n_2)!}{n_1!\, n_2!} = \frac{(15 + 7)!}{15!\, 7!} = 170{,}544$$

[4]For discussions of permutation methods applied to tests of differences, see *Permutation Statistical Methods: An Integrated Approach* by Berry, Mielke, and Johnston [14].

[5]Note that, for these data, the sample standard deviations, $s_1 = 7.4081$ and $s_2 = 7.0321$, are very similar.

possible arrangements of the Southampton and Suffolk county relief data given in Table 2.4, making an exact permutation analysis feasible. With $n_1 = 15$ and $n_2 = 7$ preserved for each arrangement, exactly 9,010 t values in the reference set of the $M = 170{,}544$ possible t values are equal to or more extreme than the observed value of $t = -2.1147$, yielding an exact two-sided probability value under the null hypothesis of

$$P(t \geq t_{\text{o}}|H_0) = \frac{\text{number of } t \text{ values } \geq t_{\text{o}}}{M} = \frac{9{,}010}{170{,}544} = 0.0528 \;,$$

where t_{o} denotes the observed value of t.

2.2.2 *Monte Carlo Permutation Statistical Tests*

When exact permutation procedures become intractable, a random subset of all possible arrangements of the observed data can be analyzed, providing approximate, but highly accurate, probability values. Resampling-approximation (hereafter, resampling) permutation tests generate and examine a Monte Carlo random subset of all possible, equally-likely arrangements of the observed response measurements. For each randomly selected arrangement of the observed data, the desired test statistic is calculated. The probability of obtaining the observed value of the test statistic, or one more extreme, is the proportion of the randomly selected test statistics with values equal to or more extreme than the value of the observed test statistic. With a sufficient number of random samples, a probability value can be computed to any reasonable accuracy. The current recommended practice is to use $L = 1{,}000{,}000$ randomly selected arrangements of the observed data to ensure a probability value with three decimal places of accuracy [71].

Meyer Dwass is usually credited with the formal development of resampling permutation tests, first presented in an article on "Modified randomization tests for nonparametric hypotheses" published in *The Annals of Mathematical Statistics* in 1957 [30].[6] Dwass provided the first rigorous investigation into the accuracy of resampling probability approximations, although Dwass relied heavily on the theoretical contributions of an article titled "On the theory of some non-parametric hypotheses" by Erich Lehmann and Charles Stein published in *The Annals of Mathematical Statistics* in 1949 [81].

Presently, Monte Carlo resampling permutation tests are the method of choice for most researchers, with exact permutation tests reserved for smaller data sets. There are three notable advantages to resampling permutation tests. First, resampling permutation tests are highly efficient given the ready availability of high-speed

[6] Also see a 1958 article in *The Journal of the American Statistical Association* by Chung and Fraser on "Randomization tests for a multivariate two-sample problem" [24].

computers and the recent development of rapid pseudorandom number generators such as the Mersenne Twister, on which resampling permutation tests are highly dependent.[7] Second, in some applications a resampling permutation test is much more efficient than an exact permutation test, even for small samples. For example, in the permutation analysis of contingency tables an exact permutation test must necessarily calculate a hypergeometric point probability value for each of, potentially, thousands of cell frequency arrangements, while a resampling permutation test need only count the number of cell arrangements as extreme or more extreme than the observed cell arrangement. Third, algorithms for exact permutation tests are non-existent or completely impractical for analyzing certain problems, such as multi-way contingency tables, while an efficient resampling algorithm is presently available for multi-way tables; see, for example, a 2007 article by Mielke, Berry, and Johnston in *Psychological Reports* [113].

A Monte Carlo Resampling Analysis Example

To illustrate a Monte Carlo resampling permutation analysis, consider Table 2.5 which contains the per capita relief expenditures in 1831, in shillings, for $N = 36$ parishes (identified only by number) in two counties in Great Britain: Oxford and Hertford. In 1831, Oxford county consisted of $n_1 = 24$ parishes with a mean relief expenditure of $\bar{x}_1 = 20.2766$ shillings and a sample standard deviation of $s_1 = 7.6408$ shillings, and Hertford county consisted of $n_2 = 12$ parishes with a mean relief expenditure of $\bar{x}_2 = 13.4720$ shillings and a sample standard deviation of $s_2 = 6.1270$ shillings.[8]

For the Oxford and Hertford county relief data given in Table 2.5, a conventional Student's two-sample t test yields $t = +2.6783$ and with

$$n_1 + n_2 - 2 = 24 + 12 - 2 = 34$$

degrees of freedom, the two-sided probability value under the null hypothesis is $P = 0.0113$. There are

$$M = \frac{(n_1 + n_2)!}{n_1!\, n_2!} = \frac{(24 + 12)!}{24!\ 12!} = 1{,}251{,}677{,}700$$

possible arrangements of the Oxford and Hertford county relief data given in Table 2.5, making an exact permutation analysis impractical. Based on $L = 1{,}000{,}000$ random arrangements of the observed data with $n_1 = 24$ and $n_2 = 12$

---

[7]Maxim Mersenne (1588–1648) was a Parisian monk, music theorist, and mathematician. Mersenne was the first to observe that if $2^n - 1$ was a prime number, then n must also be a prime number, but that the converse was not necessarily true. The Mersenne Twister pseudorandom number generator is named in his honor.

[8]Again, note that the sample standard deviations, $s_1 = 7.6408$ and $s_2 = 6.1270$, are very similar.

Table 2.5 Average per capita relief expenditures for Oxford and Hertford counties in shillings: 1831

Oxford		Hertford	
Parish	Relief	Parish	Relief
1	20.361860	2	27.974783
2	29.086095	4	6.417284
5	14.931757	7	10.484120
8	24.123211	11	10.005750
10	18.207501	13	9.769865
11	20.728732	14	15.866521
12	8.119472	15	19.342360
13	14.020071	17	17.145218
17	18.424789	20	13.134206
18	34.546600	21	10.041964
19	16.092713	22	15.083824
22	24.616592	27	6.398451
23	25.468298		
24	12.563194		
29	13.278003		
31	27.302973		
34	29.605508		
36	13.613192		
39	11.371418		
45	21.524807		
49	20.940801		
52	11.595229		
55	18.235469		
56	37.880889		

preserved for each arrangement, exactly 8,478 of the calculated t values are equal to or more extreme than the observed value of $t = +2.6783$, yielding a Monte Carlo resampling two-sided probability value under the null hypothesis of

$$P(t \geq t_{\text{o}}|H_0) = \frac{\text{number of } t \text{ values } \geq t_{\text{o}}}{L} = \frac{8{,}478}{1{,}000{,}000} = 0.0085 \,,$$

where t_{o} denotes the observed value of t.

While an exact permutation analysis is impractical for the Oxford and Hertford county relief data given in Table 2.5, it is not impossible. The exact probability value based on all $M = 1{,}251{,}677{,}700$ possible arrangements of the observed data is

$$P(t \geq t_{\text{o}}|H_0) = \frac{\text{number of } t \text{ values } \geq t_{\text{o}}}{M} = \frac{10{,}635{,}310}{1{,}251{,}677{,}700} = 0.0085 \,.$$

A Second Monte Carlo Resampling Analysis Example

For a second example of a Monte Carlo resampling permutation analysis, consider the 3×4×5 contingency table with cell frequencies given in Table 2.6. Pearson's chi-squared test statistic for an $r \times c \times s$ contingency table is given by

$$\chi^2 = N^2 \left(\sum_{i=1}^{r} \sum_{j=1}^{c} \sum_{k=1}^{s} \frac{O_{ijk}^2}{R_i C_j S_k} \right) - N \; ,$$

where R_i denotes a row marginal frequency total, $i = 1, \ldots, r$, C_j denotes a column marginal frequency total, $j = 1, \ldots, c$, S_k denotes a slice marginal frequency total, $k = 1, \ldots, s$, O_{ijk} denotes an observed cell frequency, $i = 1, \ldots, r$, $j = 1, \ldots, c$, $k = 1, \ldots, s$, and N is the total number of cell frequencies; in this case, $N = 95$. For the frequency data given in Table 2.6 with row marginal frequency totals $\{32, 32, 31\}$, column marginal frequency totals $\{25, 23, 24, 23\}$, and slice marginal frequency totals $\{19, 19, 19, 19, 19\}$, the observed value of chi-squared is $\chi^2 = 84.7379$.

The degrees of freedom for a multi-way contingency table are given by

$$df = \prod_{i=1}^{r} c_i - \sum_{i=1}^{r} (c_i - 1) - 1 \; ,$$

where r denotes the number of dimensions and c_i denotes the number of categories in each dimension, $i = 1, \ldots, r$ [112, p. 309]. Thus, for a 3×4×5 contingency table,

$$df = (3)(4)(5) - [(3-1) + (4-1) + (5-1)] - 1 = 50 \; .$$

A chi-squared value of $\chi^2 = 84.7379$ with 50 degrees of freedom yields an asymptotic probability value of $P = 0.1563 \times 10^{-2}$. In contrast, a Monte Carlo resampling approximate probability value based on $L = 1{,}000{,}000$ random

Table 2.6 Listing of the 3×4×5 cell frequencies with rows (A_1, A_2, A_3), columns (B_1, B_2, B_3, B_4), and slices (D_1, D_2, D_3, D_4, D_5) for a resampling-approximation example

	A_1				A_2				A_3			
	B_1	B_2	B_3	B_4	B_1	B_2	B_3	B_4	B_1	B_2	B_3	B_4
D_1	0	3	1	3	4	0	0	0	2	1	4	1
D_2	0	0	0	2	1	4	1	0	3	1	3	4
D_3	4	1	0	3	1	3	4	0	0	0	2	1
D_4	3	4	0	0	0	2	1	4	1	0	3	1
D_5	2	1	4	1	0	3	1	3	4	0	0	0

arrangements of the cell frequencies, given fixed marginal frequency totals, is

$$P(\chi^2 \geq \chi_o^2 \,|H_0) = \frac{\text{number of } \chi^2 \text{ values } \geq \chi_o^2}{L}$$

$$= \frac{1{,}425}{1{,}000{,}000} = 0.1425 \times 10^{-2} \, ,$$

where χ_o^2 denotes the observed value of χ^2.

2.2.3 Moment-Approximation Permutation Tests

Monte Carlo resampling permutation methods can be inefficient when desired probability values are very small, e.g., on the order of 10^{-6}, as the method requires a large number of randomly selected test statistics to approximate such a small probability value. A number of techniques have been proposed to circumvent this problem, most based on partitioning of the permutation reference set into smaller, more manageable units [83, 146]. While these partitioning methods work well for specific targeted applications, they are not sufficiently general to be readily adopted for other applications. Moreover, such techniques are most efficient when probability values are very small, e.g., 10^{-30}, which is seldom of interest to most researchers. An alternative method detailed here is based on the first three exact moments of the discrete permutation distribution.

Prior to the development of high-speed computing that made exact and Monte Carlo resampling permutation methods possible, researchers relied on moment-approximation procedures to provide approximate probability values. The moment-approximation of a test statistic requires calculation of the exact moments of the test statistic, assuming equally-likely arrangements of the observed response measurements. The moments are then used to fit a specified distribution that approximates the underlying discrete permutation distribution and provide an approximate, but often highly accurate, probability value. Historically, the beta distribution was used for the approximating distribution, but in recent years the Pearson type III distribution has largely replaced the beta distribution. For many years moment-approximation permutation tests provided an important intermediary approximation when computers lacked the speed for calculating exact permutation tests. With the advent of high-speed computing, Monte Carlo resampling permutation tests have largely replaced moment-approximation permutation procedures, although moment-approximation permutation procedures are still important in, for example, studies involving massive simulations.

The Pearson type III approximation depends on the exact mean, variance, and skewness of the test statistic under consideration, say δ, given by

$$\mu_\delta = \frac{1}{M}\sum_{i=1}^{M}\delta_i \ ,$$

$$\sigma_\delta^2 = \frac{1}{M}\sum_{i=1}^{M}\left(\delta_i - \mu_\delta\right)^2 \ ,$$

and

$$\gamma_\delta = \frac{1}{\sigma_\delta^3}\left[\frac{1}{M}\sum_{i=1}^{M}\left(\delta_i - \mu_\delta\right)^3\right] \ ,$$

respectively, where M denotes the total number of possible, equally-likely arrangements of the observed data.

In particular, the standardized statistic given by

$$T = \frac{\delta - \mu_\delta}{\sigma_\delta}$$

follows the Pearson type III distribution with density function given by

$$f(y) = \frac{(-2/\gamma_\delta)^{4/\gamma_\delta^2}}{\Gamma(4/\gamma_\delta^2)}\big[-(2+y\gamma_\delta)/\gamma_\delta\big]^{(4-\gamma_\delta^2)/\gamma_\delta^2}\exp\big[-2(2+y\gamma_\delta)/\gamma_\delta^2\big] \ ,$$

when $-\infty < y < -2/\gamma_\delta$ and $\gamma_\delta < 0$, or

$$f(y) = \frac{(2/\gamma_\delta)^{4/\gamma_\delta^2}}{\Gamma(4/\gamma_\delta^2)}\big[(2+y\gamma_\delta)/\gamma_\delta\big]^{(4-\gamma_\delta^2)/\gamma_\delta^2}\exp\big[-2(2+y\gamma_\delta)/\gamma_\delta^2\big] \ ,$$

when $-2/\gamma_\delta < y < +\infty$ and $\gamma_\delta > 0$, or

$$f(y) = (2\pi)^{-1/2}\exp\big[-y^2/2\big] \ ,$$

when $\gamma_\delta = 0$, i.e., the standard normal distribution [112, 25–26].[9]

[9]In mathematics, the gamma function $\Gamma(n)$ may be thought of as an extension of the factorial function to real and complex number arguments. If n is a positive integer, $\Gamma(n) = (n-1)!$ and $n! = \Gamma(\mathrm{n}+1)$.

If the observed standardized statistic is given by

$$T_{\text{o}} = \frac{\delta_{\text{o}} - \mu_\delta}{\sigma_\delta} ,$$

where δ_{o} denotes the observed value of the test statistic, then

$$P(\delta \leq \delta_{\text{o}}|H_0) \doteq \int_{-\infty}^{T_{\text{o}}} f(y)dy$$

and

$$P(\delta \geq \delta_{\text{o}}|H_0) \doteq \int_{T_{\text{o}}}^{+\infty} f(y)dy$$

denote approximate probability values, which are evaluated numerically over an appropriate finite interval. The Pearson type III distribution is used to approximate the permutation distribution of T because it is completely specified by the skewness of T, γ_T, and includes the normal and chi-squared distributions as special cases. Thus, these distributions are asymptotic limits of the permutation distribution for some research situations. Efficient computation expressions for μ_δ, σ_δ^2, and γ_δ under the null hypothesis are given by Mielke and Berry [112, pp. 26–29].

The Pearson type III distribution, as a three-parameter gamma distribution, has the advantage of being totally characterized by the exact mean, variance, and skewness, in the same manner that the normal distribution, as a two-parameter distribution, is fully characterized by the exact mean and variance—a property not possessed by the beta distribution. An added advantage of the Pearson type III distribution is that when the skewness parameter is zero, the distribution is normal. Because the choice of a parametric distribution, such as the beta or Pearson type III distribution, is completely arbitrary, the resulting probability value cannot be expected to replicate precisely the probability value obtained from an exact permutation analysis. Consequently, although a moment-approximation analysis is based on exact moments, the resulting probability value is only approximate.

A Moment-Approximation Analysis Example

A moment-approximation statistical test can be illustrated with an example $r \times c$ contingency table with cell frequencies given in Table 2.7. Pearson's chi-squared test statistic for an $r \times c$ contingency table is given by

$$\chi^2 = N \left(\sum_{i=1}^{r} \sum_{j=1}^{c} \frac{O_{ij}^2}{R_i C_j} \right) - N ,$$

Table 2.7 Listing of the 3×5 cell frequencies with rows (R_1, R_2, R_3) and columns (C_1, C_2, C_3, C_4, C_5) for a moment-approximation example

	A_1	A_2	A_3	A_4	A_5	Total
B_1	4	7	2	9	0	22
B_2	1	5	2	7	6	21
B_3	4	5	10	18	0	37
Total	9	17	14	34	6	80

where R_i denotes a row marginal frequency total, $i = 1, \ldots, r$, C_j denotes a column marginal frequency total, $j = 1, \ldots, c$, O_{ij} denotes an observed cell frequency, $i = 1, \ldots, r$ and $j = 1, \ldots, c$, and N is the total number of cell frequencies; in this case, $N = 80$. For the frequency data given in Table 2.7 with row marginal frequency totals $\{22, 21, 37\}$ and column marginal frequency totals $\{9, 17, 14, 34, 6\}$, the observed value of chi-squared is $\chi^2_{\text{o}} = 25.0809$, $\delta_{\text{o}} = 24.8661$, $\mu_\delta = 8.00$, $\sigma^2_\delta = 14.5148$,

$$T = \frac{\delta_{\text{o}} - \mu_\delta}{\sigma_\delta} = \frac{24.8661 - 8.00}{\sqrt{14.5148}} = +4.4270\,,$$

and the moment-approximation probability value based on the Pearson type III distribution is $P = 0.9763\times10^{-3}$.

Comparisons of the Three Permutation Approaches

The three approaches to determining permutation probability values (exact, Monte Carlo resampling, and moment-approximation) often yield similar probability values. For comparison, the exact probability value for the frequency data given in Table 2.7 based on $M = 21{,}671{,}722$ possible arrangements of the cell frequencies is $P = 0.1009\times10^{-2}$, the Monte Carlo resampling probability value based on $L = 1{,}000{,}000$ randomly selected arrangements is $P = 0.1055\times10^{-2}$, and the moment-approximation probability value based on the first three exact moments of the underlying permutation distribution is $P = 0.9763\times10^{-3}$. The difference between the moment-approximation probability value ($P = 0.9763\times10^{-3}$) and the exact probability value ($P = 0.1009\times10^{-2}$) is only 0.3270×10^{-4}, the difference between the moment-approximation probability value ($P = 0.9763\times10^{-3}$) and the Monte Carlo resampling probability value based on $L = 1{,}000{,}000$ ($P = 0.1055\times10^{-2}$) is only 0.7870×10^{-4}, and the difference between the Monte Carlo resampling probability value ($P = 0.1055\times10^{-2}$) and the exact probability value ($P = 0.1009\times10^{-2}$) is only 0.4600×10^{-4}. Finally, the asymptotic probability value of $\chi^2 = 25.0809$ with $(r - 1)(c - 1) = (3 - 1)(5 - 1) = 8$ degrees of freedom is $P = 0.1506\times10^{-2}$. The comparisons are summarized in Table 2.8.

Table 2.8 Absolute differences among probability values obtained with exact, Monte Carlo resampling, moment-approximation, and asymptotic procedures for the frequency data given in Table 2.7

	Exact	Monte Carlo	Moment	Asymptotic
Exact	–	0.4600×10^{-4}	0.3270×10^{-4}	0.4970×10^{-3}
Monte Carlo		–	0.7870×10^{-4}	0.4510×10^{-3}
Moment			–	0.5297×10^{-3}
Asymptotic				–

Table 2.9 Randomized-block example with $N = 6$ subjects and $b = 3$ blocks

	Treatment		
Subject	1	2	3
1	15	15	18
2	14	14	14
3	10	11	15
4	13	12	17
5	16	13	16
6	13	13	13

A Second Moment-Approximation Analysis Example

For a second example of a moment-approximation permutation analysis, consider the randomized-block data given in Table 2.9 with $N = 6$ subjects and $b = 3$ blocks. For the randomized-block data listed in Table 2.9, the observed value of the F-ratio is $F = 6.00$ and with $b - 1 = 2$ and $(N - 1)(b - 1) = (6 - 1)(3 - 1) = 10$ degrees of freedom, the asymptotic probability value of $F = 6.00$ is $P = 0.0194$. Alternatively, $\delta_o = 6.6667$, $\mu_\delta = 8.9444$, $\sigma_\delta^2 = 1.8920$, the observed value of test statistic T is

$$T_o = \frac{\delta_o - \mu_\delta}{\sigma_\delta} = \frac{6.6667 - 8.9444}{\sqrt{1.8920}} = -1.6560 ,$$

and the moment-approximation probability value based on the Pearson type III distribution is $P = 0.0489$.

For comparison, the number of possible arrangements for the data given in Table 2.9 is only

$$M = (N!)^b = (6!)^3 = 373{,}248{,}000 .$$

The relationships between δ and F are given by

$$F = \frac{(b-1)\left[2SS_{\text{Total}} - N(b-1)\delta\right]}{N(b-1)\delta - 2SS_{\text{Blocks}}}$$

and

$$\delta = \frac{2\left[F SS_{\text{Blocks}} + (b-1)SS_{\text{Total}}\right]}{N(b-1)(F+b-1)} ,$$

where

$$SS_{\text{Total}} = \sum_{i=1}^{N} \sum_{j=1}^{b} \left(x_{ij} - \bar{x}_{..}\right)^2 ,$$

$$SS_{\text{Blocks}} = N \sum_{j=1}^{b} \left(\bar{x}_{.j} - \bar{x}_{..}\right)^2 ,$$

$$\bar{x}_{.j} = \frac{1}{N} \sum_{i=1}^{N} x_{ij} \qquad \text{for } j = 1, \ldots, b ,$$

and

$$\bar{x}_{..} = \frac{1}{Nb} \sum_{i=1}^{N} \sum_{j=1}^{b} x_{ij} ,$$

[114]. Because both SS_{Total} and SS_{Blocks} are invariant under all M arrangements of the observed data, δ may be used as a test statistic that is equivalent to F. Thus, the exact probability value for the data given in Table 2.9 is

$$P(F \geq F_{\text{o}}|H_0) = \frac{\text{number of } F \text{ values } \geq F_{\text{o}}}{M}$$
$$= \frac{\text{number of } \delta \text{ values } \leq \delta_{\text{o}}}{M} = \frac{20{,}930{,}400}{373{,}248{,}000} = 0.0561 ,$$

where F_{o} and δ_{o} denote the observed values of F and δ, respectively.[10] For comparison, a Monte Carlo resampling probability value computed on $L = 1{,}000{,}000$ random arrangements of the observed data in Table 2.9 is

$$P(F \geq F_{\text{o}}|H_0) = \frac{\text{number of } F \text{ values } \geq F_{\text{o}}}{M}$$
$$= \frac{\text{number of } \delta \text{ values } \leq \delta_{\text{o}}}{M} = \frac{56{,}000}{1{,}000{,}000} = 0.0560 .$$

[10]Note that large values of F correspond to small values of δ.

2.3 Analyses of r-Way Contingency Tables

In this section, moment-approximation permutation statistical methods for analyzing r-way contingency tables are presented. In 1988 Mielke and Berry designed efficient cumulant methods for analyzing independence of r-way contingency tables and goodness-of-fit frequency data [110]. Because the reference set of all possible permutations of r-way contingency tables is generally very large, moment-approximation methods are usually the appropriate choice. When the frequency data are very sparse and/or the number of degrees of freedom is very small, exact tests based on efficient algorithms should be used; see, for example, three articles by Berry and Mielke in 1985 [11], 1987 [12], and 1988 [13].

2.3.1 *Tests of Independence*

Let $O_{j_1,\,\ldots,\,j_r}$ denote the observed frequency of the $(j_1, \ldots, j_r)$th cell of an r-way contingency table, where $j_i = 1, \ldots, n_i$ for $i = 1, \ldots, r$. If $\langle i \rangle_j$ denotes the jth of n_i marginal frequency totals for the ith of r dimensions in the r-way contingency table, then

$$\sum_{j=1}^{n_i} \langle i \rangle_j = N$$

for $i = 1, \ldots, r$, where N is the frequency total of the r-way contingency table. The classical Pearson chi-squared test statistic corresponding to

$$T = \sum_{j_1=1}^{n_1} \cdots \sum_{j_r=1}^{n_r} \left(O_{j_1,\,\ldots,\,j_r}^2 \bigg/ \prod_{i=1}^{r} \langle i \rangle_{j_i} \right)$$

and the modified statistic

$$S = \sum_{j_1=1}^{n_1} \cdots \sum_{j_r=1}^{n_r} \left(O_{j_1,\,\ldots,\,j_r}^{(2)} \bigg/ \prod_{i=1}^{r} \langle i \rangle_{j_i} \right)$$

are considered, where

$$c^{(m)} = \prod_{i=1}^{m} (c + 1 - i) \; .$$

Note that $\chi^2 = TN^{r-1} - N$. Statistic S possesses greater power than statistic T with properties similar to the power characteristics of the likelihood-ratio test [147].

The cumulant methods are governed by the conditional permutation distribution of the $O_{j_1,\ldots,j_r}$ values given by

$$P\left(O_{j_1,\ldots,j_r}|\langle 1\rangle_1,\ \ldots,\ \langle 1\rangle_{n_1},\ \ldots,\ \langle r\rangle_1,\ \ldots,\ \langle r\rangle_{n_r}\right)$$
$$=\prod_{i=1}^{r}\prod_{j_i=1}^{n_i}\langle i\rangle_{j_i}!\bigg/\left[(N!)^{r-1}\prod_{i=1}^{r}\prod_{j_i=1}^{n_i}O_{j_1,\ldots,j_r}!\right],$$

which is independent of any unknown probabilities under the null hypothesis [108, 110]. Thus, the marginal frequency totals, $\langle i\rangle_{j_i}$, are sufficient statistics for the marginal multinomial probabilities, $[i]_{j_i}$, under the null hypothesis. This hypergeometric distribution function provides the basis for testing the independence of categories for any r-way contingency table.

The exact mean, μ_T, variance, σ_T^2, and skewness, γ_T, of T under the conditional permutation distribution are defined in terms of the first three moments about the origin:

$$\mathrm{E}[T]=\left[\prod_{i=1}^{r}(N-n_i)+(N-1)^{r-1}\prod_{i=1}^{r}n_i\right]\bigg/\left(N^{(2)}\right)^{r-1},$$

$$\mathrm{E}[T^2]=\left\{\prod_{i=1}^{r}\left(\langle i\rangle_{4,1}+\langle i\rangle_{4,2}\right)+2N_{1,1}^{r-1}\left[2\prod_{i=1}^{r}\langle i\rangle_{3,1}+\prod_{i=1}^{r}\left(\langle i\rangle_{3,1}+\langle i\rangle_{3,2}\right)\right]\right.$$
$$\left.+\,N_{2,1}^{r-1}\left[6\prod_{i=1}^{r}\langle i\rangle_{2,1}+\prod_{i=1}^{r}\left(\langle i\rangle_{2,1}+\langle i\rangle_{2,2}\right)\right]+N_{3,1}^{r-1}\prod_{i=1}^{r}\langle i\rangle_{1,1}\right\}\bigg/N_{4,1}^{r-1},$$

$$\mathrm{E}[T^3]=\left\{\prod_{i=1}^{r}\left(\langle i\rangle_{6,3}+3\langle i\rangle_{6,4}+\langle i\rangle_{6,6}\right)+3N_{1,2}^{r-1}\left[4\prod_{i=1}^{r}\left(\langle i\rangle_{5,3}+\langle i\rangle_{5,4}\right)\right.\right.$$
$$\left.+\prod_{i=1}^{r}\left(\langle i\rangle_{5,3}+2\langle i\rangle_{5,4}+\langle i\rangle_{5,5}+\langle i\rangle_{5,6}\right)\right]+N_{2,2}^{r-1}\left[32\prod_{i=1}^{r}\langle i\rangle_{4,3}\right.$$
$$+\,18\prod_{i=1}^{r}\left(\langle i\rangle_{4,3}+\langle i\rangle_{4,4}\right)+12\prod_{i=1}^{r}\left(\langle i\rangle_{4,3}+\langle i\rangle_{4,5}\right)+3\prod_{i=1}^{r}\left(\langle i\rangle_{4,3}+\langle i\rangle_{4,4}\right.$$
$$\left.\left.+\,2\langle i\rangle_{4,5}+\langle i\rangle_{4,6}\right)\right]+N_{3,2}^{r-1}\left[68\prod_{i=1}^{r}\langle i\rangle_{3,3}+3\prod_{i=1}^{r}\left(\langle i\rangle_{3,3}+\langle i\rangle_{3,4}\right)\right.$$
$$\left.+\,18\prod_{i=1}^{r}\left(\langle i\rangle_{3,3}+\langle i\rangle_{3,5}\right)+\prod_{i=1}^{r}\left(\langle i\rangle_{3,3}+3\langle i\rangle_{3,5}+\langle i\rangle_{3,6}\right)\right]$$

$$+ N_{4,2}^{r-1}\left[28\prod_{i=1}^{r}\langle i\rangle_{2,3} + 3\prod_{i=1}^{r}\big(\langle i\rangle_{2,3} + \langle i\rangle_{2,5}\big)\right]$$

$$\left. + N_{5,2}^{r-1}\prod_{i=1}^{r}\langle i\rangle_{1,3}\right\} \Big/ N_{6,2}^{r-1} ,$$

$$N_{m,1} = \prod_{i=1}^{m}(N + i - 4) \qquad \text{for } m = 1, \ldots, 4 ,$$

$$N_{m,2} = \prod_{i=1}^{m}(N + i - 6) \qquad \text{for } m = 1, \ldots, 6 ,$$

and for $i = 1, \ldots, r$,

$$\langle i\rangle_{m,1} = \sum_{j=1}^{n_i}\langle i\rangle_j^{(m)} \big/ \langle i\rangle_j^2 \qquad \text{for } m = 1, \ldots, 4 ,$$

$$\langle i\rangle_{2,2} = n_i^{(2)} ,$$

$$\langle i\rangle_{3,2} = (n_i - 1)(N - n_i) ,$$

$$\langle i\rangle_{4,2} = \sum_{j=1}^{n_i}\big(\langle i\rangle_j - 1\big)\big(N - \langle i\rangle_j - n_i + 1\big) ,$$

$$\langle i\rangle_{m,3} = \sum_{j=1}^{n_i}\langle i\rangle_j^{(m)} \big/ \langle i\rangle_j^3 \qquad \text{for } m = 1, \ldots, 6 ,$$

$$\langle i\rangle_{m,4} = \sum_{j=1}^{n_i}\langle i\rangle_j^{(m-2)}\big(N - \langle i\rangle_j - n_i + 1\big) \big/ \langle i\rangle_j^2 \qquad \text{for } m = 3, \ldots, 6 ,$$

$$\langle i\rangle_{m,5} = (n_i - 1)\sum_{j=1}^{n_i}\langle i\rangle_j^{(m-1)} \big/ \langle i\rangle_j^2 \qquad \text{for } m = 2, \ldots, 5 ,$$

$$\langle i\rangle_{3,6} = n_i^{(3)} ,$$

$$\langle i\rangle_{4,6} = (n_i - 1)(n_i - 2)(N - n_i) ,$$

$$\langle i\rangle_{5,6} = (n_i - 2)\sum_{j=1}^{n_i}\big(\langle i\rangle_j - 1\big)\big(N - \langle i\rangle_j - n_i + 1\big)\,,$$

$$\langle i\rangle_{6,6} = \sum_{j=1}^{n_i}\big(\langle i\rangle_j - 1\big)\big(N - \langle i\rangle_j - n_i + 1\big)\big(N - 2\langle i\rangle_j - n_i + 2\big)\,.$$

The corresponding moments for S are

$$\mathrm{E}[S] = \prod_{i=1}^{r}(N - n_i)\big/\big(N^{(2)}\big)^{r-1}\,,$$

$$\mathrm{E}\big[S^2\big] = \left[\prod_{i=1}^{r}\big(\langle i\rangle_{4,1} + \langle i\rangle_{4,2}\big) + 4N_{1,1}^{r-1}\prod_{i=1}^{r}\langle i\rangle_{3,1} + 2N_{2,1}^{r-1}\prod_{i=1}^{r}\langle i\rangle_{2,1}\right]\Big/\,N_{4,1}^{r-1}\,,$$

$$\mathrm{E}\big[S^3\big] = \left\{\prod_{i=1}^{r}\big(\langle i\rangle_{6,3} + 3\langle i\rangle_{6,4} + \langle i\rangle_{6,6}\big) + 12N_{1,2}^{r-1}\prod_{i=1}^{r}\big(\langle i\rangle_{5,3} + \langle i\rangle_{5,4}\big) + N_{2,2}^{r-1}\left[6\prod_{i=1}^{r}\big(\langle i\rangle_{4,3} + \langle i\rangle_{4,4}\big) + 32\prod_{i=1}^{r}\langle i\rangle_{4,3}\right] + 32N_{3,2}^{r-1}\prod_{i=1}^{r}\langle i\rangle_{3,3} + 4N_{4,2}^{r-1}\prod_{i=1}^{r}\langle i\rangle_{2,3}\right\}\Big/\,N_{6,2}^{r-1}\,.$$

The computational expressions for μ_T, σ_T^2, and γ_T, and μ_S, σ_S^2, and γ_S given above were derived using factorial moments, recognizing the correspondence between two-way and r-way contingency table results. Verification of this correspondence involved deriving the three-way table results since the two-way table results presently exist; see discussions by Bartlett [6]; Berry and Mielke [11]; Dawson [28]; Haldane [57, 58]; Lewis, Saunders, and Westcott [82]; Mielke and Berry [109]; and Zelterman [147].

Given the exact values of μ_T, σ_T^2, and γ_T, or μ_S, σ_S^2, and γ_S, the procedure is based on the standardized statistic

$$Z = \frac{T - \mu_T}{\sigma_T} \quad \text{or} \quad Z = \frac{S - \mu_S}{\sigma_S}\,,$$

where the conditional permutation distribution of Z is approximated by the standardized Pearson type III distribution with parameter $\gamma = \gamma_T$, or $\gamma = \gamma_S$, respectively. The motivation for selecting the Pearson type III distribution is that it includes the asymptotic chi-squared and normal distributions of test statistics T and S.

2.3.2 Tests of Goodness of Fit

In this section, analogues of the cumulant methods based on T and S are presented for goodness-of-fit frequency data analyses. If $p_i > 0$ denotes the occurrence probability and O_i denotes the observed frequency for the ith of k disjoint events, then

$$\sum_{i=1}^{k} p_i = 1 \quad \text{and} \quad \sum_{i=1}^{k} O_i = N ,$$

where N is the frequency total. Also, let $E_i = Np_i$ denote the expected frequency of the ith event. Then the corresponding goodness-of-fit statistics are given by

$$T' = \sum_{i=1}^{k} \left(\frac{O_i^2}{E_i} \right) \quad \text{and} \quad S' = \sum_{i=1}^{k} \left(\frac{O_i^{(2)}}{E_i} \right) .$$

Here, $\chi^2 = T' - N$. These methods are governed by the multinomial distribution of the observed frequencies given by

$$P(O_i | p_1, \ldots, p_k, N) = N! \prod_{i=1}^{k} \left(\frac{p_i^{O_i}}{O_i!} \right) .$$

The exact mean, variance, and skewness of T' under the multinomial distribution [57] are given by

$$\mu_{T'} = k + N - 1 ,$$

$$\sigma_{T'}^2 = 2(k-1) + \left[3 - (k+1)^2 + \sum_{i=1}^{k} p_i^{-1} \right] \Big/ N ,$$

and

$$\gamma_{T'} = \frac{A}{\sigma_{T'}^3} ,$$

where

$$A = 8(k-1) - \left[2N(3k-2)(3k+8) - 2(k+3)(k^2+6k-4) - (22N-3k-22)\sum_{i=1}^{k} p_i^{-1} - \sum_{i=1}^{k} p_i^{-2} \right] \Big/ N^2 .$$

Also, the exact mean, variance, and skewness of S' are given by

$$\mu_{S'} = N - 1 ,$$

$$\sigma_{S'}^2 = \frac{2(N-1)(k-1)}{N} ,$$

and

$$\gamma_{S'} = \frac{B}{\sigma_{S'}^3} ,$$

where

$$B = 4(N-1)\left[2N(k-1) - 7k + 6 + \sum_{i=1}^{k} p_i^{-1} \right] \Big/ N^2 .$$

2.4 Permutation and Parametric Statistical Tests

Permutation statistical tests, which are based on the Fisher–Pitman permutation model, differ from traditional parametric tests, which are based on the Neyman–Pearson population model, in several ways. First, permutation tests are entirely data-dependent in that all the information required for analysis is contained within the observed data set [15, 111]. Second, permutation tests are appropriate for non-random samples, such as are common in many fields of research. Third, permutation tests are distribution-free in that they do not depend on the assumptions associated with traditional parametric tests, such as normality and homogeneity of variance. Fourth, permutation tests provide exact probability values based on the discrete permutation distribution of equally-likely test statistic values, rather than approximate probability values based on a theoretical approximating distribution, such as a normal, χ^2, t, or F distribution. Fifth, permutation tests are ideal for small data sets, whereas distribution functions often provide very poor fits.

Of these five differences, the requirements of random sampling and normality greatly limit the applications of statistical tests and measures based on the population model. Moreover, the Neyman–Pearson population model cannot be used when sample sizes are very small, e.g., clinical trials or through sub-dividing otherwise representative samples. On the other hand, since test statistics based on the Fisher–Pitman permutation model require neither random sampling nor normality and are suitable for small samples, permutation tests enjoy a decided advantage over conventional tests in many research applications. Finally, it should be noted that while conventional parametric tests are considered to be relatively robust with respect to violations of assumptions, violation of a combination of assumptions is especially problematic, e.g., random sampling and normality [59, 62, 135].

2.4.1 Permutation Tests and Random Sampling

The requirement of random sampling is fundamental to classical statistics and of paramount importance to statistical inference. Three points should be emphasized. First, permutation tests do not require random sampling [70]. Second, because permutation tests do not depend on random sampling, any inferences are only valid for the objects analyzed.[11] Third, random sampling from a completely specified population in conventional research is seldom achieved in practice.

Random sampling is the single most-important requirement in conventional statistical research, in which every element in a specified population has an equal opportunity of being selected or, alternatively, a sampling scheme that accounts for unequal but known sample probabilities. Done properly, random sampling permits the researcher to generalize results to the target population. The ultimate purpose of random sampling is to eliminate systematic bias. Four forms of bias are prevalent in sampling: frame bias, response bias, nonresponse bias, and observation bias.

Frame bias. A sampling frame is simply a complete listing of the population from which the sample of interest is to be drawn. Simply put, frame bias occurs when there is a mismatch between the sampling frame and the target population [127]. Bias in random samples can be introduced by using improper or imperfect sampling frames. Frame biases are a primary source of problems in sampling [102, p. 164]. If the sampling frame is misspecified or, as in many cases, missing altogether, it is impossible to guarantee the probability of selection for any given element. More specifically, without a random sample from a completely specified and valid sampling frame, no statistical inference about a population parameter can be made. The problem of frame bias is common when studying transient populations ranging from the homeless, migrant workers, and even wildlife populations. Of practical import for election surveys, the sampling frame often includes many adults who are not likely to vote [127].

Response bias. Missing observations due to missing cases lead to response bias. This problem is especially acute in social science research involving mailed

[11] If random sampling from a population has been accomplished, permutation tests can then provide inferences to the specified population.

questionnaires or telephone interviews where response rates are often less than 40%.[12] It is no secret that response rates for all types of surveys have been plummeting [119] and it is well documented that decreasing response rates is an increasingly important problem in the social sciences, especially in survey research. According to the General Accountability Office, responses to mail-in questionnaires and door-to-door interviews for the United States Census have been declining for years [38].

For a historical example, the *Literary Digest* poll of 1936 predicted a 3-to-2 victory for the Republican nominee, Kansas Governor Alf Landon, over the incumbent President Franklin D. Roosevelt. Roosevelt not only won, but pulled off one of the greatest landslides in political history, winning 62% of the popular vote and carrying 46 of 48 states.[13] Ten million sample ballots were mailed to prospective voters, but only 2.3 million were returned. The respondents represented only that subset of the population with a relatively intense interest in the subject at hand and, as Bryson related, "it seems clear that the minority of anti-Roosevelt voters felt more strongly about the election that did the pro-Roosevelt majority" [22, p. 185].

Nonresponse bias. Nonresponse bias occurs when the likelihood of responding to a survey is systematically related to how a respondent would have answered the survey [127]. Thus, supporters of a trailing candidate or an unpopular amendment in a political election are less likely to respond to surveys, biasing the results in favor of the leading candidate or opinion. For a political science example, in the 2012 United States presidential election campaign, it is generally agreed that Democratic candidate Barack Obama performed poorly in the first presidential debate on October 3 with Republican candidate Mitt Romney. As a result, Obama's support declined precipitously in the subsequent polls. Gelman, Goel, Rivers, and Rothschild showed that the decline was strongly correlated with changes in survey participation, i.e., nonresponse to polls, rather than changes in voter intentions [51, p. 107].

Observation bias. Missing observations due to missing values can also lead to considerable bias. In this case, respondents decline to answer one or more questions. This problem is of special concern when some questions explore especially sensitive issues, e.g., politics, criminality, drug use, religion, sexual orientation, or even amount of income. Techniques such as randomized response can overcome much of observation bias due to sensitive questions wherein a pair of questions are asked: one innocuous, the other sensitive. The randomized response procedure leaves the choice of question by a respondent to a randomization device [45, 136, 140, 143].

It is important to note that the mathematical theorems that justify most statistical procedures apply only to random samples drawn with replacement from a completely specified and valid sampling frame. For example, the model assumptions for a one-sample z test are a simple random sample of a random variable from a normal

[12]In November 2015 Higgins reported that response rates for telephone surveys had fallen to less than 10% in 2015, from more than 80% in 1970 [65, p. 30].

[13]There were only 48 states in 1936. Alaska and Hawaii were added in 1959.

distribution. Consider all possible simple random samples of size n from random variable Y. Then, if the model assumptions and the null hypothesis are both true, the sampling distribution of sample means, $\bar{Y}$, will be approximately normal with mean $\mu_{\bar{Y}}$ equal to the value specified by the null hypothesis, μ_0, and standard error $\sigma_{\bar{Y}}$ given by $\sigma_Y/\sqrt{n}$, where σ_Y denotes the population standard deviation. However, if the sample is not a simple random sample from a well-defined sampling frame, then the validity of the hypothesis test is questionable.

As noted by John Ludbrook many years ago, early statisticians such as R.A. Fisher, Frank Yates, and Oscar Kempthorne readily acknowledged that in their extensive agricultural research random samples were never drawn from, nor represented, well-defined populations. In their experiments at the Rothamsted Experimental Station, plant varieties or different fertilizers were assigned to blocks of land within a field by a process of randomization. The field was not a random sample of the population of all possible fields, or even a random sample of fields from a defined category [85, p. 675]. This holds true for contemporary research where samples of patients, laboratory animals, students, the homeless, or incarcerated criminals seldom are drawn from a well-defined population and are usually acquired in a non-random fashion, then randomized into sub-groups for intervention or treatment of one or more of the sub-groups. Moreover, a number of authors have documented that the requirement of obtaining a random sample from a well-defined population is seldom met in practice; see, for example, articles by Altman and Bland [1], Bradbury [16], Feinstein [39], Frick [46], LaFleur and Greevy [78], Ludbrook [85], Ludbrook and Dudley [91], and Still and White [133].

There are, admittedly, some applications in statistical analysis in which random sampling from a specified population is neither attempted nor considered important. The fact that medical researchers seldom use random samples often comes as a surprise to investigators who work in other domains. As Alvan Feinstein, a noted medical researcher, wrote in 1973:

> With inanimate materials, chemists achieve random samples routinely and easily as an aliquot of a homogeneous mass. With general human populations, social and political scientists given careful attention to methods of sampling and getting random selections. With medical populations, however, the investigative samples are almost never random. Why are medical researchers so delinquent? [39, p. 899].

Feinstein goes on to answer his own question.

> The answer to this question is based on the two different purposes of statistical inference. A socio-political scientist often wants to estimate a populational parameter, whereas a medical researcher usually wants to contrast a difference in two groups. A random sample is mandatory for estimating a parameter, but has not been regarded as equally imperative for contrasting a difference [39, p. 899].

Psychologists have been especially concerned with problems of random sampling. Writing in *Canadian Psychology*, psychologists Michael Hunter and Richard May noted that random sampling is of particular relevance to psychologists, "who rarely use random sampling or any other sort of probability sampling" [70, p. 385]. In 1988 psychologist William Hays wrote:

> The point is that *some* probability structure must be known or assumed to underlie the occurrence of samples if statistical inference is to proceed. This point is belabored only because it is so often overlooked, and statistical inferences are so often made with only the most casual attention to the process by which the sample was generated. The assumption of some probability structure underlying the sampling is a little "price tag" attached to a statistical inference. It is a sad fact that if one knows nothing about the probability of occurrence for particular samples of units for observation, very little of the machinery we are describing here applies. This is why our assumption of random sampling is not to be taken lightly.... Unless this assumption is at least reasonable, the probability results of inferential methods mean very little, and these methods might as well be omitted [63, p. 212].[14]

In 2001, psychologist Michael Cowles wrote:

> [T]he samples of convenience that are used in psychological research are hardly ever selected randomly in the formal sense. Undergraduate student volunteers are not labeled as automatically constituting random samples, but they are often assumed to be *unbiased* with respect to the dependent variables of interest, an assumption that has produced much criticism [26, p. 87].[15]

Finally, sampling distributions require random sampling whereas permutation distributions do not [70, p. 387].

2.4.2 Permutation Tests and Normality

The assumption of normality is so basic to classical statistics that it deserves special attention. Two points should be emphasized. First, permutation tests make no distributional assumptions and, therefore, do not depend on the assumption of normality. Second, the assumption of normality by conventional tests is always unrealistic and never justified in practice [100]. In fact, the consistent defense of the assumption of normality and the insistence on the robustness of various tests is not only unnecessary but patently risible.

In 1927 R.C. Geary famously proclaimed: "Normality is a myth; there never has, and never will be, a normal distribution" [50, p. 241], and in 1938 Joseph Berkson wrote: "we may assume that it is practically certain that any series of real observations does not actually follow a normal curve *with absolute exactitude* in all respects" [7, p. 526],[16] and The French physicist and Nobel laureate in physics, Gabriel Lippmann, once wrote in a letter to Henri Poincaré à propos the normal curve:

> Experimentalists think that it is a mathematical theorem, while mathematicians believe it to be an experimental effect.

---

[14]Emphasis in the original.

[15]Emphasis in the original.

[16]Emphasis in the original.

(Gabriel Lippman, quoted in D'Arcy Wentworth Thompson's *On Growth and Form* [134, p. 121]), and Robert Matthews once described the normal distribution as "beautiful, beguiling and thoroughly dangerous" [100, p. 193]. And in 1954 Bross pointed out that statistical methods "are based on certain assumptions—assumptions which not only can be wrong, but in many situations *are* wrong" [21, p. 815].[17] Others have empirically demonstrated the prevalence of highly skewed and heavy-tailed distributions in a variety of academic disciplines; see, for example, discussions by Schmidt and Johnson [130], Bradley [19], Saal, Downey, and Lahey [128], Bernardin and Beatty [8], Matthews [101], Micceri [107], and Murphy and Cleveland [115], the best known of which is Micceri's widely quoted 1989 article on "The unicorn, the normal curve, and other improbable creatures" in *Psychological Bulletin* [107].

A number of authors have documented that the assumption of normality is rarely satisfied in real-data situations; see, for example, articles by Bernardin and Beatty [8], Bradley [17], Bross [21], Feinstein [39], Geary [49], Micceri [107], Murphy and Cleveland [115], Saal, Downey, and Lahey [128], and Schmidt and Johnson [130]. Finally, in 1947 G.A. Barnard, writing in response to a paper by Egon Pearson on 2×2 contingency tables, noted that while it is imperative that the means and variances of samples be independently distributed, "in the case of normal distributions, and *only in this case*, the mean and variance of samples are independently distributed" [5, p. 169].[18] See also a discussion by Stephen Stigler in *The Seven Pillars of Statistical Wisdom* [132, pp. 91–92].

2.4.3 Permutation Tests and Small Sample Sizes

Permutation statistical tests have an advantage over conventional statistical tests based on the population model in that they are ideal for analyzing data from small samples. Conventional statistical approaches rely on relatively large sample sizes, although obtaining large enough samples to fit the underlying distributional assumptions is often problematic. Sample sizes may be restricted for a number of reasons: limitations due to ethical concerns, e.g., medical studies; subdividing larger samples into smaller components such as analyzing survey data from only those respondents who meet specific criteria, e.g., subdividing nationally representative data on income for comparing consumer preferences between men and women over the age of 72 with incomes above \$100,000; "large units," e.g., studying corporate response to large-scale disaster events; and meta-analyses using only published studies. In many cases, analyses are simply avoided when the required sample sizes are not available. Permutation statistics allow researchers to use all of the available data. Barry Nussbaum, chief statistician at the U.S. environmental

[17] Emphasis in the original.

[18] Emphasis in the original.

Protection Agency and president of the American Statistical Association, wrote in a 2017 article titled "Bigger isn't always better when it comes to data" that

> [B]ecause we currently have a fascination with Big Data—large volumes, velocity, variety, and, hopefully, veracity—we sometimes forget the beautiful basic utility of inferential statistics getting a lot of information from small, but well-constructed, samples [120, p. 4].

2.4.4 Permutation Tests and Data Dependency

Permutation methods are often termed "data-dependent" methods, sometimes referred to as "data at hand" methods, because all the information available for analysis is contained within the observed data set and information external to the observed data is neither necessary nor considered. As noted by Stigler [132, pp. 87–88], in 1875 Francis Galton introduced data-dependency, his first contribution to the methods of statistics [126, p. 295], which he called "statistics by intercomparison." Galton wrote:

> [W]e do not require (1) independent measurements, nor (2) arithmetical operations; we are (3) able to dispense with standards of reference, in the common acceptance of the phrase, being able to create and afterwards indirectly to define them.... Therefore it is theoretically possible, in a great degree, to replace the ordinary process of obtaining statistics by another, much simpler in conception, more convenient in certain cases, and of incomparably wider applicability.... This I suppose to be effected wholly by *intercomparison*, without the aid of any external standard [48, p. 34].[19]

Since, in data-dependent research, the computed probability values are conditioned solely on the observed data, permutation tests require no assumptions about the population(s) from which the data have been sampled [60]. Thus, permutation tests are distribution-free tests in that the tests do not assume distributional properties of the population [18, 23, 98]. With a parametric analysis, it is necessary to know the parent distribution (e.g., a normal distribution) and evaluate the data with respect to this known distribution. Conversely, a data-dependent permutation analysis generates a reference set of outcomes by way of randomization for a comparison with the observed outcome [103]. Since the randomization of objects is the basic assumption for a permutation analysis, any arrangement can be obtained by pairwise exchanges of the objects. Thus, the associated object measurements are termed "exchangeable." Hayes [61] provides an excellent discussion of exchangeability. For more rigorous presentations, see Draper et al. [29], Lehmann [80], and Lindley and Novick [84].

[19] Emphasis in the original.

2.5 Advantages of Permutation Methods

Alvan Feinstein was a strong advocate for permutation methods. Trained as a medical doctor, Feinstein is widely regarded as the founder of clinical epidemiology and patient-oriented medicine and the originator of clinimetrics: the application of mathematics to the field of medicine [10, p. 246]. In 1973 Feinstein published a formative article on "The role of randomization in sampling, testing, allocation, and credulous idolatry" [39].

Writing for a statistically unsophisticated readership, Feinstein distinguished between socio-political research where the purpose was usually to estimate a population parameter, and medical research where the purpose was typically to contrast a difference between two groups.[20] Feinstein observed that a random sample is mandatory for estimating a population parameter, but "has not been regarded as equally imperative for contrasting a difference" [39, p. 899]. Or, as May and Hunter noted,

> A major concern of surveys is external validity and generality inference, whereas comparative experiments are more concerned with internal validity and causal inference. Thus, we may need different statistical models for different research contexts [103, p. 401].

Feinstein's article is as important today as it was when published in 1973 and remains one of the most cogent and lucid expositions contrasting conventional parametric and permutation methods. While R.A. Fisher, R.C. Geary, T. Eden, F. Yates, and E.J.G. Pitman defined the field of permutation statistical methods in the 1920s and 1930s, A.R. Feinstein's 1973 article should be the *vade mecum* of every researcher interested in permutation statistical methods.

As Feinstein's focus was on medical investigations, he listed the major violations of the assumptions underlying tests of two groups:

1. The groups studied in modern clinical or epidemiologic research are seldom selected as random samples.
2. For the many clinical and epidemiologic research projects that are performed as surveys, the subjects are not randomly assigned.
3. The distribution of the target variable is usually unknown in the parent population.
4. It is usually known that the target variable does not have a Gaussian distribution, and often departs from it dramatically.
5. It is usually known that the variances of the two samples are not remotely similar.

[20] The 1973 Feinstein article was the 23rd in a series of informative summary articles on statistical methods for clinical researchers published in *Clinical Pharmacology and Therapeutics*. A collection of 29 of the articles written by Feinstein is available in *Clinical Biostatistics* where this article was retitled "Permutation tests and 'statistical significance' " [40].

Feinstein then compared, in meticulous detail, the classical approaches embodied in the two-sample t test and the chi-squared test of independence for 2×2 contingency tables. For his example data, he noted that the probability values obtained from the classical approach differed substantially from those obtained from the corresponding permutation tests.[21] Regarding the chi-squared test of independence, Feinstein observed that the corresponding permutation test provided an exact answer to the research question that was "precise, unambiguous, unencumbered by any peculiar expectations about fractional people, and unembroiled in any controversy about the Yates' correction [for continuity]" [39, p. 910].

Feinstein put forth some advantages and disadvantages of permutation tests that were insightful for the time and foreshadowed later research. In terms of permutation tests, he listed five advantages:

1. The result of a permutation test is a direct, exact probability value for the random likelihood of the observed difference.
2. Permutation tests do not require any unwarranted inferential estimations of means, variances, pooled variances, or other parameters of an unobserved, hypothetical parent population. The tests are based solely on the evidence that was actually obtained.[22]
3. The investigator is not forced into making any erroneous assumptions either that the contrasted groups were chosen as random samples from a parent population, or that treatments under study were randomly allocated to the two groups.
4. The investigator is not forced into making any erroneous or unconfirmable assumptions about a Gaussian (or any other) distribution for the parent population, or about equal variances in the contrasted groups.
5. A permutation test can be applied to groups of any size, no matter how large or small. There are no degrees of freedom to be considered. In the case of a contingency table, there is no need to worry about the magnitude of the expected value, no need to calculate expectations based on fractions of people, and no need to worry about applying, or not applying, Yates' correction for continuity.

Feinstein observed that while there were definite advantages to permutation tests, there were also disadvantages. The first three (of four) he considered as features that contributed to "the existing state of statistical desuetude" and labeled them inertia, ideology, and information [39, p. 911]:

1. Inertia: It is easier for many teachers to continue the inertia of teaching what they were taught years ago than to revise the contents of their lectures.

---

[21] Here, Feinstein utilized permutation tests as the gold standard against which to evaluate classical tests, referencing a 1963 article by McHugh [104] and 1966 articles by Baker and Collier [3], and Edgington [33].

[22] In this second advantage, Feinstein clearly described the data-dependent nature of permutation tests, anticipating by many years later research on permutation methods.

2. Ideology: Investigators who ideologically believe that the goal of science is to estimate parameters and variances will have no enthusiasm for tests that do not include or rely on these estimations.
3. Information: Many investigators have a deep-seated horror of doing anything that might entail losing information.
4. Calculation: Permutation tests are notoriously difficult to calculate.

Feinstein elaborated on items 3 (Information) and 4 (Calculation). Regarding Item 3, he emphasized that a loss of information would occur if raw data were converted into ordinal data for the sake of a non-parametric test that analyzes ranks rather than the observed raw scores. He explained that since ranks are used in nearly all non-parametric tests and since all non-parametric tests depend on random permutations, a statistician may erroneously conclude that all non-parametric tests create a loss of information.[23] He retorted that that conclusion was specious as "the non-parametric permutation tests illustrated here make use of the original values of the [observed] data, not the ranks" [39, p. 911]. In his own words:

> Many statisticians have a deep-seated horror of doing anything that may entail "losing information." This type of "loss" would occur if dimensional data were converted into ordinal ranks for the sake of a non-parametric test that uses the ranks rather than the observed values. Since ranks are used in almost all of the tests popularly known as *non-parametric*, and since all of these tests depend on the principle of random permutations, a statistician may erroneously conclude that all non-parametric tests create a loss of information. The conclusion is wrong because the non-parametric tests illustrated here make use of the original values of the data, not the ranks [39, p. 911].[24]

Regarding Item 4, Feinstein observed that every permutation test must be computed entirely from the individual values of the observed data. Thus, each application is a unique test and precludes the compilation of tables that can be used repeatedly [39, p. 912]; a point made earlier, and most emphatically, by James Bradley [18]. He followed this with the prescient observation that "in the era of the digital computer. . . these calculational difficulties will ultimately disappear" [39, p. 912]. Feinstein further observed that in situations where the sample sizes were large, the exact permutation test could be "truncated" into a Monte Carlo (resampling) type of test.

In a strongly worded conclusion, Feinstein argued that the ultimate value of permutation tests was that their intellectual directness, precision, and simplicity would free both the investigator and the statistician from "a deleterious pre-occupation with sampling distributions, pooled variances, and other mathematical distractions" [39, p. 914]. Finally, Feinstein noted that "an investigator who comprehends the

[23]In the literature of mathematical statistics there are examples of distributions where a non-parametric test that "throws away information" is clearly superior to a parametric test; see, for example, articles by Festinger in 1946 [41], Pitman in 1948 [124], Whitney in 1948 [144], and van den Brink and van den Brink in 1989 [141].

[24]Emphasis in the original.

principles of his statistical tests will be less inclined to give idolatrous worship to a numerical 'significance' that has no scientific connotation" [39, p. 914].[25]

Finally, it should be mentioned that numerous statistical tests and measures have been developed over the past 100 years for which the standard errors are either unknown or intractable. Many of these tests and measures have been very well constructed and are generally quite useful, but their utility is constrained by the lack of a known standard error. The absence of standard errors is of no consequence to permutation statistical methods. Thus, an added advantage to permutation statistical methods is the ability to generate exact probability values for these otherwise limited tests and measures.

2.6 Calculation Efficiency

While permutation statistical tests do not require random sampling, normality, homogeneity, or large sample sizes, and are also completely data-dependent, a potential drawback is the amount of computation required, with exact permutation tests formerly being unrealistic for many statistical analyses. Even Monte Carlo resampling permutation tests often require the enumeration of millions of random arrangements of the observed data in order to guarantee sufficient accuracy. For many years, exact tests were considered to be impractical, but modern computers make it possible to generate hundreds of millions of permutations in just a few minutes. In addition, Monte Carlo permutation methods can be inefficient due to millions of calls to a pseudorandom number generator (PRNG). The development of the high-speed Mersenne Twister PRNG by Matsumoto and Nishimura in 1998 greatly increased the accuracy and speed of Monte Carlo resampling permutation methods [99]. It was not too many years ago that 5,000 or 10,000 random samples were considered to be sufficient for resampling permutation methods, due to the slow speeds of computers. Presently, it is common to see 1,000,000 random samples, which generally ensure three decimal places of accuracy, and even 100,000,000 random samples, which generally ensure four decimal places of accuracy [71].

Four innovations mitigate this problem. First, high-speed computing makes possible exact permutation statistical tests in which all possible arrangements of the observed data are generated and examined. Second, examination of all combinations of arrangements of the observed data, instead of all permutations, yields the same exact probability values with considerable savings in computation time. Third, mathematical recursion with an arbitrary initial value greatly simplifies difficult computations, such as large factorial expressions. Fourth, calculation of only the variable components of the selected test statistic greatly simplifies calculation.

[25] See also an informative and engaging 2012 article on this topic by Megan Higgs in *American Scientist* [66].

2.6.1 High-Speed Computing

As Berry, Johnston, and Mielke observed in 2014 [10, pp. 364–365], one has only to observe the hordes of the digitally distracted trying to navigate a crowded sidewalk with their various smart-phones, pads, pods, and tablets to realize that computing power, speed, and accessibility have finally arrived. As Martin Hilbert documented, in 1986 just one percent of the world's capacity to store information was in digital format, but by year 2000 digital represented 25 percent of the total world's memory [67]. The year 2002 marked the start of the digital age, as 2002 was the year that humankind first stored more information in digital than in analog form. By 2007 over 97 percent of the world's storage capacity was digital [67, p. 9]. Moreover, it was estimated in 2012 that ninety percent of the data stored in the world had been created in just the previous two years. Prior to 2001, data storage was measured in bytes, kilobytes (10^3), and occasionally in megabytes (10^6); now data storage is measured in gigabytes (10^9), terabytes (10^{12}), petabytes (10^{15}), exabytes (10^{18}), zettabytes (10^{21}), and even yottabytes (10^{24}).

In 2000, the Intel Pentium processor contained 42 million transistors and ran at 1.5 GHz. In the spring of 2010, Intel released the Itanium processor, code-named Tukwila after a town in the state of Washington, containing 1.4 billion transistors and running at 2.53 GHz. On 4 June 2013 Intel announced the Haswell processor, named after a small town of 65 people in southeastern Colorado with 1.4 billion 3-D chips and running at 3.50 GHz [142]. The latest generation of Haswell processors, the i7-4790 processor, currently executes at 4.00 GHz with turbo-boost to 4.40 GHz. In April of 2017, Intel introduced the Optane memory module which, when coupled with a seventh generation Intel Core-based system, has the potential to increase desktop computer performance by 28 percent.

While not widely available to researchers, by 2010 mainframe computers were measuring computing speeds in teraflops. To emphasize the progress of computing, in 1951 the Remington Rand Corporation introduced the UNIVAC computer running at 1,905 flops, which with ten mercury delay line memory tanks could store 20,000 bytes of information; in 2008 the IBM Corporation supercomputer, code-named Roadrunner, reached a sustained performance of one petaflops;[26] in 2010 the Cray Jaguar was named the world's fastest computer performing at a sustained speed of 1.75 petaflops with 360 terabytes of memory; and in November of 2010 China exceeded the computing speed of the Cray Jaguar by 57 percent with the introduction of China's Tianhe-1A supercomputer performing at 2.67 petaflops [93].

In October of 2011, China broke the petaflops barrier again with the introduction of the Sunway Bluelight MPP [4]. In late 2011 the IBM Yellowstone supercomputer was installed at the National Center for Atmospheric Research (NCAR) Wyoming Supercomputer Center in Cheyenne, Wyoming. After months of testing, the Wyoming Supercomputer Center officially opened on Monday, 15 October 2012.

[26] One petaflops indicates a quadrillion operations per second, or a 1 with 15 zeroes following it.

Yellowstone was a 1.6 petaflops machine with 149.2 terabytes of memory and 74,592 processor cores and replaced an IBM Bluefire supercomputer installed in 2008 that had a peak speed of 76 teraflops. Also in late 2011, IBM unveiled the Blue Gene\P and \Q supercomputing processing systems that can achieve 20 petaflops. At the same time, IBM filed a patent for a massive supercomputing system capable of 107 petaflops.

From a more general perspective, in 1977 the Tandy Corporation released the TRS-80, the first fully assembled personal computer, distributed through Radio Shack stores. The TRS-80 had 4MB of RAM and ran at 1.78 MHz. By way of comparison, in 2010 the Apple iPhone had 131,072 times the memory of the TRS-80 and was approximately 2,000 times faster, running at one GHz. In 2012, Sequoia, an IBM Blue Gene/Q supercomputer was installed at Lawrence Livermore National Laboratory (LLNL) in Livermore, California. In June of 2012 Sequoia officially became the most powerful supercomputer in the world. Sequoia is capable of 16.32 petaflops—more than 16 quadrillion calculations a second—which was 55 percent faster than Japan's K supercomputer, ranked number 2, and more than five times faster than China's Tianhe-1A, which was the fastest supercomputer in the world in 2010.

Finally, high-speed computers have dramatically changed the field of computational statistics. The future of high-speed computing appears very promising for exact and Monte Carlo resampling permutation statistical methods. Combined with other efficiencies, it can safely be said that permutation methods have the potential to provide exact or resampling probability values in an efficient manner for a wide variety of statistical applications.

2.6.2 Analysis with Combinations

Although permutation statistical methods are known by the attribution "permutation," they are, in fact, not based on all possible permutations of the observed data. Instead exact permutation methods are typically based on all possible *combinations* of the observed data.[27] Conversely, a so-called combination lock is not based on combinations of numbers or letters, but is instead based on all possible *permutations* of the numbers or letters. A simple example will illustrate. Consider $N = 8$ objects that are to be divided into two groups A and B, where $n_A = n_B = 4$. The purpose is to compare differences between the two groups, such as a mean or median difference. Let the eight objects be designated $\{a, b, c, d, e, f, g, h\}$. For group A, the first object can be chosen in eight different ways, the second object in seven ways, the third in six ways, and the fourth object in five ways. Once these four members of Group A are chosen, the membership of Group B is fixed, since the remaining four objects are assigned to Group B.

[27] In keeping with convention, "permutation methods" is used throughout this book.

Of the $8{\times}7{\times}6{\times}5 = 1{,}680$ ways in which the four objects can be arranged for Group A, each individual quartet of objects will appear in a series of permutations. Thus, the quartet $\{a, b, c, d\}$ can be permuted as $\{a, b, d, c\}, \{b, a, c, d\}, \{c, d, b, a\}$, and so on. The number of different permutations for a group of four different objects is $4! = 4{\times}3{\times}2{\times}1 = 24$. Thus, each distinctive quartet will appear in 24 ways among the 1,680 possible arrangements. Therefore, 1,680 divided by 24 yields 70 distinctive quartets that could be formed by dividing eight objects into two groups of four objects each. The number of quartets can conveniently be expressed as

$$\frac{(n_A + n_B)!}{n_A!\, n_B!} = \frac{(4+4)!}{4!\, 4!} = \frac{40{,}320}{576} = 70\ .$$

Now, half of these arrangements are similar but opposite. Thus the quartet $\{a, b, c, d\}$ might be in Group A and the quartet $\{e, f, g, h\}$ might be in Group B, or vice versa, yielding the same absolute difference. Consequently, there are really only $70/2 = 35$ distinctly different pairs of quartets to be considered. The 35 possible arrangements for objects $\{a, b, c, d, e, f, g, h\}$ are listed in Table 2.10 in Gray-code order.[28] The next (36th) possible arrangement would be $\{a, b, c, h\}$ in Group A and $\{d, e, f, g\}$ in Group B, which is simply the reverse of arrangement 35, i.e., $\{d, e, f, g\}$ in Group A and $\{a, b, c, h\}$ in Group B, yielding the same absolute mean or median difference. A substantial amount of calculation can be eliminated by considering all possible combinations instead of all possible permutations, with no loss of accuracy. In this case, a decrease from 1,680 to 35 arrangements to be considered, a reduction of approximately 98%.

Example Permutation Analysis

Consider a sample of $N = 8$ objects with values $\{38, 39, 40, 43, 48, 49, 52, 57\}$. The $N = 8$ objects are divided into two groups, A and B with $n_A = 4$ objects in Group A and $n_B = 4$ objects in Group B. The objects in Group A have values of $\{43, 49, 52, 57\}$ and the objects in Group B have values of $\{38, 39, 40, 48\}$, yielding means $\bar{x}_A = 50.25$ and $\bar{x}_B = 41.25$, and a mean difference of $\bar{x}_A - \bar{x}_B = 50.25 - 41.25 = +9.00$. Now consider the data from a permutation perspective. Table 2.11 lists the 35 possible arrangements of the $N = 8$ values with $n_A = n_B = 4$ preserved for each arrangement, the mean values, $\bar{x}_A$ and $\bar{x}_B$, and the 35 mean differences, $\bar{x}_A - \bar{x}_B$.

Inspection of Table 2.11 shows that a mean difference of $\bar{x}_A - \bar{x}_B = 50.25 - 41.25 = +9.00$ or greater in favor of Group A occurs only twice in the 35 possible arrangements, i.e., row 1 with mean difference +11.50 and row 2 with mean difference +9.00, indicated by asterisks. If Table 2.11 were to be completed

[28] Gray code, after Frank Gray, or reflected binary code (RBC), is an encoding of numbers such that adjacent numbers have a single digit differing by 1.

Table 2.10 Listing of the 35 arrangements of objects $\{a, b, c, d, e, f, g, h\}$ into two groups of four objects each

Number	Group A	Group B	Number	Group A	Group B
1	a, b, c, d	e, f, g, h	19	b, c, d, g	a, e, f, h
2	a, b, c, e	d, f, g, h	20	a, b, e, g	c, d, f, h
3	a, b, d, e	c, f, g, h	21	a, c, e, g	b, d, f, h
4	a, c, d, e	b, f, g, h	22	b, c, e, g	a, d, f, h
5	b, c, d, e	a, f, g, h	23	a, d, e, g	b, c, f, h
6	a, b, c, f	d, e, g, h	24	b, d, e, g	a, c, f, h
7	a, b, d, f	c, e, g, h	25	c, d, e, g	a, b, f, h
8	a, c, d, f	b, e, g, h	26	a, b, f, g	c, d, e, h
9	b, c, d, f	a, e, g, h	27	a, c, f, g	b, d, e, h
10	a, b, e, f	c, d, g, h	28	b, c, f, g	a, d, e, h
11	a, c, e, f	b, d, g, h	29	a, d, f, g	b, c, e, h
12	b, c, e, f	a, d, g, h	30	b, d, f, g	a, c, e, h
13	a, d, e, f	b, c, g, h	31	c, d, f, g	a, b, e, h
14	b, d, e, f	a, c, g, h	32	a, e, f, g	b, c, d, h
15	c, d, e, f	a, b, g, h	33	b, e, f, g	a, c, d, h
16	a, b, c, g	d, e, f, h	34	c, e, f, g	a, b, d, h
17	a, b, d, g	c, e, f, h	35	d, e, f, g	a, b, c, h
18	a, c, d, g	b, e, f, h			

to form all 70 arrangements, a mean difference of 9.00 or greater would also occur twice. Thus, for a two-sided test the exact probability is $P = 4/70 = 0.0571$, and for a one-sided test the exact probability is $P = 2/70 = 0.0286$.

2.6.3 *Mathematical Recursion*

Mathematical recursion, in a statistical context, is a process in which an initial probability value of a test statistic is calculated, then successive probability values are generated from the initial value by a recursive process.[29] The initial value need not be an actual probability value, but can be a completely arbitrary positive value by which the resultant relative probability values are adjusted for the initializing value at the conclusion of the recursion process. This section demonstrates a recursion procedure with an initial probability value using the data on convicted and non-convicted monozygotic and dizygotic twins discussed in Sect. 2.2.1. The following

[29] A recursive process is one in which items are defined in terms of items of similar kind. Using a recursive relation, a class of items can be constructed from one or a few initial values (a base) and a small number of relationships (rules). For example, given the base, $F_0 = 0$ and $F_1 = F_2 = 1$, the Fibonacci series $\{0, 1, 1, 2, 3, 5, 8, 13, 21, \ldots\}$ can be constructed by the recursive rule $F_n = F_{n-1} + F_{n-2}$ for $n > 2$.

Table 2.11 Means and mean differences for 35 arrangements of eight observations divided into two groups of four objects each

Number	Group *A*	Group *B*	$\bar{x}_A$	$\bar{x}_B$	$\bar{x}_A - \bar{x}_B$
1*	48, 49, 52, 57	38, 39, 40, 43	51.50	40.00	+11.50
2*	43, 49, 52, 57	38, 39, 40, 48	50.25	41.25	+9.00
3	43, 48, 52, 57	38, 39, 40, 49	50.00	41.50	+8.50
4	40, 49, 52, 57	38, 39, 43, 48	49.50	42.00	+7.50
5	39, 49, 52, 57	38, 40, 43, 48	49.25	42.25	+7.00
6	40, 48, 52, 57	38, 39, 43, 49	49.25	42.25	+7.00
7	43, 48, 49, 57	38, 39, 40, 52	49.25	42.25	+7.00
8	38, 49, 52, 57	39, 40, 43, 48	49.99	42.50	+6.50
9	39, 48, 52, 57	38, 40, 43, 49	49.00	42.50	+6.50
10	38, 48, 52, 57	39, 40, 43, 49	48.75	42.75	+6.00
11	40, 48, 49, 57	38, 39, 43, 52	48.50	43.00	+5.50
12	39, 48, 49, 57	38, 40, 43, 52	48.25	43.25	+5.00
13	40, 43, 52, 57	38, 39, 48, 49	48.00	43.50	+4.50
14	38, 48, 49, 57	39, 40, 43, 52	48.00	43.50	+4.50
15	39, 43, 52, 57	38, 40, 48, 49	47.75	43.75	+4.00
16	38, 43, 52, 57	39, 40, 48, 49	47.50	44.00	+3.50
17	40, 43, 49, 57	38, 39, 48, 52	47.25	44.25	+3.00
18	39, 40, 52, 57	38, 43, 48, 49	47.00	44.50	+2.50
19	39, 43, 49, 57	38, 40, 48, 52	47.00	44.50	+2.50
20	40, 43, 48, 57	38, 39, 49, 52	47.00	44.50	+2.50
21	39, 43, 48, 57	38, 40, 49, 52	46.75	44.75	+2.00
22	38, 40, 52, 57	39, 43, 48, 49	46.75	44.75	+2.00
23	38, 43, 49, 57	39, 40, 48, 52	46.75	44.75	+2.00
24	38, 39, 52, 57	40, 43, 48, 49	46.50	45.00	+1.50
25	38, 43, 48, 57	39, 40, 49, 52	46.50	45.00	+1.50
26	39, 40, 49, 57	38, 43, 48, 52	46.25	45.25	+1.00
27	38, 40, 49, 57	39, 43, 48, 52	46.00	45.50	+0.50
28	39, 40, 48, 57	38, 43, 49, 52	46.00	45.50	+0.50
29	38, 40, 48, 57	39, 43, 49, 52	45.75	45.75	0.00
30	38, 39, 49, 57	40, 43, 48, 52	45.75	45.75	0.00
31	38, 39, 48, 57	40, 43, 49, 52	45.50	46.00	−0.50
32	39, 40, 43, 57	38, 48, 49, 52	44.75	46.75	−2.00
33	38, 40, 43, 57	39, 48, 49, 52	44.50	47.00	−2.50
34	38, 39, 43, 57	40, 48, 49, 52	44.25	47.25	−3.00
35	38, 39, 40, 57	43, 48, 49, 52	43.50	48.00	−4.50

section demonstrates a recursion procedure with an arbitrary initial value using the same data.

Mathematical recursion is so fundamental to permutation statistical methods that a detailed example of a recursion process is important to illustrate the procedure.

Perhaps no better description of the statistical recursion procedure exists than that provided by Frank Yates. In 1934 Yates succinctly described the recursion process:

> In cases where N is not too large the distribution with any particular numerical values of the marginal totals can be computed quite quickly, using a table of factorials to determine some convenient term, and working out the rest of the distribution term by term, by simple multiplications and divisions. If a table of factorials is not available we may start with any convenient term as unity, and divide by the sum of the terms so obtained [145, p. 219],

where N denotes the total number of observations.

A Recursion Example

Consider a 2×2 contingency table using the notation in Table 2.12. Denote by a dot $(\cdot)$ the partial sum of all rows or all columns, depending on the position of the $(\cdot)$ in the subscript list. If the $(\cdot)$ is in the first subscript position, the sum is over all rows and if the $(\cdot)$ is in the second subscript position, the sum is over all columns. Thus, $n_{i.}$ denotes the marginal frequency total of the ith row, $i = 1, \ldots, r$, summed over all columns, $n_{.j}$ denotes the marginal frequency total of the jth column, $j = 1, \ldots, c$, summed over all rows, and $N = n_{11} + n_{12} + n_{21} + n_{22}$ denotes the table frequency total. The probability value corresponding to any set of cell frequencies in a 2×2 contingency table, $n_{11}, n_{12}, n_{21}, n_{22}$, is the hypergeometric point probability value given by

$$P = \binom{n_{.1}}{n_{11}}\binom{n_{.2}}{n_{12}}\binom{N}{n_{1.}}^{-1} = \frac{n_{1.}!\,n_{2.}!\,n_{.1}!\,n_{.2}!}{N!\,n_{11}!\,n_{12}!\,n_{21}!\,n_{22}!}\;.$$

Since the exact probability value of a 2×2 contingency table with fixed marginal frequency totals and one degree of freedom is equivalent to the probability value of any one cell, determining the probability value of the cell containing n_{11} is sufficient. If

$$P\{n_{11}+1|n_{1.}, n_{.1}, N\} = P\{n_{11}|n_{1.}, n_{.1}, N\} \times f(n_{11})\;,$$

then solving for $f(n_{11})$ produces

$$f(n_{11}) = \frac{P\{n_{11}+1|n_{1.}, n_{.1}, N\}}{P\{n_{11}|n_{1.}, n_{.1}, N\}}$$

$$= \frac{n_{11}!\,n_{12}!\,n_{21}!\,n_{22}!}{(n_{11}+1)!\,(n_{12}-1)!\,(n_{21}-1)!\,(n_{22}+1)!}$$

and, after cancelling, yields

$$f(n_{11}) = \frac{n_{12}\,n_{21}}{(n_{11}+1)(n_{22}+1)}\;. \tag{2.1}$$

To illustrate mathematical recursion with an initial probability value, consider again the data on monozygotic and dizygotic twins given in Table 2.1 on p. 23 and replicated in Table 2.13 for convenience. The $M = 13$ exhaustive $2{\times}2$ contingency tables from the twin data are listed in Table 2.3 on p. 24, along with the associated hypergeometric point probability values, and are replicated in Table 2.14 for convenience.

Table 2.12 Conventional notation for a $2{\times}2$ contingency table

	Category		
Category	1	2	Total
1	n_{11}	n_{12}	$n_{1.}$
2	n_{21}	n_{22}	$n_{2.}$
Total	$n_{.1}$	$n_{.2}$	N

Table 2.13 Convictions of like-sex twins of criminals

Twin type	Convicted	Not convicted	Total
Monozygotic	10	3	13
Dizygotic	2	15	17
Total	12	18	30

Table 2.14 Listing of the 13 possible $2{\times}2$ contingency tables from the twin data with associated hypergeometric probability values

Table 1		Probability	Table 2		Probability
0	13	$7.1543{\times}10^{-5}$	1	12	$1.8601{\times}10^{-3}$
12	5		11	6	
Table 3		Probability	Table 4		Probability
2	11	$1.7538{\times}10^{-2}$	3	10	$8.0384{\times}10^{-2}$
10	7		9	8	
Table 5		Probability	Table 6		Probability
4	9	$2.0096{\times}10^{-1}$	5	8	$2.8938{\times}10^{-1}$
8	9		7	10	
Table 7		Probability	Table 8		Probability
6	7	$2.4554{\times}10^{-1}$	7	6	$1.2277{\times}10^{-1}$
6	11		5	12	
Table 9		Probability	Table 10		Probability
8	5	$3.5414{\times}10^{-2}$	9	4	$5.6212{\times}10^{-3}$
4	13		3	14	
Table 11		Probability	Table 12		Probability
10	3	$4.4970{\times}10^{-4}$	11	2	$1.5331{\times}10^{-5}$
2	15		1	16	
Table 13		Probability			
12	1	$1.5030{\times}10^{-7}$			
0	17				

To begin a recursion procedure it is necessary to have an initial value, in this case the probability of zero monozygotic convicted twins (Table 1 in Table 2.14) given by $P\{n_{11} = 0|n_{1.}, n_{.1}, N\}$. Thus, define

$$P\{0|13, 12, 30\} = \frac{n_{1.}!\, n_{2.}!\, n_{.1}!\, n_{.2}!}{N!\, n_{11}!\, n_{12}!\, n_{21}!\, n_{22}!}$$

$$= \frac{13!\; 17!\; 12!\; 18!}{30!\; 0!\; 20!\; 5!\; 17!} = 7.1543\times10^{-5}$$

as the initial value.

The usual procedure in such cases is to estimate the larger factorial expressions using Stirling's series approximation given by[30]

$$n! \simeq n^n e^{-n}\sqrt{2\pi n}\, \exp\left(\frac{1}{12n} - \frac{1}{360n^3} + \frac{1}{1{,}260n^5} - \frac{1}{1{,}680n^7} + \cdots\right) .$$

Then, the probability values for $n_{11} = 1, \ldots, 12$ are generated recursively utilizing the recursion equation

$$P\{n_{11} + 1|n_{1.}, n_{.1}, N\} = P\{n_{11}|n_{1.}, n_{.1}, N\} \times \frac{n_{12}\, n_{21}}{(n_{11} + 1)(n_{22} + 1)} . \tag{2.2}$$

Thus,

$$P\{n_{11} = 1|13, 12, 30\} = 7.1543\times10^{-5} \times \frac{(13)(12)}{(1)(6)} = 1.8601\times10^{-3} ,$$

$$P\{n_{11} = 2|13, 12, 30\} = 1.8601\times10^{-3} \times \frac{(12)(11)}{(2)(7)} = 1.7538\times10^{-2} ,$$

$$P\{n_{11} = 3|13, 12, 30\} = 1.7538\times10^{-2} \times \frac{(11)(10)}{(3)(8)} = 8.0384\times10^{-2} ,$$

$$P\{n_{11} = 4|13, 12, 30\} = 8.0384\times10^{-2} \times \frac{(10)(9)}{(4)(9)} = 2.0096\times10^{-1} ,$$

$$P\{n_{11} = 5|13, 12, 30\} = 2.0096\times10^{-1} \times \frac{(9)(8)}{(5)(10)} = 2.8938\times10^{-1} ,$$

$$P\{n_{11} = 6|13, 12, 30\} = 2.8938\times10^{-1} \times \frac{(8)(7)}{(6)(11)} = 2.4554\times10^{-1} ,$$

$$P\{n_{11} = 7|13, 12, 30\} = 2.4554\times10^{-1} \times \frac{(7)(6)}{(7)(12)} = 1.2277\times10^{-1} ,$$

$$P\{n_{11} = 8|13, 12, 30\} = 1.2277\times10^{-1} \times \frac{(6)(5)}{(8)(13)} = 3.5414\times10^{-2} ,$$

[30] Attribution of the series is generally given to James Stirling, but more likely was first determined by Abraham de Moivre [116, p. 25].

$$P\{n_{11} = 9|13, 12, 30\} = 3.5414\times10^{-2} \times \frac{(5)(4)}{(9)(14)} = 5.6213\times10^{-3} ,$$

$$P\{n_{11} = 10|13, 12, 30\} = 5.6213\times10^{-3} \times \frac{(4)(3)}{(10)(15)} = 4.4970\times10^{-4} ,$$

$$P\{n_{11} = 11|13, 12, 30\} = 4.4970\times10^{-4} \times \frac{(3)(2)}{(11)(16)} = 1.5331\times10^{-5} ,$$

and

$$P\{n_{11} = 12|13, 12, 30\} = 1.5331\times10^{-5} \times \frac{(2)(1)}{(12)(17)} = 1.5030\times10^{-7} .$$

2.6.4 Recursion with an Arbitrary Initial Value

It is not necessary to provide an actual probability value to initialize a recursion procedure. Any arbitrary positive value can serve as an initial value with a compensatory adjustment made at the conclusion of the recursion process. Recursion with an arbitrary initial value was used extensively by Frank Yates during his 25-year tenure as head of the Statistical Department at the Rothamsted Experimental Station, but the technique can be traced back at least to Lambert Adolphe Jacques Quetelet who used a recursion procedure to generate the binomial probability distribution with $p = 0.5$ and published the technique in a volume with the imposing title *Letters Addressed to H.R.H. the Grand Duke of Saxe Coburg and Gotha on the Theory of Probabilities as Applied to the Moral and Political Sciences* in 1846 [125]. To illustrate the use of an arbitrary origin in a recursion procedure, consider Table 1 in Table 2.14 and set relative probability value $H\{n_{11} = 0|13, 12, 30\}$ to a small arbitrarily chosen value, say 1.00; thus, $H\{n_{11} = 0|13, 12, 30\} = 1.00$. Then following Eq. (2.2), a recursion procedure produces

$$H\{n_{11} = 1|13, 12, 30\} = 1.0000 \times \frac{(13)(12)}{(1)(6)} = 26.0000 ,$$

$$H\{n_{11} = 2|13, 12, 30\} = 26.0000 \times \frac{(12)(11)}{(2)(7)} = 245.1429 ,$$

$$H\{n_{11} = 3|13, 12, 30\} = 245.1429 \times \frac{(11)(10)}{(3)(8)} = 1{,}123.5714 ,$$

$$H\{n_{11} = 4|13, 12, 30\} = 1{,}123.5714 \times \frac{(10)(9)}{(4)(9)} = 2{,}808.9286 ,$$

$$H\{n_{11} = 5|13, 12, 30\} = 2{,}808.9286 \times \frac{(9)(8)}{(5)(10)} = 4{,}044.8571 ,$$

$$H\{n_{11} = 6|13, 12, 30\} = 4{,}044.8571 \times \frac{(8)(7)}{(6)(11)} = 3{,}432.0000\,,$$

$$H\{n_{11} = 7|13, 12, 30\} = 3{,}432.0000 \times \frac{(7)(6)}{(7)(12)} = 1{,}716.0000\,,$$

$$H\{n_{11} = 8|13, 12, 30\} = 1{,}716.0000 \times \frac{(6)(5)}{(8)(13)} = 495.0000\,,$$

$$H\{n_{11} = 9|13, 12, 30\} = 495.0000 \times \frac{(5)(4)}{(9)(14)} = 78.5714\,,$$

$$H\{n_{11} = 10|13, 12, 30\} = 78.5714 \times \frac{(4)(3)}{(10)(15)} = 6.2857\,,$$

$$H\{n_{11} = 11|13, 12, 30\} = 6.2857 \times \frac{(3)(2)}{(11)(16)} = 0.2143\,,$$

and

$$H\{n_{11} = 12|13, 12, 30\} = 0.2143 \times \frac{(2)(1)}{(12)(17)} = 0.0021\,.$$

for a total of

$$T = \sum_{i=0}^{12} H\{n_{11} = i|13, 12, 30\} = 1.00 + 26.00 + \cdots + 0.0021 = 13{,}977.5735\,.$$

The desired exact probability values are then obtained by dividing each relative probability value, $H\{n_{11}|n_{1.}, n_{.1}, N\}$, by the recursively obtained total, T. For example,

$$P\{n_{11} = 0|13, 12, 30\} = \frac{1.0000}{13{,}977.5735} = 7.1543\times 10^{-5}\,,$$

$$P\{n_{11} = 1|13, 12, 30\} = \frac{26.0000}{13{,}977.5735} = 1.8601\times 10^{-3}\,,$$

$$P\{n_{11} = 2|13, 12, 30\} = \frac{245.1429}{13{,}977.5735} = 1.7538\times 10^{-2}\,,$$

$$P\{n_{11} = 3|13, 12, 30\} = \frac{1{,}123.5714}{13{,}977.5735} = 8.0384\times 10^{-2}\,,$$

$$P\{n_{11} = 4|13, 12, 30\} = \frac{2{,}808.9286}{13{,}977.5735} = 2.0096\times 10^{-1}\,,$$

$$P\{n_{11} = 5|13, 12, 30\} = \frac{4{,}044.8571}{13{,}977.5735} = 2.8938\times 10^{-1}\,,$$

$$P\{n_{11} = 6|13, 12, 30\} = \frac{3{,}432.0000}{13{,}977.5735} = 2.4554\times 10^{-1}\,,$$

$$P\{n_{11} = 7|13, 12, 30\} = \frac{1{,}716.0000}{13{,}977.5735} = 1.2277\times 10^{-1}\,,$$

$$P\{n_{11} = 8|13, 12, 30\} = \frac{495.0000}{13{,}977.5735} = 3.5414\times10^{-2} ,$$

$$P\{n_{11} = 9|13, 12, 30\} = \frac{78.5714}{13{,}977.5735} = 5.6212\times10^{-3} ,$$

$$P\{n_{11} = 10|13, 12, 30\} = \frac{6.2857}{13{,}977.5735} = 4.4970\times10^{-4} ,$$

$$P\{n_{11} = 11|13, 12, 30\} = \frac{0.2143}{13{,}977.5735} = 1.5331\times10^{-5} ,$$

and

$$P\{n_{11} = 12|13, 12, 30\} = \frac{0.0021}{13{,}977.5735} = 1.5030\times10^{-7} .$$

In this manner, the entire analysis is conducted utilizing an arbitrary initial value and a recursion procedure, thereby eliminating all factorial expressions. When the number of potential contingency tables given by $\max(n_{11}) - \min(n_{11}) + 1$ is large, the computational savings can be substantial.

2.6.5 *Variable Components of a Test Statistic*

Under permutation, only the variable components of the test statistic need be calculated for each arrangement of the observed data. As this is often only a very small piece of the desired test statistic, calculations can often be reduced by several factors; see, for example, a discussion by Scheffé in 1959 [129, pp. 314–317]. To illustrate, consider the expression for a conventional two-sample t test,

$$t = \frac{\bar{x}_1 - \bar{x}_2}{\sqrt{\dfrac{(n_1 - 1)s_1^2 + (n_2 - 1)s_2^2}{n_1 + n_2 - 2}\left(\dfrac{1}{n_1} + \dfrac{1}{n_2}\right)}} ,$$

where n_1 and n_2 denote the sample sizes, s_1^2 and s_2^2 denote the estimated population variances, and $\bar{x}_1$ and $\bar{x}_2$ denote the sample means for samples 1 and 2, respectively. In computing the permutation probability value of Student's two-sample t test, given the total of all response measurements

$$T = \sum_{i=1}^{n_1} x_{1i} + \sum_{i=1}^{n_2} x_{2i} ,$$

where x_{1i} and x_{2i} denote the response measurements in samples 1 and 2, respectively, only the sum of the response measurements in the smaller of the two samples need be calculated for each arrangement of the observed response measurements, i.e., $\sum_{i=1}^{n_1} x_{1i}$, where x_{1i} denotes a response measurement in sample 1 and $n_1 \leq n_2$. Computing only the variable components of the test statistic thus eliminates a great deal of calculation for each random arrangement of the observed data, a time-saving technique utilized by Pitman in his 1937 permutation analysis of two independent samples [121].

For a second example, in 1933 Thomas Eden and Frank Yates substantially reduced calculations in a randomized-block analysis of Yeoman II wheat shoots by recognizing that the block and total sums of squares would be constant for all of their 1,000 random samples and, consequently, the value of z for each sample would be uniquely defined by the treatment (between) sum of squares, i.e., the treatment sum of squares was sufficient for a permutation test of a randomized-block analysis of variance [31].[31]

For a third example, consider Cohen's unweighted kappa measure of inter-rater agreement given by

$$\kappa = \frac{\displaystyle\sum_{i=1}^{r} O_{ii} - \sum_{i=1}^{r} E_{ii}}{\displaystyle N - \sum_{i=1}^{r} E_{ii}} , \tag{2.3}$$

where O_{ii} and E_{ii} for $i = 1, \ldots, r$ denote the observed and expected cell frequencies, respectively, on the principal diagonal of an $r \times r$ contingency (agreement) table [25]. Since the E_{ii}, $i = 1, \ldots, r$, are based on N and the row and column marginal frequency totals, the variable components of κ in Eq. (2.3) is simply the sum of the observed cell frequencies, $\sum_{i=1}^{r} O_{ii}$, on the principal diagonal for each arrangement of the cell frequencies, given fixed marginal frequency totals.

For a fourth example, consider Pearson's product-moment correlation coefficient between variables x and y given by

$$r_{xy} = \frac{\displaystyle\sum_{i=1}^{N} x_i y_i - \left(\sum_{i=1}^{N} x_i \sum_{i=1}^{N} y_i \right) \Big/ N}{\sqrt{\left[\displaystyle\sum_{i=1}^{N} x_i^2 - \left(\sum_{i=1}^{N} x_i \right)^2 \Big/ N \right] \left[\displaystyle\sum_{i=1}^{N} y_i^2 - \left(\sum_{i=1}^{N} y_i \right)^2 \Big/ N \right]}} ,$$

[31] The letter F for the analysis of variance (variance-ratio) test statistic was introduced in 1934 by George Snedecor at Iowa State University, much to the displeasure of R.A. Fisher [131, p. 15]. Prior to 1934 the test statistic was indicated by z, the letter originally assigned to it by Fisher.

where N is the number of bivariate measurements. N and the summations

$$\sum_{i=1}^{N} x_i\ , \quad \sum_{i=1}^{N} x_i^2\ , \quad \sum_{i=1}^{N} y_i\ , \quad \text{and} \quad \sum_{i=1}^{N} y_i^2$$

are invariant under permutation. Thus, it is sufficient to calculate only $\sum_{i=1}^{N} x_i y_i$ for all permutations of the observed data, eliminating a great deal of unnecessary calculation. In addition, it is only necessary to permute either variable x or variable y, leaving the other variable fixed.

These two features, mathematical recursion with an arbitrary initial value and computation of only the variable components of the test statistic under permutation, combined with powerful resampling algorithms and high-speed computing, produce a highly efficient permutation statistical approach that, today, makes permutation analyses both feasible and practical for many research applications.

2.7 Coda

Chapter 2 introduced two models of statistical inference: the population model and the permutation model. The permutation model included three types of permutation tests: exact, Monte Carlo resampling, and moment approximation, each of which was detailed and illustrated. Emphasized were the data-dependency of permutation statistical tests and freedom from the usual assumptions of normality and homogeneity of variance. Mathematical recursion, the use of arbitrary initial values, the use of all combinations of observed values instead of all permutations, and analysis of only the variable components of tests and measures illustrated the computational efficiency of permutation statistical tests.

Chapter 3 applies statistical permutation methods to measures of association designed for two nominal-level variables. Included in Chap. 3 are the traditional chi-squared-based measures: Pearson's ϕ^2, Tschuprov's T^2, Cramér's V^2, and Pearson's C. Alternatives to the four measures are proposed that make the measures maximum-corrected and provide proper norming between the usual limits of 0 and 1. Also considered in Chap. 3 are permutation-based goodness-of-fit tests.

References

1. Altman, D.G., Bland, J.M.: Measurement in medicine: The analysis of method comparison studies. Statistician **32**, 307–317 (1983)
2. Bakeman, R., Robinson, B.F., Quera, V.: Testing sequential association: Estimating exact *p* values using sampled permutations. Psychol. Methods **1**, 4–15 (1996)
3. Baker, F.B., Collier, Jr., R.O.: Some empirical results on variance ratios under permutation in the completely randomized design. J. Am. Stat. Assoc. **61**, 813–820 (1966)

4. Barboza, D., Markoff, J.: Power in numbers: China aims for high-tech primacy. NY Times **161**, D2–D3 (6 Dec 2011)
5. Barnard, G.A.: 2 × 2 tables. A note on E. S. Pearson's paper. Biometrika **34**, 168–169 (1947)
6. Bartlett, M.S.: Properties of sufficiency and statistical tests. P. Roy. Soc. Lond. A Mat. **160**, 268–282 (1937)
7. Berkson, J.: Some difficulties of interpretation encountered in the application of the chi-square test. J. Am. Stat. Assoc. **33**, 526–536 (1938)
8. Bernardin, H.J., Beatty, R.W.: Performance Appraisal: Assessing Human Behavior at Work. Kent, Boston (1984)
9. Berry, K.J., Johnston, J.E., Mielke, P.W.: Permutation methods. Comput. Stat. **3**, 527–542 (2011)
10. Berry, K.J., Johnston, J.E., Mielke, P.W.: A Chronicle of Permutation Statistical Methods: 1920–2000 and Beyond. Springer–Verlag, Cham, CH (2014)
11. Berry, K.J., Mielke, P.W.: Subroutines for computing exact chi-square and Fisher's exact probability tests. Educ. Psychol. Meas. **45**, 153–159 (1985)
12. Berry, K.J., Mielke, P.W.: Exact chi-square and Fisher's exact probability test for 3 by 2 cross-classification tables. Educ. Psychol. Meas. **47**, 631–636 (1987)
13. Berry, K.J., Mielke, P.W.: Monte Carlo comparisons of the asymptotic chi-square and likelihood-ratio tests with the nonasymptotic chi-square test for sparse *R* by *C* tables. Psychol. Bull. **103**, 256–264 (1988)
14. Berry, K.J., Mielke, P.W., Johnston, J.E.: Permutation Statistical Methods: An Integrated Approach. Springer–Verlag, Cham, CH (2016)
15. Biondini, M.E., Mielke, P.W., Berry, K.J.: Data-dependent permutation techniques for the analysis of ecological data. Vegetatio **75**, 161–168 (1988). [The name of the journal was changed to *Plant Ecology* in 1997]
16. Bradbury, I.: Analysis of variance versus randomization—A comparison. Brit. J. Math. Stat. Psy. **40**, 177–187 (1987)
17. Bradley, I.: Analysis of variance versus randomization tests—a comparison. Brit. J. Math. Stat. Psy. **40**, 177–187 (1987)
18. Bradley, J.V.: Distribution-Free Statistical Tests. Prentice–Hall, Englewood Cliffs, NJ (1968)
19. Bradley, J.V.: A common situation conducive to bizarre distribution shapes. Am. Stat. **31**, 147–150 (1977)
20. Brillinger, D.R., Jones, L.V., Tukey, J.W.: The role of statistics in weather resources management. Tech. Rep. II, Weather Modification Advisory Board, United States Department of Commerce, Washington, DC (1978)
21. Bross, I.D.J.: Is there an increased risk? Fed. Proc. **13**, 815–819 (1954)
22. Bryson, M.C.: The Literary Digest poll: Making of a statistical myth. Am. Stat. **30**, 184–185 (1976)
23. Chen, R.S., Dunlap, W.P.: SAS procedures for approximate randomization tests. Beh. Res. Meth. Ins. C **25**, 406–409 (1993)
24. Chung, J.H., Fraser, D.A.S.: Randomization tests for a multivariate two-sample problem. J. Am. Stat. Assoc. **53**, 729–735 (1958)
25. Cohen, J.: A coefficient of agreement for nominal scales. Educ. Psychol. Meas. **20**, 37–46 (1960)
26. Cowles, M.: Statistics in Psychology: An Historical Perspective, 2nd edn. Lawrence Erlbaum, Mahwah, NJ (2001)
27. Curran-Everett, D.: Explorations in statistics: Standard deviations and standard errors. Adv. Physiol. Educ. **32**, 203–208 (2008)
28. Dawson, R.B.: A simplified expression for the variance of the χ^2 function on a contingency table. Biometrika **41**, 280 (1954)
29. Draper, D., Hodges, J.S., Mallows, C.L., Pregibon, D.: Exchangeability and data analysis. J. R. Stat. Soc. A Stat. **156**, 9–37 (1993)
30. Dwass, M.: Modified randomization tests for nonparametric hypotheses. Ann. Math. Stat. **28**, 181–187 (1957)

31. Eden, T., Yates, F.: On the validity of Fisher's z test when applied to an actual example of non-normal data. J. Agric. Sci. **23**, 6–17 (1933)
32. Edgington, E.S.: Randomization tests. J. Psychol. **57**, 445–449 (1964)
33. Edgington, E.S.: Statistical inference and nonrandom samples. Psychol. Bull. **66**, 485–487 (1966)
34. Edgington, E.S.: Approximate randomization tests. J. Psychol. **72**, 143–149 (1969)
35. Edgington, E.S.: Statistical Inference: The Distribution-free Approach. McGraw–Hill, New York (1969)
36. Edgington, E.S.: Randomization Tests. Marcel Dekker, New York (1980)
37. Edgington, E.S., Onghena, P.: Randomization Tests, 4th edn. Chapman & Hall/CRC, Boca Raton, FL (2007)
38. Editorial: Save the census. NY Times **166**, A18 (17 July 2017)
39. Feinstein, A.R.: Clinical Biostatistics XXIII: The role of randomization in sampling, testing, allocation, and credulous idolatry (Part 2). Clin. Pharmacol. Ther. **14**, 898–915 (1973)
40. Feinstein, A.R.: Clinical Biostatistics. C. V. Mosby, St. Louis (1977)
41. Festinger, L.: The significance of differences between means without reference to the frequency distribution function. Psychometrika **11**, 97–105 (1946)
42. Fisher, R.A.: Statistical Methods for Research Workers. Oliver and Boyd, Edinburgh (1925)
43. Fisher, R.A.: The Design of Experiments. Oliver and Boyd, Edinburgh (1935)
44. Fisher, R.A.: The logic of inductive inference (with discussion). J. R. Stat. Soc. **98**, 39–82 (1935)
45. Fox, J.A., Tracy, P.E.: Randomized Response: A Method for Sensitive Surveys. Sage, Beverly Hills, CA (1986)
46. Frick, R.W.: Interpreting statistical testing: Process and propensity, not population and random sampling. Beh. Res. Meth. Ins. C **30**, 527–535 (1998)
47. Friedman, M.: A comparison of alternative tests of significance for the problem of m rankings. Ann. Math. Stat. **11**, 86–92 (1940)
48. Galton, F.: Statistics by intercomparison, with remarks on the law of frequency of error. Philos. Mag. 4 **49**(322), 33–46 (1875)
49. Geary, R.C.: Some properties of correlation and regression in a limited universe. Metron **7**, 83–119 (1927)
50. Geary, R.C.: Testing for normality. Biometrika **34**, 209–242 (1947)
51. Gelman, A., Goel, S., Rivers, D., Rothschild, D.: The mythical swing voter. Quart. J. Pol. Sci. **11**, 103–130 (2016)
52. Good, I.J.: Further comments concerning the lady tasting tea or beer: P-values and restricted randomization. J. Stat. Comput. Simul. **40**, 263–267 (1992)
53. Good, P.I.: Permutation, Parametric and Bootstrap Tests of Hypotheses. Springer–Verlag, New York (1994)
54. Good, P.I.: Permutation Tests: A Practical Guide to Resampling Methods for Testing Hypotheses. Springer–Verlag, New York (1994)
55. Good, P.I.: Resampling Methods: A Practical Guide to Data Analysis. Birkhäuser, Boston (1999)
56. Good, P.I.: Permutation Tests: A Practical Guide to Resampling Methods for Testing Hypotheses, 2nd edn. Springer–Verlag, New York (2000)
57. Haldane, J.B.S.: The exact value of the moments of the distribution of χ^2, used as a test of goodness of fit, when expectations are small. Biometrika **29**, 133–143 (1937). [Correction: Biometrika **31**, 220 (1939)]
58. Haldane, J.B.S.: The mean and variance of χ^2, when used as a test of goodness of fit, when expectations are small. Biometrika **31**, 346–355 (1940)
59. Havlicek, L.L., Peterson, N.L.: Robustness of the t test: A guide for researchers on effect of violations of assumptions. Psych. Rep. **34**, 1095–1114 (1974)
60. Hayes, A.F.: Permustat: Randomization tests for the Macintosh. Beh. Res. Meth. Ins. C **28**, 473–475 (1996)

61. Hayes, A.F.: Permutation test is not distribution-free: Testing $H_0: \rho = 0$. Psychol. Method **1**, 184–198 (1996)
62. Hayes, A.F.: Randomization tests and the equality of variance assumption when comparing group means. Anim. Behav. **59**, 653–656 (2000)
63. Hays, W.L.: Statistics. Hold, Rinehart and Winston, New York (1988)
64. Henley, S.: Nonparametric Geostatistics. Applied Science, London (1981)
65. Higgins, T.: The polling industry cuts the cord. Bloomberg Businessweek **November 23–29**, 30 (2015)
66. Higgs, M.D.: Do we really need the *S*-word? Am. Sci. **101**, 6–8 (2013). http://www.americanscientist.org/issues/pub/2013/1/do-we-really-need-the-s-word (2013). Accessed 4 Jan 2013
67. Hilbert, M.: How much information is there in the "information society"? Significance **9**, 8–12 (2012)
68. Howell, D.C.: Statistical Methods for Psychology, 6th edn. Wadsworth, Belmont, CA (2007)
69. Hubbard, R.: Alphabet soup: Blurring the distinctions between p's and α's in psychological research. Theor. Psychol. **14**, 295–327 (2004)
70. Hunter, M.A., May, R.B.: Some myths concerning parametric and nonparametric tests. Can. Psychol. **34**, 384–389 (1993)
71. Johnston, J.E., Berry, K.J., Mielke, P.W.: Permutation tests: Precision in estimating probability values. Percept. Motor Skill **105**, 915–920 (2007)
72. Kempthorne, O.: The Design and Analysis of Experiments. Wiley, New York (1952)
73. Kempthorne, O.: The randomization theory of experimental inference. J. Am. Stat. Assoc. **50**, 946–967 (1955)
74. Kempthorne, O.: Some aspects of experimental inference. J. Am. Stat. Assoc. **61**, 11–34 (1966)
75. Kempthorne, O.: Why randomize? J. Stat. Plan. Infer. **1**, 1–25 (1977)
76. Kennedy, P.E.: Randomization tests in econometrics. J. Bus. Econ. Stat. **13**, 85–94 (1995)
77. Lachin, J.M.: Statistical properties of randomization in clinical trials. Control Clin. Trials **9**, 289–311 (1988)
78. LaFleur, B.J., Greevy, R.A.: Introduction to permutation and resampling-based hypothesis tests. J. Clin. Child Adolesc. **38**, 286–294 (2009)
79. Lange, J.: Crime as Destiny: A Study of Criminal Twins. Allen & Unwin, London (1931). [Translated by C. Haldane]
80. Lehmann, E.L.: Testing Statistical Hypotheses, 2nd edn. Wiley, New York (1986)
81. Lehmann, E.L., Stein, C.M.: On the theory of some non-parametric hypotheses. Ann. Math. Stat. **20**, 28–45 (1949)
82. Lewis, T., Saunders, I.W., Westcott, M.: The moments of the pearson chi-squared statistic and the minimum expected value in two-way tables. Biometrika **71**, 515–522 (1984). [Correction: Biometrika **76**, 407 (1989)]
83. Liang, F., Liu, C., Carroll, R.J.: Stochastic approximation in Monte Carlo computation. J. Am. Stat. Assoc. **102**, 305–320 (2007)
84. Lindley, D.V., Novick, M.R.: The role of exchangeability in inference. Ann. Stat. **9**, 45–58 (1981)
85. Ludbrook, J.: Advantages of permutation (randomization) tests in clinical and experimental pharmacology and physiology. Clin. Exp. Pharmacol. P **21**, 673–686 (1994)
86. Ludbrook, J.: Issues in biomedical statistics: Comparing means by computer-intensive tests. Aust. NZ J. Surg. **65**, 812–819 (1995)
87. Ludbrook, J.: The Wilcoxon–Mann–Whitney test condemned. Brit. J. Surg. **83**, 136–137 (1996)
88. Ludbrook, J.: Statistical techniques for comparing measures and methods of measurement: A critical review. Clin. Exp. Pharmacol. P **29**, 527–536 (2002)
89. Ludbrook, J., Dudley, H.A.F.: Issues in biomedical statistics: Analyzing 2×2 tables of frequencies. Aust. NZ J. Surg. **64**, 780–787 (1994)

90. Ludbrook, J., Dudley, H.A.F.: Issues in biomedical statistics: Statistical inference. Aust. NZ J. Surg. **64**, 630–636 (1994)
91. Ludbrook, J., Dudley, H.A.F.: Why permutation tests are superior to t and F tests in biomedical research. Am. Stat. **52**, 127–132 (1998)
92. Ludbrook, J., Dudley, H.A.F.: Discussion of "Why permutation tests are superior to t and F tests in biomedical research" by J. Ludbrook and H.A.F. Dudley. Am. Stat. **54**, 87 (2000)
93. Lyons, D.: In race for fastest computer, China outpaces U.S. Newsweek **158**, 57–59 (5 Dec 2011)
94. Manly, B.F.J.: Randomization and Monte Carlo Methods in Biology. Chapman & Hall, London (1991)
95. Manly, B.F.J.: Randomization and Monte Carlo Methods in Biology, 2nd edn. Chapman & Hall, London (1997)
96. Manly, B.F.J.: Randomization, Bootstrap and Monte Carlo Methods in Biology, 3rd edn. Chapman & Hall/CRC, Boca Raton, FL (2007)
97. Manly, B.F.J., Francis, R.I.C.: Analysis of variance by randomization when variances are unequal. Aust. NZ J. Stat. **41**, 411–429 (1999)
98. Marascuilo, L.A., McSweeney: Nonparametric and Distribution-free methods in the Social Sciences. Brooks–Cole, Monterey, CA (1977)
99. Matsumoto, M., Nishimura, T.: Mersenne twister: A 623-dimensionally equidistributed uniform pseudo-random number generator. ACM T Model Comput. S **8**, 3–30 (1998)
100. Matthews, R.: Beautiful, but dangerous. Significance **13**, 30–31 (2016)
101. Matthews, R.: Chancing It: The Laws of Chance and How They Can Work for You. Profile Books, London (2016)
102. Maxim, P.S.: Quantitative Research Methods in the Social Sciences. Oxford, New York (1999)
103. May, R.B., Hunter, M.A.: Some advantages of permutation tests. Can. Psychol. **34**, 401–407 (1993)
104. McHugh, R.B.: Comment on "Scales and statistics: Parametric and nonparametric" by N.H. Anderson. Psychol. Bull. **60**, 350–355 (1963)
105. Mehta, C.R., Patel, N.R.: Algorithm 643: FEXACT. A FORTRAN subroutine for Fisher's exact test on unordered $r \times c$ contingency tables. ACM T Math. Software **12**, 154–161 (1986)
106. Mehta, C.R., Patel, N.R.: A hybrid algorithm for Fisher's exact test in unordered $r \times c$ contingency tables. Commun. Stat. Theor. M **15**, 387–403 (1986)
107. Micceri, T.: The unicorn, the normal curve, and other improbable creatures. Psychol. Bull. **105**, 156–166 (1989)
108. Mielke, P.W.: Some exact and nonasymptotic analyses of discrete goodness-of-fit and r-way contingency tables. In: Johnson, N.L., Balakrishnan, N. (eds.) Advances in the Theory and Practice of Statistics: A Volume in Honor of Samuel Kotz, pp. 179–192. Wiley, New York (1997)
109. Mielke, P.W., Berry, K.J.: Non-asymptotic inferences based on the chi-square statistic for r by c contingency tables. J. Stat. Plan Infer. **12**, 41–45 (1985)
110. Mielke, P.W., Berry, K.J.: Cumulant methods for analyzing independence of r-way contingency tables and goodness-of-fit frequency data. Biometrika **75**, 790–793 (1988)
111. Mielke, P.W., Berry, K.J.: Data-dependent analyses in psychological research. Psychol. Rep. **91**, 1225–1234 (2002)
112. Mielke, P.W., Berry, K.J.: Permutation Methods: A Distance Function Approach, 2nd edn. Springer–Verlag, New York (2007)
113. Mielke, P.W., Berry, K.J., Johnston, J.E.: Resampling programs for multiway contingency tables with fixed marginal frequency totals. Psychol. Rep. **101**, 18–24 (2007)
114. Mielke, P.W., Iyer, H.K.: Permutation techniques for analyzing multi-response data from randomized block experiments. Commun. Stat. Theor. M **11**, 1427–1437 (1982)
115. Murphy, K.R., Cleveland, J.: Understanding Performance Appraisal: Social, Organizational, and Goal-based Perspectives. Sage, Thousand Oaks, CA (1995)

116. Namias, V.: A simple derivatin of Stirling's asymptotic series. Am. Math. Monthly **93**, 25–29 (1986)
117. Neyman, J., Pearson, E.S.: On the use and interpretation of certain test criteria for purposes of statistical inference: Part I. Biometrika **20A**, 175–240 (1928)
118. Neyman, J., Pearson, E.S.: On the use and interpretation of certain test criteria for purposes of statistical inference: Part II. Biometrika **20A**, 263–294 (1928)
119. Nussbaum, B.D.: To ask or not to ask? It depends on the question. AmstatNews **481**, 3–4 (July 2017)
120. Nussbaum, B.D.: Bigger isn't always better when it comes to data. AmstatNews **479**, 3–4 (May 2017)
121. Pitman, E.J.G.: Significance tests which may be applied to samples from any populations. Suppl. J. R. Stat. Soc. **4**, 119–130 (1937)
122. Pitman, E.J.G.: Significance tests which may be applied to samples from any populations: II. The correlation coefficient test. Suppl. J. R. Stat. Soc. **4**, 225–232 (1937)
123. Pitman, E.J.G.: Significance tests which may be applied to samples from any populations: III. The analysis of variance test. Biometrika **29**, 322–335 (1938)
124. Pitman, E.J.G.: Lecture notes on non-parametric statistical inference (1948). [Unpublished lecture notes for a course given at Columbia University in 1948]
125. Quetelet, L.A.J.: Lettres à S. A. R. le Duc Régnant de Saxe–Cobourg et Gotha, sur la Théorie des Probabilitiés Appliquée aux Sciences Morales et Politiques. Hayez, Bruxelles (1846). [English translation, *Letters Addressed to H.R.H. the Grand Duke of Saxe Coburg and Gotha on the Theory of Probabilities as Applied to the Moral and Political Sciences*, by O.G. Downes and published by Charles & Edwin Layton, London, 1849]
126. Rew, H.: Francis galton. J. R. Stat. Soc. **85**, 293–298 (1922)
127. Rothschild, D., Goel, S.: If a poll's margin of error is plus or minus 3 points, think 7. NY Times **166**(57,377), A20 (6 October 2016)
128. Saal, F.E., Downey, R.G., Lahey, M.A.: Rating the ratings: Assessing the quality of rating data. Psychol. Bull. **88**, 413–428 (1980)
129. Scheffé, H.: The Analysis of Variance. Wiley, New York (1959)
130. Schmidt, F.L., Johnson, R.H.: Effect of race on peer ratings in an industrial situation. J. Appl. Psychol. **57**, 237–241 (1973)
131. Snedecor, G.W.: Calculation and Interpretation of Analysis of Variance and Covariance. Collegiate Press, Ames, IA (1934)
132. Stigler, S.M.: The Seven Pillars of Statistical Wisdom. Harvard University Press, Cambridge, MA (2016)
133. Still, A.W., White, A.P.: The approximate randomization test as an alternative to the F test in analysis of variance. Brit. J. Math. Stat. Psy. **34**, 243–252 (1981)
134. Thompson, D.W.: On Growth and Form: The Complete Revised Edition. Dover, New York (1992)
135. Trachtman, J.N., Giambalvo, V., Dippner, R.S.: On the assumptions concerning the assumptions of a t test. J. Gen. Psych. **99**, 107–116 (1978)
136. Tracy, P.E., Fox, J.A.: The validity of randomized response for sensitive measurements. Am. Soc. Rev. **46**, 187–200 (1981)
137. Tukey, J.W.: Data analysis and behavioral science (1962). [Unpublished manuscript]
138. Tukey, J.W.: The future of data analysis. Ann. Math. Stat. **33**, 1–67 (1962)
139. Tukey, J.W.: Randomization and re-randomization: The wave of the past in the future. In: Statistics in the Pharmaceutical Industry: Past, Present and Future. Philadelphia Chapter of the American Statistical Association (June 1988). [Presented at a Symposium in Honor of Joseph L. Ciminera held in June 1988 at Philadelphia, Pennsylvania]
140. Umesh, U.N., Peterson, R.A.: A critical evaluation of the randomized response method. Sociol. Method Res. **20**, 104–138 (1991)
141. van den Brink, W.P., van den Brink, S.G.L.: A comparison of the power of the t test, Wilcoxon's test, and the approximate permutation test for the two-sample location problem. Brit. J. Math. Stat. Psy. **42**, 183–189 (1989)

142. Vuong, A.: A new chip off the old block. Denver Post **120**, 1A, 16A (2 June 2013)
143. Warner, S.L.: Randomized response: A survey technique for eliminating evasive answer bias. J. Am. Stat. Assoc. **60**, 63–69 (1965)
144. Whitney, D.R.: A Comparison of the Power of Non-parametric Tests and Tests Based on the Normal Distribution Under Nonnormal Alternatives (1948). [Unpublished Ph.D. dissertation at The Ohio State University, Columbus, Ohio]
145. Yates, F.: Contingency tables involving small numbers and the χ^2 test. Suppl. J. R. Stat. Soc. **1**, 217–235 (1934)
146. Yu, K., Liang, F., Ciampa, J., Chatterjee, N.: Efficient p-value evaluation for resampling-based tests. Biostatistics **12**, 582–593 (2011)
147. Zelterman, D.: Goodness-of-fit tests for large sparse multinomial distributions. J. Am. Stat. Assoc. **82**, 624–629 (1987)

Chapter 3
Nominal-Level Variables, I

The relationships between nominal-level (categorical) variables are often difficult to analyze because discrete, unordered categories usually contain a very limited amount of usable information. Examples of nominal-level variables are: Gender (Female, Male), Political Affiliation (Democrat, Republican, Independent, Libertarian), and Marital Status (Single, Married, Widowed, Separated, Divorced). Measures of association for two nominal-level variables are of two types: those based on Pearson's chi-squared test statistic, e.g., maximum-corrected measures such as Pearson's ϕ^2, and those based on criteria other than Pearson's chi-squared test statistic, e.g., proportional-reduction-in-error measures such as Goodman and Kruskal's λ_a and λ_b measures, which are based on category modal values.

This third chapter of *The Measurement of Association* applies exact and Monte Carlo permutation statistical methods to measures of association that are based on Pearson's chi-squared test statistic. Also included are several measures that are not based directly on Pearson's chi-squared test statistic but are approximately distributed as chi-squared. The chapter begins with an examination of four measures based on Pearson's chi-squared test statistic that are notoriously difficult to interpret because they do not norm properly between the terminal values of 0 and 1: Pearson's ϕ^2, Tschuprov's T^2, Cramér's V^2, and Pearson's C. A chi-squared-based alternative to the four conventional measures is proposed that norms properly between 0, corresponding to independence, and 1, corresponding to perfect association, making intermediate values interpretable. The discussion of the four chi-squared-based measures of association is followed by a discussion of permutation-based goodness-of-fit tests. Chapter 3 concludes with an examination of the relationship between Pearson's chi-squared and Pearson's product-moment correlation coefficient for $r \times c$ contingency tables. Measures of association for nominal-level variables that are based on criteria other than Pearson's chi-squared test statistic are discussed in Chap. 4. Examples of the measures of nominal association that are based on criteria other than chi-squared are Goodman and Kruskal's λ_a and λ_b, Cohen's unweighted

K. J. Berry et al., *The Measurement of Association*,
https://doi.org/10.1007/978-3-319-98926-6_3

kappa coefficient, McNemar's Q and Cochran's Q tests of change, Leik and Gove's d_N^c measure of nominal association, and Fisher's exact probability test.

3.1 Chi-squared-Based Measures

It is well known that values of chi-squared and sample size are positively and proportionately related, i.e., for a chi-squared test of independence, if all cell frequencies are doubled in size, the calculated value of chi-squared will also be doubled. Because of this relationship, a number of measures of association based on Pearson's chi-squared have been proposed, purportedly to implement measures of association with proper norming, i.e., provide values between 0 and 1, where 0 indicates independence and 1 indicates perfect association between the two variables. Four popular measures based on chi-squared are Pearson's ϕ^2, Tschuprov's T^2, Cramér's V^2, and Pearson's C.[1,2]

3.1.1 *Pearson's ϕ^2 Measure of Association*

Pearson's mean-square measure of nominal-level association, ϕ^2, is used almost exclusively for 2×2 contingency tables, such as depicted in Table 3.1.[3] Denote by a dot $(\cdot)$ the partial sum of all rows or all columns, depending on the position of the $(\cdot)$ in the subscript list. If the $(\cdot)$ is in the first subscript position, the sum is over all rows and if the $(\cdot)$ is in the second subscript position, the sum is over all columns. Thus, $n_{i.}$ denotes the marginal frequency total of the ith row, $i = 1, \ldots, r$, summed over all columns, $n_{.j}$ denotes the marginal frequency total of the jth column, $j = 1, \ldots, c$, summed over all rows, and $N = n_{11} + n_{12} + n_{21} + n_{22}$ denotes the table frequency total. Then, in terms of chi-squared, Pearson's ϕ^2 measure of nominal association is given by:

$$\phi^2 = \frac{\chi^2}{N} , \tag{3.1}$$

[1] While Pearson's ϕ^2, Cramér's V^2, and Pearson's C are still occasionally found in the contemporary literature, Tschuprov's T^2 has fallen into desuetude.

[2] Tschuprov's measure of association is commonly known as T or T^2, but Tschuprov actually labeled it φ^2, and Cramér's measure of association is commonly known as V or V^2, but Cramér also labeled it φ^2.

[3] In some references, Pearson's ϕ^2 is defined for other contingency tables. It is discussed here in the context of 2×2 contingency tables because ϕ^2 is not equal to unity when there is perfect association in larger frequency tables, although there are exceptions for certain configurations of 2×c contingency tables.

Table 3.1 Conventional notation for a 2×2 contingency table

	Category		
Category	1	2	Total
1	n_{11}	n_{12}	$n_{1.}$
2	n_{21}	n_{22}	$n_{2.}$
Total	$n_{.1}$	$n_{.2}$	N

where N denotes the total of the cell frequencies in the observed contingency table. This statement is not entirely true, however, although it is standard in myriad textbooks and articles, where it is often argued that when the observed cell frequencies are doubled, chi-squared is also doubled and therefore the observed value of chi-squared should be divided by N to give a suitable measure of contextuality; see, for example, a 1968 article by Frederick Mosteller [77, pp. 2–3]. In fact, the N in the denominator of Eq. (3.1) represents the maximum possible value of χ^2 for a 2×2 contingency table when and only when the marginal frequency distributions are equivalent, e.g., $\{5, 5\}$ and $\{5, 5\}$, $\{6, 4\}$ and $\{6, 4\}$, or $\{6, 4\}$ and $\{4, 6\}$.

Let chi-squared for a contingency table with $r = 2$ rows, $c = 2$ columns, and N cases be defined in the conventional textbook fashion as:

$$\chi^2 = \sum_{i=1}^{r} \sum_{j=1}^{c} \frac{\left(O_{ij} - E_{ij}\right)^2}{E_{ij}} , \tag{3.2}$$

where O_{ij} denotes the observed cell frequencies and E_{ij} denotes the expected cell values given by:

$$E_{ij} = \frac{n_{i.}n_{.j}}{N} \qquad \text{for } i = 1, \ldots, r \text{ and } j = 1, \ldots, c .$$

Now, let the four marginal frequency totals be identical, as displayed in Table 3.2. For the notation in Table 3.2, each expected value is given by:

$$E_{ij} = \frac{\left(\frac{N}{2}\right)\left(\frac{N}{2}\right)}{N} = \frac{N}{4}$$

and, therefore, following Eq. (3.2),

$$\chi^2 = \frac{\left(\frac{N}{4}\right)^2 + \left(\frac{-N}{4}\right)^2 + \left(\frac{-N}{4}\right)^2 + \left(\frac{N}{4}\right)^2}{\frac{N}{4}} = \left(\frac{N^2}{4}\right)\left(\frac{4}{N}\right) = N .$$

An example will confirm that N is the maximum value for a 2×2 contingency table with identical marginal frequency distributions. Consider the 2×2 contingency

Table 3.2 Example 2×2 contingency table with identical marginal frequency distributions

	Category		
Category	1	2	Total
1	$\frac{N}{2}$	0	$\frac{N}{2}$
2	0	$\frac{N}{2}$	$\frac{N}{2}$
Total	$\frac{N}{2}$	$\frac{N}{2}$	N

Table 3.3 Example 2×2 contingency table

	A_1	A_2	Total
B_1	0	4	4
B_2	6	0	6
Total	6	4	10

table in Table 3.3 and let N denote the total of the cell frequencies, R_i denote a row total for $i = 1, 2$, C_j denote a column total for $j = 1, 2$, and O_{ij} denote a cell frequency for $i, j = 1, 2$. Then, the expected cell values are

$$E_{11} = \frac{n_{1.}n_{.1}}{N} = \frac{(4)(6)}{10} = 2.40\,, \qquad E_{12} = \frac{n_{1.}n_{.2}}{N} = \frac{(4)(4)}{10} = 1.60\,,$$

$$E_{21} = \frac{n_{2.}n_{.1}}{N} = \frac{(6)(6)}{10} = 3.60\,, \qquad E_{22} = \frac{n_{2.}n_{.2}}{N} = \frac{(6)(4)}{10} = 2.40\,,$$

following Eq. (3.2) on p. 75 the observed value of chi-squared is

$$\begin{aligned} \chi^2 &= \sum_{i=1}^{r}\sum_{j=1}^{c} \frac{\left(O_{ij} - E_{ij}\right)^2}{E_{ij}} \\ &= \frac{(0-2.40)^2}{2.40} + \frac{(4-1.60)^2}{1.60} + \frac{(6-3.60)^2}{3.60} + \frac{(0-2.40)^2}{2.40} \\ &= 2.40 + 3.60 + 1.60 + 2.40 = 10.00\,, \end{aligned}$$

and the observed value of Pearson's mean-square measure of contingency is therefore

$$\phi^2 = \frac{\chi^2}{N} = \frac{10.00}{10} = 1.00\,.$$

If the marginal frequency distributions of a 2×2 contingency table are not equivalent, e.g., $\{7, 3\}$ and $\{8, 2\}$, Pearson's ϕ^2 measure of nominal association will necessarily be less than 1.00. To illustrate the limiting value of Pearson's ϕ^2, consider the frequency data given in Table 3.4 with observed row and column marginal frequency distributions $\{6, 4\}$ and $\{5, 5\}$, respectively. In this case, the max-

Table 3.4 Example 2×2 contingency table

	A_1	A_2	Total
B_1	5	1	6
B_2	0	4	4
Total	5	5	10

Table 3.5 Example 2×2 contingency table with (0, 1) coding for variables x and y

	y		
x	0	1	Total
0	2	3	5
1	1	4	5
Total	3	7	10

imum value of chi-squared, given the observed marginal frequency distributions, is $\chi^2_{\max} = 6.6667$ and the maximum value of Pearson's ϕ^2 is only

$$\phi^2_{\max} = \frac{\chi^2_{\max}}{N} = \frac{6.6667}{10} = 0.6667 \; .$$

More positively, as noted by Yule and Filon, a singular advantage of Pearson's ϕ^2 over other measures of nominal association is that it is based on departure from independence [104, p. 83].

Pearson's ϕ^2 and r^2_{xy}

It is well known that Pearson's ϕ^2 is equivalent to Pearson's squared product-moment correlation coefficient, r^2_{xy}, when the two variables, x and y, are dummy-coded (0, 1). Some textbooks even go so far as to label Pearson's ϕ^2 as r^2_ϕ [87, p. 232]. To illustrate the equivalency between Pearson's ϕ^2 and Pearson's r^2_{xy}, consider the 2×2 contingency table given in Table 3.5, where the row and column variables are both dummy-coded (0, 1), the row variable is denoted as x, and the column variable is denoted as y. For the frequency data given in Table 3.5, the observed value of chi-squared is $\chi^2 = 0.4762$ and the observed value of Pearson's ϕ^2 is

$$\phi^2 = \frac{\chi^2}{N} = \frac{0.4762}{10} = 0.0476 \; .$$

The frequency data given in Table 3.5 can be recoded as in Table 3.6, where Objects 1 and 2, coded (0, 0), represent the two objects in row 1 and column 1; Objects 3 through 5, coded (0, 1), represent the three objects in row 1 and column 2; Object 6, coded (1, 0), represents the single object in row 2 and column 1; and Objects 7 through 10, coded (1, 1), represent the four objects in row 2 and column 2 of Table 3.5.

Table 3.6 Example dummy-coded values from the cell frequencies in the 2×2 contingency table in Table 3.5

	Variable	
Object	x	y
1	0	0
2	0	0
3	0	1
4	0	1
5	0	1
6	1	0
7	1	1
8	1	1
9	1	1
10	1	1

For the binary-coded data listed in Table 3.6,

$$N = 10, \quad \sum_{i=1}^{N} x_i = \sum_{i=1}^{N} x_i^2 = 5, \quad \sum_{i=1}^{N} y_i = \sum_{i=1}^{N} y_i^2 = 7, \quad \sum_{i=1}^{N} x_i y_i = +4 \,,$$

and the Pearson product-moment correlation coefficient for variables x and y is

$$r_{xy}^2 = \frac{\left(N \sum_{i=1}^{N} x_i y_i - \sum_{i=1}^{N} x_i \sum_{i=1}^{N} y_i \right)^2}{\left[N \sum_{i=1}^{N} x_i^2 - \left(\sum_{i=1}^{N} x_i \right)^2 \right] \left[N \sum_{i=1}^{N} y_i^2 - \left(\sum_{i=1}^{N} y_i \right)^2 \right]}$$

$$= \frac{\left[(10)(+4) - (5)(7)\right]^2}{\left[(10)(5) - 5^2\right]\left[(10)(7) - 7^2\right]} = 0.0476 \,,$$

which is identical to the value for Pearson's ϕ^2 measure calculated from chi-squared.

3.1.2 Tschuprov's T^2 Measure of Association

Compare Eq. (3.1) on p. 74 for Pearson's ϕ^2, that is,

$$\phi^2 = \frac{\chi^2}{N} \,,$$

Table 3.7 Example 3×3 contingency table with equivalent marginal frequency distributions

	A_1	A_2	A_3	Total
B_1	20	0	0	20
B_2	0	30	0	30
B_3	0	0	50	50
Total	20	30	50	100

with the equation for Tschuprov's T^2, which was specifically designed for square contingency tables of any size,[4] such as 3×3 or 4×4, and given by:

$$T^2 = \frac{\chi^2}{N\sqrt{(r-1)(c-1)}}\,, \tag{3.3}$$

where r and c denote the number of rows and columns in the observed contingency table, respectively [93, pp. 50–53]. It is obvious from Eq. (3.3) that Tschuprov's T^2 and Pearson's ϕ^2 are equivalent for 2×2 contingency tables.

The denominator for T^2 in Eq. (3.3) represents the maximum value of χ^2 for an $r \times c$ contingency table where $r = c$ and the marginal frequency distributions are equivalent, e.g., $\{4, 5, 6\}$ and $\{4, 5, 6\}$, $\{4, 5, 6\}$ and $\{6, 5, 4\}$, or $\{4, 5, 6\}$ and $\{5, 6, 4\}$, or any permutation of the marginal frequency totals as the order of the categories does not matter. An example will make this point clear. Consider the 3×3 contingency table in Table 3.7 with observed row marginal frequency distribution $\{20, 30, 50\}$ and observed column marginal frequency distribution $\{20, 30, 50\}$, and let R_i denote a row marginal frequency total, $i = 1, 2, 3$; C_j denote a column marginal frequency total, $j = 1, 2, 3$; O_{ij} denote a cell frequency, $i, j = 1, 2, 3$; and let N denote the total of the cell frequencies. Then, the observed value of Pearson's χ^2 is

$$\begin{aligned}
\chi^2 &= N\left(\sum_{i=1}^{r}\sum_{j=1}^{c}\frac{O_{ij}^2}{R_iC_j}\right) - N \\
&= 100\left[\frac{20^2}{(20)(20)} + \frac{0^2}{(20)(30)} + \frac{0^2}{(20)(50)} + \frac{0^2}{(30)(20)} + \frac{30^2}{(30)(30)}\right. \\
&\quad \left. + \frac{0^2}{(30)(50)} + \frac{0^2}{(50)(20)} + \frac{0^2}{(50)(30)} + \frac{50^2}{(50)(50)}\right] - 100 \\
&= 100(1+0+0+0+1+0+0+0+1) - 100 = 200
\end{aligned}$$

[4] There are a number of spellings of Tschuprov in the literature, possibly due to different translators. Alexander (Aleksandr) Alexandrovich (Aleksandrovich) Tschuprov (Tschuprow, Tchouprow, or Čhuprov) (1874–1926) was a Russian statistician noted for his contributions to mathematical statistics, probability sampling, and demography.

Table 3.8 Example 3×3 contingency table with unequal marginal frequency distributions

	A_1	A_2	A_3	Total
B_1	20	0	0	20
B_2	0	20	10	30
B_3	0	0	50	50
Total	20	20	60	100

and the observed value of Tschuprov's T^2 is

$$T^2 = \frac{\chi^2}{N\sqrt{(r-1)(c-1)}} = \frac{200}{100\sqrt{(3-1)(3-1)}} = \frac{200}{100(2)} = 1.00 \,.$$

However, if the marginal frequency distributions of a square $r \times c$ contingency table are not equivalent, Tschuprov's T^2 must necessarily be less than 1.00. Consider the frequency data given in Table 3.8 with observed row and column marginal frequency distributions, {20, 30, 50} and {20, 20, 60}, respectively.

In this case, given the observed marginal frequency distributions, the maximum value of χ^2 is $\chi^2_{\max} = 155.5556$ and the maximum value of T^2 is only

$$T^2_{\max} = \frac{\chi^2_{\max}}{N\sqrt{(r-1)(c-1)}} = \frac{155.5556}{100\sqrt{(3-1)(3-1)}} = 0.7778 \,.$$

3.1.3 Cramér's V^2 Measure of Association

Next, consider Cramér's V^2, which was designed for $r \times c$ contingency tables, is not restricted to contingency tables where $r = c$, and is given by:

$$V^2 = \frac{\chi^2}{N\,[\min(r-1, c-1)]} \tag{3.4}$$

[36, pp. 280–283]. It is obvious from Eq. (3.4) that Cramér's V^2, Tschuprov's T^2, and Pearson's ϕ^2 are equivalent for 2×2 contingency tables, and V^2 and T^2 are equivalent for any contingency table where $r = c$.

The denominator in Eq. (3.4) represents the maximum value of χ^2 for an $r \times c$ contingency table. Consider the 2×3 contingency table given in Table 3.9 and let N denote the sum of the cell frequencies; R_i denote a row total, $i = 1, 2$; C_j denote a column total, $j = 1, 2, 3$; and O_{ij} denote a cell frequency for $i = 1, 2$ and

Table 3.9 Example 2×3 contingency table

	A_1	A_2	A_3	Total
B_1	5	0	1	6
B_2	0	5	0	5
Total	5	5	1	11

Table 3.10 Example 2×3 contingency table

	A_1	A_2	A_3	Total
B_1	4	0	2	6
B_2	0	4	2	6
Total	4	4	4	12

$j = 1, 2, 3$. Then, the observed value of Pearson's χ^2 is

$$\begin{aligned}\chi^2 &= N\left(\sum_{i=1}^{r}\sum_{j=1}^{c}\frac{O_{ij}^2}{R_iC_j}\right) - N \\ &= 11\left[\frac{5^2}{(6)(5)} + \frac{0^2}{(6)(5)} + \frac{1^2}{(6)(5)} + \frac{0^2}{(5)(5)} + \frac{5^2}{(5)(5)} + \frac{0^2}{(5)(1)}\right] - 11 \\ &= 11(0.8333 + 0 + 0.1667 + 0 + 1 + 0) - 11 = 11.00\end{aligned}$$

and the observed value of Cramér's V^2 is

$$V^2 = \frac{\chi^2}{N[\min(r-1, c-1)]} = \frac{11.00}{11[\min(2-1, 3-1)]} = \frac{11.00}{11} = 1.00 \, .$$

On the other hand, consider the 2×3 contingency table in Table 3.10, where the observed value of Pearson's chi-squared is $\chi^2 = 8.00$, which is the maximum value of χ^2 for a 2×3 contingency table with marginal frequency distributions $\{6, 6\}$ and $\{4, 4, 4\}$. Consequently, the observed value of Cramér's V^2 is only $V^2 = 8/12 = 0.6667$ since $N = 12$ and $\min(r-1, c-1) = \min(2-1, 3-1) = 1$. Thus, Cramér's V^2, like Pearson's ϕ^2 and Tschuprov's T^2, standardizes Pearson's chi-squared to the maximum value of a contingency table other (usually) than the table being analyzed.

Nonetheless, the three measures of association, Pearson's ϕ^2, Tschuprov's T^2, and Cramér's V^2, were designed to be expressed as:

$$\phi^2 = T^2 = V^2 = \frac{\chi^2}{\chi^2_{\max}} \, ,$$

where $\chi^2_{\max}$ represents the maximum chi-squared value for an idealized contingency table, but not necessarily the contingency table under consideration.

3.1.4 Limitations of ϕ^2, T^2, and V^2

Measures of association based on Pearson's chi-squared test statistic have been heavily criticized in recent years. Wickens observed that Cramér's V^2 lacks an intuitive interpretation other than as a scaling of Pearson's chi-squared test statistic, which limits its usefulness [97, p. 226]. Costner noted that V^2 and other measures based on Pearson's chi-squared lack any interpretation at all for values other than the limiting values 0 and 1, or for the maximum possible value given the observed marginal frequency distributions [34].[5] Agresti and Finlay also noted that Cramér's V^2 is very difficult to interpret and recommended other measures [3, p. 284]. Blalock observed that "all measures based on chi square are somewhat arbitrary in nature, and their interpretations leave a lot to be desired…they all give greater weight to those columns or rows having the smallest marginals rather than to those with the largest marginals" [18, 19, p. 306]. Ferguson discussed the problem of using idealized marginal frequencies [42, p. 422], and Guilford noted that measures such as Pearson's ϕ^2, Tschuprov's T^2, and Cramér's V^2 necessarily underestimate the magnitude of association present [49, p. 342]. Berry, Martin, and Olson considered these issues with respect to 2×2 contingency tables [15, 16], and Berry, Johnston, and Mielke discussed in some detail the problems with using ϕ^2, T^2, and V^2 as measures of effect size [14].

3.1.5 Pearson's C Measure of Association

A fourth measure based on chi-squared is Pearson's coefficient of contingency, C, first proposed because it can be shown that if a bivariate normal distribution with correlation parameter ρ^2 is classified into a contingency table, then C^2 approaches ρ^2 as the number of categories in the contingency table increases.[6]

Pearson's coefficient of contingency is given by:

$$C = \sqrt{\frac{\chi^2}{\chi^2 + N}}$$

and was originally designed to measure the degree of association between two categorical variables that have been cross-classified into an $r \times c$ contingency table where $r = c$. Since χ^2, C, and ϕ^2 were all developed by Karl Pearson at University

[5]Some authors have defended Cramér's V^2, observing that it can be interpreted as the average of the squared product-moment correlation coefficients calculated on the $(r-1)(c-1)$ possible orthonormalized 2×2 tables embedded in the $r \times c$ contingency table, but this hardly seems helpful to a typical reader.

[6]Pearson actually labeled the test statistic as C_1, "the first coefficient of contingency."

Table 3.11 Example 2×2 contingency table

	A_1	A_2	Total
B_1	4	2	6
B_2	2	2	4
Total	6	4	10

College London, it is not surprising that C and ϕ^2 are related as they are both based on chi-squared. For the example 2×2 contingency table given in Table 3.11, the observed value of chi-squared is $\chi^2 = 0.2778$, the observed value of Pearson's mean-square contingency coefficient is

$$\phi^2 = \frac{\chi^2}{N} = \frac{0.2778}{10} = 0.0278$$

and the observed value of Pearson's coefficient of contingency is

$$C = \sqrt{\frac{\chi^2}{\chi^2 + N}} = \sqrt{\frac{0.2778}{0.2778 + 10}} = \sqrt{0.0270} = 0.1644 .$$

Then, the relationships between C and ϕ^2 for a 2×2 contingency table are given by:

$$C = \sqrt{\frac{\phi^2}{1 + \phi^2}} = \sqrt{\frac{0.0278}{1 + 0.0278}} = \sqrt{0.0270} = 0.1644$$

and

$$\phi^2 = \frac{C^2}{1 - C^2} = \frac{0.1644^2}{1 - 0.1644^2} = 0.0278 .$$

Because Pearson's C always has an upper limit less than unity, it is common to correct C by dividing the observed value of C by the maximum value of C for the size of the contingency table under consideration. For convenience, let $r = c = k$, then it follows that the maximum value that chi-squared can attain for any $k \times k$ contingency table with equivalent row and column marginal frequency distributions is

$$\chi^2_{\text{max}} = N(k - 1) .$$

Then, the maximum value of Pearson's C is

$$C_{\text{max}} = \sqrt{\frac{\chi^2}{\chi^2_{\text{max}} + N}} = \sqrt{\frac{N(k-1)}{N(k-1) + N}} = \sqrt{\frac{k-1}{k}} .$$

Table 3.12 Values of C_{max} for various $k \times k$ contingency tables

$k \times k$	C_{max}	$k \times k$	C_{max}
2×2	0.7071	8×8	0.9354
3×3	0.8165	9×9	0.9428
4×4	0.8660	10×10	0.9487
5×5	0.8944	11×11	0.9535
6×6	0.9129	12×12	0.9574
7×7	0.9258	13×13	0.9608

Table 3.13 Example data for Pearson's coefficient of contingency, C, with equivalent row and column marginal frequency distributions, {60, 50, 50, 40} and {60, 50, 50, 40}, respectively

	A_1	A_2	A_3	A_4	Total
B_1	60	0	0	0	60
B_2	0	50	0	0	50
B_3	0	0	50	0	50
B_4	0	0	0	40	40
Total	60	50	50	40	200

Table 3.12 lists various $k \times k$ contingency tables and associated values of C_{max}. While the upper limit of C_{max} increases as k increases, the upper limit is always less than unity. For this reason, Pearson's C is somewhat difficult to interpret, unless a correction is introduced by dividing C by C_{max} for the observed number of rows and columns. However, even then C is being standardized by a maximum value calculated on an idealized $k \times k$ contingency table with equivalent marginal frequency distributions, rather than the marginal frequency distributions of the contingency table actually observed.

An example illustrates how C_{max} corrects C for table size. Consider the frequency data given in Table 3.13 with equivalent row and column marginal frequency distributions, {60, 50, 50, 40} and {60, 50, 50, 40}, respectively, where the observed value of chi-squared is $\chi^2 = N(k-1) = 200(4-1) = 600$, the observed value of Pearson's C is

$$C = \sqrt{\frac{\chi^2}{\chi^2 + N}} = \sqrt{\frac{600}{600 + 200}} = \sqrt{0.75} = 0.8660\,,$$

the maximum value of C_{max} for a 4×4 contingency table is

$$C_{max} = \sqrt{\frac{k-1}{k}} = \sqrt{\frac{4-1}{4}} = \sqrt{0.75} = 0.8660\,,$$

and the ratio of C to C_{max} is

$$\frac{C}{C_{max}} = \frac{0.8660}{0.8660} = 1.00\,.$$

While the ratio of C to $C_{\max}$ ensures proper norming, at the same time the limitations of Pearson's C as a measure of association are also revealed. The utility of Pearson's C in research is highly qualified because $C_{\max}$, which is required for proper norming, is defined only for square contingency tables with equivalent row and column marginal frequency totals and is clearly not appropriate for non-square contingency tables.

3.1.6 *Proper Norming*

For proper norming, with a measure of association that varies over the range of probability values from 0 to 1, the computed χ^2 test statistic should be standardized by the maximum value of χ^2 obtained from the observed contingency table, not some idealized contingency table. Fortunately, it is not difficult to generate the maximum value of χ^2 for any $r \times c$ contingency table. First, generate an $r \times c$ contingency table with cell frequencies chosen to provide the maximum value of chi-squared, then calculate chi-squared on that table to obtain $\chi^2_{\max}$. In a permutation context, this is quite easily done as, under permutation, a complete empirically generated reference set of $r \times c$ contingency tables is generated, all belonging to the same Fréchet class, and all possible values of chi-squared are calculated and included in the reference set. The chi-squared test statistic with the largest value in the reference set is $\chi^2_{\max}$.

3.2 Maximum Arrangement of Cell Frequencies

The determination of the maximum arrangement of cell frequencies in an $r \times c$ contingency table requires a different approach than a simple 2×2 contingency table. In this section, a step-by-step procedure is described to generate an arrangement of cell frequencies in an $r \times c$ contingency table that provides the maximum value of a test statistic, such as Cramér's V^2.[7]

STEP 1: List the observed marginal frequency totals of an $r \times c$ contingency table with empty cell frequencies.

STEP 2: If any pair of marginal frequency totals, one from each set of marginal frequency totals, are equal to each other, enter that value in the table as n_{ij} and subtract the value from the two associated marginal frequency totals. For example, if the marginal frequency total for Row 2 is equal to the marginal frequency total for Column 3, enter the marginal frequency total in the table as n_{23} and subtract the value of n_{23} from the marginal frequency totals of Row 2 and Column 3.

[7]The procedure is adapted from an algorithm by Leik and Gove [64, pp. 288–289].

Table 3.14 Example 3×3 contingency table with row marginal frequency distribution {20, 30, 40} and column marginal frequency distribution {30, 50, 10}

	A_1	A_2	A_3	Total
B_1	8	6	6	20
B_2	10	17	3	30
B_3	12	27	1	40
Total	30	50	10	90

Table 3.15 Empty 3×3 contingency table with row marginal frequency distribution {20, 30, 40} and column marginal frequency distribution {30, 50, 10}

	A_1	A_2	A_3	Total
B_1	—	—	—	20
B_2	—	—	—	30
B_3	—	—	—	40
Total	30	50	10	90

Repeat STEP 2 until no two marginal frequency totals are equal. If all marginal frequency totals have been reduced to zero, go to STEP 5; otherwise, go to STEP 3.

STEP 3: Find the largest remaining marginal frequency totals in each set and enter the smaller of the two values in n_{ij}. Then, subtract that (smaller) value from the two marginal frequency totals. Go to STEP 4.

STEP 4: If all marginal frequency totals have been reduced to zero, go to STEP 5; otherwise, go to STEP 2.

STEP 5: Set any remaining n_{ij} values to zero, $i = 1, \ldots, r$ and $j = 1, \ldots, c$.

To illustrate the maximum-generating procedure, consider the 3×3 contingency table given in Table 3.14 with observed row marginal frequency distribution $\{20, 30, 40\}$ and observed column marginal frequency distribution $\{30, 50, 10\}$. Then, the procedure is:

STEP 1: List the observed row and column marginal frequency totals, leaving the cell frequencies empty, as in Table 3.15.

STEP 2: For the two sets of marginal frequency totals given in Table 3.15, two are equal to 30, one for Row 2 and one for Column 1. Set $n_{21} = 30$ and subtract 30 from the two associated marginal frequency totals. The adjusted row and column marginal frequency totals are now $\{20, 0, 40\}$ and $\{0, 50, 10\}$, respectively. No other two marginal frequency totals are identical, so go to STEP 3.

STEP 3: The two largest remaining marginal frequency totals are 40 in Row 3 and 50 in Column 2. Set $n_{32} = 40$, the smaller of the two marginal frequency totals, and subtract 40 from the two adjusted marginal frequency totals. The adjusted row and column marginal frequency totals are now $\{20, 0, 0\}$ and $\{0, 10, 10\}$, respectively. Go to STEP 4.

STEP 4: All marginal frequency totals have not yet been reduced to zero, so go to STEP 2.

STEP 2: No two marginal frequency totals are identical, so go to STEP 3.

STEP 3: The two largest marginal frequency totals are 20 in Row 1 and 10 in either Column 2 or Column 3. As it does not matter which of the two column marginals is chosen, choose Column 3 and set $n_{13} = 10$, the smaller of the two marginal

Table 3.16 Example 3×3 contingency table with row marginal frequency distribution {20, 30, 40} and column marginal frequency distribution {30, 50, 10}

	A_1	A_2	A_3	Total
B_1	0	10	10	20
B_2	30	0	0	30
B_3	0	40	0	40
Total	30	50	10	90

frequency totals and subtract 10 from the two adjusted marginal frequency totals. The adjusted row and column marginal frequency totals are now $\{10, 0, 0\}$ and $\{0, 10, 0\}$. Go to STEP 4.

STEP 4: All marginal frequency totals have not yet been reduced to zero, so go to STEP 2.

STEP 2: Two marginal frequency totals are equal to 10, one for Row 1 and one for Column 2. Set $n_{12} = 10$ and subtract 10 from the two adjusted marginal frequency totals. The adjusted row and column marginal frequency totals are now $\{0, 0, 0\}$ and $\{0, 0, 0\}$. All adjusted marginal frequency totals are now zero, so go to STEP 5.

STEP 5: Set any remaining n_{ij} values to zero; in this case, n_{11}, n_{22}, n_{23}, n_{31}, and n_{33} are set equal to zero.

The completed contingency table is listed in Table 3.16. There may be alternative cell locations for the non-zero entries, meaning that more than one arrangement of cell frequencies may satisfy the conditions, but the four non-zero cell frequency values $\{10, 10, 30, 40\}$ must be included in the 3×3 contingency table.

For the frequency data in the 3×3 contingency table given in Table 3.16, the observed value of Pearson's χ^2 is $\chi^2 = 12.9060$, the observed value of both Tschuprov's T^2 and Cramér's V^2 is

$$T^2 = V^2 = \frac{\chi^2}{N\sqrt{(r-1)(c-1)}} = \frac{12.9060}{90\sqrt{(3-1)(3-1)}} = 0.0717 \,,$$

and the observed values of Pearson's C and $C_{\max}$ are $C = 0.1254$ and $C_{\max} = 0.8165$, yielding a corrected value for C of $C/C_{\max} = 0.1254/0.8165 = 0.1536$. On the other hand, the maximum value of Pearson's chi-squared for the frequency data given in Table 3.16 is $\chi^2_{\max} = 126.00$, and the value of the ratio of the observed chi-squared value to the maximum chi-squared value is only

$$\frac{\chi^2}{\chi^2_{\max}} = \frac{12.9060}{126.00} = 0.1025 \,,$$

indicating that the observed value of $\chi^2 = 12.9060$ is approximately 10 % of the maximum possible value of $\chi^2 = 126.00$, given the observed row and column marginal frequency distributions, {20, 30, 40} and {30, 50, 10}, respectively.

3.2.1 Application to $r \times c \times s$ Contingency Tables

The procedure to find the cell configuration that will yield the maximum value of chi-squared is not restricted to two-way contingency tables. A procedure for a three-way contingency table illustrates application to higher dimensions.

STEP 1: List the observed marginal frequency totals of an $r \times c \times s$ contingency table with empty cell frequencies.

STEP 2: If any triplet of marginal frequency totals, one from each set of marginal frequency totals, are equal to each other, enter that value in the table as n_{ijk} and subtract the value from the three associated marginal frequency totals. For example, if the marginal frequency total for Row 2 is equal to the marginal frequency total for Column 3 and is also equal to the marginal frequency total for Slice 1, enter the marginal frequency total in the three-way contingency table as n_{231} and subtract the value of n_{231} from the associated marginal frequency totals of Row 2, Column 3, and Slice 1.

Repeat STEP 2 until no three marginal frequency totals are equal. If all marginal frequency totals have been reduced to zero, go to STEP 5; otherwise, go to STEP 3.

STEP 3: Find the largest remaining marginal frequency totals in each set and enter the smaller of the three values in n_{ijk}. Then, subtract that (smallest) value from the three marginal frequency totals. Go to STEP 4.

STEP 4: If all marginal frequency totals have been reduced to zero, go to STEP 5; otherwise, go to STEP 2.

STEP 5: Set any remaining n_{ijk} values to zero, $i = 1, \ldots, r$, $j = 1, \ldots, c$, and $k = 1, \ldots, s$.

To illustrate, consider a $3 \times 3 \times 3$ contingency table with observed row marginal frequency distribution {20, 30, 40}, observed column marginal frequency distribution {30, 50, 10}, and observed slice marginal frequency distribution {30, 30, 30}, such as depicted in Fig. 3.1. Then, the procedure is:

STEP 1: List the observed row, column, and slice marginal frequency totals, leaving the cell frequencies empty, as in Fig. 3.1.

STEP 2: For the three sets of marginal frequency totals given in Fig. 3.1, three are equal to 30, one for Row 2, one for Column 1, and one for Slice 1. Set $n_{211} = 30$ and subtract 30 from the three marginal frequency totals. The adjusted row, column, and slice marginal frequency totals are now {20, 0, 40}, {0, 50, 10}, and {0, 30, 30}, respectively.[8] No other three marginal frequency totals are identical, so go to STEP 3.

STEP 3: The three largest remaining marginal frequency totals are 40 in Row 3, 50 in Column 2, and 30 in either Slice 2 or Slice 3. As it does not matter

[8]In this case, all three slice marginal frequency totals are equal to 30. It does not matter which slice marginal frequency total is reduced by 30. In this example, 30 was subtracted from slice 1.

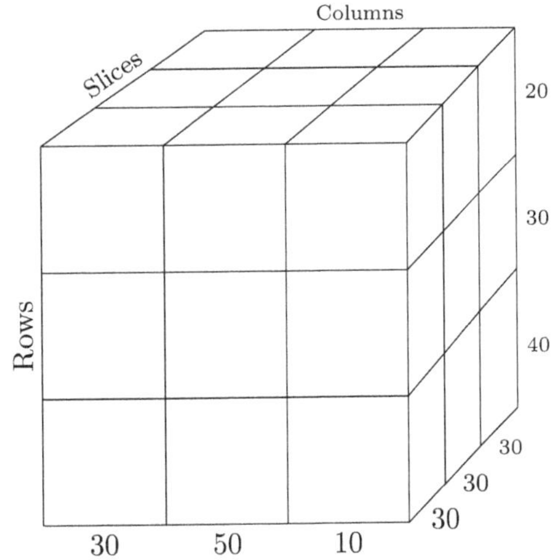

Fig. 3.1 Three-dimensional graphic depicting row marginal frequency totals {20, 30, 40}, column marginal frequency totals {30, 50, 10}, and slice marginal frequency totals {30, 30, 30}

which slice marginal is chosen, choose Slice 2 and set $n_{322} = 30$, the smallest of the three adjusted marginal frequency totals, and subtract 30 from the three adjusted marginal frequency totals. The adjusted row, column, and slice marginal frequency totals are now {20, 0, 10}, {0, 20, 10}, and {0, 0, 30}, respectively. Go to STEP 4.

STEP 4: All marginal frequency totals have not yet been reduced to zero, so go to STEP 2.

STEP 2: No three marginal frequency totals are identical, so go to STEP 3.

STEP 3: The three largest marginal frequency totals are 20 in Row 1, 20 in Column 2, and 30 in Slice 3. Set $n_{123} = 10$, the smallest of the three marginal frequency totals and subtract 10 from the three adjusted marginal frequency totals. The adjusted row, column, and slice marginal frequency totals are now {10, 0, 10}, {0, 10, 10}, and {0, 0, 20}, respectively. Go to STEP 4.

STEP 4: All marginal frequency totals have not yet been reduced to zero, so go to STEP 2.

STEP 2: For the three sets of marginal frequency totals, four are equal to 10, two for Rows 1 and 3, two for Columns 2 and 3, and one is equal to 20 for Slice 3. Set $n_{333} = 10$ and subtract 10 from the three adjusted marginal frequency totals. The adjusted row, column, and slice marginal frequency totals are now {0, 0, 10}, {0, 0, 10}, and {0, 0, 10}, respectively. Go to STEP 4.

STEP 4: All marginal frequency totals have not yet been reduced to zero, so go to STEP 2.

STEP 2: For the three sets of marginal frequency totals, three are equal to 10, one for row 3, one for column 3, and one for slice 3. Set $n_{333} = 10$ and subtract 10 from the three adjusted marginal frequency totals. The adjusted row, column, and slice marginal frequency totals are now {0, 0, 0}, {0, 0, 0}, and {0, 0, 0}, respectively. All adjusted marginal frequency totals are now zero, so go to STEP 5.

Table 3.17 Listing of the 3×3×3 cell frequencies with rows (A_1, A_2, A_3), columns (B_1, B_2, B_3), and slices (D_1, D_2, D_3)

	A_1			A_2			A_3		
	B_1	B_2	B_3	B_1	B_2	B_3	B_1	B_2	B_3
D_1	0	0	0	30	0	0	0	0	0
D_2	0	0	0	0	0	0	0	30	0
D_3	0	20	0	0	0	0	0	0	10

STEP 5: Set any remaining n_{ijk} values to zero, $i = 1, \ldots, r$, $j = 1, \ldots, c$, and $k = 1, \ldots, s$.

The completed contingency table is given in Table 3.17. There may be alternative cell locations for the non-zero entries, meaning that more than one arrangement of cell frequencies may satisfy the conditions, but the four non-zero cell frequency values {20, 30, 30, 10} must be included in the 3×3×3 contingency table.

A χ^2 value for an $r \times c \times s$ contingency table is given by:

$$\chi^2 = N^2 \left(\sum_{i=1}^{r} \sum_{j=1}^{c} \sum_{k=1}^{s} \frac{O_{ij}^2}{R_i C_j S_k} \right) - N \,,$$

where R_i denotes a row marginal frequency total, $i = 1, \ldots, r$, C_j denotes a column marginal frequency total, $j = 1, \ldots, c$, S_k denotes a slice marginal frequency total, $k = 1, \ldots, s$, O_{ijk} denotes an observed cell frequency, $i = 1, \ldots, r$, $j = 1, \ldots, c$, $k = 1, \ldots, s$, and N is the total of all cell frequencies; in this case, $N = 90$. The maximum value of chi-squared for the 3×3×3 contingency table given in Table 3.17 is

$$\chi^2_{\max} = 90^2 \left[\frac{20^2}{(20)(50)(30)} + \frac{30^2}{(30)(30)(30)} + \frac{30^2}{(40)(50)(30)} + \frac{10^2}{(40)(10)(30)} \right.$$
$$\left. + \frac{0^2}{(20)(30)(30)} + \frac{0^2}{(20)(50)(30)} + \cdots + \frac{0^2}{(40)(10)(30)} \right] - 90$$
$$= (8{,}100)(0.0700) - 90 = 477.00 \,.$$

To illustrate the procedure, consider the 3×4×5 contingency table given in Table 3.18 with observed row marginal frequency distribution {32, 32, 31}, observed column marginal frequency distribution {25, 23, 24, 23}, and observed slice marginal frequency distribution {19, 19, 19, 19, 19}. For the frequency data in the 3×4×5 contingency table given in Table 3.18 with $N = 95$ observations, the observed value of Pearson's chi-squared is $\chi^2 = 84.7379$, the maximum value of chi-squared is $\chi^2_{\max} = 474.9616$, and the ratio of the observed chi-squared value to the maximum chi-squared value is

$$\frac{\chi^2}{\chi^2_{\max}} = \frac{84.7379}{474.9616} = 0.1784 \,,$$

Table 3.18 Listing of the 3×4×5 cell frequencies with rows (A_1, A_2, A_3), columns (B_1, B_2, B_3, B_4), and slices $(D_1, D_2, D_3, D_4, D_5)$ for a resampling-approximation example

	A_1				A_2				A_3			
	B_1	B_2	B_3	B_4	B_1	B_2	B_3	B_4	B_1	B_2	B_3	B_4
D_1	0	3	1	3	4	0	0	0	2	1	4	1
D_2	0	0	0	2	1	4	1	0	3	1	3	4
D_3	4	1	0	3	1	3	4	0	0	0	2	1
D_4	3	4	0	0	0	2	1	4	1	0	3	1
D_5	2	1	4	1	0	3	1	3	4	0	0	0

indicating that the observed value of $\chi^2 = 84.7379$ is approximately 18 % of the maximum possible value of chi-squared, given the observed row, column, and slice marginal frequency distributions, $\{32, 32, 31\}$, $\{25, 23, 24, 23\}$, and $\{19, 19, 19, 19, 19\}$, respectively.

3.3 Measures of Effect Size

The fact that a chi-squared statistical test produces low probability values indicates only that there are differences among the response measurement scores between the two variables that (possibly) cannot be attributed to error. The obtained probability value does not indicate whether these differences are of any practical value.[9]

Statisticians and quantitative methodologists have raised a number of issues and concerns with null hypothesis statistical testing (NHST). A brief overview is provided by Cowles:

> The main criticisms [of NHST], endlessly repeated, are easily listed. NHST does not offer any way of testing the alternative or research hypothesis; the null hypothesis is usually false and when differences or relationships are trivial, large samples will lead to its rejection; the method discourages replication and encourages one-shot research; the inferential model depends on assumptions about hypothetical populations and data that cannot be verified; and there are more [35, p. 83].

In addition, there are literally hundreds of articles and chapters dealing with the problems of NHST, far too many to be summarized here. However, a brief overview of the limitations of null hypothesis statistical testing will suffice for these purposes.[10]

First, the null hypothesis is almost never literally true, so rejection of the null hypothesis is relatively uninformative; see, for example, articles by Baken [6],

---

[9] In the literature, "practical value" is often referred to as "practical significance," as contrasted with "statistical significance" [60].

[10] A comprehensive bibliography for the limitations of null hypothesis statistical testing has been compiled by William Thompson [91].

Carver [28, 29], Levine, Weber, Hullett, Park, and Massi Lindsey [66], Levine, Weber, Park, and Hullett [67], McLean and Ernest [71], and Nix and Barnette [79, 80]. This is especially true with null hypotheses for measures of association and correlation. For example, rejection of the null hypothesis of no correlation in the population between variables x and y (H_0: $\rho_{xy} = 0$), where x is, say, Years of Education, and y is, say, Yearly Income, is meaningless. Otherwise, the proportion of young adults ages 18–22 attending college would be only a fraction of what it is.

Second, tests of significance are highly dependent on sample sizes. When sample sizes are small, important effects can be non-significant, and when sample sizes are large, even trivial effects can produce very small probability values; see, for example, articles by Daniel [38] and Levine and Hullett [65].

Third, the requirement of obtaining a random sample from a well-defined population is seldom met in practice; see, for example, articles by Altman and Bland [5], Bradbury [22], Feinstein [41], Frick [44], LaFleur and Greevy [62], Ludbrook [69], Ludbrook and Dudley [70], and Still and White [90].

Fourth, the assumption of normality is rarely satisfied in real-data situations; see, for example, articles by Bernardin and Beatty [12], Bradley [23], Bross [24], Feinstein [41], Geary [45], Micceri [72], Murphy and Cleveland [78], Saal, Downey, and Lahey [84], and Schmidt and Johnson [86].[11]

Moreover, a test statistic such as chi-squared and its associated probability value provides no information as to the size of treatment effects, only whether they are statistically significant [59, p. 135]. As Kirk explained in 1996 [60, p. 747], the one individual most responsible for bringing the shortcomings of hypothesis testing to the attention of researchers was the psychologist Jacob Cohen with two articles with unconventional titles in *American Psychologist*: "Things I have learned (so far)" in 1990 [32] and "The earth is round ($p < .05$)" in 1994 [33]. As a result of the identified challenges with NHST and the reporting of probability values, various measures of effect size have been designed to reflect the substantive importance and practical value of differences between the variables. In the context of Pearson's chi-squared, these measures are Pearson's ϕ^2, Tschuprov's T^2, Cramér's V^2, and Pearson's C.

Recent trends in the literature have stressed the importance of reporting a measure of effect size along with a test of significance when analyzing experimental data [30, 54, 60, 99]. As far back as 1957, I. Richard Savage criticized authors for confining their interests to tests of significance and ignoring the magnitudes of the differences [85, p. 332]. In 1958, Bolles and Messick suggested that tests of significance be supplemented with "indices of utility"[20]. In 1963, William Hays challenged researchers to report measures of effect size in addition to the usual tests of significance [53]. The challenge by Hays was reiterated by Vaughan and Corballis in 1969 [94] who expressed concerns about the lack of attention paid to the problems described by Hays, and by Keppel in 1982 who urged researchers to

[11] William Thompson has compiled an extensive list of quotes from various authors detailing the limits of null hypothesis statistical testing [92].

always report an index of the strength of association along with a test of statistical significance [58]. The demand for the reporting of measures of effect size was largely led by academic psychologists [100]. However, in February of 2016, the American Statistical Association released a statement advocating eliminating the uncritical use of significance levels, such as 0.05 and 0.01, suggesting instead reporting actual probability values such as $P = 0.0320$ along with confidence intervals and measures of effect size [96].

For many years, statisticians and psychometricians who were Fellows of the American Psychological Association, Division 5, urged the editors of APA journals to mandate the reporting of effect sizes. The fourth edition of the *Publication Manual of the American Psychological Association* strongly encouraged reporting measures of effect size in conjunction with probability values. In 1999, the American Psychological Association Task Force on Statistical Inference, under the leadership of Leland Wilkinson, noted that "reporting and interpreting effect sizes in the context of previously reported effects is essential to good research" [100, p. 599]. Consequently, a number of editors of academic journals, both APA and others, began requiring measures of effect size as a condition of publication. In recent years, there has been increased emphasis on reporting measures of effect size in addition to tests of significance in a number of academic disciplines, recognizing that determination of a significant treatment effect does not necessarily translate into a substantial effect. As a result, numerous journals now require the reporting of measures of effect size as part of their editorial policies [26, 27].

While the chi-squared-based measures, Pearson's ϕ^2, Tschuprov's T^2, Cramér's V^2, and Pearson's C, are often presented as measures of effect size, because their upper limit is usually less than unity for any realized contingency table, they systematically underestimate the true measure of effect size. Let R denote an unbiased measure of effect size defined as:

$$R = \frac{\chi^2}{\chi^2_{\text{max}}}$$

for any contingency table composed of two or more nominal-level variables. To illustrate the advantage of the R measure of effect size, consider the 2×2 contingency table in Table 3.19, where the observed value of Pearson's chi-squared is $\chi^2 = 0.2667$, the maximum value of chi-squared given the observed row and column marginal frequency distributions, $\{15, 5\}$ and $\{10, 10\}$, respectively, is $\chi^2_{\text{max}} = 0.3333$, and the observed value of the R measure of effect size is $R = \chi^2/\chi^2_{\text{max}} = 0.2667/0.3333 = 0.80$, indicating that the observed chi-squared value

Table 3.19 Example 2×2 contingency table

	A_1	A_2	Total
B_1	8	7	15
B_2	2	3	5
Total	10	10	20

Table 3.20 Example 2×4 contingency table

	A_1	A_2	A_3	A_4	Total
B_1	6	1	2	6	15
B_2	1	8	9	7	25
Total	7	9	11	13	40

is 80 % of the maximum possible chi-squared value, given the observed marginal frequency distributions. In contrast, $\phi^2 = T^2 = V^2 = 0.0133$, $C = 0.1147$, $C_{\max} = 0.7071$, and $C/C_{\max} = 0.1147/0.7071 = 0.1622$.

Consider a second example with a larger contingency table, such as the 2×4 contingency table given in Table 3.20. For the frequency data given in Table 3.20, Pearson's ϕ^2, Tschuprov's T^2, and Pearson's C are not appropriate for the 2×4 contingency table as $r \neq c$.[12] The observed value of Pearson's chi-squared is $\chi^2 = 11.7873$, the maximum value of chi-squared given the observed row and column marginal frequency distributions, $\{15, 25\}$ and $\{7, 9, 11, 13\}$, respectively, is $\chi^2_{\max} = 33.9048$, and the observed value of the R measure of effect size is

$$R = \frac{\chi^2}{\chi^2_{\max}} = \frac{11.7873}{33.9048} = 0.3476 \, ,$$

indicating that the observed value of χ^2 is approximately 35 % of the maximum possible chi-squared value, given the observed marginal frequency distributions. In contrast, Cramér's $V^2 = 0.2947$.

3.4 Likelihood-Ratio Tests

It is common to see likelihood-ratio tests of independence instead of tests based on chi-squared in the research literature. Likelihood-ratio tests are preferred by many researchers as it is believed that likelihood-ratio tests are less affected by small sample sizes than chi-squared tests when there are two or more degrees of freedom. In addition, likelihood-ratio tests are widely used in log-linear models for the analysis of contingency tables. The likelihood-ratio test for an $r \times c$ contingency table is given by:

$$G^2 = 2N \ln(N) + 2\sum_{i=1}^{r}\sum_{j=1}^{c} n_{ij} \ln(n_{ij}) - 2\sum_{i=1}^{r} R_i \ln(R_i) - 2\sum_{j=1}^{c} C_j \ln(C_j) \, ,$$

[12] Technically, Pearson's ϕ^2 can be calculated on $2\times c$ contingency tables, where it has the potential to norm properly between the limiting values of 0 and 1. In this case, $\phi^2 = 0.2947$, the same as Cramér's V^2.

where n_{ij} denotes a cell frequency and R_i and C_j denote the row and column frequency totals, respectively, for $i = 1, \ldots, r$ and $j = 1, \ldots, c$; however, the likelihood-ratio is usually expressed more succinctly for calculation purposes as:

$$G^2 = 2\sum_{i=1}^{r}\sum_{j=1}^{c} O_{ij} \ln\left(\frac{O_{ij}}{E_{ij}}\right) ,$$

where O_{ij} and E_{ij} denote the observed and expected cell frequencies, respectively, for $i = 1, \ldots, r$ and $j = 1, \ldots, c$. To illustrate the likelihood-ratio test, consider the frequency data given in Table 3.21, where the expected cell frequency values are

$$E_{11} = \frac{(26)(30)}{60} = 13.00 , \quad E_{12} = \frac{(26)(20)}{60} = 8.6667 ,$$

$$E_{13} = \frac{(26)(10)}{60} = 4.3333 , \quad E_{21} = \frac{(34)(30)}{60} = 17.00 ,$$

$$E_{22} = \frac{(34)(20)}{60} = 11.3333 , \quad E_{23} = \frac{(34)(10)}{60} = 5.6667 ,$$

and the observed value of G^2 is

$$\begin{aligned} G^2 &= 2\sum_{i=1}^{r}\sum_{j=1}^{c} O_{ij} \ln\left(\frac{O_{ij}}{E_{ij}}\right) \\ &= 2\left[20 \ln\left(\frac{20}{13}\right) + 5 \ln\left(\frac{5}{8.6667}\right) + 1 \ln\left(\frac{1}{4.3333}\right) + 10 \ln\left(\frac{10}{17}\right)\right. \\ &\quad \left. + 15 \ln\left(\frac{15}{11.3333}\right) + 9 \ln\left(\frac{9}{5.6667}\right)\right] = 14.9219 . \end{aligned}$$

Unfortunately, no maximum value for G^2 has been determined and the algorithmic procedure detailed in Sect. 3.2 for the maximum value of chi-squared is not appropriate for the likelihood-ratio test, as the procedure will always yield some cell frequencies that are zero and ln(0) is $-\infty$. For the same reason, G^2 is one of the very few statistical measures that is not amenable to permutation methods. In generating the reference set of all possible arrangements of cell frequencies, some arrangements will necessarily include one or more cell frequencies equal to zero.

Table 3.21 Example 2×3 contingency table

	A_1	A_2	A_3	Total
B_1	20	5	1	26
B_2	10	15	9	34
Total	30	20	10	60

3.5 Multi-way Contingency Tables

The analysis of multi-way contingency tables composed of disjoint, unordered categories has become increasingly important in contemporary research [2, 46, 57, 61, 81, 83, 95, 97, 98]. In particular, a great deal of attention has been given in recent years to log-linear analysis of multi-way contingency tables [2, 17, 47, 48, 50, 51]. Each log-linear model for a contingency table contains a set of expected values that satisfies the model perfectly, and the model goodness of fit is typically tested with either Pearson's chi-squared test statistic (χ^2) or Wilks' likelihood-ratio test statistic (G^2), both of which are asymptotically distributed as chi-squared with appropriate degrees of freedom. However, these asymptotic tests require fairly large expected cell values, while permutation tests are ideal when expected cell values are small. Small expected cell values are common in sparse multi-way contingency tables, resulting in discretely distributed test statistic values that are poorly approximated by a continuous chi-squared distribution. Contingency tables are considered to be sparse when a substantial proportion of table cells contain small observed frequencies, Sparse tables occur when (1) the sample size is small, (2) there are a large number of cells in the contingency table, (3) the number of variables is large, or (4) one or more variables contain numerous unordered categories [1, p. 244]. In this section, Monte Carlo resampling permutation methods are presented that provide approximate probability values for the chi-squared and likelihood-ratio test statistics for sparse multi-way contingency tables [68].

3.5.1 *Method*

Following the notation of Mielke and Berry [73, 75, pp. 283–285], consider an r-way contingency table with $n_1 \times n_2 \times \cdots \times n_r$ cells, where $n_r \geq 2$ is the number of disjoint, unordered categories for variables $i = 1, \ldots, r$, the observed frequency of the $(j_1, \ldots, j_r)$th cell is denoted by $O_{j_1, \ldots, j_r}$, $\langle i \rangle_{ji}$ is the fixed marginal frequency total in the j_ith category of the ith variable for $j_i = 1, \ldots, n_i$, and

$$N = \sum_{j_i=1}^{n_i} \langle i \rangle_{j_i}$$

is the frequency total for the r-way contingency table. The notation accommodates all contingency tables for $r \geq 2$. The Pearson chi-squared and Wilks likelihood-ratio test statistics for the independence of r variables are then given by:

$$\chi^2 = N^{r-1} \left[\sum_{i=1}^{r} \sum_{j_i=1}^{n_i} \left(O^2_{j_1, \ldots, j_r} \Big/ \prod_{k=1}^{r} \langle k \rangle_{j_k} \right) \right] - N \tag{3.5}$$

and

$$G^2 = 2\sum_{i=1}^{r}\sum_{j_i=1}^{n_i} O_{j_1,\ldots,j_r} \ln\left(N^{r-1}O_{j_1,\ldots,j_r} \Big/ \prod_{k=1}^{r}\langle k\rangle_{j_k}\right) , \tag{3.6}$$

respectively [75, p. 309].

Under the null hypothesis that the r variables of an r-way contingency table are mutually independent, the conventional asymptotic method to obtain a probability value uses a large sample approximation, which assumes that all expected cell frequencies are at least five [4, p. 227]. The asymptotic distribution of χ^2 and G^2 under the null hypothesis is chi-squared with

$$\prod_{i=1}^{r} n_i - \sum_{i=1}^{r}(n_i - 1) - 1$$

degrees of freedom (df).

As either N or r increases in an r-way contingency table, the number of possible cell arrangements becomes exceedingly large; consequently, only a random sample of size L drawn from all possible arrangements is typically examined. The resulting probability values are based on Monte Carlo procedures and are variously termed "resampling" or "randomization" tests. The Monte Carlo resampling permutation method to obtain probability values calculates the χ^2 and G^2 test statistic values for L cell arrangements of the r-way contingency table, given fixed marginal frequency totals. The accuracy of the resampling probability value is a function of the true probability value and the number of random samples. When the true probability value is not too extreme, $L = 1{,}000{,}000$ random samples generally ensures three decimal places of accuracy [56]. A Monte Carlo resampling algorithm for r-way contingency tables provides L random arrangements of cell frequencies, given fixed marginal frequency totals [76].

If χ^2_{o} denotes the value of χ^2 calculated on the observed r-way contingency table, the resampling probability value of χ^2_{o} under the null hypothesis is given by:

$$P\left\{\chi^2_{\text{o}}|N, \langle i\rangle_{j_i}\right\} = \frac{1}{L}\sum_{k=1}^{L}\phi\left(\chi^2_k\right) ,$$

where χ^2_k denotes the kth of L random χ^2 values and

$$\phi\left(\chi^2_k\right) = \begin{cases} 1 & \text{if } \chi^2_k \geq \chi^2_{\text{o}} , \\ 0 & \text{otherwise} . \end{cases}$$

Analogously, if G^2_{o} denotes the value of G^2 calculated on the observed r-way contingency table, the resampling probability value of G^2_{o} under the null hypothesis is given by:

$$P\left\{G_o^2|N, \langle i\rangle_{ji}\right\} = \frac{1}{L}\sum_{k=1}^{L}\phi(G_k^2) ,$$

where G_k^2 denotes the kth of L random G^2 values and

$$\phi(G_k^2) = \begin{cases} 1 & \text{if } G_k^2 \geq G_o^2 , \\ 0 & \text{otherwise} . \end{cases}$$

The probability values of the asymptotic and Monte Carlo resampling methods are essentially equivalent when all cell frequencies are large. However, given the small expected cell values that commonly occur in r-way contingency tables, probability values obtained with the asymptotic method may differ considerably from probability values obtained with either an exact or Monte Carlo resampling permutation method.

3.5.2 Example

In this section, the calculation of Monte Carlo resampling probability values for χ^2 and G^2 is illustrated with an example data set. To simplify the presentation, the example analysis is confined to a three-way contingency table.

A health-care facility evaluates prospective residents using the third version of the Test of Nonverbal Intelligence (TONI-3) as a test to evaluate incoming residents and assign them to an appropriate level of care: Independent Living, Assisted Living, or Continuous Care [25]. In addition, administrators of the facility gather basic demographic information on prospective residents, including marital status and religious preference. TONI-3 is a norm-referenced measure of intelligence, aptitude, abstract reasoning, and problem solving that is completely nonverbal and largely motor-free, requiring only a gesture to indicate response choices, such as pointing or nodding. TONI-3 is particularly well-suited for individuals who have disorders of communication or thinking, such as aphasia, speech problems, deafness, stroke, or other neurological impairments. The hypothesis to be tested is: Level of Care is independent of Marital Status and Religious Preference.

Consider the sparse $3{\times}4{\times}5$ contingency table given in Table 3.22 with $N = 32$ residents. For consistency with the notation in the previous section, j_1 denotes Level of Care with 1 indicating Independent Living, 2 indicating Assisted Living, and 3 indicating Continuous Care; j_2 denotes Religious Preference with 1 indicating Protestant, 2 indicating Catholic, 3 indicating Jewish, and 4 indicating Other; and j_3 denotes Marital Status with 1 indicating Single, 2 indicating Married, 3 indicating Widowed, 4 indicating Divorced, and 5 indicating Separated.

Table 3.22 Example of a sparse three-way contingency table data with three levels of variable j_1, four levels of variable j_2, and five levels of variable j_3

		j_3				
j_1	j_2	1	2	3	4	5
1	1	0	0	0	1	0
	2	0	1	0	0	0
	3	2	0	0	0	2
	4	1	0	1	1	0
2	1	1	1	0	0	1
	2	0	0	2	1	0
	3	0	0	1	2	0
	4	0	1	0	0	0
3	1	0	0	1	0	0
	2	1	0	0	1	3
	3	0	1	0	0	0
	4	0	4	0	0	1

For the frequency data given in Table 3.22, the observed value of chi-squared is $\chi_o^2 = 67.41$, the asymptotic probability value based on

$$\prod_{i=1}^{r} n_i - \sum_{i=1}^{r} (n_i - 1) - 1$$
$$= (3)(4)(5) - [(3-1) + (4-1) + (5-1)] - 1 = 50$$

degrees of freedom is $P = 0.0508$, and the Monte Carlo resampling probability value based on $L = 1{,}000{,}000$ random samples is $P = 0.0407$. Analogously, for the frequency data given in Table 3.22, $G_0^2 = 66.28$, the asymptotic probability value based on 50 degrees of freedom is $P = 0.0613$, and the Monte Carlo resampling probability value based on $L = 1{,}000{,}000$ random samples is $P = 0.0315$.

Illustration of the Resampling Procedure

To illustrate the Monte Carlo resampling process, consider the 3-way contingency table in Table 3.22 and summarized in two 2-way subtables in Table 3.23, where the marginal frequency distributions of variables j_1, j_2, and j_3 are denoted by $\langle 1\rangle_{j_1}$, $\langle 2\rangle_{j_2}$, and $\langle 3\rangle_{j_3}$, respectively. The Monte Carlo resampling procedure can be illustrated with just seven steps.

STEP 1: The $3\times4\times5 = 60$ cells are each initialized to zero.

STEP 2: Each observed marginal frequency distribution is converted to a cumulative probability distribution. Thus, for variable j_1 the observed marginal

Table 3.23 Subtables of the frequency data given in Table 3.22 with variable j_1 cross-classified with variable j_2 and variable j_1 cross-classified with variable j_3

	j_1			
j_2	1	2	3	$\langle 2 \rangle_{j_2}$
1	1	3	2	6
2	1	3	5	9
3	4	3	1	8
4	3	1	5	9
$\langle 1 \rangle_{j_1}$	9	10	13	32

	j_1			
j_3	1	2	3	$\langle 3 \rangle_{j_3}$
1	3	1	1	5
2	1	2	5	8
3	1	3	1	5
4	2	3	2	7
5	2	1	4	7
$\langle 1 \rangle_{j_1}$	9	10	13	32

frequency totals $\langle 1 \rangle_{j_1} = \{9, 10, 13\}$ in Table 3.23 are converted to cumulative probability values as follows:

$$\frac{9}{32} = 0.2813\,, \quad \frac{9+10}{32} = 0.5938\,, \quad \text{and} \quad \frac{9+10+13}{32} = 1.0000\,.$$

For variable j_2, the observed marginal frequency totals are $\langle 2 \rangle_{j_2} = \{6, 9, 8, 9\}$ and the cumulative probability distribution is 0.1875, 0.4688, 0.7188, and 1.0000. For variable j_3, the observed marginal frequency totals are $\langle 3 \rangle_{j_3} = \{5, 8, 5, 7, 7\}$ and the cumulative probability distribution is 0.1563, 0.4063, 0.5625, 0.7813, and 1.0000.

STEP 3: A total of $r = 3$ uniform pseudorandom numbers, U_1, U_2, and U_3, are generated on [0, 1).

STEP 4: The pseudorandom numbers, U_1, U_2, and U_3, are located in the three cumulative probability distributions as follows. Suppose that $U_1 = 0.30$, $U_2 = 0.50$, and $U_3 = 0.70$. Since $0.2813 \leq U_1 = 0.30 < 0.5938$, $0.4688 \leq U_2 = 50 < 0.7188$, and $0.5625 \leq U_3 = 70 < 0.7813$, the frequency O_{234} is increased by 1 and the corresponding marginal frequency totals of 10, 8, and 7 are each reduced by 1, i.e., to 9, 7, and 6, respectively.

STEP 5: The cumulative probability distributions are recalculated on the modified marginal frequency totals and the process is repeated until all $N = 32$ observations have been randomly assigned to a new 3×4×5 contingency table.

STEP 6: The test statistics of interest, χ^2 and G^2, are calculated on the random table.

STEP 7: The randomization procedure is repeated L times.

Illustration of the Chi-squared Calculations

To illustrate the computation of χ^2_o, consider the portion of Eq. (3.5) enclosed in square brackets. Using the observed cell frequency values in Table 3.22, i.e., O_{j_1,j_2,j_3}, and the marginal frequency totals in Table 3.23, i.e., $\langle 1 \rangle_{j_1}$, $\langle 2 \rangle_{j_2}$, and $\langle 3 \rangle_{j_3}$

for $j_1 = \{1, 2, 3\}$, $j_{21} = \{1, 2, 3, 4\}$, and $j_{31} = \{1, 2, 3, 4, 5\}$, the calculation of χ_o^2 proceeds as follows:

$$\sum_{i=1}^{r}\sum_{j_i=1}^{n_i}\left(O_{j_1,\ldots,j_r}^2\Big/\prod_{k=1}^{r}\langle k\rangle_{j_k}\right)$$
$$= \frac{0^2}{(9)(6)(5)} + \frac{0^2}{(9)(6)(8)} + \frac{1^2}{(9)(6)(5)} + \cdots + \frac{1^2}{(13)(9)(7)} = 0.0971\,,$$

corresponding to cells 111, 112, 113, ..., 345. Then, Eq. (3.5) yields $\chi_o^2 = 32^{3-1}(0.0971) - 32 = 67.41$.

Illustration of the Likelihood-Ratio Calculations

Following the same pattern as in the χ^2 calculations, i.e., cells 111, 112, 113, ..., 345, G_o^2 in Eq. (3.6) is obtained from the observed cell frequency values in Table 3.22 and the marginal frequency totals in Table 3.23 as follows:

$$\sum_{i=1}^{r}\sum_{j_i=1}^{n_i} O_{j_1,\ldots,j_r}\ln\left(N^{r-1}O_{j_1,\ldots,j_r}\Big/\prod_{k=1}^{r}\langle k\rangle_{j_k}\right)$$
$$= 0\ln\left[\frac{(32^{3-1})(0)}{(9)(6)(5)}\right] + 0\ln\left[\frac{(32^{3-1})(0)}{(9)(6)(8)}\right] + 0\ln\left[\frac{(32^{3-1})(0)}{(13)(9)(7)}\right]$$
$$+ \cdots + 1\ln\left[\frac{(32^{3-1})(1)}{(9)(6)(5)}\right] = 33.14\,.$$

Then, Eq. (3.6) yields $G_o^2 = 2(33.14) = 66.28$.[13]

The example analyses illustrate the advantage of a Monte Carlo resampling approach over a conventional asymptotic approach for sparse multi-way contingency tables. For both χ^2 and G^2 in the example analyses, the asymptotic probability values, i.e., $P = 0.0508$ and $P = 0.0613$, respectively, are somewhat greater than the resampling probability values, i.e., $P = 0.0407$ and $P = 0.0315$, respectively.

[13] Since the natural logarithm of zero is $-\infty$, for this example $\ln(0)$ has been set to zero.

3.6 Chi-squared Goodness-of-Fit Tests

Although chi-squared tests for goodness of fit are generally not considered to be measures of association, in a sense they are, since, like chi-squared tests of independence, they measure the departure between the observed and expected category frequencies. Consequently, a chi-squared measure of goodness of fit can easily be created to yield a maximum-corrected measure of effect size [55]. Consider the Pearson chi-squared goodness-of-fit statistic given by:

$$\chi^2 = \sum_{i=1}^{k} \frac{O_i^2}{E_i} - N ,$$

where k is the number of disjoint, unordered categories, O_i and E_i are the observed and expected category frequencies, respectively, for $i = 1, \ldots, k$, and N is the total sample size. The maximum value for a chi-squared goodness-of-fit test can be shown to be given by:

$$\chi^2_{\max} = \frac{N(N-q)}{q} ,$$

where $q = \min(E_1, E_2, \ldots, E_k)$ [55, p. 413]. In the case of tied values, any of the smallest frequency values will suffice for q. Then, a maximum-corrected measure of effect size for the chi-squared goodness-of-fit test is given by:

$$R = \frac{\chi^2}{\chi^2_{\max}} = \frac{q\,\chi^2}{N(N-q)} .$$

Since $0 \leq R \leq 1$, interpretation of intermediate values is straightforward as the proportion of the maximum departure between the observed and expected values [55, p. 413].

In 1988, Jacob Cohen developed statistic **w**, an unstandardized measure of effect size for a chi-squared goodness-of-fit test given by:

$$\mathbf{w} = \sqrt{\frac{1}{N} \sum_{i=1}^{k} \frac{(O_i - E_i)^2}{E_i}} = \sqrt{\frac{\chi^2}{N}} = \phi ,$$

where $0 \leq \mathbf{w} \leq \infty$ [31, pp. 216–218]. Because **w** is not maximum corrected, it does not norm between 0 and 1. Consequently, **w** is difficult to interpret [31, p. 224]. The relationships between test statistics R and **w** are given by:

$$R = \frac{q}{N-q}\mathbf{w}^2 \quad \text{and} \quad \mathbf{w} = \left(\frac{N-q}{q}R\right)^{1/2} ,$$

where $q = \min(E_1, E_2, \ldots, E_k)$.

Table 3.24 Example goodness-of-fit frequencies with $k = 4$ categories and $N = 40$ observations

	Category				
	A	*B*	*C*	*D*	Total
Observed	24	8	6	2	40
Expected	8	10	10	12	40

3.6.1 Chi-squared Goodness-of-Fit Example

To illustrate the calculation of test statistic R, consider the frequency data given in Table 3.24 where $k = 4$, $N = 40$, and $q = \min(8, 10, 10, 12) = 8$. For the frequency data given in Table 3.24, the observed value of Pearson's chi-squared is

$$\chi^2 = \sum_{i=1}^{k} \frac{O_i^2}{E_i} - N = \frac{24^2}{8} + \frac{8^2}{10} + \frac{6^2}{10} + \frac{2^2}{12} - 40 = 42.3333$$

and the maximum value of chi-squared is

$$\chi^2_{\max} = \frac{N(N-q)}{q} = \frac{40(40-8)}{8} = 160 \; .$$

Then, the observed value of the maximum-corrected measure of effect size for the Pearson chi-squared goodness-of-fit test is

$$R = \frac{\chi^2}{\chi^2_{\max}} = \frac{42.3333}{160} = 0.2646 \; ,$$

indicating that the observed value of chi-squared is approximately 26 % of the maximum possible χ^2 value, given the expected values.

Many researchers prefer the likelihood-ratio test over the chi-squared test for testing goodness of fit. Consider Wilks' likelihood-ratio goodness-of-fit test given by:

$$G^2 = 2 \sum_{i=1}^{k} O_i \ln\left(\frac{O_i}{E_i}\right) \; ,$$

where k is the number of disjoint, unordered categories and O_i and E_i are the observed and expected category frequencies, respectively, for $i = 1, \ldots, k$, and all O_i are greater than zero. The maximum value for G^2 can be shown to be

$$G^2_{\max} = -2N \ln\left(\frac{q}{N}\right) \; ,$$

where $q = \min(E_1, E_2, \ldots, E_k)$ and N is the total sample size [55, p. 413]. In the case of tied values, any of the smallest frequency values will suffice for q. Then, a maximum-corrected measure of effect size for the likelihood-ratio goodness-of-fit test is given by:

$$R = \frac{G^2}{G^2_{\text{max}}} = \frac{G^2}{-2N \ln\left(\frac{q}{N}\right)} .$$

Since $0 \leq R \leq 1$, interpretation of intermediate values is straightforward as the proportion of the maximum departure between the observed and expected values [55, p. 413].

3.6.2 Likelihood-Ratio Goodness-of-Fit Example

To illustrate the calculation of test statistic R, consider the frequency data given in Table 3.24, replicated as Table 3.25 for convenience. For the frequency data given in Table 3.25, $k = 4$, $N = 40$, the observed value of G^2 is

$$G^2 = 2\sum_{i=1}^{k} O_i \ln\left(\frac{O_i}{E_i}\right)$$

$$= 2\left[24 \ln\left(\frac{24}{8}\right) + 8 \ln\left(\frac{8}{10}\right) + 6 \ln\left(\frac{6}{10}\right) + 2 \ln\left(\frac{2}{12}\right)\right] = 35.8661 ,$$

and the maximum value of G^2 is

$$G^2_{\text{max}} = -2N \ln\left(\frac{q}{N}\right) = -2(40) \ln\left(\frac{8}{40}\right) = 128.7550 .$$

Then, the observed value of the maximum-corrected measure of effect size for Wilks' likelihood-ratio goodness-of-fit test is

$$R = \frac{G^2}{G^2_{\text{max}}} = \frac{35.8661}{128.7550} = 0.2786 ,$$

indicating that the observed value of G^2 is approximately 28 % of the maximum possible G^2 value, given the expected values. As noted previously, the

Table 3.25 Example goodness-of-fit frequencies with $k = 4$ categories (A, B, C, D) and $N = 40$ observations

	Category				
	A	B	C	D	Total
Observed	24	8	6	2	40
Expected	8	10	10	12	40

likelihood-ratio for goodness of fit is not amenable to permutation methods. In generating the reference set of all possible arrangements of cell frequencies, some arrangements will necessarily include one or more cell frequencies equal to zero and $\ln(0)$ is $-\infty$.

3.7 Other Goodness-of-Fit Tests

Besides goodness-of-fit tests based on the chi-squared and likelihood-ratio test statistics, a number of other goodness-of-fit tests have been developed. While these alternative tests are not directly based on Pearson's chi-squared test statistic, most are distributed as chi-squared with defined degrees of freedom. In this section, goodness-of-fit tests for unordered equiprobable categories are described and compared. Included in this section are Fisher's exact test, exact chi-squared, exact likelihood-ratio, exact Freeman–Tukey, and exact Cressie–Read goodness-of-fit tests for k disjoint, unordered categories with equal probabilities under the null hypothesis. As noted previously, exact tests are free from any asymptotic assumptions; consequently, they are ideal for sparse tables where expected values may be small.

Consider the random assignment of N objects to k unordered, mutually exclusive, exhaustive, equiprobable categories, i.e., the probability for each of the k categories is $p_i = 1/k$ for $i = 1, \ldots, k$ under the null hypothesis. Then, the probability that O_i objects occur in the ith of k categories is the multinomial probability given by:

$$P(O_i|p_i, N) = P(O_1, \ldots, O_k|p_1, \ldots, p_k, N) = \left(N! \Big/ \prod_{i=1}^{k} O_i!\right) \prod_{i=1}^{k} p_i^{O_i} ,$$

where

$$\sum_{i=1}^{k} p_i = 1 \quad \text{and} \quad \sum_{i=1}^{k} O_i = N .$$

Fisher's exact goodness-of-fit test is the sum of all distinct $P(O_i|N, p_i)$ values that are equal to or less than the observed value of $P(O_i|N, p_i)$ associated with a set of observations, $O_1, \ldots, O_k$ [74]. The Pearson [82] chi-squared goodness-of-fit test statistic for N objects in k disjoint, unordered categories is given by:

$$\chi^2 = \sum_{i=1}^{k} \frac{(O_i - E_i)^2}{E_i}$$

and Wilks' [101, 102] likelihood-ratio test statistic is given by:

$$G^2 = 2 \sum_{i=1}^{k} O_i \ln\left(\frac{O_i}{E_i}\right) ,$$

where the expected frequency of the ith category under the null hypothesis of equal category probabilities is given by:

$$E_i = \frac{N}{k} \qquad \text{for } i = 1, \ldots, k .$$

Two other tests that have received attention are the Freeman–Tukey [43] goodness-of-fit test given by:

$$T^2 = \sum_{i=1}^{k} \left[\sqrt{O_i} + \sqrt{O_i + 1} - \sqrt{4N/k + 1} \right]^2$$

and the Cressie–Read [37] goodness-of-fit test given by:

$$I(\lambda) = \frac{2}{\lambda(\lambda + 1)} \sum_{i=1}^{k} O_i \left[\left(\frac{k\, O_i}{N} \right)^{\lambda} - 1 \right] .$$

Cressie and Read demonstrated that $I(\lambda)$ with λ set to 2/3 was optimal both in terms of attained significance level and small sample properties.

Under the null hypothesis, the χ^2, G^2, T^2, and $I(2/3)$ goodness-of-fit test statistics are distributed as chi-squared with $k - 1$ degrees of freedom. However, when N is small or k is large, the expected frequencies are often small and the chi-squared approximation to these tests is, therefore, suspect. Based on early work by Bartlett [7, 8, 9, 10, 11], Box [21], and Lawley [63], Williams [103] introduced a correction to Wilks' G^2 given by:

$$Q = 1 + \frac{1}{6N(k-1)} \sum_{i=1}^{k} \frac{1 - p_i}{p_i} . \tag{3.7}$$

A further correction to Wilks' G^2 by Smith, Rae, Manderscheid, and Silbergeld [88] is given by:

$$Q' = 1 + \frac{1}{6N^2(k-1)} \sum_{i=1}^{k} \frac{(1 - p_i)(1 + Np_i)}{p_i^2} . \tag{3.8}$$

Under the null hypothesis of equal category probabilities, i.e., $p_i = 1/k$ for $i = 1, \ldots, k$, Eq. (3.7) reduces to

$$Q = 1 + \frac{k+1}{6N}$$

and Eq. (3.8) reduces to

$$Q' = 1 + \frac{k+1}{6N} + \frac{k^2}{6N^2} .$$

Both the Williams [103] corrected test statistic given by:

$$G_W^2 = \frac{G^2}{Q}$$

and the Smith et al. [89] corrected test statistic given by:

$$G_S^2 = \frac{G^2}{Q'}$$

are distributed as chi-squared with $k - 1$ degrees of freedom.

3.7.1 Partition Theory

In general, for an exact goodness-of-fit test with N objects in k categories there are

$$M = \binom{N+k-1}{k-1}$$

distinct, ordered configurations to be examined. Under the null hypothesis that the probabilities of all k categories are equal, a vastly reduced number of distinct partitions of the data can be considered using a further condensation of the M ordered configurations. The condensation is based on a 1748 result by Leonhard Euler that provides a generating function for the number of decompositions of N integer summands without regard to order using the recurrence relation:

$$p(N) = \sum_{j=1} (-1)^{j-1} p\left[N - \frac{3j^2 \pm j}{2}\right] ,$$

where $p(0) = 1$ and j is a positive integer satisfying $2 \leq 3j^2 \pm j \leq 2N$ [40, pp. 256–282]. Note that if $N = 1$, then $j = 1$ with only the minus ($-$) sign allowed; if $2 \leq N \leq 4$, then $j = 1$ with both the plus ($+$) and minus ($-$) signs allowed;

if $5 \leq N \leq 6$, then $j = 1$ with both the plus (+) and minus (−) signs allowed and $j = 2$ with only the minus (−) sign allowed; and so forth.[14] G.H. Hardy and S. Ramanujan [52, p. 79] provided the asymptotic formula for $p(N)$ given by:

$$p(N) \sim \frac{1}{4N\sqrt{3}} \exp\left(\pi\sqrt{2N/3}\right)$$

as $N \to \infty$.

3.7.2 Algorithm

Given k disjoint, unordered categories and observed categorical frequencies $O_1, \ldots, O_k$, an algorithmic procedure generates all $p(N)$ partitions, computes the exact probability for each partition, calculates the observed χ^2, G^2, G^2_W, G^2_S, T^2, and $I(2/3)$ test statistic values, and calculates the number of ways that each partition can occur, i.e., the partition weights [13]. The partition weights are multinomial and are given by:

$$W = \frac{k!}{\displaystyle\prod_{i=1}^{m} f_i!} ,$$

where f_i is the frequency for each of m distinct integers comprising a partition. For example, if the observed partition is {3 2 2 1 0 0} where $N = 8$ objects, $k = 6$ categories, and $m = 4$ distinct integers (3, 2, 1, 0), then $f_1 = 1$, $f_2 = 2$, $f_3 = 1$, $f_4 = 2$, and

$$W = \frac{6!}{1!\,2!\,1!\,2!} = \frac{720}{4} = 180\,.$$

If $k < N$, the number of distinct partitions is reduced to eliminate those partitions where the number of partition values exceeds k. For example, if $k = 3$ and $N = 5$, then the two partitions {2 1 1 1} and {1 1 1 1 1} cannot be considered as the respective number of partitions, four and five, both exceed $k = 3$. The sum of the values of W for the included distinct partitions is equal to M.

The exact probability values for the Fisher exact, χ^2, G^2, T^2, and $I(2/3)$ goodness-of-fit tests are obtained by comparing observed values to partition probability values. In the case of Fisher's exact test, partition probability values equal

[14] In order to maintain consistency with the mathematical notation first employed by Euler, $p(N)$ denotes the number of partitions of N into distinct parts and should not be confused with the common statistical use of p, which usually indicates a probability value.

to or less than the observed partition probability value are weighted and summed. For the exact χ^2, G^2, T^2, and $I(2/3)$ goodness-of-fit tests, partition probability values associated with partition test statistics equal to or greater than the observed test statistic values are weighted and summed. Under the null hypothesis, G^2_W and G^2_S are simple scalar functions of G^2; consequently, the exact probability values for G^2_W and G^2_S are identical to the probability value for G^2.

3.7.3 Examples

Three examples illustrate the application of the goodness-of-fit tests. The first example is based on $N = 8$ events in $k = 8$ categories, i.e., $N = k$; the second example is based on $N = 45$ events in $k = 20$ categories, i.e., $N > k$; and the third example is based on $N = 10$ events in $k = 50$ categories, i.e., $N < k$.

Example 1

This first example illustrates the application of goodness-of-fit tests when $N = k$. Consider an example application in which $N = 8$ learning-disabled elementary school children are classified into $k = 8$ disjoint, unordered categories of learning disability with categorical frequencies $O_1 = O_2 = 3$, $O_3 = 2$, and $O_4 = O_5 = O_6 = O_7 = O_8 = 0$. The null hypothesis specifies that the k expected category probabilities are equally likely, i.e., $p_i = 1/k = 1/8 = 0.125$ for $i = 1, \ldots, 8$. Table 3.26 lists the $p(8) = 22$ distinct partitions of the $N = 8$ events into the $k = 8$ categories, the partition probabilities, the multinomial weight for each partition, and the weighted partition probability values.

Partition number 10 in Table 3.26 (identified with an asterisk) corresponds to the observed categorical frequencies. Table 3.27 illustrates the calculation of exact cumulative partition probability values for Fisher's exact, Pearson's chi-squared (χ^2), and Wilks' likelihood-ratio (G^2) goodness-of-fit tests. The partition probability values for Fisher's exact test are accumulated according to the magnitudes of the partition probability values. Thus, the cumulative probability value for Fisher's exact goodness-of-fit test is the sum of the partition probability values equal to or less than the observed partition probability value. The χ^2 (G^2) partition probability values are accumulated according to the magnitudes of the associated χ^2 (G^2) test statistic values. Thus, the cumulative probability value for the χ^2 (G^2) goodness-of-fit test is the sum of the partition probability values associated with the χ^2 (G^2) test statistic values equal to or greater than the observed χ^2 (G^2) test statistic value. The T^2 and $I(2/3)$ partition probability values are accumulated in like manner to the χ^2 and G^2 tests. The probability values for Fisher's exact, χ^2, and G^2 goodness-of-fit tests are indicated by asterisks in Table 3.27.

Table 3.26 Partitions, exact partition probability values, multinomial weights, and exact weighted probability values for $N = 8$ events and $k = 8$ categories

Number	Partition	Partition probability	Multinomial weight	Weighted probability
1	1 1 1 1 1 1 1 1	0.2403×10^{-2}	1	0.2403×10^{-2}
2	2 1 1 1 1 1 1 1	0.1202×10^{-2}	56	0.6729×10^{-1}
3	2 2 1 1 1 1 0 0	0.6008×10^{-3}	420	0.2523
4	2 2 2 1 1 0 0 0	0.3004×10^{-3}	560	0.1682
5	2 2 2 2 0 0 0 0	0.1502×10^{-3}	70	0.1051×10^{-1}
6	3 1 1 1 1 1 0 0	0.4005×10^{-3}	168	0.6729×10^{-1}
7	3 2 1 1 1 0 0 0	0.2003×10^{-3}	1,120	0.2243
8	3 2 2 1 0 0 0 0	0.1001×10^{-3}	840	0.8411×10^{-1}
9	3 3 1 1 0 0 0 0	0.6676×10^{-4}	420	0.2804×10^{-1}
10*	3 3 2 0 0 0 0 0	0.3338×10^{-4}	168	0.5608×10^{-2}
11	4 1 1 1 1 0 0 0	0.1001×10^{-3}	280	0.2804×10^{-1}
12	4 2 1 1 0 0 0 0	0.5007×10^{-4}	840	0.4206×10^{-1}
13	4 2 2 0 0 0 0 0	0.2503×10^{-4}	168	0.4206×10^{-2}
14	4 3 1 0 0 0 0 0	0.1669×10^{-4}	336	0.5608×10^{-2}
15	4 4 0 0 0 0 0 0	0.4172×10^{-5}	28	0.1168×10^{-3}
16	5 1 1 1 0 0 0 0	0.2003×10^{-4}	280	0.5608×10^{-2}
17	5 2 1 0 0 0 0 0	0.1001×10^{-4}	336	0.3365×10^{-2}
18	5 3 0 0 0 0 0 0	0.3338×10^{-5}	56	0.1869×10^{-3}
19	6 1 1 0 0 0 0 0	0.3338×10^{-5}	168	0.5608×10^{-3}
20	6 2 0 0 0 0 0 0	0.1669×10^{-5}	56	0.9346×10^{-4}
21	7 1 0 0 0 0 0 0	0.4768×10^{-6}	56	0.2670×10^{-4}
22	8 0 0 0 0 0 0 0	0.5960×10^{-7}	8	0.4768×10^{-6}

* The row containing the observed categorical frequencies is identified with an asterisk

Fisher's exact goodness-of-fit probability value is $P = 0.2538 \times 10^{-1}$, the observed Pearson uncorrected chi-squared test statistic is $\chi^2 = 14.00$ with an exact probability value of $P = 0.6744 \times 10^{-1}$, the observed Wilks likelihood-ratio test statistic is $G^2 = 15.96$ with an exact probability value of $P = 0.2538 \times 10^{-1}$, the observed Williams likelihood-ratio test statistic is $G^2_W = 13.44$ with an exact probability value of $P = 0.2538 \times 10^{-1}$, the observed Smith et al. likelihood-ratio test statistic is $G^2_S = 11.78$ with an exact probability value of $P = 0.2538 \times 10^{-1}$,[15] the observed Freeman–Tukey test statistic is $T^2 = 12.94$ with an exact probability value of $P = 0.1977 \times 10^{-1}$, and the observed Cressie–Read test statistic is $I(2/3) = 13.78$ with an exact probability value of 0.2538×10^{-1}.

Given the different criteria used for determining the Fisher exact, Pearson χ^2, and Wilks G^2 probability values in Table 3.27, the exact probability values for the three tests will sometimes differ, e.g., Fisher's exact test and Pearson's χ^2 on the

[15] As scalar functions of G^2, G^2_W, and G^2_S yield identical probability values to G^2.

Table 3.27 Exact probability (P) values for Fisher's exact, Pearson's chi-squared, and Wilks' likelihood-ratio tests

	Chi-squared (χ^2)		Likelihood-ratio (G^2)	
Exact P value	Statistic	P value	Statistic	P value
0.4768×10^{-6}	56.00	0.4768×10^{-6}	33.27	0.4768×10^{-6}
0.2718×10^{-4}	42.00	0.2718×10^{-4}	27.24	0.2718×10^{-4}
0.1206×10^{-3}	32.00	0.1206×10^{-3}	24.27	0.1206×10^{-3}
0.3076×10^{-3}	30.00	0.6814×10^{-3}	22.69	0.3076×10^{-3}
0.8683×10^{-3}	26.00	0.8683×10^{-3}	22.18	0.4244×10^{-3}
0.9851×10^{-3}	24.00	0.9851×10^{-3}	21.50	0.9851×10^{-3}
0.4350×10^{-2}	22.00	0.4350×10^{-2}	18.87	0.4350×10^{-2}
0.9957×10^{-2}	20.00	0.9957×10^{-2}	17.68	0.9957×10^{-2}
0.1556×10^{-1}	18.00	0.1556×10^{-1}	16.64	0.1416×10^{-1}
0.1977×10^{-1}	16.00	0.1977×10^{-1}	16.09	0.1977×10^{-1}
$0.2538\times10^{-1}*$	14.00	0.2538×10^{-1}	15.96	$0.2538\times10^{-1}*$
0.6744×10^{-1}	14.00	$0.6744\times10^{-1}*$	13.86	0.6744×10^{-1}
0.9547×10^{-1}	12.00	0.9547×10^{-1}	13.18	0.9547×10^{-1}
0.1796	12.00	0.1235	12.14	0.1796
0.2076	10.00	0.2076	11.09	0.2076
0.2181	8.00	0.2181	11.09	0.2181
0.4424	8.00	0.4424	9.36	0.4424
0.6107	6.00	0.6107	8.32	0.6107
0.6780	6.00	0.6780	6.59	0.6780
0.9303	4.00	0.9303	5.55	0.9303
0.9976	2.00	0.9976	2.77	0.9976
1.0000	0.00	1.0000	0.00	1.0000

$*$ Observed probability values are identified with asterisks

one hand and Pearson's χ^2 and Wilks' G^2 on the other hand, and sometimes agree, e.g., Fisher's exact test and Wilks' G^2. While exact and resampling-approximation probability values are the *sine qua non* for statistical inference in this book, it is sometimes informative to compare exact probability values with asymptotic probability values, which are more common in the literature. Table 3.28 lists the exact and asymptotic probability values for the Fisher exact, Pearson χ^2, Wilks G^2, Williams G^2_W, Smith et al. G^2_S, Freeman–Tukey T^2, and Cressie–Read $I(2/3)$ test statistics.

Example 1 illustrates the analysis of data with $N = 8$ observations in $k = 8$ unordered equiprobable categories; thus, the expected value for each category is $E_i = N/k = 8/8 = 1.00$ for $i = 1, \ldots, 8$. As can be seen in Table 3.28, Fisher's exact, G^2, G^2_W, G^2_S, and $I(2/3)$ yield identical exact probability values of $P = 0.2538\times10^{-1}$, while the uncorrected χ^2 exact probability value is substantially larger at $P = 0.6744\times10^{-1}$. In contrast, the exact probability value for T^2 is considerably lower at $P = 0.1977\times10^{-1}$. In contrast, the asymptotic

Table 3.28 Test statistics, exact probability values, and asymptotic probability values for the Fisher exact, Pearson χ^2, Wilks G^2, Williams G^2_W, Smith et al. G^2_S, Freeman–Tukey T^2, and Cressie–Read $I(2/3)$ tests for Example 1

Test	Statistic	Probability	
		Exact	Asymptotic
Fisher exact test	–	0.2538×10^{-1}	–
Pearson χ^2	14.00	0.6744×10^{-1}	0.5118×10^{-1}
Wilks G^2	15.96	0.2538×10^{-1}	0.2552×10^{-1}
Williams G^2_W	13.44	0.2538×10^{-1}	0.6216×10^{-1}
Smith et al. G^2_S	11.78	0.2538×10^{-1}	0.1078
Freeman–Tukey T^2	12.94	0.1977×10^{-1}	0.7349×10^{-1}
Cressie–Read $I(2/3)$	13.78	0.2538×10^{-1}	0.5524×10^{-1}

probability values for χ^2 and G^2 are good approximations to the corresponding exact probability values, while the asymptotic probability values for G^2_W and G^2_S provide increasingly conservative estimates of the corresponding exact probability values. The asymptotic probability values for both T^2 and $I(2/3)$ are much too conservative with asymptotic probability values of $P = 0.7349\times10^{-1}$ and $P = 0.5524\times10^{-1}$, respectively.

Example 2

This second example illustrates the application of goodness-of-fit tests when $N > k$. Consider $N = 45$ patients with a history of substance abuse classified into $k = 20$ substance types, with categorical frequencies $O_1 = O_2 = O_3 = 6$, $O_4 = 5$, $O_5 = 4$, $O_6 = 3$, $O_7 = 2$, and $O_8 = \cdots = O_{20} = 1$. For this second example, only 81,801 of the $p(45) = 89{,}134$ partitions are relevant to the analysis as it is not possible to distribute all $N = 45$ events into the $k = 20$ categories and have all categories contain two or fewer observations. The null hypothesis specifies that the k expected category probabilities are equally likely, i.e., $p_i = 1/k = 1/20 = 0.05$ for $i = 1, \ldots, 20$.

Fisher's exact goodness-of-fit probability value is $P = 0.6927\times10^{-1}$, the observed Pearson uncorrected chi-squared test statistic is $\chi^2 = 32.78$ with an exact probability value of $P = 0.2864\times10^{-1}$, the observed Wilks likelihood-ratio test statistic is $G^2 = 28.07$ with an exact probability value of $P = 0.1667$, the observed Williams likelihood-ratio test statistic is $G^2_W = 26.04$ with an exact probability value of $P = 0.1289$, the observed Smith et al. likelihood-ratio test statistic is $G^2_S = 25.27$ with an exact probability value of $P = 0.1667$, the observed Freeman–Tukey test statistic is $T^2 = 22.28$ with an exact probability value of $P = 0.3579$, and the observed Cressie–Read test statistic is $I(2/3) = 30.70$ with an exact probability value of $P = 0.3701\times10^{-1}$. Table 3.29 lists the exact and asymptotic

Table 3.29 Test statistics, exact probability values, and asymptotic probability values for the Fisher exact, Pearson χ^2, Wilks G^2, Williams G^2_W, Smith et al. G^2_S, Freeman–Tukey T^2, and Cressie–Read $I(2/3)$ tests for Example 2

		Probability	
Test	Statistic	Exact	Asymptotic
Fisher exact test	–	0.6927×10^{-1}	–
Pearson χ^2	32.78	0.2864×10^{-1}	0.2550×10^{-1}
Wilks G^2	28.07	0.1667	0.8212×10^{-1}
Williams G^2_W	26.04	0.1667	0.1290
Smith et al. G^2_S	25.27	0.1667	0.1518
Freeman–Tukey T^2	22.28	0.3579	0.2704
Cressie–Read $I(2/3)$	30.70	0.3701×10^{-1}	0.4359×10^{-1}

probability values for the Fisher exact, Pearson χ^2, Wilks G^2, Williams G^2_W, Smith et al. G^2_S, Freeman–Tukey T^2, and Cressie–Read $I(2/3)$ test statistics.

Example 2 illustrates the analysis of data with $N = 45$ observations in $k = 20$ unordered equiprobable categories; thus, the expected value for each category is $E_i = N/k = 45/20 = 2.25$ for $i = 1, \ldots, 20$. As can be seen in Table 3.29, G^2, G^2_W, G^2_S, and T^2 all yield very conservative exact probability values. In comparison, the asymptotic probability values for χ^2 and $I(2/3)$ are good approximations to the corresponding exact probability values, while the asymptotic probability values for G^2, G^2_W, and T^2 provide poor approximations to the corresponding exact probability values. On the other hand, the asymptotic probability value for G^2_S of $P = 0.1518$ is a good approximation to the exact G^2_S probability value of $P = 0.1667$. As in Example 1, the asymptotic probability values for G^2_W and G^2_S result in pronounced increases over the value for G^2 with the added corrections of Williams [103] and Smith et al. [88].

Example 3

This third example illustrates the application of goodness-of-fit tests when $N < k$. Consider that a patient is asked to check any of $k = 50$ symptoms experienced in the past six months, resulting in $N = 10$ selections for categorical frequencies of $O_1 = 4$, $O_2 = 3$, $O_3 = 2$, $O_4 = 1$, and $O_5 = \cdots = O_{50} = 0$. In this example, all of the $p(10) = 42$ partitions are relevant to the analysis, given that $N < k$. The null hypothesis specifies that the k expected category probabilities are equally likely, i.e., $p_i = 1/k = 1/50 = 0.02$ for $i = 1, \ldots, 50$.

Fisher's exact probability value is 0.1795×10^{-5}, the observed Pearson uncorrected chi-squared test statistic is $\chi^2 = 140.00$ with an exact probability value of $P = 0.3788\times10^{-4}$, the observed Wilks likelihood-ratio test statistic is $G^2 = 52.64$ with an exact probability value of $P = 0.1795\times10^{-5}$, the observed Williams likelihood-ratio test statistic is $G^2_W = 28.46$ with an exact probability value

Table 3.30 Test statistics, exact probability values, and asymptotic probability values for the Fisher exact, Pearson χ^2, Wilks G^2, Williams G_W^2, Smith et al. G_S^2, Freeman–Tukey T^2, and Cressie–Read $I(2/3)$ tests for Example 3

		Probability	
Test	Statistic	Exact	Asymptotic
Fisher exact test	–	0.1795×10^{-5}	–
Pearson χ^2	140.00	0.3788×10^{-4}	0.1077×10^{-9}
Wilks G^2	52.64	0.1795×10^{-5}	0.3351
Williams G_W^2	28.46	0.1795×10^{-5}	0.9917
Smith et al. G_S^2	8.75	0.1795×10^{-5}	1.0000
Freeman–Tukey T^2	23.87	0.1795×10^{-5}	0.9991
Cressie–Read $I(2/3)$	89.87	0.8356×10^{-5}	0.3339×10^{-3}

of $P = 0.1795\times10^{-5}$, the observed Smith et al. likelihood-ratio test statistic is $G_S^2 = 8.75$ with an exact probability value of 0.1795×10^{-5}, the observed Freeman–Tukey test statistic is $T^2 = 23.87$ with an exact probability value of $P = 0.1795\times10^{-5}$, and the observed Cressie–Read test statistic is $I(2/3) = 89.87$ with an exact probability value of $P = 0.8356\times10^{-5}$. Table 3.30 lists the exact and asymptotic probability values for the Fisher exact, Pearson χ^2, Wilks G^2, Williams G_W^2, Smith et al. G_S^2, Freeman–Tukey T^2, and Cressie–Read $I(2/3)$ test statistics.

Example 3 illustrates the analysis of very sparse data with $N = 10$ observations in $k = 50$ unordered equiprobable categories; thus, the expected value for each category is only $E_i = N/k = 10/50 = 0.20$ for $i = 1, \ldots, 50$. As can be seen in Table 3.30, Fisher's exact test, G^2, G_W^2, G_S^2, and T^2 yield identical exact probability values of $P = 0.1795\times10^{-5}$ and the exact probability values for χ^2 and $I(2/3)$ are not far removed at $P = 0.3788\times10^{-4}$ and $P = 0.8356\times10^{-5}$, respectively. On the other hand, the asymptotic probability values range from $P = 0.1077\times10^{-9}$ for χ^2 to $P = 1.0000$ for G_S^2. The asymptotic probability value for $I(2/3)$ of $P = 0.3339\times10^{-3}$ is the only asymptotic probability value that even remotely approximates the corresponding exact probability value of $P = 0.8356\times10^{-5}$.

In general, asymptotic goodness-of-fit probability values are heavily influenced by small sample sizes leading to sparse tables with low expected values. As is evident in Example 3, asymptotic probability values are of little use for very sparse tables. Moreover, asymptotic probability values provide conservative estimates of the corresponding exact probability values in some cases, and in other cases, liberal estimates. As asymptotic goodness-of-fit probability values are neither dependable nor reliable for sparse tables, exact probability values are recommended. Other things being equal, Fisher's exact test is probably the best choice of the exact tests since the probability value is based solely on the underlying exact probability structure.

3.7.4 Computational Efficiency

The use of a partition algorithmic procedure based on $p(N)$ with equal category probabilities is highly efficient when compared with the calculation of test statistic values based on all M possible configurations. Table 3.31 compares the $p(N)$ partitions with the M possible configurations for $1 \leq N = k \leq 20$. For example, with $N = 15$ observations in $k = 15$ categories, there are only $p(15) = 176$ partitions, but

$$M = \binom{N+k-1}{k-1} = \binom{15+15-1}{15-1} = \binom{29}{14} = 77{,}558{,}760$$

total configurations to be analyzed. When k is much larger than N, the efficiency of the partition procedure is increased.

Table 3.31 Comparison of $p(N)$ partitions and M configurations when $1 \leq N = k \leq 20$

N	$p(N)$	M
1	1	1
2	2	3
3	3	10
4	5	35
5	7	126
6	11	462
7	15	1,716
8	22	6,435
9	30	24,310
10	42	92,378
11	56	352,716
12	77	1,352,078
13	101	5,200,300
14	135	20,058,300
15	176	77,558,760
16	231	300,540,195
17	297	1,166,803,110
18	385	4,537,567,650
19	490	17,672,631,900
20	627	68,923,264,410

3.8 Chi-squared and Correlation for $r \times c$ Tables

Although the relationship between Pearson's chi-squared and the Pearson product-moment correlation coefficient is well known and easily demonstrated for a 2×2 contingency table with dummy coding as shown in Sect. 3.1, that is,

$$r_{xy}^2 = \frac{\chi^2}{N} \quad \text{and} \quad \chi^2 = Nr_{xy}^2 \ ,$$

it is not widely recognized that Pearson's chi-squared test statistic and Pearson's product-moment correlation coefficient are also related for larger contingency tables. In an appendix to his 1988 textbook titled simply *Statistics*, psychologist William Hays provided an excellent presentation of the Gram–Schmidt orthonormalization technique, on which this discussion is primarily based [53, pp. 890–895]. See also a 2000 article by Dunlap, Brody, and Greer [39]. An advantage of the Gram–Schmidt orthonormalization algorithm is that it guarantees the existence of an orthonormal basis for any inner-product space.

The Gram–Schmidt orthonormalization process requires an initial set of vectors, $\mathbf{X}$, which includes the unit vector $\mathbf{x}_0$, i.e., $\mathbf{x}_0' = [1 \ 1 \ 1 \cdots]$. Choose vector $\mathbf{x}_0$ to serve as an initial vector, $\mathbf{v}_0$, in the set $\mathbf{V}$. Then, vector $\mathbf{v}_1$ is given by:

$$\mathbf{v}_1 = \mathbf{x}_1 - b_{1,0}\mathbf{v}_0 \ ,$$

where

$$b_{1,0} = \frac{(\mathbf{x}_1, \mathbf{v}_0)}{\|\mathbf{v}_0\|^2} \ ,$$

$(\mathbf{x}_1, \mathbf{v}_0)$ is the Euclidean inner product (dot product) of vectors $\mathbf{x}_1$ and $\mathbf{v}_0$, and $\|\mathbf{v}_0\|^2$ is the inner product of vector $\mathbf{v}_0$ with itself. Vector $\mathbf{v}_1$ is now orthogonal to the unit vector $\mathbf{v}_0$, i.e., the correlation between vectors $\mathbf{v}_0$ and $\mathbf{v}_1$ is zero, within rounding error. Now, consider vector $\mathbf{x}_2$ in $\mathbf{X}$ and find vector $\mathbf{v}_2$ given by:

$$\mathbf{v}_2 = \mathbf{x}_2 - b_{2,0}\mathbf{v}_0 - b_{2,1}\mathbf{v}_1 \ ,$$

where

$$b_{2,0} = \frac{(\mathbf{x}_2, \mathbf{v}_0)}{\|\mathbf{v}_0\|^2} \ , \quad b_{2,1} = \frac{(\mathbf{x}_2, \mathbf{v}_1)}{\|\mathbf{v}_1\|^2} \ ,$$

$(\mathbf{x}_2, \mathbf{v}_0)$ is the inner product of vectors $\mathbf{x}_2$ and $\mathbf{v}_0$, $\|\mathbf{v}_0\|^2$ is the inner product of vector $\mathbf{v}_0$ with itself, $(\mathbf{x}_2, \mathbf{v}_1)$ is the inner product of vectors $\mathbf{x}_2$ and $\mathbf{v}_1$, and $\|\mathbf{v}_1\|^2$ is the inner product of vector $\mathbf{v}_1$ with itself. Vector $\mathbf{v}_2$ is orthogonal to vectors $\mathbf{v}_0$ and $\mathbf{v}_1$, i.e., the inter-correlations among vectors $\mathbf{v}_0$, $\mathbf{v}_1$, and $\mathbf{v}_2$ are zero, within rounding error.

Vector $\mathbf{v}_3$ is given by:

$$\mathbf{v}_3 = \mathbf{x}_3 - b_{3,0}\mathbf{v}_0 - b_{3,1}\mathbf{v}_1 - b_{3,2}\mathbf{v}_2 ,$$

where

$$b_{3,0} = \frac{(\mathbf{x}_3, \mathbf{v}_0)}{\|\mathbf{v}_0\|^2} , \quad b_{3,1} = \frac{(\mathbf{x}_3, \mathbf{v}_1)}{\|\mathbf{v}_1\|^2} , \quad b_{3,2} = \frac{(\mathbf{x}_3, \mathbf{v}_2)}{\|\mathbf{v}_2\|^2} ,$$

$(\mathbf{x}_3, \mathbf{v}_0)$ is the inner product of vectors $\mathbf{x}_3$ and $\mathbf{v}_0$, $\|\mathbf{v}_0\|^2$ is the inner product of vector $\mathbf{v}_0$ with itself, $(\mathbf{x}_3, \mathbf{v}_1)$ is the inner product of vectors $\mathbf{x}_3$ and $\mathbf{v}_1$, $\|\mathbf{v}_1\|^2$ is the inner product of vector $\mathbf{v}_1$ with itself, $(\mathbf{x}_3, \mathbf{v}_2)$ is the inner product of vectors $\mathbf{x}_3$ and $\mathbf{v}_2$, and $\|\mathbf{v}_2\|^2$ is the inner product of vector $\mathbf{v}_2$ with itself. Vector $\mathbf{v}_3$ is orthogonal to vectors $\mathbf{v}_0$, $\mathbf{v}_1$, and $\mathbf{v}_2$, i.e., the inter-correlations among vectors $\mathbf{v}_0$, $\mathbf{v}_1$, $\mathbf{v}_2$, and $\mathbf{v}_3$ are zero, within rounding error. The process continues until all vectors in $\mathbf{X}$ have been used or until each additional vector in $\mathbf{X}$ yields a $\mathbf{v}$ vector consisting of all zeroes.

The standard deviation of each row vector is given by:

$$S_v = \left(\frac{1}{N} \sum_{i=1}^{r} n_i v_i^2 \right)^{1/2} ,$$

where v_i is the ith element in vector $\mathbf{v}$ for $v = 1, \ldots, r-1$. Next, compute the values for the orthonormal row weights given by:

$$\mathbf{c}_i = \frac{1}{S_v}\mathbf{v}_i$$

for $i = 1, \ldots, r-1$. The purpose is to standardize the $\mathbf{c}_i$ vectors, $i = 1, \ldots, r-1$, so that the variances of the $r-1$ $\mathbf{c}_i$ values will be 1.00 and any pair of $\mathbf{c}$ vectors will have a product-moment correlation coefficient of 0.00.

The process is repeated for columns with

$$S_v = \left(\frac{1}{N} \sum_{j=1}^{c} n_i v_j^2 \right)^{1/2}$$

for $v = 1, \ldots, c-1$ and the values for the orthonormal column weights are given by:

$$\mathbf{d}_j = \frac{1}{S_v}\mathbf{v}_j$$

for $j = 1, \ldots, c-1$.

Table 3.32 Example $r \times c$ contingency table with $r = 4$ rows and $c = 3$ columns

	Column			
Row	1	2	3	Total
1	122	70	8	200
2	141	39	15	195
3	106	79	18	203
4	92	104	3	199
Total	461	292	44	797

3.8.1 Example Orthonormalization Analysis

To illustrate the Gram–Schmidt orthonormalization process, consider the $r \times c$ contingency table given in Table 3.32 with $r = 4$ rows and $c = 3$ columns. It is possible to code the 4×3 contingency table given in Table 3.32 with dummy variables representing row membership into new uncorrelated variables, each of which has a mean of 0.00 and a variance of 1.00. Similarly, dummy variables representing column membership can also be transformed in the same manner.

Orthonormal Row Weights

Consider the **X** matrix coded with dummy variables given by:

$$\mathbf{X} = \begin{bmatrix} 1 & 1 & 0 & 0 & 0 \\ 1 & 0 & 1 & 0 & 0 \\ 1 & 0 & 0 & 1 & 0 \\ 1 & 0 & 0 & 0 & 1 \end{bmatrix} ,$$

which is then divided into vectors $\mathbf{x}_0, \mathbf{x}_1, \ldots, \mathbf{x}_4$:

$$\mathbf{x}_0 = \begin{bmatrix} 1 \\ 1 \\ 1 \\ 1 \end{bmatrix} , \quad \mathbf{x}_1 = \begin{bmatrix} 1 \\ 0 \\ 0 \\ 0 \end{bmatrix} , \quad \mathbf{x}_2 = \begin{bmatrix} 0 \\ 1 \\ 0 \\ 0 \end{bmatrix} , \quad \mathbf{x}_3 = \begin{bmatrix} 0 \\ 0 \\ 1 \\ 0 \end{bmatrix} , \quad \mathbf{x}_4 = \begin{bmatrix} 0 \\ 0 \\ 0 \\ 1 \end{bmatrix} .$$

Choose $\mathbf{v}_0 = \mathbf{x}_0$ to serve as an initial vector and, given the observed row marginal frequency distribution in Table 3.32, {200, 195, 203, 199}, the inner product of vectors $\mathbf{x}_1$ and $\mathbf{v}_0$ is

$$(\mathbf{x}_1, \mathbf{v}_0) = (200 \times 1 \times 1) + (195 \times 1 \times 0) + (203 \times 1 \times 0) + (100 \times 1 \times 0) = 200 ,$$

the inner product of vector $\mathbf{v}_0$ with itself is

$$\|\mathbf{v}_0\|^2 = (200 \times 1 \times 1) + (195 \times 1 \times 1) + (203 \times 1 \times 1) + (199 \times 1 \times 1) = 797 ,$$

$$b_{1,0} = \frac{(\mathbf{x}_1, \mathbf{v}_0)}{\|\mathbf{v}_0\|^2} = \frac{200}{797} ,$$

and vector $\mathbf{v}_1$ is

$$\mathbf{v}_1 = \mathbf{x}_1 - b_{1,0}\mathbf{v}_0 = \begin{bmatrix} 1 \\ 0 \\ 0 \\ 0 \end{bmatrix} - \frac{200}{797} \begin{bmatrix} 1 \\ 1 \\ 1 \\ 1 \end{bmatrix} = \begin{bmatrix} +0.749059 \\ -0.250941 \\ -0.250941 \\ -0.250941 \end{bmatrix} .$$

Next, consider vector $\mathbf{x}_2$ where

$$\mathbf{x}_2 = \begin{bmatrix} 0 \\ 1 \\ 0 \\ 0 \end{bmatrix} .$$

The inner product of vectors $\mathbf{x}_2$ and $\mathbf{v}_0$ is

$$(\mathbf{x}_2, \mathbf{v}_0) = (200 \times 1 \times 0) + (195 \times 1 \times 1) + (203 \times 1 \times 0) + (199 \times 1 \times 0) = 195 ,$$

the inner product of vectors $\mathbf{x}_2$ and $\mathbf{v}_1$ is

$$(\mathbf{x}_2, \mathbf{v}_1) = [200 \times 0 \times (+0.749059)] + [195 \times 1 \times (-0.250941)] + [203 \times 0 \times (-0.250941)] + [199 \times 0 \times (-0.250941)] = -48.933501 ,$$

the inner product of vector $\mathbf{v}_1$ with itself is

$$\|\mathbf{v}_1\|^2 = [200 \times (+0.749059)^2] + [195 \times (-0.250941)^2] + [203 \times (-0.250941)^2] + [199 \times (-0.250941)^2] = 149.811794 ,$$

$$b_{2,0} = \frac{(\mathbf{x}_2, \mathbf{v}_0)}{\|\mathbf{v}_0\|^2} = \frac{195}{797}, \quad \text{and} \quad b_{2,1} = \frac{(\mathbf{x}_2, \mathbf{v}_1)}{\|\mathbf{v}_1\|^2} = \frac{-48.933501}{149.811794} .$$

Then, vector $\mathbf{v}_2$ is

$$\mathbf{v}_2 = \mathbf{x}_2 - b_{2,0}\mathbf{v}_0 - b_{2,1}\mathbf{v}_1 = \begin{bmatrix} 0 \\ 1 \\ 0 \\ 0 \end{bmatrix} - \frac{195}{797} \begin{bmatrix} 1 \\ 1 \\ 1 \\ 1 \end{bmatrix}$$

$$- \frac{-48.933501}{149.811794} \begin{bmatrix} +0.749059 \\ -0.250941 \\ -0.250941 \\ -0.250941 \end{bmatrix} = \begin{bmatrix} 0.000000 \\ +0.673367 \\ -0.326633 \\ -0.326633 \end{bmatrix} .$$

Next, consider vector $\mathbf{x}_3$ where

$$\mathbf{x}_3 = \begin{bmatrix} 0 \\ 0 \\ 1 \\ 0 \end{bmatrix} .$$

The inner product of vectors $\mathbf{x}_3$ and $\mathbf{v}_0$ is

$$(\mathbf{x}_3, \mathbf{v}_0) = (200 \times 1 \times 0) + (195 \times 1 \times 0) + (203 \times 1 \times 1) + (199 \times 1 \times 0) = 203 ,$$

the inner product of vectors $\mathbf{x}_3$ and $\mathbf{v}_1$ is

$$(\mathbf{x}_3, \mathbf{v}_1) = [200 \times 0 \times (+0.749059)] + [195 \times 0 \times (-0.250941)] + [203 \times 1 \times (-0.250941)] + [199 \times 0 \times (-0.250941)] = -50.941029 ,$$

the inner product of vectors $\mathbf{x}_3$ and $\mathbf{v}_2$ is

$$(\mathbf{x}_3, \mathbf{v}_2) = (200 \times 0 \times 0) + [195 \times 0 \times (+0.673367)] + [203 \times 1 \times (-0.327733)] + [199 \times 0 \times (-0.326633)] = -66.306499 ,$$

the inner product of vector $\mathbf{v}_2$ with itself is

$$\|\mathbf{v}_2\|^2 = (200 \times 0) + [195 \times (+0.673367)^2] + [203 \times (-0.326633)^2] + [199 \times (-0.326633)^2] = 131.306533 ,$$

$$b_{3,0} = \frac{(\mathbf{x}_3, \mathbf{v}_0)}{\|\mathbf{v}_0\|^2} = \frac{203}{797}, \quad b_{3,1} = \frac{(\mathbf{x}_3, \mathbf{v}_1)}{\|\mathbf{v}_1\|^2} = \frac{-50.941029}{149.811794},$$

and

$$b_{3,2} = \frac{(\mathbf{x}_3, \mathbf{v}_2)}{\|\mathbf{v}_2\|^2} = \frac{-66.306499}{131.306533} \ .$$

Then, vector $\mathbf{v}_3$ is

$$\mathbf{v}_3 = \mathbf{x}_3 - b_{3,0}\mathbf{v}_0 - b_{3,1}\mathbf{v}_1 - b_{3,2}\mathbf{v}_2 = \begin{bmatrix} 0 \\ 0 \\ 1 \\ 0 \end{bmatrix} - \frac{203}{797} \begin{bmatrix} 1 \\ 1 \\ 1 \\ 1 \end{bmatrix}$$

$$- \frac{-50.941029}{149.811794} \begin{bmatrix} +0.749059 \\ -0.250941 \\ -0.250941 \\ -0.250941 \end{bmatrix} - \frac{-66.306499}{131.306533} \begin{bmatrix} 0.000000 \\ +0.673367 \\ -0.326633 \\ -0.326633 \end{bmatrix}$$

$$= \begin{bmatrix} 0.000000 \\ 0.000000 \\ +0.495025 \\ -0.504975 \end{bmatrix} .$$

The standard deviations of the row vectors are given by:

$$S_v = \left(\frac{1}{N} \sum_{i=1}^{r} n_i v_i^2 \right)^{1/2} .$$

for $v = 1, \ldots, r - 1$. Thus,

$$S_1 = \left\{ \frac{1}{797} \Big[(200)(+0.749059)^2 + (195)(-0.250941)^2 + (203)(-0.250941)^2 + (199)(-0.250941)^2 \Big] \right\}^{1/2} = 0.433555 \ ,$$

$$S_2 = \left\{ \frac{1}{797} \Big[(200)(0)^2 + (195)(-0.673367)^2 + (203)(-0.326633)^2 + (199)(-0.326633)^2 \Big] \right\}^{1/2} = 0.405895 \ ,$$

and

$$S_3 = \left\{ \frac{1}{797} \Big[(200)(0)^2 + (195)(0)^2 + (203)(-0.495025)^2 + (199)(-0.504975)^2 \Big] \right\}^{1/2} = 0.355085 \; .$$

The standard deviations of the row vectors, S_1, S_2, and S_3, are used to calculate the orthonormal row weights, $\mathbf{c}_1$, $\mathbf{c}_2$, and $\mathbf{c}_3$, where

$$\mathbf{c}_1 = \frac{1}{S_1}\mathbf{v}_1 = \frac{1}{0.433555}\begin{bmatrix} +0.749059 \\ -0.250941 \\ -0.250941 \\ -0.250941 \end{bmatrix} = \begin{bmatrix} +1.727715 \\ -0.578799 \\ -0.578799 \\ -0.578799 \end{bmatrix} ,$$

$$\mathbf{c}_2 = \frac{1}{S_2}\mathbf{v}_2 = \frac{1}{0.405895}\begin{bmatrix} 0 \\ +0.673367 \\ -0.326633 \\ -0.326633 \end{bmatrix} = \begin{bmatrix} 0.000000 \\ +1.658967 \\ -0.804723 \\ -0.804723 \end{bmatrix} ,$$

and

$$\mathbf{c}_3 = \frac{1}{S_3}\mathbf{v}_3 = \frac{1}{0.355085}\begin{bmatrix} 0.000000 \\ 0.000000 \\ +0.495025 \\ -1.422124 \end{bmatrix} = \begin{bmatrix} 0.000000 \\ 0.000000 \\ +1.394102 \\ -1.422124 \end{bmatrix} .$$

Orthonormal Column Weights

In a similar fashion, the orthonormal weights are calculated for the columns of data given in Table 3.32, where there are only $c = 3$ columns and, thus, only $c - 1 = 2$ orthonormal column weights to be determined. Consider Table 3.32 on p. 118, replicated in Table 3.33 for convenience. The $\mathbf{X}$ matrix for columns, coded with dummy variables, is given by:

$$\mathbf{X} = \begin{bmatrix} 1 & 1 & 0 & 0 \\ 1 & 0 & 1 & 0 \\ 1 & 0 & 0 & 1 \end{bmatrix}$$

Table 3.33 Example $r \times c$ contingency table with $r = 4$ rows and $c = 3$ columns

Row	Column 1	2	3	Total
1	122	70	8	200
2	141	39	15	195
3	106	79	18	203
4	92	104	3	199
Total	461	292	44	797

then divided into vectors $\mathbf{x}_0$, $\mathbf{x}_1$, $\mathbf{x}_2$, and $\mathbf{x}_3$:

$$\mathbf{x}_0 = \begin{bmatrix} 1 \\ 1 \\ 1 \end{bmatrix}, \quad \mathbf{x}_1 = \begin{bmatrix} 1 \\ 0 \\ 0 \end{bmatrix}, \quad \mathbf{x}_2 = \begin{bmatrix} 0 \\ 1 \\ 0 \end{bmatrix}, \quad \mathbf{x}_3 = \begin{bmatrix} 0 \\ 0 \\ 1 \end{bmatrix}.$$

The unit vector $\mathbf{v}_0$ is

$$\mathbf{v}_0 = \mathbf{x}_0 = \begin{bmatrix} 1 \\ 1 \\ 1 \end{bmatrix}$$

and given the observed column marginal frequency distribution $\{461, 292, 44\}$, the inner product of vectors $\mathbf{x}_1$ and $\mathbf{v}_0$ is

$$(\mathbf{x}_1, \mathbf{v}_0) = (461 \times 1 \times 1) + (292 \times 1 \times 0) + (44 \times 1 \times 0) = 461 ,$$

the inner product of vector $\mathbf{v}_0$ with itself is

$$\|\mathbf{v}_0\|^2 = (461 \times 1 \times 1) + (292 \times 1 \times 1) + (44 \times 1 \times 1) = 797 ,$$

$$b_{1,0} = \frac{(\mathbf{x}_0, \mathbf{v}_0)}{\|\mathbf{v}_0\|^2} = \frac{461}{797} ,$$

and vector $\mathbf{v}_1$ is

$$\mathbf{v}_1 = \mathbf{x}_1 - b_{1,0}\mathbf{v}_0 = \begin{bmatrix} 1 \\ 0 \\ 0 \end{bmatrix} - \frac{461}{797} \begin{bmatrix} 1 \\ 1 \\ 1 \end{bmatrix} = \begin{bmatrix} +0.421581 \\ -0.578419 \\ -0.578419 \end{bmatrix} .$$

Next, consider vector $\mathbf{x}_2$ where

$$\mathbf{x}_2 = \begin{bmatrix} 0 \\ 1 \\ 0 \end{bmatrix} .$$

The inner product of vectors $\mathbf{x}_2$ and $\mathbf{v}_0$ is

$$(\mathbf{x}_2, \mathbf{v}_0) = (461 \times 1 \times 0) + (292 \times 1 \times 1) + (44 \times 1 \times 0) = 292 ,$$

the inner product of vectors $\mathbf{x}_2$ and $\mathbf{v}_1$ is

$$(\mathbf{x}_2, \mathbf{v}_1) = [461 \times 0 \times (+0.421581)] + [292 \times 1 \times (-0.578410)] + [44 \times 0 \times (-0.578419)] = 168.898369 ,$$

the inner product of vector $\mathbf{v}_1$ with itself is

$$\|\mathbf{v}_1\|^2 = \left[461 \times (+0.421581)^2\right] + \left[292 \times (-0.578419)^2\right] + \left[44 \times (-0.578419)^2\right] = 194.348808 ,$$

$$b_{2,0} = \frac{(\mathbf{x}_2, \mathbf{v}_0)}{\|\mathbf{v}_0\|^2} = \frac{292}{797}, \quad \text{and} \quad b_{2,1} = \frac{(\mathbf{x}_2, \mathbf{v}_1)}{\|\mathbf{v}_1\|^2} = \frac{168.898369}{194.348808} .$$

Then, vector $\mathbf{v}_2$ is

$$\mathbf{v}_2 = \mathbf{x}_2 - b_{2,0}\mathbf{v}_0 - b_{2,1}\mathbf{v}_1 = \begin{bmatrix} 0 \\ 1 \\ 0 \end{bmatrix} - \frac{292}{797}\begin{bmatrix} 1 \\ 1 \\ 1 \end{bmatrix} - \frac{168.898369}{194.348808}\begin{bmatrix} +0.421581 \\ -0.578419 \\ -0.578419 \end{bmatrix} = \begin{bmatrix} 0 \\ +0.131952 \\ -0.869048 \end{bmatrix} .$$

The standard deviations of the column vectors are given by:

$$S_v = \left(\frac{1}{N}\sum_{j=1}^{c} n_j v_j^2\right)^{1/2}$$

for $v = 1, \ldots, c-1$. Thus,

$$S_1 = \left\{\frac{1}{797}\left[(461)(+0.421581)^2 + (292)(-0.578419)^2 + (44)(-0.578491)^2\right]\right\}^{1/2} = 0.493812$$

and

$$S_2 = \left\{ \frac{1}{797} \Big[(461)(0)^2 + (292)(-0.130952)^2 + (44)(-0.869048)^2 \Big] \right\}^{1/2} = 0.219038 \; .$$

The standard deviations of the column vectors, S_1 and S_2, are used to calculate the orthonormal column weights, $\mathbf{d}_1$ and $\mathbf{d}_2$, where

$$\mathbf{d}_1 = \frac{1}{S_1}\mathbf{v}_1 = \frac{1}{0.493812}\begin{bmatrix} +0.421581 \\ -0.578419 \\ -0.578419 \end{bmatrix} = \begin{bmatrix} +0.853727 \\ -1.171334 \\ -1.171334 \end{bmatrix}$$

and

$$\mathbf{d}_2 = \frac{1}{S_2}\mathbf{v}_2 = \frac{1}{0.219038}\begin{bmatrix} 0.000000 \\ +0.130952 \\ -0.869048 \end{bmatrix} = \begin{bmatrix} 0.000000 \\ +0.597853 \\ -3.967570 \end{bmatrix} .$$

The $\mathbf{c}_1$, $\mathbf{c}_2$, and $\mathbf{c}_3$ orthonormal row weights and the $\mathbf{d}_1$ and $\mathbf{d}_2$ orthonormal column weights are thus

$$\mathbf{c}_1 = \begin{bmatrix} +1.727715 \\ -0.578799 \\ -0.578799 \\ -0.578799 \end{bmatrix} , \quad \mathbf{c}_2 = \begin{bmatrix} 0.000000 \\ +1.658967 \\ -0.804723 \\ -0.804723 \end{bmatrix} , \quad \mathbf{c}_3 = \begin{bmatrix} 0.000000 \\ 0.000000 \\ +1.394102 \\ -1.422124 \end{bmatrix} ,$$

$$\mathbf{d}_1 = \begin{bmatrix} +0.853727 \\ -1.171334 \\ -1.171334 \end{bmatrix} , \quad \text{and} \quad \mathbf{d}_2 = \begin{bmatrix} 0.000000 \\ +0.597853 \\ -3.967570 \end{bmatrix} .$$

Correlation and Chi-squared

The orthonormal row and column weights can be arranged into an inter-correlation matrix in which the entries are zero-order correlation coefficients, as given in Table 3.34. For example, the zero-order correlation between the values for c_1 and d_1 is given by:

$$r_{kl} = \frac{1}{N}\sum_{i=1}^{r}\sum_{j=1}^{c} n_{ij} c_{ik} d_{jl} \; .$$

Table 3.34 Inter-correlation matrix for vectors **c** and **d**

	c_1	c_2	c_3	d_1	d_2
c_1	1	0	0	+0.037016	+0.029256
c_2		1	0	+0.189495	−0.029256
c_3			1	+0.043041	−0.132012
d_1				1	0
d_2					1

Thus,

$$\begin{aligned} r_{11} = \frac{1}{797}\big[&(122)(+1.727715)(+0.853727) + (70)(+1.727715)(-1.171334) \\ &+ (8)(+1.727715)(-1.171334) + (141)(-0.578799)(+0.853727) \\ &+ (39)(-0.578799)(-1.171334) + (15)(-0.578799)(-1.171334) \\ &+ (106)(-0.578799)(+0.853727) + (79)(-0.578799)(-1.171334) \\ &+ (18)(-0.578799)(-1.171334) + (92)(-0.578799)(+0.853727) \\ &+ (104)(-0.578799)(-1.171334) + (3)(-0.578799)(-1.171334)\big] \\ &= +0.037016\,. \end{aligned}$$

Given the zero-order correlation coefficients for vectors **c** and **d** listed in Table 3.34, the squared multiple correlation coefficient predicting d_1 from c_1, c_2, and c_3 is given by:

$$\begin{aligned} R^2_{d_1\cdot c_1,c_2,c_3} = r^2_{11} + r^2_{21} + r^2_{31} = (+0.037016)^2 \\ + (+0.189495)^2 + (+0.043041)^2 = 0.039131 \end{aligned}$$

since r_{11}, r_{21}, and r_{31} are independent, and the squared multiple correlation coefficient predicting d_2 from c_1, c_2, and c_3 is given by:

$$\begin{aligned} R^2_{d_2\cdot c_1,c_2,c_3} = r^2_{12} + r^2_{22} + r^2_{32} = (+0.029256)^2 \\ + (-0.101686)^2 + (-0.132012)^2 = 0.028623 \end{aligned}$$

since r_{12}, r_{22}, and r_{32} are independent.

Then,

$$\frac{\chi^2}{N} = R^2_{d_1\cdot c_1,c_2,c_3} + R^2_{d_2\cdot c_1,c_2,c_3} = 0.039131 + 0.028623 = 0.067754\,,$$

$$\chi^2 = N\left(R^2_{d_1\cdot c_1,c_2,c_3} + R^2_{d_2\cdot c_1,c_2,c_3}\right) = (797)(0.039131 + 0.028623) = 54.00\,,$$

and Cramér's V^2 is the average of $R^2_{d_1 \cdot c_1,c_2,c_3}$ and $R^2_{d_2 \cdot c_1,c_2,c_3}$ given by:

$$V^2 = \frac{R^2_{d_1 \cdot c_1,c_2,c_3} + R^2_{d_2 \cdot c_1,c_2,c_3}}{c-1} = \frac{0.039131 + 0.028623}{3-1} = 0.033877 \, .$$

In the same manner, the values of χ^2/N, χ^2, and V^2 can be obtained from the sum of the squared multiple correlation coefficients predicting rows from columns. Thus,

$$R^2_{c_1 \cdot d_1,d_2} = r^2_{11} + r^2_{12} = (+0.037016)^2 + (+0.029256)^2 = 0.002226 \, ,$$

$$R^2_{c_2 \cdot d_1,d_2} = r^2_{21} + r^2_{22} = (+0.189495)^2 + (-0.101686)^2 = 0.046248 \, ,$$

$$R^2_{c_3 \cdot d_1,d_2} = r^2_{31} + r^2_{32} = (+0.043041)^2 + (-0.132012)^2 = 0.019280 \, ,$$

$$\frac{\chi^2}{N} = R^2_{c_1 \cdot d_1,d_2} + R^2_{c_2 \cdot d_1,d_2} + R^2_{c_3 \cdot d_1,d_2} = 0.002226 + 0.046247 + 0.019280 = 0.067754 \, ,$$

$$\chi^2 = N\left(R^2_{c_1 \cdot d_1,d_2} + R^2_{c_2 \cdot d_1,d_2} + R^2_{c_3 \cdot d_1,d_2}\right) = (797)(0.002226 + 0.046247 + 0.019280) = 54.00 \, ,$$

and Cramér's V^2 is the average of $R^2_{c_1 \cdot d_1,d_2}$, $R^2_{c_2 \cdot d_1,d_2}$, and $R^2_{c_3 \cdot d_1,d_2}$ given by:

$$V^2 = \frac{R^2_{c_1 \cdot d_1,d_2} + R^2_{c_2 \cdot d_1,d_2} + R^2_{c_3 \cdot d_1,d_2}}{r-1} = \frac{0.002226 + 0.046248 + 0.019280}{4-1} = 0.033877 \, .$$

3.8.2 *Analysis with Shadow Tables*

Consider the frequency data given in the 4×3 contingency table in Table 3.33 on p. 123, but rearranged into a series of independent 2×2 contingency tables or the so-called shadow tables. Then, it can be shown that: (1) the sum of the partial chi-squared values calculated on the $(r-1)(c-1)$ possible shadow tables is equal to the chi-squared value calculated on the full $r \times c$ contingency table; (2) the

Table 3.35 Cell frequencies and orthonormal vectors representing rows and columns

			d_1'	+0.853727	−1.171334	−1.171334
c_1	c_2	c_3	d_2'	0.000000	+0.597853	−3.967570
+1.727715	0.000000	0.000000		122	70	8
−0.578799	+1.658967	0.000000		141	39	15
−0.578799	−0.804723	+1.394102		106	79	18
−0.578799	−0.804723	−1.422124		92	104	3

Table 3.36 Shadow Table $(1, 1)$ with associated c_1 and d_1' orthonormal weights

	d_1'	
c_1	+0.853727	−1.171334
+1.727715	122	78
−0.578799	339	258

sum of all the squared product-moment correlation coefficients calculated on the $(r-1)(c-1)$ shadow tables is equal to the value of chi-squared calculated on the full $r \times c$ contingency table, divided by N; and (3) the squared Cramér's coefficient V^2 is equal to the average of the squared product-moment correlation coefficients calculated on the $(r-1)(c-1)$ possible orthonormalized 2×2 shadow tables.

Table 3.35 displays the frequencies of the 4×3 contingency table in Table 3.33 on p. 123 along with the **c** and **d** orthonormal vectors representing rows and columns. Table 3.36 contains the first of the $(r-1)(c-1) = (4-1)(3-1) = 6$ possible shadow tables. Shadow Table $(1, 1)$ in Table 3.36 is constructed from the frequency data given in Table 3.35 as follows. The cell value in row 1 and column 1 of Shadow Table $(1, 1)$ in Table 3.36 containing 122 observations is simply transferred from $n_{11} = 122$ in the 4×3 contingency table in Table 3.35. The cell value in row 1 and column 2 of Shadow Table $(1, 1)$ in Table 3.36 containing 78 observations is the sum of $n_{12} = 70$ and $n_{13} = 8$ in the 4×3 contingency table in Table 3.35. The cell value in row 2 and column 1 of Shadow Table $(1, 1)$ in Table 3.36 containing 339 observations is the sum of $n_{21} = 141$, $n_{31} = 106$, and $n_{41} = 92$ in the 4×3 contingency table in Table 3.35. And, the cell value in row 2 and column 2 of Shadow Table $(1, 1)$ in Table 3.36 containing 258 observations is the sum of $n_{22} = 39$, $n_{23} = 15$, $n_{32} = 79$, $n_{33} = 18$, $n_{42} = 104$, and $n_{43} = 3$ in the 4×3 contingency table in Table 3.35.

Given

$$r_{kl} = \frac{1}{N} \sum_{i=1}^{r} \sum_{j=1}^{c} n_{ij} c_{ik} d_{jl} \ , \tag{3.9}$$

the product-moment correlation coefficient between c_1 and d_1' for Shadow Table (1, 1) in Table 3.36 is

$$r_{11} = \frac{1}{797}\big[(122)(+1.727715)(+0.853727) + (78)(+1.727715)(-1.171334) + (339)(-0.578799)(+0.853727) + (258)(-0.578799)(-1.171334)\big] = +0.037016\,,$$

and the chi-squared statistic for the frequency data given in Shadow Table (1, 1) in Table 3.36 is

$$\chi^2_{11} = Nr^2_{11} = (797)(+0.037016)^2 = 1.092044\,.$$

Alternatively, consider Shadow Table (1, 1) in Table 3.36 complete with marginal frequency totals as given in Table 3.37 and define Pearson's χ^2 in the conventional manner as:

$$\chi^2 = N\left(\sum_{i=1}^{r}\sum_{j=1}^{c}\frac{O_{ij}^2}{R_i C_j}\right) - N\,,$$

where O_{ij} denotes an observed cell frequency and R_i and C_j denote the row and column marginal frequency totals, respectively, for $i = 1, \ldots, r$ and $j = 1, \ldots, c$. Then,

$$\chi^2_{11} = 797\left[\frac{122^2}{(200)(461)} + \frac{78^2}{(200)(336)} + \frac{339^2}{(597)(461)} + \frac{258^2}{(597)(36)}\right] - 797 = (797)(1.001370) - 797 = 1.092044$$

and

$$r_{11} = \sqrt{\frac{\chi^2}{N}} = \sqrt{\frac{1.092044}{797}} = 0.037016\,.$$

Table 3.38 contains the second of six possible 2×2 shadow tables obtained from the frequency data given in Table 3.35. Shadow Table (1, 2) in Table 3.38 is constructed from the frequency data given in Table 3.35 as follows. The cell value in

Table 3.37 Shadow Table (1, 1) with cell frequencies and marginal frequency totals

	A_1	A_2	Total
B_1	122	78	200
B_2	339	258	597
Total	461	336	797

Table 3.38 Shadow Table (1, 2) with associated c_1 and d'_2 orthonormal weights

	d'_2	
c_1	+0.597853	−3.967570
+1.727715	70	8
−0.578799	222	36

row 1 and column 2 of Shadow Table (1, 2) in Table 3.38 containing 70 observations is simply transferred from $n_{12} = 70$ in the 4×3 contingency table in Table 3.35. The cell value in row 1 and column 2 of Shadow Table (1, 2) in Table 3.38 containing 8 observations is transferred from $n_{22} = 8$ in the 4×3 contingency table in Table 3.35. The cell value in row 2 and column 1 of Shadow Table (1, 2) in Table 3.38 containing 222 observations is the sum of $n_{22} = 39$, $n_{32} = 79$, and $n_{42} = 104$ in the 4×3 contingency table in Table 3.35. And, the cell value in row 2 and column 2 of Shadow Table (1, 2) in Table 3.38 containing 36 observations is the sum of $n_{23} = 15$, $n_{33} = 18$, and $n_{43} = 3$ in the 4×3 contingency table in Table 3.35.

Following Eq. (3.9) on p. 128, the product-moment correlation coefficient between c_1 and d'_2 for Shadow Table (1, 2) in Table 3.38 is

$$r_{12} = \frac{1}{797}\big[(70)(+1.727715)(+0.597853) + (8)(+1.727715)(-3.967570)$$
$$+ (222)(-0.578799)(+0.597853) + (36)(-0.578799)(-3.967570)\big]$$
$$= +0.029256\,,$$

and the chi-squared statistic for the frequency data given in Shadow Table (1, 2) in Table 3.38 is

$$\chi^2_{12} = Nr^2_{12} = (797)(+0.029256)^2 = 0.682155\,.$$

Table 3.39 contains the third of six possible 2×2 shadow tables obtained from the frequency data given in Table 3.35. Following Eq. (3.9) on p. 128, the Pearson product-moment correlation coefficient between c_2 and d'_1 for Shadow Table (2, 1) in Table 3.39 is

$$r_{21} = \frac{1}{797}\big[(141)(+1.658967)(+0.853727) + (54)(+1.658967)(-1.171334)$$
$$+ (198)(-0.804723)(+0.853727) + (204)(-0.804723)(-1.171334)\big]$$
$$= +0.189495\,,$$

Table 3.39 Shadow Table (2, 1) with associated c_2 and d'_1 orthonormal weights

	d'_1	
c_2	+0.853727	−1.171334
+1.658967	141	54
-0.804723	198	204

Table 3.40 Shadow Table (2, 2) with associated c_2 and d_2' orthonormal weights

c_2	d_2' +0.597853	−3.967570
+1.658967	39	15
-0.804723	183	21

and the chi-squared statistic for the frequency data given in Shadow Table (2, 1) in Table 3.39 is

$$\chi^2_{21} = Nr^2_{21} = (797)(+0.189495)^2 = 28.618962 .$$

Table 3.40 contains the fourth of six possible 2×2 shadow tables obtained from the frequency data given in Table 3.35. Following Eq. (3.9) on p. 128, the product-moment correlation coefficient between c_2 and d_2' for Shadow Table (2, 2) in Table 3.40 is

$$r_{22} = \frac{1}{797}\big[(39)(+1.658967)(+0.597853) + (15)(+1.658967)(-3.967570) + (183)(-0.804723)(+0.597853) + (21)(-0.804723)(-3.967570)\big] = -0.101686 ,$$

and the chi-squared statistic for the frequency data given in Shadow Table (2, 2) in Table 3.40 is

$$\chi^2_{22} = Nr^2_{22} = (797)(-0.101686)^2 = 8.241027 .$$

Table 3.41 contains the fifth of six possible 2×2 shadow tables obtained from the frequency data given in Table 3.35. Following Eq. (3.9) on p. 128, the product-moment correlation coefficient between c_3 and d_1' for Shadow Table (3, 1) in Table 3.41 is

$$r_{31} = \frac{1}{797}\big[(106)(+1.394102)(+0.853727) + (97)(+1.394102)(-1.171334) + (92)(-1.422124)(+0.853727) + (107)(-1.422124)(-1.171334)\big] = +0.043041 ,$$

Table 3.41 Shadow Table (3, 1) with associated c_3 and d_1' orthonormal weights

c_3	d_1' +0.853727	−1.171334
+1.394102	106	97
-0.422124	92	107

Table 3.42 Shadow Table (3, 2) with associated c_3 and d_2' orthonormal weights

	d_2'	
c_3	+0.597853	−3.967570
+1.394102	79	18
-0.422124	104	3

and the chi-squared statistic for the frequency data given in Shadow Table (3, 1) in Table 3.41 is

$$\chi^2_{31} = Nr^2_{31} = (797)(+0.043041)^2 = 1.476433 .$$

Table 3.42 contains the sixth of six possible 2×2 shadow tables obtained from the frequency data given in Table 3.35. Following Eq. (3.9) on p. 128, the product-moment correlation coefficient between c_3 and d_2' for Shadow Table (3, 2) in Table 3.42 is

$$r_{32} = \frac{1}{797}\big[(79)(+1.394102)(+0.597853) + (18)(+1.394102)(-3.967570)$$
$$+ (104)(-1.422124)(+0.597853) + (3)(-1.422124)(-3.967570)\big]$$
$$= -0.132012 ,$$

and the chi-squared statistic for the frequency data given in Shadow Table (3, 2) in Table 3.42 is

$$\chi^2_{32} = Nr^2_{32} = (797)(-0.132012)^2 = 13.889429 .$$

3.8.3 Summary

To summarize the Gram–Schmidt orthonormalization procedure, consider first that the sum of the partial chi-squared values calculated on the $(r-1)(c-1) = (4-1)(3-1) = 6$ shadow tables is equal to the chi-squared value computed on the full $r \times c$ contingency table. Thus,

$$\chi^2 = 1.092044 + 0.682156 + 28.618962 + 8.241027 + 1.476433$$
$$+ 13.889429 = 54.00$$

Table 3.43 Example $r \times c$ contingency table with $r = 4$ rows and $c = 3$ columns

	Column			
Row	1	2	3	Total
1	122	70	8	200
2	141	39	15	195
3	106	79	18	203
4	92	104	3	199
Total	461	292	44	797

and the chi-squared value for the full 4×3 contingency table given in Table 3.33 on p. 123, replicated in Table 3.43 for convenience, is

$$\chi^2 = N\left(\sum_{i=1}^{r}\sum_{j=1}^{c}\frac{O_{ij}^2}{R_iC_j}\right) - N$$
$$= 797\left[\frac{122}{(200)(461)} + \frac{70}{(200)(292)} + \frac{8}{(200)(44)} + \frac{141}{(195)(461)}\right.$$
$$+ \frac{39}{(195)(292)} + \frac{15}{(195)(44)} + \frac{106}{(203)(461)} + \frac{79}{(203)(292)}$$
$$\left. + \frac{18}{(203)(44)} + \frac{92}{(199)(461)} + \frac{104}{(199)(292)} + \frac{3}{(199)(44)}\right] - 797$$
$$= 54.00\,.$$

Second, the sum of all the squared correlation coefficients calculated on the $(r - 1)(c - 1) = (4 - 1)(3 - 1) = 6$ shadow tables is equal to the chi-squared value calculated on the full $r \times c$ contingency table, divided by N. Thus, since the r_{ij} values are independent for $i = 1, \ldots, r - 1$ and $j = 1, \ldots, c - 1$,

$$R^2 = \sum_{i=1}^{r-1}\sum_{j=1}^{c-1} r_{ij}^2 = (+0.037016)^2 + (+0.029256)^2 + (+0.189495)^2$$
$$+ (-0.101686)^2 + (+0.043041)^2 + (-0.132012)^2$$
$$= 0.067754$$

and

$$R^2 = \frac{\chi^2}{N} = \frac{54.00}{797} = 0.067754\,.$$

Third, Cramér's squared coefficient, V^2, is equal to the average of the squared correlation coefficients calculated on the $(r - 1)(c - 1) = (4 - 1)(3 - 1) = 6$

orthonormalized shadow tables. Let $L = \min(r-1, c-1) = \min(4-1)(3-1) = 2$ and determine the sum of the squared correlation coefficients from either

$$\sum_{i=1}^{r-1}\sum_{j=1}^{c-1} r_{ij}^2 \quad \text{or} \quad \frac{1}{N}\sum_{i=1}^{r-1}\sum_{j=1}^{c-1} \chi_{ij}^2 .$$

Thus, Cramér's V^2, the average of the $(r-1)(c-1)$ squared correlation coefficients, is given by:

$$V^2 = \frac{1}{L}\sum_{i=1}^{r-1}\sum_{j=1}^{c-1} r_{ij}^2 = \frac{1}{2}(0.067754) = 0.033877$$

or, more conventionally,

$$V^2 = \frac{1}{NL}\sum_{i=1}^{r-1}\sum_{j=1}^{c-1} \chi_{ij}^2 = \frac{1}{(797)(2)}(54.00) = 0.033877 ,$$

where r_{ij}^2 and χ_{ij}^2 are calculated on the $(r-1)(c-1)$ orthonormalized shadow tables, $i = 1, \ldots, r-1$ and $j = 1, \ldots, c-1$.

3.9 Coda

Chapter 3 considered permutation statistical methods applied to measures of association for two nominal-level variables based on Pearson's chi-squared test statistic. Included in Chap. 3 were detailed discussions of Pearson's ϕ^2, Tschuprov's T^2, Cramér's V^2, and Pearson's C. A chi-squared-based alternative was proposed that corrected the four measures and normed properly between 0 and 1. The chapter continued with a presentation of permutation-based goodness-of-fit tests including the Fisher exact probability test, the Wilks G^2 test, the Williams G_W^2 test, the Smith et al. G_S^2 test, the Freeman–Tukey T^2 test, and the Cressie–Read $I(2/3)$ test. For each test, examples illustrating the various measures and either exact or Monte Carlo resampling probability values based on the appropriate permutation analysis were provided. The chapter concluded with an oft-neglected topic: the relationship between chi-squared and Pearson's product-moment correlation for $r \times c$ contingency tables.

Chapter 4 applies exact and Monte Carlo permutation statistical methods to measures of association for two nominal-level variables that are not based on Pearson's chi-squared test statistic. Included in Chap. 4 are discussions of Goodman and Kruskal's asymmetric λ_a, λ_b, t_a, and t_b measures, Cohen's unweighted chance-corrected κ coefficient of chance-corrected inter-rater agreement, McNemar's and

Cochran's Q measures of change, Leik and Gove's d_N^c measure, Mielke and Siddiqui's exact probability for the matrix occupancy problem, and Fisher's exact probability test, extended to cover a variety of larger contingency tables.

References

1. Agresti, A.: Categorical Data Analysis. Wiley, New York (1990)
2. Agresti, A.: Categorical Data Analysis, 2nd edn. Wiley, New York (2002)
3. Agresti, A., Finlay, B.: Statistical Methods for the Social Sciences. Prentice–Hall, Upper Saddle River, NJ (1997)
4. Agresti, A., Finlay, B.: Statistical Methods for the Social Sciences, 4th edn. Pearson, Essex, UK (2009)
5. Altman, D.G., Bland, J.M.: Measurement in medicine: The analysis of method comparison studies. Statistician **32**, 307–317 (1983)
6. Bakan, D.: The test of significance in psychological research. Psychol. Bull. **66**, 423–437 (1966)
7. Bartlett, M.S.: Properties of sufficiency and statistical tests. P. Roy. Soc. Lond. A Mat. **160**, 268–282 (1937)
8. Bartlett, M.S.: Approximate confidence intervals. Biometrika **40**, 12–19 (1953)
9. Bartlett, M.S.: Approximate confidence intervals: Ii. More than one unknown parameter. Biometrika **40**, 306–317 (1953)
10. Bartlett, M.S.: A note on the multiplying factors for various χ^2 approximations. J. R. Stat. Soc. B Meth. **16**, 296–298 (1954)
11. Bartlett, M.S.: Approximate confidence intervals: Iii. A bias correction. Biometrika **42**, 201–204 (1955)
12. Bernardin, H.J., Beatty, R.W.: Performance Appraisal: Assessing Human Behavior at Work. Kent, Boston (1984)
13. Berry, K.J., Johnston, J.E., Mielke, P.W.: Exact goodness-of-fit tests for unordered equiprobable categories. Percept. Motor Skill **98**, 909–918 (2004)
14. Berry, K.J., Johnston, J.E., Mielke, P.W.: Exact and resampling probability values for measures associated with ordered R by C contingency tables. Psychol. Rep. **99**, 231–238 (2006)
15. Berry, K.J., Martin, T.W., Olson, K.F.: A note on fourfold point correlation. Educ. Psychol. Meas. **34**, 53–56 (1974)
16. Berry, K.J., Martin, T.W., Olson, K.F.: Testing theoretical hypotheses: A PRE statistic. Social Forces **53**, 190–196 (1974)
17. Bishop, Y.M., Fienberg, S.E., Holland, P.W.: Discrete Multivariate Analysis: Theory and Practice. MIT Press, Cambridge, MA (1975)
18. Blalock, H.M.: Probabilistic interpretations for the mean square contingency. J. Am. Stat. Assoc. **53**, 102–105 (1958)
19. Blalock, H.M.: Social Statistics, 2nd edn. McGraw–Hill, New York (1979)
20. Bolles, R., Messick, S.: Statistical utility in experimental inference. Psychol. Rep. **4**, 223–227 (1958)
21. Box, G.E.P.: A general distribution theory for a class of likelihood criteria. Biometrika **36**, 317–346 (1949)
22. Bradbury, I.: Analysis of variance versus randomization—A comparison. Brit. J. Math. Stat. Psy. **40**, 177–187 (1987)
23. Bradley, I.: Analysis of variance versus randomization tests—a comparison. Brit. J. Math. Stat. Psy. **40**, 177–187 (1987)
24. Bross, I.D.J.: Is there an increased risk? Fed. Proc. **13**, 815–819 (1954)
25. Brown, L., Sherbenou, R.J., Johnson, S.K.: Manual of Test of Nonverbal Intelligence, 3rd edn. PRO-ED, Austin, TX (1997)

26. Capraro, R.M., Capraro, M.M.: Treatments of effect sizes and statistical significance tests in textbooks. Educ. Psychol. Meas. **62**, 771–782 (2002)
27. Capraro, R.M., Capraro, M.M.: Exploring the APA fifth edition *Publication Manual's* impact on the analytic preferences of journal editorial board members. Educ. Psychol. Meas. **63**, 554–565 (2003)
28. Carver, R.P.: The case against statistical significance testing. Harvard Educ. Rev. **48**, 378–399 (1978)
29. Carver, R.P.: The case against statistical significance testing, revisited. J. Exp. Educ. **61**, 287–292 (1993)
30. Cohen, J.: A coefficient of agreement for nominal scales. Educ. Psychol. Meas. **20**, 37–46 (1960)
31. Cohen, J.: Statistical Power Analysis for the Behavioral Sciences, 2nd edn. Erlbaum, Hillsdale, NJ (1988)
32. Cohen, J.: Things I have learned (so far). Am. Psychol. **45**, 1304–1312 (1990)
33. Cohen, J.: The earth is round ($p < .05$). Am. Psychol. **49**, 997–1003 (1994)
34. Costner, H.L.: Criteria for measures of association. Am. Sociol. Rev. **30**, 341–353 (1965)
35. Cowles, M.: Statistics in Psychology: An Historical Perspective, 2nd edn. Lawrence Erlbaum, Mahwah, NJ (2001)
36. Cramér, H.: Mathematical Methods of Statistics. Princeton University Press, Princeton, NJ (1946)
37. Cressie, N., Read, T.R.C.: Multinomial goodness-of-fit tests. J. R. Stat. Soc. B Meth. **46**, 440–464 (1984)
38. Daniel, W.W.: Statistical significance versus practical significance. Sci. Educ. **61**, 423–427 (1977)
39. Dunlap, W.P., Brody, C.J., Greer, T.: Canonical correlation and chi-square: Relationships and interpretation. J. Gen. Psych. **127**, 341–353 (2000)
40. Euler, L.: Introduction to Analysis of the Infinite. Springer–Verlag, New York (1748/1988). [English translation by J.D. Blanton]
41. Feinstein, A.R.: Clinical Biostatistics XXIII: The role of randomization in sampling, testing, allocation, and credulous idolatry (Part 2). Clin. Pharmacol. Ther. **14**, 898–915 (1973)
42. Ferguson, G.A.: Statistical Analysis in Psychology and Education, 5th edn. McGraw–Hill, New York (1981)
43. Freeman, M.F., Tukey, J.W.: Transformations related to the angular and the square root. Ann. Math. Stat. **21**, 607–611 (1950)
44. Frick, R.W.: Interpreting statistical testing: Process and propensity, not population and random sampling. Beh. Res. Meth. Ins. C **30**, 527–535 (1998)
45. Geary, R.C.: Some properties of correlation and regression in a limited universe. Metron **7**, 83–119 (1927)
46. Gilbert, N.: Analyzing Tabular Data: Log-linear and Logistic Models for Social Researchers. UCL Press, London (1993)
47. Goodman, L.A.: The multivariate analysis of qualitative data: Interactions among multiple classifications. J. Am. Stat. Assoc. **65**, 226–256 (1970)
48. Goodman, L.A.: The analysis of multidimensional contingency tables: Stepwise procedures and direct estimation methods for building models for multiple classifications. Technometrics **13**, 33–61 (1971)
49. Guilford, J.P.: Fundamental Statistics in Psychology and Education. McGraw–Hill, New York (1950)
50. Haberman, S.J.: Analysis of Qualitative Data: Introductory Topics, vol. 1. Academic Press, New York (1978)
51. Haberman, S.J.: Analysis of Qualitative Data: New Developments, vol. 2. Academic Press, New York (1979)
52. Hardy, G.H., Ramanujan, S.: Asymptotic formulae in combinatory analysis. P. Lond. Math. Soc. **17**, 75–115 (1918)
53. Hays, W.L.: Statistics. Holt, Rinehart and Winston, New York (1963)

54. Henson, R.K., Smith, A.D.: State of the art in statistical significance and effect size reporting: A review of the APA Task Force report and current trends. J. Res. Dev. Educ. **33**, 285–296 (2000)
55. Johnston, J.E.: Amenity, community, and ranching: Rancher's beliefs, behaviors, and attitudes regarding ranching in the West. Unpublished dissertation, Colorado State University (2006)
56. Johnston, J.E., Berry, K.J., Mielke, P.W.: Permutation tests: Precision in estimating probability values. Percept. Motor Skill **105**, 915–920 (2007)
57. Kennedy, J.J.: Analyzing Qualitative Data: Introductory Log-linear Analysis for Behavioral Research. Praeger, New York (1983)
58. Keppel, G.: Design and Analysis: A Researcher's Handbook, 2nd edn. Prentice–Hall, Englewood Cliffs, NJ (1982)
59. Kirk, R.E.: Experimental Design: Procedures for the Behavioral Sciences. Brooks/Cole, Belmont, CA (1968)
60. Kirk, R.E.: Practical significance: A concept whose time has come. Educ. Psychol. Meas. **56**, 746–759 (1996)
61. Kroonenberg, P.M.: Applied Multiway Data Analysis. Wiley, Hoboken, NJ (2008)
62. LaFleur, B.J., Greevy, R.A.: Introduction to permutation and resampling-based hypothesis tests. J. Clin. Child Adolesc. **38**, 286–294 (2009)
63. Lawley, D.N.: A general method for approximating to the distribution of likelihood ratio criteria. Biometrika **43**, 295–303 (1956)
64. Leik, R.K., Gove, W.R.: Integrated approach to measuring association. In: Costner, H.L. (ed.) Sociological Methodology, pp. 279–301. Jossey Bass, San Francisco, CA (1971)
65. Levine, T.R., Hullett, C.R.: Eta squared, partial eta squared, and misreporting of effect size in communication research. Hum. Commun. Res. **28**, 612–625 (2002)
66. Levine, T.R., Weber, R., Hullett, C.R., Park, H.S., Massi Lindsey, L.L.: A critical assessment of null hypothesis significance testing in quantitative communication research. Hum. Commun. Res. **34**, 171–187 (2008)
67. Levine, T.R., Weber, R., Park, H.S., Hullett, C.R.: A communication researchers' guide to null hypothesis significance testing and alternatives. Hum. Commun. Res. **34**, 188–209 (2008)
68. Long, M.A., Berry, K.J., Mielke, P.W.: Multiway contingency tables: Monte Carlo resampling probability values for the chi-squared and likelihood-ratio tests. Psychol. Rep. **107**, 501–510 (2010)
69. Ludbrook, J.: Advantages of permutation (randomization) tests in clinical and experimental pharmacology and physiology. Clin. Exp. Pharmacol. P. **21**, 673–686 (1994)
70. Ludbrook, J., Dudley, H.A.F.: Why permutation tests are superior to t and F tests in biomedical research. Am. Stat. **52**, 127–132 (1998)
71. McLean, J.E., Ernest, J.M.: The role of statistical significance testing in educational research. J. Health. Soc. Beh. **5**, 15–22 (1998)
72. Micceri, T.: The unicorn, the normal curve, and other improbable creatures. Psychol. Bull. **105**, 156–166 (1989)
73. Mielke, P.W., Berry, K.J.: Cumulant methods for analyzing independence of r-way contingency tables and goodness-of-fit frequency data. Biometrika **75**, 790–793 (1988)
74. Mielke, P.W., Berry, K.J.: Exact goodness-of-fit probability tests for analyzing categorical data. Educ. Psychol. Meas. **53**, 707–710 (1993)
75. Mielke, P.W., Berry, K.J.: Permutation Methods: A Distance Function Approach, 2nd edn. Springer–Verlag, New York (2007)
76. Mielke, P.W., Berry, K.J., Johnston, J.E.: Resampling programs for multiway contingency tables with fixed marginal frequency totals. Psychol. Rep. **101**, 18–24 (2007)
77. Mosteller, F.: Association and estimation in contingency tables. J. Am. Stat. Assoc. **63**, 1–28 (1968)
78. Murphy, K.R., Cleveland, J.: Understanding Performance Appraisal: Social, Organizational, and Goal-based Perspectives. Sage, Thousand Oaks, CA (1995)
79. Nix, T.W., Barnette, J.J.: The data analysis dilemma: Ban or abandon. A review of null hypothesis significance testing. Res. Schools **5**, 3–14 (1998)

80. Nix, T.W., Barnette, J.J.: A review of hypothesis testing revisited: Rejoinder to Thompson, Knapp, and Levin. Res. Schools **5**, 55–57 (1998)
81. Olzak, L.A., Wickens, T.D.: The interpretation of detection data through direct multivariate frequency analysis. Psychol. Bull. **93**, 574–585 (1983)
82. Pearson, K.: On the criterion that a given system of deviations from the probable in the case of a correlated system of variables is such that it can be reasonably supposed to have arisen from random sampling. Philos. Mag. 5 **50**, 157–175 (1900)
83. Rao, J.N.K., Scott, A.J.: On chi-squared tests for multiway contingency tables with cell proportions estimated from survey data. Ann. Stat. **12**, 46–60 (1984)
84. Saal, F.E., Downey, R.G., Lahey, M.A.: Rating the ratings: Assessing the quality of rating data. Psychol. Bull. **88**, 413–428 (1980)
85. Savage, I.R.: Nonparametric statistics. J. Am. Stat. Assoc. **52**, 331–344 (1957)
86. Schmidt, F.L., Johnson, R.H.: Effect of race on peer ratings in an industrial situation. J. Appl. Psychol. **57**, 237–241 (1973)
87. Siegel, S., Castellan, N.J.: Nonparametric Statistics for the Behavioral Sciences, 2nd edn. McGraw–Hill, New York (1988)
88. Smith, P.J., Rae, D.S., Manderscheid, R.W., Silbergeld, S.: Approximating the moments and distribution of the likelihood ratio statistic for multinomial goodness of fit. J. Am. Stat. Assoc. **76**, 737–740 (1981)
89. Smith, W.B.: Herman Otto Hartley (1912–1980). Am. Stat. **35**, 142–143 (1981)
90. Still, A.W., White, A.P.: The approximate randomization test as an alternative to the *F* test in analysis of variance. Brit. J. Math. Stat. Psy. **34**, 243–252 (1981)
91. Thompson, W.L.: 402 citations questioning the indiscriminate use of null hypothesis significance tests in observational studies (2001). http://www.warnercnr.colostate.edu/~anderson/thompson1.html (2001). Accessed 18 June 2015
92. Thompson, W.L.: Problems with the hypothesis testing approach (2001). http://www.warnercnr.colostate.edu/~gwhite/fw663/testing.pdf (2001) Accessed 18 June 2015
93. Tschuprov, A.A.: Principles of the Mathematical Theory of Correlation. Hodge, London (1939). [Translated by M. Kantorowitsch]
94. Vaughan, G.M., Corballis, M.C.: Beyond tests of significance: Estimating strength of effects in selected ANOVA designs. Psychol. Bull. **79**, 391–395 (1969)
95. Vokey, J.R.: Multiway frequency analysis for experimental psychologists. Can. J. Exp. Psychol. **57**, 257–264 (2003)
96. Wasserstein, R., Lazar, N.A.: The ASA's statement on p-values: Context, process, and purpose. Am. Stat. **70**, 129–133 (2016)
97. Wickens, T.D.: Multiway Contingency Tables Analysis for the Social Sciences. Erlbaum, Hillsdale, NJ (1989)
98. Wickens, T.D.: Analysis of contingency tables with between-subjects variability. Psychol. Bull. **113**, 191–204 (1993)
99. Wilcox, R.R., Muska, J.: Measuring effect size: A non-parametric analogue of $\hat{\omega}^2$. Brit. J. Math. Stat. Psy. **52**, 93–110 (1999)
100. Wilkinson, L.: Statistical methods in psychology journals: Guidelines and explanations. Am. Psychol. **54**, 594–604 (1999)
101. Wilks, S.S.: The likelihood test of independence in contingency tables. Ann. Math. Stat. **6**, 190–196 (1935)
102. Wilks, S.S.: The large-sample distribution of the likelihood ratio for testing composite hypotheses. Ann. Math. Stat. **9**, 60–62 (1938)
103. Williams, D.A.: Improved likelihood-ratio tests for complete contingency tables. Biometrika **63**, 33–37 (1976)
104. Yule, G.U., Filon, L.N.G.: Karl Pearson. 1857–1936. Obit. Notices Fellows Roy. Soc. **2**, 73–110 (1936)

Chapter 4
Nominal-Level Variables, II

Chapter 3 of *The Measurement of Association* applied permutation statistical methods to measures of association based on Pearson's chi-squared test statistic for two nominal-level (categorical) variables, e.g., Pearson's ϕ^2, Tschuprov's T^2, Cramér's V^2, and Pearson's C. This fourth chapter of *The Measurement of Association* continues the examination of measures of association designed for nominal-level variables, but concentrates on exact and Monte Carlo permutation statistical methods for measures of nominal association that are based on criteria other than Pearson's chi-squared test statistic. First, two asymmetric measures of nominal-level association proposed by Goodman and Kruskal in 1954, λ and t, are described [37]. Next, Cohen's unweighted kappa coefficient, κ, provides an introduction to the measurement of agreement, in contrast to measures of association [23]. Also included in Chap. 4 are McNemar's [63] and Cochran's [22] Q tests that measure the degree to which response measurements change over time, Leik and Gove's [52] d_N^c measure of nominal association, and a solution to the matrix occupancy problem proposed by Mielke and Siddiqui [68]. Fisher's [32] exact probability test is the iconic permutation test for contingency tables. While Fisher's exact test is typically limited to 2×2 contingency tables, for which it was originally intended, in this chapter Fisher's exact test is extended to 2×c, 3×3, 2×2×2, and other larger contingency tables.

Some measures designed for ordinal-level variables also serve as measures of association for nominal-level variables when $r = 2$ rows and $c = 2$ columns, i.e., a 2×2 contingency table. Other measures were originally designed for 2×2 contingency tables with nominal-level variables. Included in measures of association for 2×2 contingency tables are percentage differences, Yule's Q and Y measures [90], the odds ratio, and Somers' asymmetric measures, d_{yx} and d_{xy} [78]. These measures are more appropriately described and discussed in Chaps. 9 and 10, which are devoted to measures of association for analyzing 2×2 contingency tables, where the level of measurement is often irrelevant.

K. J. Berry et al., *The Measurement of Association*,
https://doi.org/10.1007/978-3-319-98926-6_4

Table 4.1 Notation for a 2×2 contingency table

	A_1	A_2	Total
B_1	n_{11}	n_{12}	R_1
B_2	n_{21}	n_{22}	R_2
Total	C_1	C_2	N

4.1 Hypergeometric Probability Values

Exact permutation statistical methods, especially when applied to contingency tables, are heavily dependent on hypergeometric probability values.[1] In this section, a brief introduction to hypergeometric probability values illustrates their calculation and interpretation. For 2×2 contingency tables, the calculation of hypergeometric probability values is easily demonstrated. Consider the 2×2 contingency table in Table 4.1 where $n_{11}, \ldots, n_{22}$ denote the four cell frequencies, R_1 and R_2 denote the two row marginal frequency totals, C_1 and C_2 denote the two column marginal frequency totals, and

$$N = \sum_{i=1}^{2} \sum_{j=1}^{2} n_{ij} \ .$$

Because the contingency table given in Table 4.1 is a 2×2 table and, consequently, has only one degree of freedom, the probability of any one cell frequency constitutes the probability of the entire contingency table. Thus, the hypergeometric point probability value for the cell containing n_{11} is given by:

$$p(n_{11}|R_1, C_1, N) = \binom{C_1}{n_{11}}\binom{C_2}{n_{12}}\binom{N}{R_1}^{-1} = \binom{R_1}{n_{11}}\binom{R_2}{n_{21}}\binom{N}{C_1}^{-1} = \frac{R_1!\ R_2!\ C_1!\ C_2!}{N!\ n_{11}!\ n_{12}!\ n_{21}!\ n_{22}!} \ . \tag{4.1}$$

To illustrate the calculation of a hypergeometric point probability value for a 2×2 contingency table, consider the frequency data given in Table 4.2 with $N = 20$ observations. Following Eq. (4.1)

$$p(n_{11}|R_1, C_1, N) = \frac{R_1!\ R_2!\ C_1!\ C_2!}{N!\ n_{11}!\ n_{12}!\ n_{21}!\ n_{22}!} = \frac{11!\ 9!\ 12!\ 8!}{20!\ 9!\ 2!\ 3!\ 6!} = 0.0367 \ .$$

The calculation of hypergeometric probability values for $r \times c$ contingency tables is more complex than for simple 2×2 contingency tables. Consider the

[1] While exact permutation statistical methods for $r \times c$ contingency tables depend on hypergeometric probability values for each of the M possible arrangements of cell frequencies, Monte Carlo resampling permutation statistical methods do not rely on hypergeometric probability values.

Table 4.2 Example 2×2 contingency table

	A_1	A_2	Total
B_1	9	2	11
B_2	3	6	9
Total	12	8	20

Table 4.3 Notation for a 4×3 contingency table

	A_1	A_2	A_3	Total
B_1	n_{11}	n_{12}	n_{13}	R_1
B_2	n_{21}	n_{22}	n_{23}	R_2
B_3	n_{31}	n_{32}	n_{33}	R_3
B_4	n_{41}	n_{42}	n_{43}	R_4
Total	C_1	C_2	C_3	N

4×3 contingency table given in Table 4.3 where $n_{11}, \ldots, n_{43}$ denote the 12 cell frequencies, $R_1, \ldots, R_4$ denote the four row marginal frequency totals, C_1, C_2, and C_3 denote the three column marginal frequency totals, and

$$N = \sum_{i=1}^{4} \sum_{j=1}^{3} n_{ij} \; .$$

When there are only two rows, as in the previous 2×2 example, each column probability value is binomial, but with four rows each column probability value is multinomial. It is well known that a multinomial probability value can be obtained from an inter-connected series of binomial expressions. For example, for column A_1 in Table 4.3,

$$\binom{C_1}{n_{11}}\binom{C_1 - n_{11}}{n_{21}}\binom{C_1 - n_{11} - n_{21}}{n_{31}} = \frac{C_1!}{n_{11}!\,(C_1 - n_{11})!} \times \frac{(C_1 - n_{11})!}{n_{21}!\,(C_1 - n_{11} - n_{21})!} \times \frac{(C_1 - n_{11} - n_{21})!}{n_{31}!\,(C_1 - n_{11} - n_{21} - n_{31})!} = \frac{C_1!}{n_{11}!\,n_{21}!\,n_{31}!\,n_{41}!} \;,$$

for column A_2 in Table 4.3,

$$\binom{C_2}{n_{12}}\binom{C_2 - n_{12}}{n_{22}}\binom{C_2 - n_{12} - n_{22}}{n_{32}} = \frac{C_2!}{n_{12}!\,(C_2 - n_{12})!} \times \frac{(C_2 - n_{12})!}{n_{22}!\,(C_2 - n_{12} - n_{22})!} \times \frac{(C_2 - n_{12} - n_{22})!}{n_{32}!\,(C_2 - n_{12} - n_{22} - n_{32})!} = \frac{C_2!}{n_{12}!\,n_{22}!\,n_{32}!\,n_{42}!} \;,$$

for column A_3 in Table 4.3,

$$\binom{C_3}{n_{13}}\binom{C_3 - n_{13}}{n_{23}}\binom{C_3 - n_{13} - n_{23}}{n_{33}} = \frac{C_3!}{n_{13}!\,(C_3 - n_{13})!}$$
$$\times \frac{(C_3 - n_{13})!}{n_{23}!\,(C_3 - n_{13} - n_{23})!} \times \frac{(C_3 - n_{13} - n_{23})!}{n_{33}!\,(C_3 - n_{13} - n_{23} - n_{33})!}$$
$$= \frac{C_3!}{n_{13}!\,n_{23}!\,n_{33}!\,n_{43}!}\ ,$$

and for the row marginal frequency distribution in Table 4.3,

$$\binom{N}{R_1}\binom{N - R_1}{R_2}\binom{N - R_1 - R_2}{R_3} = \frac{N!}{R_1!\,(N - R_1)!}$$
$$\times \frac{(N - R_1)!}{R_2!\,(N - R_1 - R_2)!} \times \frac{(N - R_1 - R_2)!}{R_3!\,(N - R_1 - R_2 - R_3)!}$$
$$= \frac{N!}{R_1!\,R_2!\,R_3!\,R_4!}\ .$$

Thus, for an $r\times c$ contingency table,

$$p(n_{ij}|R_i, C_j, N) = \frac{\left(\prod_{i=1}^{r} R_i!\right)\left(\prod_{j=1}^{c} C_j!\right)}{N!\prod_{i=1}^{r}\prod_{j=1}^{c} n_{ij}!}\ . \tag{4.2}$$

In this form, Eq. (4.2) can easily be generalized to more complex multi-way contingency tables [64].

To illustrate the calculation of a hypergeometric point probability value for an $r\times c$ contingency table, consider the sparse frequency data given in Table 4.4 with $N = 14$ observations. Following Eq. (4.2)

$$p(n_{ij}|R_i, C_j, N) = \frac{\left(\prod_{i=1}^{r} R_i!\right)\left(\prod_{j=1}^{c} C_j!\right)}{N!\prod_{i=1}^{r}\prod_{j=1}^{c} n_{ij}!}$$
$$= \frac{3!\ 4!\ 3!\ 4!\ 5!\ 5!\ 5!}{14!\ 2!\ 1!\ 0!\ 0!\ 1!\ 3!\ 0!\ 3!\ 0!\ 3!\ 0!\ 1!} = 0.1903\times 10^{-3}\ .$$

Table 4.4 Example 4×3 contingency table

	A_1	A_2	A_3	Total
B_1	2	1	0	3
B_2	0	1	3	4
B_3	0	3	0	3
B_4	3	0	1	4
Total	5	5	4	14

While this section illustrates the calculation of a hypergeometric point probability value, for an exact permutation test of an $r \times c$ contingency table it is necessary to calculate the selected measure of association for the observed cell frequencies and, then, exhaustively enumerate all possible, equally-likely arrangements of the N objects in the rc cells, given the observed marginal frequency distributions.

For each arrangement in the reference set of all permutations of cell frequencies, a measure of association, say, T, is calculated and the exact hypergeometric point probability value, $p(n_{ij}|R_i, C_j, N)$ for $i = 1, \ldots, r$ and $j = 1, \ldots, c$, is calculated. If T_o denotes the value of the observed test statistic, i.e., measure of association, the exact two-sided probability value of T_o is the sum of the hypergeometric point probability values associated with the values of T computed on all possible arrangements of cell frequencies that are equal to or greater than T_o.

When the number of possible arrangements of cell frequencies is very large, exact tests are impractical and Monte Carlo permutation statistical methods become necessary. Monte Carlo permutation statistical methods generate a random sample of all possible arrangements of cell frequencies, drawn with replacement, given the observed marginal frequency distributions. The resampling two-sided probability value is simply the proportion of the T values computed on the randomly selected arrangements that are equal to or greater than T_o. In the case of Monte Carlo resampling, hypergeometric probability values are not involved—simply the proportion of the values of the measures of association (T values) equal to or greater than the value of the observed measure of association (T_o).

4.2 Goodman and Kruskal's λ_a and λ_b Measures

A common problem that many researchers confront is the analysis of a cross-classification table where both variables are categorical, as categorical variables usually do not contain as much information as ordinal- or interval-level variables [54]. As noted in Chap. 3, the usual measures of association based on chi-squared, such as Pearson's ϕ^2, Tschuprov's T^2, Cramér's V^2, and Pearson's C, have proven to be less than satisfactory due to difficulties in interpretation; see, for example, discussions by Agresti and Finlay [2, p. 284], Berry, Martin, and

Table 4.5 Notation for the cross-classification of two categorical variables, A_j for $j = 1, \ldots, c$ and B_i for $i = 1, \ldots, r$

	A				
B	a_1	a_2	$\cdots$	a_c	Total
b_1	n_{11}	n_{12}	$\cdots$	n_{1c}	$n_{1.}$
b_2	n_{21}	n_{22}	$\cdots$	n_{2c}	$n_{2.}$
$\vdots$	$\vdots$	$\vdots$	$\ddots$	$\vdots$	$\vdots$
b_r	n_{r1}	n_{r2}	$\cdots$	n_{rc}	$n_{r.}$
Total	$n_{.1}$	$n_{.2}$	$\cdots$	$n_{.c}$	N

Olson [11], Berry, Johnston, and Mielke [8, 9], Blalock [18, p. 306], Costner [27], Ferguson [30, p. 422], Guilford [42, p. 342], and Wickens [86, p. 226].

In 1954, Leo Goodman and William Kruskal proposed several new measures of association [37].[2] Among the measures were two asymmetric proportional-reduction-in-error (PRE) prediction measures for the analyses of a random sample of two categorical variables: λ_a, for when A was considered to be the dependent variable, and λ_b, for when B was considered to be the dependent variable [37].[3]

Consider an $r \times c$ contingency table such as depicted in Table 4.5, where a_j for $j = 1, \ldots, c$ denotes the c categories for dependent variable A, b_i for $i = 1, \ldots, r$ denotes the r categories for independent variable B, n_{ij} denotes a cell frequency for $i = 1, \ldots, r$ and $j = 1, \ldots, c$, and N denotes the total of cell frequencies in the table. Denote by a dot $(\cdot)$ the partial sum of all rows or all columns, depending on the position of the $(\cdot)$ in the subscript list. If the $(\cdot)$ is in the first subscript position, the sum is over all rows and if the $(\cdot)$ is in the second subscript position, the sum is over all columns. Thus, $n_{i.}$ denotes the marginal frequency total of the ith row, $i = 1, \ldots, r$, summed over all columns, and $n_{.j}$ denotes the marginal frequency total of the jth column, $j = 1, \ldots, c$ summed over all rows.

Given the notation in Table 4.5, let

$$W = \sum_{i=1}^{r} \max(n_{i1}, n_{i2}, \ldots, n_{ic})$$

and

$$X = \max(n_{.1}, n_{.2}, \ldots, n_{.c}) .$$

Then, λ_a, with variable A the dependent variable, is given by:

$$\lambda_a = \frac{W - X}{N - X} .$$

[2]This formative 1954 article by Goodman and Kruskal [37] was followed by three subsequent articles on measures of association for cross-classifications in 1959, 1963, and 1972 [38, 39, 40]

[3]These same statistics, λ_a and λ_b, were independently developed by Louis (Eliyahu) Guttman in 1941 [43].

In like manner, let

$$Y = \sum_{j=1}^{c} \max(n_{1j}, n_{2j}, \ldots, n_{rj})$$

and

$$Z = \max(n_{1.}, n_{2.}, \ldots, n_{r.}) \; .$$

Then, λ_b, with variable B the dependent variable, is given by:

$$\lambda_b = \frac{Y - Z}{N - Z} \; .$$

Both λ_a and λ_b are proportional-reduction-in-error (PRE) measures. Consider λ_a and two possible scenarios:

Case 1: Knowledge of only the disjoint categories of dependent variable A.
Case 2: Knowledge of the disjoint categories of variable A, and also knowledge of the disjoint categories of independent variable B.

For Case 1, it is expedient for a researcher to guess the category of dependent variable A that has the largest marginal frequency total (mode), which in this case is $X = \max(n_{.1}, \ldots, n_{.c})$. Then, the probability of error is $N - X$; label these "errors of the first kind" or E_1. For Case 2, it is expedient for a researcher to guess the category of dependent variable A that has the largest cell frequency (mode) in each category of the independent variable B, which in this case is

$$W = \sum_{i=1}^{r} \max(n_{i1}, n_{i2}, \ldots, n_{ic}) \; .$$

The probability of error is then $N - W$; label these "errors of the second kind" or E_2. Then, λ_a may be expressed as:

$$\lambda_a = \frac{E_1 - E_2}{E_1} = \frac{N - X - (N - W)}{N - X} = \frac{W - X}{N - X} \; .$$

As noted by Goodman and Kruskal in 1954, a problem was immediately observed with the interpretations of both λ_a and λ_b. Since both measures were based on the modal values of the categories of the independent variable, when the modal values all occurred in the same category of the dependent variable λ_a and λ_b returned results of zero [37, p. 742]. Thus, while λ_a and λ_b were equal to zero under independence, λ_a and λ_b could also be equal to zero for cases other than independence. This made both λ_a and λ_b difficult to interpret; consequently, λ_a and λ_b are seldom found in the contemporary literature. The problem is easy to illustrate

Table 4.6 Example 2×2 contingency table with variables A and B independent

	A_1	A_2	Total
B_1	36	24	60
B_2	24	16	40
Total	60	40	100

Table 4.7 Example 2×2 contingency table with variables A and B not independent

	A_1	A_2	Total
B_1	32	28	60
B_2	28	12	40
Total	60	40	100

with simple 2×2 contingency tables. Consider first the 2×2 contingency table given in Table 4.6 where the cell frequencies indicate independence between variables A and B. For the frequency data given in Table 4.6,

$$W = \sum_{i=1}^{r} \max(n_{i1}, \ldots, n_{ic}) = \max(36, 24) + \max(24, 16) = 36 + 24 = 60 ,$$

$$X = \max(n_{.1}, \ldots, n_{.c}) = \max(60, 40) = 60 ,$$

and the observed value of λ_a is

$$\lambda_a = \frac{W - X}{N - X} = \frac{60 - 60}{100 - 60} = 0.00 .$$

Now, consider the 2×2 contingency table given in Table 4.7 where the cell frequencies do not indicate independence between variables A and B. For the frequency data given in Table 4.7,

$$W = \sum_{i=1}^{r} \max(n_{i1}, \ldots, n_{ic}) = \max(32, 28) + \max(28, 12) = 32 + 28 = 60 ,$$

$$X = \max(n_{.1}, \ldots, n_{.c}) = \max(60, 40) = 60 ,$$

and the observed value of λ_a is

$$\lambda_a = \frac{W - X}{N - X} = \frac{60 - 60}{100 - 60} = 0.00 .$$

Finally, consider the 2×2 contingency table given in Table 4.8, where the cell frequencies indicate perfect association between variables A and B. For the

Table 4.8 Example 2×2 contingency table with variables A and B in perfect association

	A_1	A_2	Total
B_1	60	0	60
B_2	0	40	40
Total	60	40	100

frequency data given in Table 4.8,

$$W = \sum_{i=1}^{r} \max(n_{i1}, \ldots, n_{ic}) = \max(60, 0) + \max(0, 40) = 60 + 40 = 100 ,$$

$$X = \max(n_{.1}, \ldots, n_{.c}) = \max(60, 40) = 60 ,$$

and the observed value of λ_a is

$$\lambda_a = \frac{W - X}{N - X} = \frac{100 - 60}{100 - 60} = 1.00 .$$

Thus, as Goodman and Kruskal explained in 1954 [37, p. 742]:

1. λ_a is indeterminate if and only if the population lies in one column; that is, it appears in one category of variable A.
2. Otherwise, the value of λ_a lies between the limits 0 and 1.
3. λ_a is 0 if and only if knowledge of the B classification is of no help in predicting the A classification.
4. λ_a is 1 if and only if knowledge of an object's B category completely specifies its A category, i.e., if each row of the cross-classification table contains at most one non-zero value.
5. In the case of statistical independence, λ_a, when determinate, is zero. The converse need not hold: λ_a may be zero without statistical independence holding.
6. λ_a is unchanged by any permutation of rows or columns.

4.2.1 Example λ_a and λ_b Analyses

For a more realistic application of Goodman and Kruskal's λ_a and λ_b measures of nominal association, consider the 3×4 contingency table given in Table 4.9, where for λ_a

$$W = \sum_{i=1}^{r} \max(n_{i1}, \ldots, n_{ic}) = \max(5, 0, 15, 0) + \max(5, 5, 15, 5)$$

$$+ \max(5, 20, 5, 10) = 15 + 15 + 20 = 50 ,$$

$$X = \max(n_{.1}, \ldots, n_{.c}) = \max(15, 25, 35, 15) = 35 ,$$

Table 4.9 Example 3×4 contingency table for Goodman and Kruskal's λ_a and λ_b

	A_1	A_2	A_3	A_4	Total
B_1	5	0	15	0	20
B_2	5	5	15	5	30
B_3	5	20	5	10	40
Total	15	25	35	15	90

and the observed value of λ_a is

$$\lambda_a = \frac{W - X}{N - X} = \frac{50 - 35}{90 - 35} = 0.2727 \; .$$

The exact probability value of an observed value of λ_a under the null hypothesis is given by the sum of the hypergeometric point probability values associated with values of λ_a equal to or greater than the observed λ_a value. For the frequency data given in Table 4.9, there are only $M = 3{,}453{,}501$ possible, equally-likely arrangements in the reference set of all permutations of cell frequencies given the observed row and column marginal frequency distributions, $\{20, 30, 40\}$ and $\{15, 25, 35, 15\}$, respectively, making an exact permutation analysis possible. The exact upper-tail probability value of the observed λ_a value is $P = 0.2715$, i.e., the sum of the hypergeometric point probability values associated with values of $\lambda_a = 0.2727$ or greater.

The frequency data given in Table 4.9 can also be considered with variable B as the dependent variable. Thus, for λ_b

$$Y = \sum_{j=1}^{c} \max(n_{1j}, \; \ldots, \; n_{rj}) = \max(5, 5, 5) + \max(0, 5, 20)$$

$$+ \max(15, 15, 5) + \max(0, 5, 10) = 5 + 20 + 15 + 10 = 50 \; ,$$

$$Z = \max(n_{1.}, \ldots, n_{r.}) = \max(20, 30, 40) = 40 \; ,$$

and the observed value of λ_b is

$$\lambda_b = \frac{Y - Z}{N - Z} = \frac{50 - 40}{90 - 40} = 0.20 \; .$$

For the frequency data given in Table 4.9, there are only $M = 3{,}453{,}501$ possible, equally-likely arrangements in the reference set of all permutations of cell frequencies given the observed row and column marginal frequency distributions, $\{20, 30, 40\}$ and $\{15, 25, 35, 15\}$, respectively, making an exact permutation analysis feasible. The exact upper-tail probability value of the observed λ_b value is $P = 0.7669$, i.e., the sum of the hypergeometric point probability values associated with values of $\lambda_b = 0.20$ or greater.

Table 4.10 Notation for the cross-classification of two categorical variables, A_j for $j = 1, \ldots, c$ and B_i for $i = 1, \ldots, r$

	A				
B	a_1	a_2	$\cdots$	a_c	Total
b_1	n_{11}	n_{12}	$\cdots$	n_{1c}	$n_{1.}$
b_2	n_{21}	n_{22}	$\cdots$	n_{2c}	$n_{2.}$
$\vdots$	$\vdots$	$\vdots$	$\ddots$	$\vdots$	$\vdots$
b_r	n_{r1}	n_{r2}	$\cdots$	n_{rc}	$n_{r.}$
Total	$n_{.1}$	$n_{.2}$	$\cdots$	$n_{.c}$	N

4.3 Goodman and Kruskal's t_a and t_b Measures

As noted, *vide supra*, in 1954 Leo Goodman and William Kruskal proposed several new measures of association. Among the measures was an asymmetric proportional-reduction-in-error (PRE) prediction measure, t_a, for the analysis of a random sample of two categorical variables [37]. Consider two cross-classified unordered polytomies, A and B, with variable A the dependent variable and variable B the independent variable. Table 4.5 on p. 144, replicated in Table 4.10 for convenience, provides notation for the cross-classification, where a_j for $j = 1, \ldots, c$ denotes the c categories for dependent variable A, b_i for $i = 1, \ldots, r$ denotes the r categories for independent variable B, N denotes the total of cell frequencies in the table, $n_{i.}$ denotes a marginal frequency total for the ith row, $i = 1, \ldots, r$, summed over all columns, $n_{.j}$ denotes a marginal frequency total for the jth column, $j = 1, \ldots, c$, summed over all rows, and n_{ij} denotes a cell frequency for $i = 1, \ldots, r$ and $j = 1, \ldots, c$.

Goodman and Kruskal's t_a statistic is a measure of the relative reduction in prediction error where two types of errors are defined. The first type is the error in prediction based solely on knowledge of the distribution of the dependent variable, termed "errors of the first kind" (E_1) and consisting of the expected number of errors when predicting the c dependent variable categories ($a_1, \ldots, a_c$) from the observed distribution of the marginals of the dependent variable ($n_{.1}, \ldots, n_{.c}$). The second type is the error in prediction based on knowledge of the distributions of both the independent and dependent variables, termed "errors of the second kind" (E_2) and consisting of the expected number or errors when predicting the c dependent variable categories ($a_1, \ldots, a_c$) from knowledge of the r independent variable categories ($b_1, \ldots, b_r$).

To illustrate the two error types, consider predicting category a_1 only from knowledge of its marginal distribution, $n_{.1}, \ldots, n_{.c}$. Clearly, $n_{.1}$ out of the N total cases are in category a_1, but exactly which $n_{.1}$ of the N cases is unknown. The probability of incorrectly identifying one of the N cases in category a_1 by chance alone is given by:

$$\frac{N - n_{.1}}{N} \ .$$

Since there are $n_{.1}$ such classifications required, the number of expected incorrect classifications is

$$\frac{n_{.1}(N - n_{.1})}{N}$$

and, for all c categories of variable A, the number of expected errors of the first kind is given by:

$$E_1 = \sum_{j=1}^{c} \frac{n_{.j}(N - n_{.j})}{N} \ .$$

Likewise, to predict $n_{11}, \ldots, n_{1c}$ from the independent category b_1, the probability of incorrectly classifying one of the $n_{1.}$ cases in cell n_{11} by chance alone is

$$\frac{n_{1.} - n_{11}}{n_{1.}} \ .$$

Since there are n_{11} such classifications required, the number of incorrect classifications is

$$\frac{n_{11}(n_{1.} - n_{11})}{n_{1.}}$$

and, for all cr cells, the number of expected errors of the second kind is given by:

$$E_2 = \sum_{j=1}^{c} \sum_{i=1}^{r} \frac{n_{ij}(n_{i.} - n_{ij})}{n_{i.}} \ .$$

Goodman and Kruskal's t_a statistic is then defined as:

$$t_a = \frac{E_1 - E_2}{E_1} \ .$$

An efficient computation form for Goodman and Kruskal's t_a is given by:

$$t_a = \frac{N \displaystyle\sum_{i=1}^{r} \sum_{j=1}^{c} \frac{n_{ij}^2}{n_{i.}} - \sum_{j=1}^{c} n_{.j}^2}{N^2 - \displaystyle\sum_{j=1}^{c} n_{.j}^2} \ . \tag{4.3}$$

A computed value of t_a indicates the proportional reduction in prediction error given knowledge of the distribution of independent variable B over and above knowledge of only the distribution of dependent variable A. As defined, t_a is a point estimator of Goodman and Kruskal's population parameter τ_a for the population from which the sample of N cases was obtained. If variable B is considered the dependent variable and variable A the independent variable, then Goodman and Kruskal's test statistic t_b and associated population parameter τ_b are analogously defined.

While parameter τ_a norms properly from 0 to 1, possesses a clear and meaningful proportional-reduction-in-error interpretation [27], and is characterized by high intuitive and factorial validity [45], test statistic t_a poses difficulties whenever the null hypothesis posits that $H_0\colon \tau_a = 0$ [61]. The problem is that the sampling distribution of t_a is not asymptotically normal under the null hypothesis $H_0\colon \tau_a = 0$. Consequently, the applicability of Goodman and Kruskal's t_a to typical tests of null hypotheses has been severely circumscribed.

Although t_a was developed by Goodman and Kruskal in 1954, it was not until 1963 that the asymptotic normality for t_a was established and an asymptotic variance was given for t_a, but only for $0 < \tau_a < 1$ [39]. Unfortunately, the asymptotic variance for t_a given in 1963 was later found to be incorrect, and it was not until 1972 that the correct asymptotic variance for t_a was obtained, but again, only for $0 < \tau_a < 1$.

In 1971, Richard Light and Barry Margolin developed R^2, an analysis-of-variance technique for categorical response variables, called CATANOVA for CATegorical ANalysis Of VAriance [55]. Light and Margolin apparently were unaware that R^2 was identical to Goodman and Kruskal's t_a and that they had asymptotically solved the longstanding problem of testing $H_0\colon \tau_a = 0$. The identity between R^2 and t_a was first recognized by Särndal in 1974 [75] and later discussed by Margolin and Light [61], where they showed that $t_a(N-1)(r-1)$ was distributed as chi-squared with $(r-1)(c-1)$ degrees of freedom under $H_0\colon \tau_a = 0$ as $N \to \infty$ [13].

4.3.1 Example Analysis for t_a

Consider the same 3×4 contingency table analyzed with Goodman and Kruskal's λ_a, replicated in Table 4.11 for convenience. Following Eq. (4.3), the observed value of Goodman and Kruskal's t_a is

$$t_a = \frac{N \displaystyle\sum_{i=1}^{r} \sum_{j=1}^{c} \frac{n_{ij}^2}{n_{i.}} - \sum_{j=1}^{c} n_{.j}^2}{N^2 - \displaystyle\sum_{j=1}^{c} n_{.j}^2}$$

$$= \frac{90\left(\dfrac{5^2}{20} + \dfrac{0^2}{20} + \cdots + \dfrac{10^2}{40}\right) - (15^2 + 25^2 + 35^2 + 15^2)}{90^2 - (15^2 + 25^2 + 35^2 + 15^2)} = 0.1659\ .$$

Table 4.11 Example 3×4 contingency table

	A_1	A_2	A_3	A_4	Total
B_1	5	0	15	0	20
B_2	5	5	15	5	30
B_3	5	20	5	10	40
Total	15	25	35	15	90

The exact probability value of an observed t_a under the null hypothesis is given by the sum of the hypergeometric point probability values associated with values of t_a equal to or greater than the observed value of t_a. For the frequency data given in Table 4.11, there are only $M = 3{,}453{,}501$ possible, equally-likely arrangements in the reference set of all permutations of cell frequencies given the observed row and column marginal frequency distributions, $\{20, 30, 40\}$ and $\{15, 25, 35, 15\}$, respectively, making an exact permutation analysis possible. The exact upper-tail probability value of the observed t_a value is $P = 0.3828$, i.e., the sum of the hypergeometric point probability values associated with values of $t_a = 0.1659$ or greater.

4.3.2 Example Analysis for t_b

Now, consider variable B as the dependent variable. A convenient computing formula for t_b is

$$t_b = \frac{N \displaystyle\sum_{j=1}^{c} \sum_{i=1}^{r} \frac{n_{ij}^2}{n_{.j}} - \sum_{i=1}^{r} n_{i.}^2}{N^2 - \displaystyle\sum_{i=1}^{r} n_{i.}^2} .$$

Thus, for the frequency data given in Table 4.11 the observed value of t_b is

$$t_b = \frac{90 \left(\dfrac{5^2}{15} + \dfrac{0^2}{25} + \cdots + \dfrac{10^2}{40} \right) - (20^2 + 30^2 + 40^2)}{90^2 - (20^2 + 30^2 + 40^2)} = 0.2022 .$$

For the frequency data given in Table 4.11, there are only $M = 3{,}453{,}501$ possible, equally-likely arrangements in the reference set of all permutations of cell frequencies given the observed row and column marginal frequency distributions, $\{20, 30, 40\}$ and $\{15, 25, 35, 15\}$, respectively, making an exact permutation analysis feasible. The exact upper-tail probability value of the observed t_b value is $P =$

0.5187, i.e., the sum of the hypergeometric point probability values associated with values of $t_b = 0.2022$ or greater.

4.4 An Asymmetric Test of Homogeneity

Oftentimes a research question involves determining if the proportions of items in a set of mutually exclusive categories are the same for two or more groups. When independent random samples are drawn from each of $g \geq 2$ groups and then classified into $r \geq 2$ mutually exclusive categories, the appropriate test is a test of homogeneity of the g distributions. In a test of homogeneity, one of the marginal distributions is known prior to collecting the data, i.e., the row or column marginal frequency totals indicating the numbers in each of the g groups. This is termed *product* multinomial sampling, since the sampling distribution is the product of g multinomial distributions and the null hypothesis is that the g multinomial distributions are identical [19, 49, 61].

A test of homogeneity is quite different from a test of independence, where a single sample is drawn and then classified on both variables. In a test of independence, both sets of marginal frequency totals are known only after the data have been collected [62]. This is termed *simple* multinomial sampling, since the sampling distribution is a multinomial distribution [19, 49]. The most widely used test of homogeneity is the Pearson [69] chi-squared test of homogeneity with degrees of freedom given by $df = (r - 1)(g - 1)$. The Pearson chi-squared test of homogeneity tests the null hypothesis that there is no difference in the proportions of subjects in a set of mutually exclusive categories between two or more populations [60].

Pearson's chi-squared test of homogeneity is a symmetrical test, yielding only a single value for an $r \times g$ contingency table. In contrast, an asymmetrical test yields two values depending on which variable is considered to be the dependent variable. As noted by Berkson, if the differences are all in one direction, a symmetrical test such as chi-squared is insensitive to this fact [6, p. 536].

A symmetrical test of homogeneity, by its nature, excludes known information about the data—which variable is the independent variable and which variable is the dependent variable. While it is sometimes necessary to reduce the level of measurement when distributional requirements cannot be met, in general it is not advisable to use a statistical test that discounts important information [29, p. 911]. For example, a researcher should not discard the magnitude of a set of scores and use a signed-ranks test instead of a Fisher–Pitman test, nor should a researcher subsequently ignore the ranks and reduce the analysis to a simple sign test. In the same fashion, given the problem of examining the contingency of two ordered polytomies, the use of a chi-squared-based measure of association does not take into consideration the inherent ordering of the categories [7].

Consider two cross-classified unordered polytomies, A and B, with B the dependent variable. Let $b_1, \ldots, b_r$ represent the $r \geq 2$ categories of the dependent

Table 4.12 Notation for the cross-classification of two categorical variables, A_j for $j = 1, \ldots, g$ and B_i for $i = 1, \ldots, r$

	A				
B	a_1	a_2	$\cdots$	a_g	Total
b_1	n_{11}	n_{12}	$\cdots$	n_{1g}	$n_{1.}$
b_2	n_{21}	n_{22}	$\cdots$	n_{2g}	$n_{2.}$
$\vdots$	$\vdots$	$\vdots$	$\ddots$	$\vdots$	$\vdots$
b_r	n_{r1}	n_{r2}	$\cdots$	n_{rg}	$n_{r.}$
Total	$n_{.1}$	$n_{.2}$	$\cdots$	$n_{.g}$	N

variable, $a_1, \ldots, a_g$ represent the $g \geq 2$ categories of the independent variable, n_{ij} indicate the cell frequency in the ith row and jth column, $i = 1, \ldots, r$ and $j = 1, \ldots, g$, and N denote the total sample size. Denote by a dot $(\cdot)$ the partial sum of all rows or all columns, depending on the position of the $(\cdot)$ in the subscript list. If the $(\cdot)$ is in the first subscript position, the sum is over all rows and if the $(\cdot)$ is in the second subscript position, the sum is over all columns. Thus, $n_{1.}, \ldots, n_{r.}$ denotes the marginal frequency totals of row variable B summed over all columns and $n_{.1}, \ldots, n_{.g}$ denotes the marginal frequency totals of column variable A summed over all rows. The cross-classification of variables A and B is displayed in Table 4.12.

Although never advanced as a test of homogeneity, the asymmetrical test t_b, first introduced by Goodman and Kruskal in 1954 [37], is an attractive alternative to the symmetrical chi-squared test of homogeneity. The test statistic is given by:

$$t_b = \frac{N \displaystyle\sum_{j=1}^{g} \sum_{i=1}^{r} \frac{n_{ij}^2}{n_{.j}} - \sum_{i=1}^{r} n_{i.}^2}{N^2 - \displaystyle\sum_{i=1}^{r} n_{i.}^2} ,$$

where B is the dependent variable and the associated population parameter is denoted as τ_b. If variable A is considered the dependent variable, the test statistic is given by:

$$t_a = \frac{N \displaystyle\sum_{i=1}^{r} \sum_{j=1}^{g} \frac{n_{ij}^2}{n_{i.}} - \sum_{j=1}^{g} n_{.j}^2}{N^2 - \displaystyle\sum_{j=1}^{g} n_{.j}^2}$$

and the associated population parameter is τ_a.

Test statistic t_b takes on values between 0 and 1; t_b is 0 if and only if there is homogeneity over the r categories of the dependent variable (B) for all g groups, and t_b is 1 if and only if knowledge of variable A_j for $j = 1, \ldots, g$ completely determines knowledge of variable B_i for $i = 1, \ldots, r$. In like fashion, test statistic t_a is 0 if and only if there is homogeneity over the g categories of the dependent variable (A) for all r groups, and t_a is 1 if and only if knowledge of variable B_i for $i = 1, \ldots, r$ completely determines knowledge of variable A_j for $j = 1, \ldots, g$.

While no general equivalence exists for test statistics t_b, t_a, and χ^2, certain relationships hold among t_b, t_a, and χ^2 under special conditions. If $g = 2$, $\chi^2 = Nt_b$, and if $g > 2$ and $n_{.j} = N/g$ for $j = 1, \ldots, g$, $\chi^2 = N(g-1)t_b$. Similarly, if $r = 2$, $\chi^2 = Nt_a$, and if $r > 2$ and $n_{i.} = N/r$ for $i = 1, \ldots, r$, $\chi^2 = N(r-1)t_a$. It follows that if $r = g = 2$, $t_b = t_a = \chi^2/N$, which is the Pearson mean-squared contingency coefficient, ϕ^2. Finally, as $N \to \infty$, $t_b(N-1)(r-1)$ and $t_a(N-1)(g-1)$ are distributed as chi-squared with $(r-1)(g-1)$ degrees of freedom.

There are three methods to determine the probability value of a computed t_b or t_a test statistic: exact, Monte Carlo resampling, and asymptotic procedures. The following discussions consider only t_b, but the methods are analogous for t_a.

Exact Probability Values Under the null hypothesis, H_0: $\tau_b = 0$, each of the M possible arrangements of the N cases over the rg categories of the contingency table is equally probable with fixed marginal frequency distributions. For each arrangement of the observed data in the reference set of all possible arrangements, the desired test statistic is calculated. The exact probability value of an observed t_b test statistic is the sum of the hypergeometric point probability values associated with values of t_b or greater.

Resampling Probability Values An exact test is computationally not practical except for fairly small samples. An alternative method that avoids the computational demands of an exact test is a resampling permutation approximation. Under the null hypothesis, H_0: $\tau_b = 0$, resampling permutation tests generate and examine a Monte Carlo random subset of all possible, equally-likely arrangements of the observed data. For each randomly selected arrangement of the observed data, the desired test statistic is calculated. The Monte Carlo resampling probability value of an observed t_b test statistic is simply the proportion of the randomly selected values of t_b equal to or greater than the observed value of t_b.

Asymptotic Probability Values Under the null hypothesis, H_0: $\tau_b = 0$, as $N \to \infty$, $t_b(N-1)(g-1)$ is distributed as chi-squared with $(r-1)(g-1)$ degrees of freedom [61]. The asymptotic probability value is the proportion of the appropriate chi-squared distribution equal to or greater than the observed value of $t_b(N-1)(g-1)$.

4.4.1 Example 1

Consider a sample of $N = 80$ seventh grade female students, all from complete families with three children, stratified by Resident Type (Rural, Suburban, or Urban). Each subject is categorized into one of four Personality Characteristics

Table 4.13 Example data set of residence type (A) and personality type (B)

	Residence (A)			
Personality (B)	Rural	Suburb	Urban	Total
Domineering	15	15	15	45
Assertive	15	0	0	15
Submissive	0	15	0	15
Passive	0	0	5	5
Total	30	30	20	80

(Domineering, Assertive, Submissive, or Passive) in a classroom setting by a panel of trained observers. The data are given in Table 4.13. The null hypothesis posits that the proportions of the $r = 4$ observed Personality Types are the same for each of the $g = 3$ Residence Types. Thus, Residence Type (A) is the independent variable and Personality Type (B) is the dependent variable.

For the frequency data given in Table 4.13,

$$t_b = \frac{N \sum_{j=1}^{g} \sum_{i=1}^{r} \frac{n_{ij}^2}{n_{.j}} - \sum_{i=1}^{r} n_{i.}^2}{N^2 - \sum_{i=1}^{r} n_{i.}^2}$$

$$= \frac{80\left(\frac{15^2}{30} + \frac{15^2}{30} + \cdots + \frac{5^2}{20}\right) - (45^2 + 15^2 + 15^2 + 5^2)}{80^2 - (45^2 + 15^2 + 15^2 + 5^2)} = 0.2308\ .$$

There are only $M = 359{,}961$ possible, equally-likely arrangements in the reference set of all permutations of cell frequencies given the observed row and column marginal frequency distributions, $\{45, 15, 15, 5\}$ and $\{30, 30, 20\}$, respectively, making an exact permutation analysis reasonable. The exact upper-tail probability value for the observed value of t_b is $P = 0.1728$, i.e., the sum of the hypergeometric point probability values associated with values of $t_b = 0.2308$ or greater.

In dramatic contrast, the Pearson chi-squared test of homogeneity yields a computed value of $\chi^2 = 66.6667$ for the frequency data given in Table 4.13 and the exact Pearson χ^2 probability value is $P = 0.1699\times10^{-12}$. For comparison, the asymptotic Pearson χ^2 probability value based on $(r-1)(g-1) = (4-1)(3-1) = 6$ degrees of freedom is $P = 0.1969\times10^{-11}$.

The Pearson χ^2 test of homogeneity is a symmetrical test and does not distinguish between independent and dependent variables, thus excluding important information. Because the Pearson χ^2 test of homogeneity considers both variables A and B, some insight can be gained by calculating a value for t_a. For the frequency data given in Table 4.13,

$$t_a = \frac{N \sum_{i=1}^{r} \sum_{j=1}^{g} \frac{n_{ij}^2}{n_{i.}} - \sum_{j=1}^{g} n_{.j}^2}{N^2 - \sum_{j=1}^{g} n_{.j}^2}$$

$$= \frac{80\left(\frac{15^2}{45} + \frac{15^2}{45} + \cdots + \frac{5^2}{5}\right) - (30^2 + 30^2 + 20^2)}{80^2 - (30^2 + 30^2 + 20^2)} = 0.4286\,,$$

which is considerably larger than the value for t_b of 0.2308. There are only $M = 359{,}961$ possible, equally-likely arrangements in the reference set of all permutations of cell frequencies given the observed row and column marginal frequency distributions, $\{45, 15, 15, 5\}$ and $\{30, 30, 20\}$, respectively, making an exact permutation analysis feasible. The exact upper-tail probability value for the observed value of t_a is $P = 0.0073$, i.e., the sum of the hypergeometric point probability values associated with values of $t_a = 0.4286$ or greater.

Clearly, the Pearson χ^2 test of homogeneity is detecting the substantial departure from homogeneity of the row proportions. This is reflected in the relatively low probability value for t_a ($P = 0.0073$) where the column variable (A) is considered to be the dependent variable. As the dependent variable of interest is variable B, the Pearson χ^2 test of homogeneity yields a misleading result with an asymptotic probability value of $P = 0.1969 \times 10^{-11}$ compared with the exact probability value for t_b of $P = 0.1728$.

Table 4.14 displays the conditional column proportions obtained from the sample cell frequencies of Table 4.13. In Table 4.14, variable B is the dependent variable and the conditional column proportions are given by $p_{i|j} = n_{ij}/n_{.j}$, e.g., $p_{1|1} = 15/30 = 0.5000$. Table 4.15 displays the conditional row proportions obtained from the sample cell frequencies of Table 4.13. In Table 4.15, variable A is the dependent variable and the conditional row proportions are given by $p_{j|i} = n_{ij}/n_{i.}$, e.g., $p_{1|1} = 15/45 = 0.3333$.

Table 4.14 Conditional column proportions for residence type (A) and personality type (B)

	Residence (A)		
Personality (B)	Rural	Suburb	Urban
Domineering	0.5000	0.5000	0.7500
Assertive	0.5000	0.0000	0.0000
Submissive	0.0000	0.5000	0.0000
Passive	0.0000	0.0000	0.2500
Total	1.0000	1.0000	1.0000

Table 4.15 Conditional row proportions for residence type (A) and personality type (B)

	Residence (A)			
Personality (B)	Rural	Suburb	Urban	Total
Domineering	0.3333	0.3333	0.3333	1.0000
Assertive	1.0000	0.0000	0.0000	1.0000
Submissive	0.0000	1.0000	0.0000	1.0000
Passive	0.0000	0.0000	1.0000	1.0000

Even the most casual inspection of Tables 4.14 and 4.15 reveals the relative homogeneity extant among the proportions in the columns of Table 4.14, compared with the lack of homogeneity among the proportions in the rows of Table 4.15. Compare, for example, the Domineering (0.3333, 0.3333, 0.3333) and Assertive (1.0000, 0.0000, 0.0000) row proportions in Table 4.15. It is this departure from homogeneity in the row proportions that contributes to the low probability value, i.e., $P = 0.1969 \times 10^{-11}$, associated with the Pearson χ^2 test of homogeneity.

4.4.2 Example 2

To clarify the utility of a test of homogeneity based on Goodman and Kruskal's t_b test statistic, consider a simplified example. Suppose that a researcher wishes to conduct a test of homogeneity with respect to Voting Behavior on three categories of Marital Status. The null hypothesis posits that the proportions of the $r = 3$ observed categories of Marital Status (independent variable) are the same for each of the $g = 3$ categories of Voting Behavior (dependent variable). The researcher obtains three independent simple random samples of 80 individuals from each of the three categories of Marital Status—Single, Married, and Divorced—in a local election. Table 4.16 contains the raw frequency data and conditional row proportions where independent variable Marital Status (Single, Married, Divorced) is cross-classified with dependent variable Voting Behavior (Republican, Democrat, Independent).

Table 4.16 Example data set of marital status (A) and voting behavior (B) with row proportions in parentheses

	Voting Behavior (B)			
Marital Status (A)	Republican	Democrat	Independent	Total
Single	50 (0.625)	20 (0.250)	10 (0.125)	80 (1.000)
Married	50 (0.625)	20 (0.250)	10 (0.125)	80 (1.000)
Divorced	50 (0.625)	20 (0.250)	10 (0.125)	80 (1.000)
Total	150	60	30	240

Because the frequency data given in Table 4.16 correspond to the expected values for each of the nine cells, Pearson's chi-squared test of homogeneity is $\chi^2 = 0.00$ with a probability value under the null hypothesis of $P = 1.00$. In contrast, Goodman and Kruskal's test statistic, with variable B (Voting Behavior) the dependent variable is $t_b = 1.00$ with a probability value under the null hypothesis of $P = 0.00$.

4.5 The Measurement of Agreement

The measurement of agreement is a special case of measuring association between two or more variables. A number of statistical research problems require the measurement of agreement, rather than association or correlation. Agreement indices measure the extent to which a set of response measurements are identical to another set, i.e., agree, rather than the extent to which one set of response measurements is a linear function of another set of response measurements, i.e., correlated.

The usual research situation involving a measure of agreement arises when several judges or raters assign objects to a set of disjoint, unordered categories. In 1957, W.S. Robinson published an article in *American Sociological Review* on "The statistical measurement of agreement" [73]. In this formative article, Robinson developed the idea of agreement, as contrasted with correlation, and showed that a simple modification of the intraclass correlation coefficient was an appropriate measure of statistical agreement, which he called A, presumably for agreement [73, p. 20]. Robinson explained that statistical agreement requires that paired values be identical, while correlation requires only that the paired values be linked by some mathematical function [73, p. 19]. Thus, agreement is a more restrictive measure than is correlation. Robinson argued that the distinction between agreement and correlation leads to the conclusion that a logically correct estimate of the reliability of a test is given by the intraclass correlation coefficient rather than the Pearsonian (interclass) correlation coefficient and that the concept of agreement, rather than correlation, is the proper basis of reliability theory [73, p. 18]. The 1957 Robinson article, which was quite mathematical, was followed by a more interpretive article in 1959 in the same journal on "The geometric interpretation of agreement" [74].

A measure of inter-rater agreement should, as a minimum, embody seven basic attributes [16]. First, it is generally agreed that a measure of agreement should be chance corrected, i.e., any agreement coefficient should reflect the amount of agreement in excess of what would be expected by chance. Several researchers have advocated chance-corrected measures of agreement, including Brennan and Prediger [20], Cicchetti, Showalter, and Tyrer [21], Cohen [23], Conger [26], and Krippendorff [50]. Although some investigators have argued against chance-corrected measures of agreement, e.g., Armitage, Blendis, and Smyllie [3] and Goodman and Kruskal [37], supporters of chance-corrected measures of agreement far outweigh detractors.

Second, as noted by Bartko [4, 5], Bartko and Carpenter [5], Krippendorff [50], and Robinson [72], a measure of inter-rater agreement possesses an added advantage if it is directly applicable to the assessment of reliability. Robinson, in particular, was emphatic that reliability could not simply be measured by some function of Pearsonian product-moment correlation, such as in the split-half or test–retest methods, and argued that the concept of agreement should be the basis of reliability theory, not correlation [73, p. 18].

Third, a number of researchers have commented on the simplicity of Euclidean distance for measures of inter-rater agreement, noting that the squaring of differences between scale values is questionable at best, while acknowledging that squared differences allow for familiar interpretations of coefficients [34, 50]. Moreover, Graham and Jackson noted that squaring of differences between values, i.e., quadratic weighting, results in a measure of association, not agreement [41]. Thus, Euclidean distance is a desired property for measures of inter-rater agreement.

Fourth, every measure of agreement should have a statistical base [5]. A measure of agreement without a proper test of significance is severely limited in application to practical research situations. Asymptotic analyses are interesting and useful, under large sample conditions, but often limited in their practical utility when sample sizes are small.

Fifth, a measure of agreement that analyzes multivariate data has a decided advantage over univariate measures of agreement. Thus, if one observer locates a set of objects in an r-dimensional space, a multivariate measure of agreement can ascertain the degree to which a second observer locates the same set of objects in the defined r-dimensional space.

Sixth, a measure of agreement should be able to analyze data at any level of measurement. Cohen's kappa measure of inter-rater agreement is, at the present time, the most widely used measure of agreement. Extensions of Cohen's kappa to incompletely ranked data by Iachan [46] and to continuous categorical data by Conger [26] have been established. An extension of Cohen's kappa measure of agreement to fully ranked ordinal data and to interval data was provided by Berry and Mielke in 1988 [16].

Seventh, a measure of agreement should be able to evaluate information from more than two raters or judges. Fleiss proposed a measure of agreement for multiple raters on a nominal scale [33]. Williams presented a measure that was limited to comparisons of the joint agreement of several raters with another rater singled out as being of special interest [88]. Landis and Koch considered agreement among several raters in terms of a majority opinion [51]. Light focused on an extension of Cohen's [23] kappa measure of inter-rater agreement to multiple raters that was based on the average of all pairwise kappa values [54].

Unfortunately, the measure proposed by Fleiss was dependent on the average proportion of raters who agree on the classification of each observation. The limitation in the measure proposed by Williams appears to be overly restrictive, and the formulation by Landis and Koch becomes computationally prohibitive if either the number of observers or the number of response categories is large. Moreover, the extension of kappa proposed by Fleiss did not reduce to Cohen's kappa when the number of raters was two. Finally, Hubert [44] and Conger [25] provided critical summaries of the problem of extending Cohen's kappa measure of inter-rater agreement to multiple raters for categorical data.

4.5.1 Robinson's Measure of Agreement

An early measure of maximum-corrected agreement was developed by W.S. Robinson in 1957 [73, 74]. Assume that $k = 2$ judges independently rate N objects. Robinson argued that the Pearson product-moment (interclass) correlation calculated between the ratings of two judges was an inadequate measure of agreement because it measures the degree to which the paired values of the two variables are proportional, when expressed as deviations from their means, rather than identical [73, p. 19]. Robinson proposed a new measure of agreement based on the intraclass correlation coefficient that he called A. Consider two sets of ratings such as given in Table 4.17, where there are $N = 3$ pairs of values. Robinson defined A as:

$$A = 1 - \frac{D}{D_{\max}} ,$$

where D (for Disagreement) is given by:

$$D = \sum_{i=1}^{N} (X_{1i} - \bar{X}_i)^2 + \sum_{i=1}^{N} (X_{2i} - \bar{X}_i)^2$$

and

$$X_{1i} = \text{ the value of } X_1 \text{ for the } i\text{th pair of ratings} ,$$

$$X_{2i} = \text{ the value of } X_2 \text{ for the } i\text{th pair of ratings} ,$$

$$\bar{X}_i = \text{ the mean of } X_1 \text{ and } X_2 \text{ for the } i\text{th pair of ratings} .$$

Robinson noted that, by itself, D is not a very useful measure because it involves the units of X_1 and X_2. To find a relative, rather than an absolute, measure of agreement, Robinson standardized D by its range of possible variation, given by:

$$D_{\max} = \sum_{i=1}^{N} (X_{1i} - \bar{X})^2 + \sum_{i=1}^{N} (X_{2i} - \bar{X})^2 ,$$

Table 4.17 Example data for Robinson's A coefficient of agreement

X_1	X_2
1	2
3	7
8	12

Table 4.18 Illustration of the calculation of Robinson's D coefficient of agreement

X_{1i}	X_{2i}	$\bar{X}_i$	$(X_{1i} - \bar{X}_i)^2$	$(X_{2i} - \bar{X}_i)^2$
1	2	1.50	0.25	0.25
3	7	5.00	4.00	4.00
8	12	10.00	4.00	4.00
12	21		8.25	8.25

where the common mean is given by:

$$\bar{X} = \frac{\sum_{i=1}^{N} X_{1i} + \sum_{i=1}^{N} X_{2i}}{2N} .$$

Example

Consider the data listed in Table 4.17 on p. 162 with $N = 3$ paired observations and $k = 2$ sets of ratings, replicated in Table 4.18 for convenience. Then,

$$D = \sum_{i=1}^{N} (X_{1i} - \bar{X}_i)^2 + \sum_{i=1}^{N} (X_{2i} - \bar{X}_i)^2 = 8.25 + 8.25 = 16.50 .$$

Define the common mean as:

$$\bar{X} = \frac{\sum_{i=1}^{N} X_{1i} + \sum_{i=1}^{N} X_{2i}}{2N} = \frac{12 + 21}{(2)(3)} = 5.50 ,$$

then the maximum value of D is illustrated in Table 4.19. The maximum value of D is then

$$D_{\max} = \sum_{i=1}^{N} (X_{1i} - \bar{X})^2 + \sum_{i=1}^{N} (X_{2i} - \bar{X})^2 = 32.75 + 56.75 = 89.50$$

Table 4.19 Illustration of calculation of Robinson's maximum value of D

X_{1i}	X_{2i}	$\bar{X}_i$	$(X_{1i} - \bar{X}_i)^2$	$(X_{2i} - \bar{X}_i)^2$
1	2	5.50	20.25	12.25
3	7	5.50	6.25	2.25
8	12	5.50	6.25	42.25
12	21		32.75	56.75

Table 4.20 The $M = 6$ possible arrangements of the X_{1i} values, $i = 1, 2, 3$, with associated values of Robinson's D and A

Arrangement	X_1	D	A
1*	1, 3, 8	16.50	0.8156
2	3, 1, 8	26.50	0.7039
3	1, 8, 3	41.50	0.5363
4	3, 8, 1	61.50	0.3128
5	8, 1, 3	76.50	0.1453
6	8, 3, 1	86.50	0.0335

and Robinson's A is

$$A = 1 - \frac{D}{D_{\max}} = 1 - \frac{16.50}{89.50} = 0.8156 .$$

The sums,

$$\sum_{i=1}^{N} X_{1i} = 12 \quad \text{and} \quad \sum_{i=1}^{N} X_{2i} = 21 ,$$

are invariant under permutation. Therefore, $\bar{X} = 5.50$ and $D_{\max} = 89.50$ are also invariant under permutation. Moreover,

$$\sum_{i=1}^{N} (X_{1i} - \bar{X}_i)^2 = \sum_{i=1}^{N} (X_{2i} - \bar{X}_i)^2$$

for all arrangements of the observed data. Thus, for an exact permutation analysis, it is only required to calculate either

$$\sum_{i=1}^{N} (X_{1i} - \bar{X}_i)^2 \quad \text{or} \quad \sum_{i=1}^{N} (X_{2i} - \bar{X}_i)^2 .$$

In addition, it is only necessary to shuffle either the X_{1i} values or the X_{2i} values, $i = 1, 2, 3$, while holding the X_{2i} or X_{1i} values, respectively, constant.

For the data listed in Table 4.18, there are only $M = 6$ possible, equally-likely arrangements of the observed data. Since $M = 6$ is a very small number, it will be illustrative to list the shuffled X_{1i} values and the associated D and A values in Table 4.20, where the arrangement with the observed values in Table 4.18 is indicated with an asterisk. The exact upper-tail probability of the observed value of

Table 4.21 Example data for the intraclass correlation coefficient

X_{1i}	X_{2i}	X_{1i}^2	X_{2i}^2	$X_{1i}X_{2i}$
1	2	1	4	2
3	7	9	49	21
8	12	64	144	96
2	1	4	1	2
7	3	49	9	21
12	8	144	64	96
33	33	271	271	238

$A = 0.8156$ under the null hypothesis is given by:

$$P(A \geq A_\text{o}|H_0) = \frac{\text{number of } A \text{ values } \geq A_\text{o}}{M} = \frac{1}{6} = 0.1667\,,$$

where A_o denotes the observed value of Robinson's A. Alternatively,

$$P(D \leq D_\text{o}|H_0) = \frac{\text{number of } D \text{ values } \leq D_\text{o}}{M} = \frac{1}{6} = 0.1667\,,$$

where D_o denotes the observed value of Robinson's D.

The Intraclass Correlation Coefficient

It is well known that the intraclass correlation coefficient (r_I) between N pairs of observations on two variables is by definition the ordinary Pearson product-moment (interclass) correlation between $2N$ pairs of observations, the first N of which are the original observations, and the second N the original observations with X_{1i} replacing X_{2i} and vice versa for $i = 1, \ldots, N$ [31, Sect. 38]. Thus, the intraclass correlation between the values of X_{1i} and X_{2i} for $i = 1, \ldots, N$ given in Table 4.18 on p. 162 is the Pearson product-moment correlation between the six pairs of values, as illustrated in Table 4.21.

For the data given in Table 4.21 with $N = 6$ pairs of observations, the intraclass correlation coefficient is

$$r_\text{I} = r_{12} = \frac{N \displaystyle\sum_{i=1}^{N} X_{1j}X_{2i} - \sum_{i=1}^{N} X_{1i} \sum_{i=1}^{N} X_{2i}}{\sqrt{\left[N \displaystyle\sum_{i=1}^{N} X_{1i}^2 - \left(\sum_{i=1}^{N} X_{1i}\right)^2\right]\left[N \displaystyle\sum_{i=1}^{N} X_{2i}^2 - \left(\sum_{i=1}^{N} X_{2i}\right)^2\right]}}$$

$$= \frac{(6)(238) - (33)(33)}{\sqrt{\left[(6)(271) - (33)^2\right]\left[(6)(271) - (33)^2\right]}} = +0.6313\,. \qquad (4.4)$$

It is obvious from Eq. (4.4) that certain computational simplifications follow from the reversal of the variable values, i.e., the row and column marginal frequency distributions for the new variables are identical and, therefore, the means and variances of the new variables are identical [73, p. 20].

For the case of two variables, the relationships between Robinson's coefficient of agreement and the coefficient of intraclass correlation are given by:

$$r_{\mathrm{I}} = 2A - 1 \quad \text{and} \quad A = \frac{r_{\mathrm{I}} + 1}{2} \, .$$

Thus, in the case of two variables the intraclass correlation is a simple linear function of the coefficient of agreement. For the example data given in Table 4.18 on p. 162,

$$r_{\mathrm{I}} = 2(0.8156) - 1 = 0.6313 \quad \text{and} \quad A = \frac{0.6313 + 1}{2} = 0.8156 \, .$$

For $k > 2$ sets of ratings, the relationships between the intraclass correlation coefficient and Robinson's A are not so simple and are given by:

$$r_{\mathrm{I}} = \frac{kA - 1}{k - 1} \quad \text{and} \quad A = \frac{r_{\mathrm{I}}(k - 1) + 1}{k} \, . \tag{4.5}$$

It is apparent from the expressions in Eq. (4.5) that the value of the intraclass coefficient depends not only upon A but also upon k, the number of observations per case. The range of Robinson's A is always from zero to unity regardless of the number of observations. Therefore, comparisons between agreement coefficients based upon different numbers of variables are commensurable [73, p. 22]. The upper limit of the intraclass correlation coefficient is always unity, but its lower limit is $-1/(k - 1)$ [31, Sect. 38]. For $k = 2$ variables, the lower limit of r_{I} is -1, but for $k = 3$ variables the lower limit is $-1/2$, for $k = 4$ the lower limit is $-1/3$, for $k = 5$ the lower limit is $-1/4$, and so on.

4.5.2 Scott's π Measure of Agreement

An early measure of chance-corrected agreement was introduced by William Scott in 1955 [76]. Assume that two judges or raters independently classify each of N observations into one of c categories. The resulting classifications can be displayed in a $c \times c$ contingency table, such as the 3×3 table in Table 4.22, with frequencies for cell entries. Denote by a dot $(\cdot)$ the partial sum of all rows or all columns, depending on the position of the $(\cdot)$ in the subscript list. If the $(\cdot)$ is in the first subscript position, the sum is over all rows and if the $(\cdot)$ is in the second subscript position, the sum is over all columns. Thus, $n_{i.}$ denotes the marginal frequency total of the ith row, $i = 1, \ldots, r$, summed over all columns; $n_{.j}$ denotes the marginal frequency total

Table 4.22 Example 3×3 cross-classification (agreement) table with frequencies for cell entries

	Column			
Row	1	2	3	Total
1	n_{11}	n_{12}	n_{13}	$n_{1.}$
2	n_{21}	n_{22}	n_{23}	$n_{2.}$
3	n_{31}	n_{32}	n_{33}	$n_{3.}$
Total	$n_{.1}$	$n_{.2}$	$n_{.3}$	N

of the jth column, $j = 1, \ldots, c$, summed over all rows; and

$$N = \sum_{i=1}^{r} \sum_{j=1}^{c} n_{ij}$$

denotes the table frequency total. In the notation of Table 4.22, Scott's coefficient of agreement for nominal-level data is given by:

$$\pi = \frac{p_{\mathrm{o}} - p_{\mathrm{e}}}{1 - p_{\mathrm{e}}} , \tag{4.6}$$

where

$$p_{\mathrm{o}} = \frac{1}{N} \sum_{i=1}^{c} n_{ii} \quad \text{and} \quad p_{\mathrm{e}} = \frac{1}{4N^2} \sum_{k=1}^{c} \left(n_{.k} + n_{k.} \right)^2 .$$

In this configuration, p_{o} is the observed proportion of observations on which the judges agree, p_{e} is the proportion of observations for which agreement is expected by chance, $p_{\mathrm{o}} - p_{\mathrm{e}}$ is the proportion of agreement beyond that expected by chance, $1 - p_{\mathrm{e}}$ is the maximum possible proportion of agreement beyond that expected by chance, and Scott's π is the proportion of agreement between the two judges, after chance agreement has been removed.

Example

For an example of Scott's π measure of inter-rater agreement, consider the frequency data given in Table 4.23, where two judges have independently classified $N = 40$ objects into four disjoint categories: A, B, C, and D. For the agreement data given in Table 4.23,

$$p_{\mathrm{o}} = \frac{1}{N} \sum_{1=1}^{c} n_{ii} = \frac{4+4+4+4}{40} = 0.40 ,$$

$$p_{\mathrm{e}} = \frac{1}{4N^2} \sum_{k=1}^{c} (n_{.k} + n_{k.})^2 = \frac{1}{(4)(40^2)} \big[(10+10)^2 + (10+10)^2$$

$$+ (10+10)^2 + (10+10)^2 \big] = 0.25 ,$$

Table 4.23 Example 4×4 cross-classification (agreement) table

	Judge 2				
Judge 1	A	B	C	D	Total
A	4	3	2	1	10
B	3	4	1	3	10
C	2	1	4	2	10
D	1	2	3	4	10
Total	10	10	10	10	40

and the observed value of Scott's π is

$$\pi = \frac{p_\mathrm{o} - p_\mathrm{e}}{1 - p_\mathrm{e}} = \frac{0.40 - 0.25}{1 - 0.25} = +0.20 \,, \qquad (4.7)$$

indicating 20% agreement above that expected by chance.

The exact probability value of an observed value of Scott's π under the null hypothesis is given by the sum of the hypergeometric point probability values associated with the π values equal to or greater than the observed π value. For the frequency data given in Table 4.23, there are only $M = 5{,}045{,}326$ possible, equally-likely arrangements in the reference set of all permutations of cell frequencies given the observed row and column marginal frequency distributions, $\{10, 10, 10, 10\}$ and $\{10, 10, 10, 10\}$, respectively, making an exact permutation analysis possible. The exact upper-tail probability value of the observed π value is $P = 0.2047$, i.e., the sum of the hypergeometric point probability values associated with values of $\pi = +0.20$ or greater.

While Scott's π is interesting from a historical perspective, π has fallen into desuetude and is no longer found in the current literature. Based as it is on joint proportions, Scott's π makes the assumption that the two judges have the same distribution of responses, as in the example data in Table 4.18 on p. 162 with identical marginal distributions, $\{10, 10, 10, 10\}$ and $\{10, 10, 10, 10\}$. Cohen's κ measure does not make this assumption and, consequently, has emerged as the preferred chance-corrected measure of inter-rater agreement for two judges/raters.

4.5.3 Cohen's κ Measure of Agreement

Currently, the most popular measure of agreement between two judges or raters is the chance-corrected measure of inter-rater agreement first proposed by Jacob Cohen in 1960 and termed kappa [23]. Cohen's kappa measures the magnitude of agreement between $b = 2$ observers on the assignment of N objects to a set of c disjoint, unordered categories. In 1968, Cohen proposed a version of kappa that allowed for weighting of the c categories [24]. Whereas the original (unweighted)

Table 4.24 Example 3×3 cross-classification table with proportions for cell entries

Row	Column 1	2	3	Total
1	p_{11}	p_{12}	p_{13}	$p_{1.}$
2	p_{21}	p_{22}	p_{23}	$p_{2.}$
3	p_{31}	p_{32}	p_{33}	$p_{3.}$
Total	$p_{.1}$	$p_{.2}$	$p_{.3}$	$p_{..}$

kappa did not distinguish among magnitudes of disagreement, weighted kappa incorporated the magnitude of each disagreement and provided partial credit for disagreements when agreement was not complete [57]. The usual approach is to assign weights to each disagreement pair with larger weights indicating greater disagreement.[4]

In both the unweighted and weighted cases, kappa is equal to +1 when perfect agreement among two or more judges occurs, 0 when agreement is equal to that expected under independence, and negative when agreement is less than expected by chance. Because weighted kappa applies to ordered categories, it is discussed in Chap. 6. Unweighted kappa is discussed here as it is typically used for unordered categorical data.

Assume that two judges or raters independently classify each of N observations into one of c mutually exclusive, exhaustive, unordered categories. The resulting classifications can be displayed in a $c \times c$ cross-classification, such as the 3×3 contingency table in Table 4.24, with proportions for cell entries. Denote by a dot $(\cdot)$ the partial sum of all rows or all columns, depending on the position of the $(\cdot)$ in the subscript list. If the $(\cdot)$ is in the first subscript position, the sum is over all rows and if the $(\cdot)$ is in the second subscript position, the sum is over all columns. Thus, $p_{i.}$ denotes the marginal proportion total of the ith row, $i = 1, \ldots, c$, summed over all columns; $p_{.j}$ denotes the marginal proportion total of the jth column, $j = 1, \ldots, c$, summed over all rows; and $p_{..} = 1.00$. In the notation of Table 4.24, Cohen's unweighted kappa coefficient for nominal-level data is given by:

$$\kappa = \frac{p_{\mathrm{o}} - p_{\mathrm{e}}}{1 - p_{\mathrm{e}}} \,, \tag{4.8}$$

where

$$p_{\mathrm{o}} = \sum_{i=1}^{c} p_{ii} \quad \text{and} \quad p_{\mathrm{e}} = \sum_{i=1}^{c} p_{i.}p_{.i} \,.$$

[4]Some authors prefer to define kappa in terms of agreement weights, instead of disagreement weights, e.g., Fleiss [33] and Vanbelle and Albert [83].

Cohen's kappa can also be defined in terms of raw frequency values, making calculations somewhat more straightforward. Thus,

$$\kappa = \frac{\sum_{i=1}^{c} O_{ii} - \sum_{i=1}^{c} E_{ii}}{N - \sum_{i=1}^{c} E_{ii}} ,$$

where O_{ii} denotes an observed cell frequency value on the principal diagonal of a $c \times c$ agreement table, E_{ii} denotes an expected cell frequency value on the principal diagonal, and

$$E_{ii} = \frac{n_{i.}n_{.i}}{N} \qquad \text{for } i = 1, \ldots, c .$$

In the configuration of Table 4.24, p_{o} is the observed proportion of observations on which the judges agree, p_{e} is the proportion of observations for which agreement is expected by chance, $p_{\text{o}} - p_{\text{e}}$ is the proportion of agreement beyond that expected by chance, $1 - p_{\text{e}}$ is the maximum possible proportion of agreement beyond that expected by chance, and Cohen's kappa test statistic is the proportion of agreement between the two judges, after chance agreement has been removed.

Example 1

To illustrate Cohen's kappa measure of chance-corrected inter-rater agreement, consider the frequency data given in Table 4.25 where two judges have independently classified $N = 5$ objects into $c = 3$ disjoint, unordered categories: A, B, and C. For the agreement data given in Table 4.25,

$$p_{\text{o}} = \sum_{i=1}^{c} p_{ii} = \frac{0}{5} + \frac{2}{5} + \frac{1}{5} = 0.60 ,$$

$$p_{\text{e}} = \sum_{i=1}^{c} p_{i.}p_{.i} = \left(\frac{1}{5}\right)\left(\frac{1}{5}\right) + \left(\frac{2}{5}\right)\left(\frac{3}{5}\right) + \left(\frac{2}{5}\right)\left(\frac{1}{5}\right) = 0.36 ,$$

and following Eq. (4.8), the observed value of Cohen's κ is

$$\kappa = \frac{p_{\text{o}} - p_{\text{e}}}{1 - p_{\text{e}}} = \frac{0.60 - 0.36}{1 - 0.36} = +0.3750 ,$$

indicating approximately 37% agreement above that expected by chance.

Table 4.25 Example 3×3 cross-classification table for Cohen's unweighted kappa

	Judge 2			
Judge 1	A	B	C	Total
A	0	1	0	1
B	0	2	0	2
C	1	0	1	2
Total	1	3	1	5

Table 4.26 Listing of the eight sets of 3×3 cell frequencies with row marginal distribution {1, 2, 2} and column marginal distribution {1, 3, 1}

Table 1			Table 2			Table 3			Table 4		
0	0	1	0	1	0	0	1	0	0	0	1
0	2	0	0	1	1	0	2	0	1	1	0
1	1	0	1	1	0	1	0	1	0	2	0
Table 5			Table 6			Table 7			Table 8		
0	1	0	0	1	0	1	0	0	1	0	0
1	0	1	0	1	1	0	1	1	0	2	0
0	2	0	0	1	1	0	2	0	0	1	1

Table 4.27 Kappa and hypergeometric probability values for the eight 3×3 contingency tables listed in Table 4.26

Table	κ	Probability
8∗	+0.6875	0.2000
3∗	+0.3750	0.1000
1	+0.0625	0.1000
6	+0.0625	0.1000
7	+0.0625	0.1000
2	−0.2500	0.1000
4	−0.2500	0.1000
5	−0.5625	0.2000

The exact probability value of an observed κ value under the null hypothesis is given by the sum of the hypergeometric point probability values associated with the κ values equal to or greater than the observed κ value. For the frequency data given in Table 4.25, there are only $M = 8$ possible, equally-likely arrangements in the reference set of all permutations of cell frequencies given the observed row and column marginal frequency distributions, $\{1, 2, 2\}$ and $\{1, 3, 1\}$, respectively, making an exact permutation analysis possible. The eight possible arrangements of cell frequencies, given the observed marginal frequency totals, are listed in Table 4.26, where Table 3 of Table 4.26 contains the $N = 5$ observed cell frequencies.

Table 4.27 lists the computed κ values and associated hypergeometric point probability values for the $M = 8$ tables given in Table 4.26, ordered from high to low by the κ values. Only two κ values are equal to or greater than the observed value of $\kappa = +0.3750$, those belonging to Tables 8 and 3 (indicated with asterisks). Thus, the exact upper-tail probability value of the observed κ value is $P = 0.2000 + 0.1000 = 0.3000$, the sum of the hypergeometric point probability

Table 4.28 Example 4×4 cross-classification table

	Judge 2				
Judge 1	A	B	C	D	Total
A	8	4	2	1	15
B	1	7	6	3	17
C	2	4	9	5	20
D	0	1	7	8	16
Total	11	16	24	17	68

values associated with values of $\kappa = +0.3750$ or greater, i.e., $\kappa_8 = +0.6875$ and $\kappa_3 = +0.3750$.

Example 2

For a second, more realistic, example of Cohen's unweighted kappa measure of chance-corrected inter-rater agreement, consider the frequency data given in Table 4.28, where two judges have independently classified $N = 68$ objects into four disjoint, unordered categories: A, B, C, and D. For the agreement data given in Table 4.28,

$$p_{\text{o}} = \sum_{i=1}^{c} p_{ii} = \frac{8}{68} + \frac{7}{68} + \frac{9}{68} + \frac{8}{68} = 0.4706 ,$$

$$\begin{aligned} p_{\text{e}} &= \sum_{i=1}^{c} p_{i.}p_{.i} \\ &= \left(\frac{15}{68}\right)\left(\frac{11}{68}\right) + \left(\frac{17}{68}\right)\left(\frac{16}{68}\right) + \left(\frac{20}{68}\right)\left(\frac{24}{68}\right) + \left(\frac{16}{68}\right)\left(\frac{17}{68}\right) \\ &= 0.2571 , \end{aligned}$$

and following Eq. (4.8), the observed value of Cohen's κ is

$$\kappa = \frac{p_{\text{o}} - p_{\text{e}}}{1 - p_{\text{e}}} = \frac{0.4706 - 0.2571}{1 - 0.2571} = +0.2873 ,$$

indicating approximately 29% agreement above that expected by chance.

The exact probability value of an observed κ value under the null hypothesis is given by the sum of the hypergeometric point probability values associated with κ values equal to or greater than the observed κ value. For the frequency data given in Table 4.28, there are $M = 181{,}260{,}684$ possible, equally-likely arrangements in the reference set of all permutations of cell frequencies, given the observed row and column marginal frequency distributions, $\{15, 17, 20, 16\}$ and $\{11, 16, 24, 17\}$, respectively, making an exact permutation analysis feasible. The exact upper-tail probability value of the observed κ value is $P = 0.1098\times10^{-3}$, i.e., the sum of the hypergeometric point probability values associated with values of $\kappa = +0.2873$ or greater.

4.5.4 Application with Multiple Judges

Cohen's κ measure of chance-corrected inter-rater agreement was originally designed for, and limited to, only $b = 2$ judges. In this section, a procedure is introduced for computing unweighted kappa with multiple judges. Although the procedure is appropriate for any number of $c \geq 2$ disjoint, unordered categories and $b \geq 2$ judges, the description of the procedure is confined to $b = 3$ independent judges and the example is limited to $b = 3$ independent judges and $c = 3$ disjoint, unordered categories to simplify presentation.

Consider $b = 3$ judges who independently classify N objects into c disjoint, unordered categories. The classification may be conceptualized as a $c\times c\times c$ contingency table with c rows, c columns, and c slices. Let n_{ijk}, R_i, C_j, and S_k denote the observed cell frequencies and the row, column, and slice marginal frequency totals for $i, j, k = 1, \ldots, c$ and let the frequency total be given by:

$$N = \sum_{i=1}^{c} \sum_{j=1}^{c} \sum_{k=1}^{c} n_{ijk} \ .$$

Cohen's unweighted kappa test statistic for a three-way contingency table is given by:

$$\kappa = 1 - \frac{N^2 \displaystyle\sum_{i=1}^{c} \sum_{j=1}^{c} \sum_{k=1}^{c} w_{ijk} n_{ijk}}{\displaystyle\sum_{i=1}^{c} \sum_{j=1}^{c} \sum_{k=1}^{c} w_{ijk} R_i C_j S_k} , \tag{4.9}$$

where w_{ijk} are disagreement "weights" assigned to each cell for $i, j, k = 1, \ldots, c$. For unweighted kappa, the disagreement weights are given by:

$$w_{ijk} = \begin{cases} 0 & \text{if } i = j = k \ , \\ 1 & \text{otherwise} \ . \end{cases}$$

Given a $c\times c\times c$ contingency table with N objects cross-classified by $b = 3$ independent judges, an exact permutation test involves generating all possible, equally-likely arrangements of the N objects to the c^3 cells, while preserving the marginal frequency distributions. For each arrangement of cell frequencies, the unweighted kappa statistic, κ, and the exact hypergeometric point probability value under the null hypothesis, $p(n_{ijk}|R_i, C_j, S_k, N)$, are calculated, where

$$p(n_{ijk}|R_i, C_j, S_k, N) = \frac{\left(\prod_{i=1}^{c} R_i!\right)\left(\prod_{j=1}^{c} C_j!\right)\left(\prod_{k=1}^{c} S_k!\right)}{(N!)^{b-1}\prod_{i=1}^{c}\prod_{j=1}^{c}\prod_{k=1}^{c} n_{ijk}!} . \tag{4.10}$$

If κ_{o} denotes the value of the observed unweighted kappa test statistic, the exact probability value of κ_{o} under the null hypothesis is given by:

$$P(\kappa_{\text{o}}) = \sum_{l=1}^{M} \Psi_l\left(n_{ijk}|R_i, C_j, S_k, N\right) ,$$

where

$$\Psi_l\left(n_{ijk}|R_i, C_j, S_k, N\right) = \begin{cases} p(n_{ijk}|R_i, C_j, S_k, N) & \text{if } \kappa \geq \kappa_{\text{o}} , \\ 0 & \text{otherwise} , \end{cases}$$

and M denotes the total number of possible, equally-likely cell frequency arrangements in the reference set of all possible arrangements of cell frequencies, given the observed marginal frequency distributions. When M is very large, as is typical with multi-way contingency tables, exact tests are impractical and Monte Carlo resampling procedures become necessary. In such cases, a random sample of the M possible, equally-likely arrangements of cell frequencies provides a comparison of κ test statistics calculated on L random multi-way tables with the κ test statistic calculated on the observed multi-way contingency table.

An efficient Monte Carlo resampling algorithm to generate random cell frequency arrangements for multi-way contingency tables with fixed marginal frequency distributions was developed by Mielke, Berry, and Johnston in 2007 [66, pp. 19–20]. For a three-way contingency table with r rows, c columns, and s slices, the resampling algorithm is given in 12 simple steps.

STEP 1. Construct an $r \times c \times s$ contingency table from the observed data.

STEP 2. Obtain the fixed marginal frequency totals $R_1, \ldots, R_r$, $C_1, \ldots, C_c$, $S_1, \ldots, S_s$, and frequency total N. Set a resampling counter $JL = 0$, and set L equal to the number of samples desired.

STEP 3. Set the resampling counter $JL = JL + 1$.

STEP 4. Set the marginal frequency counters $JR_i = R_i$ for $i = 1, \ldots, r$; $JC_j = C_j$ for $j = 1, \ldots, c$; $JS_k = S_k$ for $k = 1, \ldots, s$, and $M = N$.

STEP 5. Set $n_{ijk} = 0$ for $i = 1, \ldots, r$, $j = 1, \ldots, c$, and $k = 1, \ldots, s$, and set row, column, and slice counters *IR*, *IC*, and *IS* equal to zero.

STEP 6. Create cumulative probability distributions PR_i, PC_j, and PS_k from the adjusted marginal frequency totals JR_i, JC_j, and JS_k for $i = 1, \ldots, r$, $j = 1, \ldots, c$, and $k = 1, \ldots, s$, where

$$PR_1 = JR_1/M \quad \text{and} \quad PR_i = PR_{i-1} + JR_i/M$$

for $i = 1, \ldots, r$,

$$PC_1 = JC_1/M \quad \text{and} \quad PC_j = PC_{j-1} + JC_j/M$$

for $j = 1, \ldots, c$, and

$$PS_1 = JS_1/M \quad \text{and} \quad PS_k = PS_{k-1} + JS_k/M$$

for $k = 1, \ldots, s$.

STEP 7. Generate three uniform pseudorandom numbers U_r, U_c, and U_s over $[0, 1)$ and set row, column, and slice indices $i = j = k = 1$, respectively.

STEP 8. If $U_r \leq PR_i$, then $IR = i$, $JR_i = JR_i - 1$, and go to STEP 9; otherwise, $i = i + 1$ and repeat STEP 8.

STEP 9. If $U_c \leq PC_j$, then $IC = j$, $JC_j = JC_j - 1$, and go to STEP 10; otherwise, $j = j + 1$ and repeat STEP 9.

STEP 10. If $U_s \leq PS_k$, then $IS = k$, $JS_k = JS_k - 1$, and go to STEP 11; otherwise, $k = k + 1$ and repeat STEP 10.

STEP 11. Set $M = M - 1$ and $n_{IR,IC,IS} = n_{IR,IC,IS} + 1$. If $M > 0$, go to STEP 4; otherwise, obtain the required test statistic.

STEP 12. If $JL < L$, go to STEP 3; otherwise, stop.

At the conclusion of the resampling procedure, Cohen's κ, as given in Eq. (4.9) on p. 172, is obtained for each of the L random three-way contingency tables, given fixed marginal frequency distributions. Let κ_o denote the observed value of κ, then under the null hypothesis the resampling approximate probability value for κ_o is given by:

$$P(\kappa_o) = \frac{1}{L} \sum_{l=1}^{L} \Psi_l(\kappa) ,$$

where

$$\Psi_l(\kappa) = \begin{cases} 1 & \text{if } \kappa \geq \kappa_o , \\ 0 & \text{otherwise} . \end{cases}$$

Table 4.29 Classification of $N = 93$ objects by three independent judges into one of three disjoint, unordered categories: A, B, or C, with disagreement weights in parentheses

		Judge 3		
Judge 1	Judge 2	A	B	C
A	A	6 (0)	4 (1)	2 (1)
	B	3 (1)	5 (1)	4 (1)
	C	2 (1)	3 (1)	4 (1)
B	A	4 (1)	5 (1)	3 (1)
	B	5 (1)	8 (0)	4 (1)
	C	3 (1)	2 (1)	3 (1)
C	A	1 (1)	3 (1)	4 (1)
	B	3 (1)	2 (1)	2 (1)
	C	1 (1)	2 (1)	5 (0)

4.5.5 *Example Analysis with Multiple Judges*

The calculation of unweighted kappa and the resampling procedure for obtaining a probability value with multiple judges can be illustrated with a sparse data set. Consider $b = 3$ independent judges who classify $N = 93$ objects into one of $c = 3$ disjoint, unordered categories: A, B, or C. Table 4.29 lists the c^3 cross-classified frequencies and corresponding disagreement weights, where the cell disagreement weights are given in parentheses.

For the frequency data listed in Table 4.29, the observed value of kappa is $\kappa = +0.1007$, indicating approximately 10% agreement among the $b = 3$ judges above that expected by chance. If κ_o denotes the observed value of κ, the approximate resampling probability value based on $L = 1{,}000{,}000$ random arrangements of the observed data is

$$P(\kappa \geq \kappa_o | H_0) = \frac{\text{number of } \kappa \text{ values } \geq \kappa_o}{L} = \frac{8{,}311}{1{,}000{,}000} = 0.0083 \,.$$

4.6 McNemar's Q Test for Change

In 1947, psychologist Quinn McNemar proposed a test for change that was derived from the matched-pairs t test for proportions [63]. A typical application is to analyze binary responses, coded (0, 1), at $g = 2$ time periods for each of $N \geq 2$ subjects, such as Success and Failure, Yes and No, Agree and Disagree, or Pro and Con. If the four cells are identified as in Table 4.30, then McNemar's test for change is given by:

$$Q = \frac{(B - C)^2}{B + C} \,,$$

Table 4.30 Notation for a 2×2 cross-classification for McNemar's Q test for change

	Time 2		
Time 1	Pro	Con	Total
Pro	A	B	$A+B$
Con	C	D	$C+D$
Total	$A+C$	$B+D$	N

where $N = A + B + C + D$ and B and C represent the two cells of change, i.e., from Pro to Con and from Con to Pro.

Alternatively, McNemar's Q test can be thought of as a chi-squared goodness-of-fit test with two categories, where the observed frequencies, O_1 and O_2, correspond to cells B and C, respectively, and the expected frequencies, E_1 and E_2, are given by $E_1 = E_2 = (B + C)/2$, i.e., half the subjects are expected to change in one direction (e.g., from Pro to Con) and half in the other direction (e.g., from Con to Pro), under the null hypothesis of no change from Time 1 to Time 2. Let

$$E = \frac{B+C}{2}$$

denote an expected value where, by chance, half of the changes are from Pro to Con and half are from Con to Pro. Then, a chi-squared goodness of fit for the two categories of change is given by:

$$\chi^2 = \frac{(B-E)^2}{E} + \frac{(C-E)^2}{E} = \frac{B^2}{E} + \frac{C^2}{E} + 2E - 2B - 2C \; .$$

Substituting $(B + C)/2$ for E yields

$$\begin{aligned} &\frac{2B^2}{B+C} + \frac{2C^2}{B+C} + B + C - 2B - 2C \\ &= \frac{2B^2}{B+C} + \frac{2C^2}{B+C} - B - C \\ &= \frac{2B^2 + 2C^2 - B(B+C) - C(B+C)}{B+C} \\ &= \frac{B^2 - 2BC + C^2}{B+C} \\ &= \frac{(B-C)^2}{B+C} \; . \end{aligned}$$

4.6.1 Example 1

To illustrate McNemar's test for change, consider the frequency data given in Table 4.31, where $N = 50$ objects have been recorded as either Pro or Con on a specified issue at Time 1 and again on the same issue at Time 2. For the frequency data given in Table 4.31, the observed value of McNemar's Q test statistic is

$$Q = \frac{(B-C)^2}{B+C} = \frac{(5-25)^2}{5+25} = 13.3333 \; .$$

Alternatively, $O_1 = B = 5$, $O_2 = C = 25$, $E_1 = E_2 = (O_1 + O_2)/2 = (5+25)/2 = 15$, and

$$\chi_1^2 = \frac{(O_1 - E_1)^2}{E_1} + \frac{(O_2 - E_2)^2}{E_2} = \frac{(5-15)^2}{15} + \frac{(25-15)^2}{15} = 13.3333 \; .$$

The exact probability value of an observed value of Q, under the null hypothesis, is given by the sum of the hypergeometric point probability values associated with the Q values that are equal to or greater than the observed value of Q. For the frequency data listed in Table 4.31, there are only $M = 31$ possible, equally-likely arrangements in the reference set of all permutations of cell frequencies given the two cell frequencies of change, 5 and 25, and only 12 Q values are equal to or greater than the observed value of $Q = 13.3333$.

Since $M = 31$ is a reasonably small number of arrangements, it will be illustrative to list the complete set of Q values and the associated hypergeometric point probability values in Table 4.32, where rows with hypergeometric point probability values associated with Q values equal to or greater than the observed value of Q are indicated with asterisks. The exact upper-tail probability value of the observed value of Q is the sum of the hypergeometric point probability values that are associated with values of $Q = 13.3333$ or greater. Since the distribution of all possible Q values is symmetrical, the exact two-tailed probability value is

$$P = 2\Big(0.1327\times10^{-3} + 0.2552\times10^{-4} + 0.3781\times10^{-5} + 0.4051\times10^{-6} + 0.2794\times10^{-7} + 0.9313\times10^{-9}\Big) = 0.3429\times10^{-3} \; .$$

Table 4.31 Example frequency data for McNemar's test for change with $N = 50$ objects

	Time 2		
Time 1	Pro	Con	Total
Pro	15	5	20
Con	25	5	30
Total	40	10	50

Table 4.32 McNemar Q values and exact hypergeometric point probability values for $M = 31$ possible arrangements of the frequency data given in Table 4.31

Number	B	C	Q	Probability
1*	0	30	30.0000	0.9313×10^{-9}
2*	1	29	26.1333	0.2794×10^{-7}
3*	2	28	22.5333	0.4051×10^{-6}
4*	3	27	19.2000	0.3781×10^{-5}
5*	4	26	16.1333	0.2552×10^{-4}
6*	5	25	13.3333	0.1327×10^{-3}
7	6	24	10.8000	0.5530×10^{-3}
8	7	23	8.5333	0.1896×10^{-2}
9	8	22	6.5333	0.5451×10^{-2}
10	9	21	4.8000	0.1333×10^{-1}
11	10	20	3.3333	0.2798×10^{-1}
12	11	19	2.1333	0.5088×10^{-1}
13	12	18	1.2000	0.8055×10^{-1}
14	13	17	0.5333	0.1115
15	14	16	0.1333	0.1354
16	15	15	0.0000	0.1445
17	16	14	0.1333	0.1354
18	17	13	0.5333	0.1154
19	18	12	1.2000	0.8055×10^{-1}
20	19	11	2.1333	0.5088×10^{-1}
21	20	10	3.3333	0.2798×10^{-1}
22	21	9	4.8000	0.1333×10^{-1}
23	22	8	6.5333	0.5451×10^{-2}
24	23	7	8.5333	0.1896×10^{-2}
25	24	6	10.8000	0.5530×10^{-3}
26*	25	5	13.3333	0.1327×10^{-3}
27*	26	4	16.1333	0.2552×10^{-4}
28*	27	3	19.2000	0.3781×10^{-5}
29*	28	2	22.5333	0.4051×10^{-6}
30*	29	1	26.1333	0.2794×10^{-7}
31*	30	0	30.0000	0.9313×10^{-9}
Sum				1.0000

4.6.2 Example 2

For a second example of McNemar's Q test, consider the frequency data given in Table 4.33, where $N = 190$ objects have been recorded as either Pro or Con on a specified issue at Time 1 and again at Time 2. For the frequency data given in Table 4.33, the observed value of McNemar's Q test statistic is

$$Q = \frac{(B - C)^2}{B + C} = \frac{(59 - 37)^2}{59 + 37} = 5.0417 \; .$$

Table 4.33 Example frequency data for McNemar's test for change with $N = 190$ objects

	Time 2		
Time 1	Pro	Con	Total
Pro	73	59	132
Con	37	21	58
Total	110	80	190

Alternatively, $O_1 = B = 59$, $O_2 = C = 37$, $E_1 = E_2 = (O_1 + O_2)/2 = (59 + 37)/2 = 48$, and

$$\chi_1^2 = \frac{(O_1 - E_1)^2}{E_1} + \frac{(O_2 - E_2)^2}{E_2} = \frac{(59 - 48)^2}{48} + \frac{(37 - 48)^2}{48} = 5.0417 \ .$$

The exact probability value of an observed value of Q, under the null hypothesis, is given by the sum of the hypergeometric point probability values associated with the Q values that are equal to or greater than the observed value of Q. For the frequency data listed in Table 4.33, there are only $M = 97$ possible, equally-likely arrangements in the reference set of all permutations of cell frequencies given the two cell frequencies of change, 59 and 37, and only 76 Q values are equal to or greater than the observed value of $Q = 5.0417$. The exact upper-tail probability value of the observed Q value is $P = 0.0315$, i.e., the sum of the hypergeometric point probability values that are associated with values of $Q = 5.0417$ or greater.

4.7 Cochran's Q Test for Change

The ubiquitous dichotomous variable plays a large role and has many applications in research and measurement. Conventionally, a value of one is assigned to each test item that a subject answers correctly and a zero is assigned to each incorrect answer. A common example application occurs when subjects are placed into an experimental situation, observed as to whether or not some specified response is elicited, and scored appropriately [56].

In 1950, William Cochran published an article on "The comparison of percentages in matched samples" [22]. In this brief but formative article, Cochran described a test for equality of matched proportions that is now widely used in educational and psychological research. The matching may be based on the characteristics of different subjects or on the same subjects under different conditions. The Cochran Q test may be viewed as an extension of the McNemar [63] test to three or more treatment conditions. For a typical application, suppose that a sample of $N \geq 2$ subjects is observed in a situation wherein each subject performs individually under each of $k \geq 1$ different experimental conditions. The performance is scored as a success (1) or as a failure (0). The research question evaluates whether the true proportion of successes is constant over the k time periods.

Cochran's Q test for the analysis of k treatment conditions (columns) and N subjects (rows) is given by:

$$Q = \frac{(k-1)\left(k\sum_{j=1}^{k} C_j^2 - A^2\right)}{kA - B} , \tag{4.11}$$

where

$$C_j = \sum_{i=1}^{N} x_{ij}$$

is the number of 1s in the jth of k columns,

$$R_i = \sum_{j=1}^{k} x_{ij}$$

is the number of 1s in the ith of N rows,

$$A = \sum_{i=1}^{N} R_i , \quad B = \sum_{i=1}^{N} R_i^2 ,$$

and x_{ij} denotes the cell entry of either 0 or 1 associated with the ith of N rows and the jth of k columns. The null hypothesis stipulates that each of the

$$M = \prod_{i=1}^{N} \binom{k}{R_i}$$

distinguishable arrangements of 1s and 0s within each of the N rows occurs with equal probability, given that the values of $R_1, \ldots, R_N$ are fixed [65].

4.7.1 Example 1

For an example analysis of Cochran's Q test, consider the binary-coded data listed in Table 4.34 consisting of responses (1 or 0) for $N = 10$ subjects evaluated over

Table 4.34 Successes (1) and failures (0) of $N = 10$ subjects on a series of $k = 5$ time periods

	Time					
Subject	1	2	3	4	5	R_i
1	0	1	1	0	0	2
2	1	0	1	0	1	3
3	0	1	1	0	0	2
4	1	1	0	0	0	2
5	1	0	1	1	0	3
6	0	1	1	0	0	2
7	0	1	0	1	0	2
8	0	0	1	0	0	1
9	0	1	0	1	0	2
10	1	1	1	0	0	3
C_j	4	7	7	3	1	22

$k = 5$ time periods, where a 1 denotes success on a prescribed task and a 0 denotes failure. For the binary-coded data listed in Table 4.34,

$$\sum_{j=1}^{k} C_j^2 = 4^2 + 7^2 + 7^2 + 3^2 + 1^2 = 124 ,$$

$$A = \sum_{i=1}^{N} R_i = 2 + 3 + 2 + 2 + 3 + 2 + 2 + 1 + 2 + 3 = 22 ,$$

$$B = \sum_{i=1}^{N} R_i^2 = 2^2 + 3^2 + 2^2 + 2^2 + 3^2 + 2^2 + 2^2 + 1^2 + 2^2 + 3^2 = 52 ,$$

and, following Eq. (4.11) on p. 180, the observed value of Cochran's Q is

$$Q = \frac{(k-1)\left(k\sum_{j=1}^{k} C_j^2 - A^2\right)}{kA - B} = \frac{(5-1)[(5)(124) - 22^2]}{(5)(22) - 52} = 9.3793 .$$

For the binary-coded data listed in Table 4.34, there are

$$M = \prod_{i=1}^{N} \binom{k}{R_i} = \binom{5}{1}^1 \binom{5}{2}^6 \binom{5}{3}^3 = (5)(10^6)(10^3) = 5{,}000{,}000{,}000$$

possible, equally-likely arrangements of the observed data, making an exact permutation analysis prohibitive and a Monte Carlo resampling analysis necessary. Based on $L = 1{,}000{,}000$ random arrangements of the observed data, there are 54,486 Q values equal to or greater than the observed value of $Q = 9.3793$. If Q_o denotes the observed value of Q, the approximate resampling probability value of the observed data is

$$P(Q \geq Q_o | H_0) = \frac{\text{number of } Q \text{ values } \geq Q_o}{L} = \frac{54{,}486}{1{,}000{,}000} = 0.0545 \; .$$

For comparison, under the null hypothesis Cochran's Q is approximately distributed as chi-squared with $k-1$ degrees of freedom. The approximate probability of $Q = 9.3793$ with $k-1 = 5-1 = 4$ degrees of freedom is $P = 0.0523$.

4.7.2 Example 2

For a second example of Cochran's Q test, consider the binary-coded data listed in Table 4.35 consisting of responses (1 or 0) for $N = 9$ subjects evaluated over $k = 3$ time periods, where a 1 indicates success on a prescribed task and a 0 indicates failure. For the binary-coded data listed in Table 4.35,

$$A = \sum_{i=1}^{N} R_i = 1+1+1+1+2+1+2+1+2 = 12 \; ,$$

$$B = \sum_{i=1}^{N} R_i^2 = 1^2+1^2+1^2+1^2+2^2+1^2+2^2+1^2+2^2 = 18 \; ,$$

$$\sum_{j=1}^{g} C_j^2 = 4^2+7^2+1^2 = 66 \; ,$$

Table 4.35 Successes (1) and failures (0) of $N = 9$ subjects on a series of $k = 3$ time periods

	Time			
Subject	1	2	3	R_i
1	0	1	0	1
2	0	1	0	1
3	1	0	0	1
4	0	1	0	1
5	1	0	1	2
6	0	1	0	1
7	1	1	0	2
8	0	1	0	1
9	1	1	0	2
C_j	4	7	1	12

and, following Eq. (4.11) on p. 180, the observed value of Cochran's Q is

$$Q = \frac{(k-1)\left(k \sum_{j=1}^{k} C_j^2 - A^2\right)}{kA - B} = \frac{(3-1)[(3)(66) - 12^2]}{(3)(12) - 18} = 6.00 \, .$$

For the binary-coded data listed in Table 4.35, there are only

$$M = \prod_{i=1}^{N} \binom{k}{R_i} = \binom{3}{1}^6 \binom{3}{2}^3 = (3^6)(3^3) = 19{,}683$$

possible, equally-likely arrangements of the observed data in the reference set of all possible arrangements, making an exact permutation analysis easily accomplished. Based on $M = 19{,}683$ equally-likely, possible arrangements of the observed data, there are 1,056 Q values equal to or greater than the observed value of $Q = 6.00$. If Q_{o} denotes the observed value of Q, the exact upper-tail probability value of the observed data is

$$P(Q \geq Q_{\text{o}}|H_0) = \frac{\text{number of } Q \text{ values } \geq Q_{\text{o}}}{M} = \frac{1{,}056}{19{,}683} = 0.0537 \, .$$

For comparison, under the null hypothesis Cochran's Q is approximately distributed as chi-squared with $k - 1$ degrees of freedom. The approximate probability of $Q =$ 86.00 with $k - 1 = 3 - 1 = 2$ degrees of freedom is $P = 0.0498$.

4.8 A Measure of Effect Size for Cochran's Q Test

Measures of effect size are increasingly important in reporting research outcomes. The American Psychological Association (APA) has long recommended measures of effect size for articles published in APA journals. For example, as far back as 1994 the 4th edition of the *APA Publication Manual* strongly encouraged reporting measures of effect size in conjunction with probability values. In 1999, the APA Task Force on Statistical Inference, under the direction of Leland Wilkinson, noted that "reporting and interpreting effect sizes in the context of previously reported effects is essential to good research" [87, p. 599]. In 2016, the American Statistical Association (ASA) recommended that measures of effect size be included in future publications in ASA journals [84]. Unfortunately, measures of effect size do not exist for a number of common statistical tests. In this section, a chance-corrected measure of effect size is presented for Cochran's Q test for related proportions [9].

Consider an alternative approach to Cochran's Q test where g treatments are applied independently to each of N subjects with the result of each treatment application recorded as either 1 or 0, representing any suitable dichotomization of the treatment results, i.e., a randomized-block design where the subjects are the blocks and the treatment results are registered as either 1 or 0. Let x_{ij} denote the recorded 1 and 0 response measurements for $i = 1, \ldots, N$ and $j = 1, \ldots, g$. Then, Cochran's test statistic can be defined as:

$$Q = \frac{g-1}{2\sum_{i=1}^{N} p_i(1-p_i)} \left[2\left(\sum_{i=1}^{N} p_i\right)\left(N - \sum_{i=1}^{N} p_i\right) - N(N-1)\,\delta \right],$$

where

$$\delta = \left[g\binom{N}{2} \right]^{-1} \sum_{k=1}^{g} \sum_{i=1}^{N-1} \sum_{j=i+1}^{N} \left| x_{ik} - x_{jk} \right| \tag{4.12}$$

and

$$p_i = \frac{1}{g} \sum_{j=1}^{g} x_{ij} \qquad \text{for } i = 1, \ldots, N,$$

that is, the proportion of 1 values for the ith of N subjects. Note that in this representation the variation of Q is totally dependent on δ.

In 1979, Acock and Stavig [1] proposed a maximum value for Q given by:

$$Q_{\max} = N(g-1). \tag{4.13}$$

Acock and Stavig's maximum value of Q in Eq. (4.13) was employed by Serlin, Carr, and Marascuilo [77] to provide a measure of effect size for Cochran's Q given by:

$$\hat{\eta}_Q^2 = \frac{Q}{Q_{\max}} = \frac{Q}{N(g-1)},$$

which standardized Cochran's Q by a maximum value. Unfortunately, the value of $Q_{\max} = N(g-1)$ advocated by Acock and Stavig is achieved only when each subject g-tuple is identical and there is at least one 1 and one 0 in each g-tuple. Thus, $\hat{\eta}_Q^2$ is a "maximum-corrected" measure of effect size and $0 \leq \hat{\eta}_Q^2 \leq 1$ only under these rare conditions.

Assume $0 < p_i < 1$ for $i = 1, \ldots, N$ since $p_i = 0$ and $p_i = 1$ are uninformative. If p_i is constant for $i = 1, \ldots, N$, then $Q_{\max} = N(g-1)$. However, for the vast majority of cases when $p_i \neq p_j$ for $i \neq j$, $Q_{\max} < N(g-1)$. Thus, the routine use of setting $Q_{\max} = N(g-1)$ is problematic and leads to questionable results.

It should also be noted that $\hat{\eta}_Q^2$ is a member of the V family of measures of nominal association based on Cramér's V^2 test statistic given by:

$$V^2 = \frac{\chi^2}{\chi^2_{\max}} = \frac{\chi^2}{N\big[\min(r-1, c-1)\big]} ,$$

where r and c denote the number of rows and columns in an $r \times c$ contingency table [1]. Other members of the V family are Pearson's ϕ^2 for 2×2 contingency tables [70] and Tschuprov's T^2 for $r \times c$ contingency tables where $r = c$ [82]. The difficulties in interpreting V^2 extend to $\hat{\eta}_Q^2$.

As noted in Chap. 3, Wickens observed that Cramér's V^2 lacks an intuitive interpretation other than as a scaling of chi-squared, which limits its usefulness [86, p. 226]. Also, Costner noted that V^2 and other measures based on Pearson's chi-squared lack any interpretation at all for values other than 0 and 1, or the maximum, given the observed marginal frequency distributions [27]. Agresti and Finlay also noted that Cramér's V^2 is very difficult to interpret and recommended other measures [2, p. 284]. Blalock noted that "all measures based on chi square are somewhat arbitrary in nature, and their interpretations leave a lot to be desired...they all give greater weight to those columns or rows having the smallest marginals rather than to those with the largest marginals" [17, 18, p. 306]. Ferguson discussed the problem of using idealized marginal frequencies [30, p. 422], and Guilford noted that measures such as Pearson's ϕ^2, Tschuprov's T^2, and Cramér's V^2 necessarily underestimate the magnitude of association present [42, p. 342]. Berry, Martin, and Olson considered these issues with respect to 2×2 contingency tables [10, 12], and Berry, Johnston, and Mielke discussed in some detail the problems with using Pearson's ϕ^2, Tschuprov's T^2, and Cramér's V^2 as measures of effect size [8]. Since $\hat{\eta}_Q^2$ is simply a special case of Cramér's V^2, it presents the same problems of interpretation. For a detailed assessment of Pearson's ϕ^2, Tschuprov's T^2, and Cramér's V^2, see Chap. 3.

4.8.1 A Chance-Corrected Measure of Effect Size

Chance-corrected measures of effect size have much to commend them over maximum-corrected measures. A chance-corrected measure of effect size is a measure of agreement among the N subjects over g treatments, corrected for chance. A number of researchers have advocated chance-corrected measures of effect size, including Brennan and Prediger [20], Cicchetti, Showalter, and Tyrer [21], Conger [26], and Krippendorff [50]. A chance-corrected measure is zero under chance conditions, unity when agreement among the N subjects is perfect, and negative under conditions of disagreement. Some well-known chance-corrected measures are Scott's coefficient of inter-coder agreement [76], Kendall and Babington Smith's u measure of agreement [48], Cohen's unweighted and weighted coefficients of inter-rater agreement [23, 24], and Spearman's footrule measure [79, 80]. Under certain conditions, Spearman's rank-order correlation coefficient [79, 80] is also a chance-corrected measure of agreement, i.e., when variables x and y consist of ranks from 1 to N with no tied values, or when variable x includes tied values and variable y is a permutation of variable x, then Spearman's rank-order correlation coefficient is both a measure of correlation and a chance-corrected measure of agreement [50, p. 144].

Let x_{ij} denote the (0, 1) response measurements for $i = 1, \ldots, N$ blocks and $j = 1, \ldots, g$ treatments, then

$$\delta = \left[g \binom{N}{2} \right]^{-1} \sum_{k=1}^{g} \sum_{i=1}^{N-1} \sum_{j=i+1}^{N} \left| x_{ik} - x_{jk} \right| .$$

Under the null hypothesis that the distribution of δ assigns equal probability to each of

$$M = (g!)^N$$

possible allocations of the g dichotomous response measurements to the g treatment positions for each of the N subjects, the average value of δ is given by:

$$\mu_\delta = \frac{2}{N(N-1)} \left[\left(\sum_{i=1}^{N} p_i \right) \left(N - \sum_{i=1}^{N} p_i \right) - \sum_{i=1}^{N} p_i (1 - p_i) \right] ,$$

where

$$p_i = \frac{1}{g} \sum_{i=1}^{g} x_{ij} \qquad \text{for } i = 1, \ldots, N .$$

Then, a chance-corrected measure of effect size may be defined as:

$$\Re = 1 - \frac{\delta}{\mu_\delta} .$$

4.8.2 Example

Consider a sample of $N = 6$ psychology graduate students enrolled in a seminar designed to hone skills in assessing patients with various disorders. The seminar includes a clinical aspect whereby actors, provided with different scripts, present symptoms that the students then diagnose. There are $g = 8$ scripts for a variety

Table 4.36 Example data for Cochran's Q test of related proportions with $N = 6$ subjects and $g = 8$ treatments

	Treatment							
Subject	1	2	3	4	5	6	7	8
1	0	1	1	1	0	0	1	0
2	1	1	1	0	0	1	1	1
3	0	1	0	1	1	0	1	1
4	1	1	1	1	0	1	1	1
5	0	1	1	0	0	0	1	1
6	1	1	1	1	0	1	1	0

Table 4.37 Summations for p_i and $p_i(1 - p_i)$ for $i = 1, \ldots, N$

i	p_i	$1 - p_i$	$p_i(1 - p_i)$
1	0.5000	0.5000	0.2500
2	0.7500	0.2500	0.1875
3	0.6250	0.3750	0.2344
4	0.8750	0.1250	0.1094
5	0.5000	0.5000	0.2500
6	0.7500	0.2500	0.1875
Total	4.0000		1.2188

of symptoms including eating disorders, anxiety, depression, oppositional defiant behavior, obsessive-compulsive disorder, and post-traumatic stress disorders, any of which may be presented over the course of the seminar. The "patients" present at random intervals during the semester and the students are assessed as to whether or not the correct diagnosis was made. Table 4.36 lists the data with a 1 (0) indicating a correct (false) diagnosis. For the binary data listed in Table 4.36, Table 4.37 illustrates the calculation of

$$\sum_{i=1}^{N} p_i \quad \text{and} \quad \sum_{i=1}^{N} p_i(1 - p_i) ,$$

where

$$p_1 = \frac{1}{g} \sum_{j=1}^{g} x_{1j} = \frac{0 + 1 + 1 + 1 + 0 + 0 + 1 + 0}{8} = 0.5000 ,$$

$$p_2 = \frac{1}{g} \sum_{j=1}^{g} x_{2j} = \frac{1 + 1 + 1 + 0 + 0 + 1 + 1 + 1}{8} = 0.7500 ,$$

$$p_3 = \frac{1}{g} \sum_{j=1}^{g} x_{3j} = \frac{0 + 1 + 0 + 1 + 1 + 0 + 1 + 1}{8} = 0.6250 ,$$

$$p_4 = \frac{1}{g}\sum_{j=1}^{g} x_{4j} = \frac{1+1+1+1+0+1+1+1}{8} = 0.8750\ ,$$

$$p_5 = \frac{1}{g}\sum_{j=1}^{g} x_{5j} = \frac{0+1+1+0+0+0+1+1}{8} = 0.5000\ ,$$

and

$$p_6 = \frac{1}{g}\sum_{j=1}^{g} x_{6j} = \frac{1+1+1+1+0+1+1+0}{8} = 0.7500\ .$$

Table 4.38 illustrates the calculation of the $|x_{ik} - x_{jk}|$ values, $i = 1, \ldots, N-1$ and $j = i+1, \ldots, N$, for Treatments $1, 2, \ldots, 8$. Then,

$$\delta = \left[g\binom{N}{2}\right]^{-1} \sum_{k=1}^{g}\sum_{i=1}^{N-1}\sum_{j=i+1}^{N} |x_{ik} - x_{jk}|$$

$$= \left[8\binom{6}{2}\right]^{-1} (9+0+5+8+5+9+0+8) = 0.3667\ ,$$

$$Q = \frac{g-1}{2\displaystyle\sum_{i=1}^{N} p_i(1-p_i)} \left[2\left(\sum_{i=1}^{N} p_i\right)\left(N - \sum_{i=1}^{N} p_i\right) - N(N-1)\,\delta\right]$$

$$= \frac{8-1}{2(1.2188)}\big[2(4.00)(6-4.00) - 6(6-1)(0.3667)\big] = 14.3590\ ,$$

$$\mu_\delta = \frac{2}{N(N-1)}\left[\left(\sum_{i=1}^{N} p_i\right)\left(N - \sum_{i=1}^{N} p_i\right) - \sum_{i=1}^{N} p_i(1-p_i)\right]$$

$$= \frac{2}{6(6-1)}\big[(4.00)(6-4.00) - 1.2188\big] = 0.4521\ ,$$

and

$$\Re = 1 - \frac{\delta}{\mu_\delta} = 1 - \frac{0.3667}{0.4521} = +0.1889\ ,$$

Table 4.38 Summation totals for $|x_{ik} - x_{jk}|$ for $k = 1, 2, \ldots, 7, 8$ treatments, $i = 1, \ldots, N-1$, and $j = i + 1, \ldots, N$

	Treatment				
	1	2	...	7	8
i	$\|x_{i1} - x_{j1}\|$	$\|x_{i2} - x_{j2}\|$	...	$\|x_{i7} - x_{j7}\|$	$\|x_{i8} - x_{j8}\|$
1	$\|0-1\| = 1$	$\|1-1\| = 0$	...	$\|1-1\| = 0$	$\|0-1\| = 1$
2	$\|0-0\| = 0$	$\|1-1\| = 0$	...	$\|1-1\| = 0$	$\|0-1\| = 1$
3	$\|0-1\| = 1$	$\|1-1\| = 0$	...	$\|1-1\| = 0$	$\|0-1\| = 1$
4	$\|0-0\| = 0$	$\|1-1\| = 0$	...	$\|1-1\| = 0$	$\|0-1\| = 1$
5	$\|0-1\| = 1$	$\|1-1\| = 0$	...	$\|1-1\| = 0$	$\|0-0\| = 0$
6	$\|1-0\| = 1$	$\|1-1\| = 0$	...	$\|1-1\| = 0$	$\|1-1\| = 0$
7	$\|1-1\| = 0$	$\|1-1\| = 0$	...	$\|1-1\| = 0$	$\|1-1\| = 0$
8	$\|1-0\| = 1$	$\|1-1\| = 0$	...	$\|1-1\| = 0$	$\|1-1\| = 0$
9	$\|1-1\| = 0$	$\|1-1\| = 0$	...	$\|1-1\| = 0$	$\|1-0\| = 1$
10	$\|0-1\| = 1$	$\|1-1\| = 0$	...	$\|1-1\| = 0$	$\|1-1\| = 0$
11	$\|0-0\| = 0$	$\|1-1\| = 0$	...	$\|1-1\| = 0$	$\|1-1\| = 0$
12	$\|0-1\| = 1$	$\|1-1\| = 0$	...	$\|1-1\| = 0$	$\|1-0\| = 1$
13	$\|1-0\| = 1$	$\|1-1\| = 0$	...	$\|1-1\| = 0$	$\|1-1\| = 0$
14	$\|1-1\| = 0$	$\|1-1\| = 0$	...	$\|1-1\| = 0$	$\|1-0\| = 1$
15	$\|0-1\| = 1$	$\|1-1\| = 0$	...	$\|1-1\| = 0$	$\|1-0\| = 1$
Total	9	0	...	0	8

indicating approximately 19% agreement above that expected by chance. For comparison, the maximum-corrected measure of effect size proposed by Serlin et al. [77] is

$$\hat{\eta}_Q^2 = \frac{Q}{Q_{\max}} = \frac{Q}{N(g-1)} = \frac{14.3590}{6(8-1)} = 0.3419 .$$

4.8.3 Advantages of the $\Re$ Measure of Effect Size

Chance-corrected measures of effect size, such as $\Re$, possess distinct advantages in interpretation over maximum-corrected measures of effect size, such as $\hat{\eta}_Q^2$. The problem with $\hat{\eta}_Q^2$ lies in the manner in which $\hat{\eta}_Q^2$ is maximized. The denominator of $\hat{\eta}_Q^2$, $Q_{\max} = N(g-1)$, standardizes the observed value of Q for the sample size (N) and the number of treatments (g). Unfortunately, $N(g-1)$ does not standardize Q for the data on which Q is based, but rather standardizes Q on another unobserved hypothetical set of data.

Consider a simple example with $N = 10$ subjects and $g = 2$ treatments. The observed data are given in Table 4.39, where at Time 1 seven subjects were classified

Table 4.39 Example 2×2 cross-classification for Cochran's Q test for change

	Time 2		
Time 1	Pro	Con	Total
Pro	5	2	7
Con	0	3	3
Total	5	5	10

Table 4.40 Four possible arrangements of the data given in Table 4.39 with fixed observed row and column marginal frequency distributions, $\{7, 3\}$ and $\{5, 5\}$, respectively

	Table A		Table B		Table C		Table D	
	Pro	Con	Pro	Con	Pro	Con	Pro	Con
Pro	5	2	4	3	3	4	2	5
Con	0	3	1	2	2	1	3	0

as Pro and three subjects were classified as Con, and at Time 2 five subjects were classified as Pro and five subjects were classified as Con.

Given the observed data in Table 4.39, only four values of Q are possible. Table 4.40 displays the four possible arrangements in the reference set of all permutations of cell frequencies given the observed row and column marginal frequency distributions, $\{7, 3\}$ and $\{5, 5\}$, respectively. Table A in Table 4.40 (the observed table) yields $Q = 2.00$, Table B yields $Q = 1.00$, Table C yields $Q = 0.6667$, and Table D yields $Q = 0.50$. Thus, for the observed data given in Table 4.40, $Q = 2.00$ is the maximum value of Q possible, given the observed marginal frequency distributions. Note that $Q_{\max} = N(g-1) = 10(2-1) = 10$ cannot be achieved with these data. For the data given in Table A in Table 4.40 with $Q = 2.00$, $\hat{\eta}_Q^2$ is only 0.20, while $\mathfrak{R} = 1.00$, indicating the proper maximum-corrected effect size.

$\mathfrak{R}$ is a preferred alternative to $\hat{\eta}_Q^2$ as a measure of effect size for two reasons. First, $\mathfrak{R}$ can achieve an effect size of unity for the observed data, while this is often impossible for $\hat{\eta}_Q^2$. Second, $\mathfrak{R}$ is a chance-corrected measure of effect size, meaning that $\mathfrak{R}$ is zero under chance conditions, unity when agreement among the N subjects is perfect, and negative under conditions of disagreement. Therefore, $\mathfrak{R}$ possesses a clear interpretation corresponding to Cohen's coefficient of inter-rater agreement and other chance-corrected measures that are familiar to most researchers. On the other hand, $\hat{\eta}_Q^2$ possesses no meaningful interpretation except for the limiting values of $Q = 0$ and $Q = 1$.

4.9 Leik and Gove's d_N^c Measure of Association

In 1971, Robert Leik and Walter Gove proposed a new measure of nominal association based on pairwise comparisons of differences between observations [53]. Dissatisfied with the existing measures of nominal association, Leik and Gove suggested a proportional-reduction-in-error measure of association that was corrected for the true maximum amount of association, given the observed marginal frequency distributions. The new measure was denoted by d_N^c, where d indicated the index, following other indices such as Somers' d_{yx} and d_{xy}; the subscript N indicated the relevance of d to a nominal dependent variable; and the superscript c indicated that the measure was corrected for the constraints imposed by the marginal frequency distributions [53, p. 287].

Like d_N^c, many measures of association for two variables have been based on pairwise comparisons of differences between observations. Consider two nominal-level variables that have been cross-classified into an $r \times c$ contingency table, where r and c denote the number of rows and columns, respectively. Let $n_{i.}$, $n_{.j}$, and n_{ij} denote the row marginal frequency totals, column marginal frequency totals, and number of objects in the ijth cell, respectively, for $i = 1, \ldots, r$ and $j = 1, \ldots, c$, and let N denote the total number of objects in the $r \times c$ contingency table. If y and x represent the row and column variables, respectively, there are $N(N-1)/2$ pairs of objects in the table that can be partitioned into five mutually exclusive, exhaustive types of pairs: concordant pairs, discordant pairs, pairs tied on variable y but differing on variable x, pairs tied on variable x but differing on variable y, and pairs tied on both variables x and y.

For an $r \times c$ contingency table, concordant pairs (pairs of objects that are ranked in the same order on both variable x and variable y) are given by:

$$C = \sum_{i=1}^{r-1} \sum_{j=1}^{c-1} n_{ij} \left(\sum_{k=i+1}^{r} \sum_{l=j+1}^{c} n_{kl} \right) ,$$

discordant pairs (pairs of objects that are ranked in one order on variable x and the reverse order on variable y) are given by:

$$D = \sum_{i=1}^{r-1} \sum_{j=1}^{c-1} n_{i,c-j+1} \left(\sum_{k=i+1}^{r} \sum_{l=1}^{c-j} n_{kl} \right) ,$$

pairs of objects tied on variable x but differing on variable y are given by:

$$T_x = \sum_{i=1}^{r} \sum_{j=1}^{c-1} n_{ij} \left(\sum_{k=j+1}^{c} n_{ik} \right) ,$$

pairs of objects tied on variable y but differing on variable x are given by:

$$T_y = \sum_{j=1}^{c} \sum_{i=1}^{r-1} n_{ij} \left(\sum_{k=i+1}^{r} n_{kj} \right) ,$$

Table 4.41 Example observed values in a 3×3 contingency table with $N = 100$ observations

	x			
y	x_1	x_2	x_3	Total
y_1	15	5	0	20
y_2	15	25	10	50
y_3	0	10	20	30
Total	30	40	30	100

and pairs of objects tied on both variable x and variable y are given by:

$$T_{xy} = \frac{1}{2}\sum_{i=1}^{r}\sum_{j=1}^{c} n_{ij}\left(n_{ij} - 1\right) .$$

Then,

$$C + D + T_x + T_y + T_{xy} = \frac{N(N-1)}{2} .$$

To illustrate the calculation of Leik and Gove's d_N^c measure, consider first an example 3×3 contingency table, such as given in Table 4.41, where $N = 100$ observations are cross-classified into variable x and variable y, each with $r = c = 3$ categories labeled x_1, x_2, x_3 and y_1, y_2, y_3, respectively.

4.9.1 Observed Contingency Table

For the frequency data given in Table 4.41, consider all possible pairs of observed cell frequency values that have been partitioned into concordant pairs,

$$\begin{aligned} C &= \sum_{i=1}^{r-1}\sum_{j=1}^{c-1} n_{ij}\left(\sum_{k=i+1}^{r}\sum_{l=j+1}^{c} n_{kl}\right) \\ &= (15)(25+10+10+20) + (5)(10+20) + (15)(10+20) + (25)(20) \\ &= 2{,}075 , \end{aligned}$$

all discordant pairs of observed cell frequency values,

$$\begin{aligned} D &= \sum_{i=1}^{r-1}\sum_{j=1}^{c-1} n_{i,c-j+1}\left(\sum_{k=i+1}^{r}\sum_{l=1}^{c-j} n_{kl}\right) \\ &= (0)(15+25+0+10) + (5)(15+0) + (10)(0+10) + (25)(0) \\ &= 175 , \end{aligned}$$

all pairs of observed cell frequency values tied on variable x,

$$T_x = \sum_{j=1}^{c} \sum_{i=1}^{r-1} n_{ij} \left(\sum_{k=i+1}^{r} n_{kj} \right)$$

$$= (15)(15+0) + (15)(0) + (5)(25+10) + (25)(10) + (0)(10+20) + (10)(20) = 850 ,$$

all pairs of observed cell frequency values tied on variable y,

$$T_y = \sum_{i=1}^{r} \sum_{j=1}^{c-1} n_{ij} \left(\sum_{k=j+1}^{c} n_{ik} \right)$$

$$(15)(5+0) + (5)(0) + (15)(25+10) + (25)(10) + (0)(10+20) + (10)(20) = 1{,}050 ,$$

and all pairs of observed cell frequency values tied on both variables x and y,

$$T_{xy} = \frac{1}{2} \sum_{i=1}^{r} \sum_{j=1}^{c} n_{ij} \left(n_{ij} - 1 \right)$$

$$= \frac{1}{2} \big[(15)(15-1) + (5)(5-1) + (15)(15-1) + (25)(25-1) + (10)(10-1) + (10)(10-1) + (20)(20-1) \big] = 800 .$$

Then,

$$C + D + T_x + T_y + T_{xy} = \frac{N(N-1)}{2}$$

and, for the observed frequency data given in Table 4.41,

$$2{,}075 + 175 + 850 + 1{,}050 + 800 = \frac{100(100-1)}{2} = 4{,}950 .$$

4.9.2 Expected Contingency Table

Now, consider Table 4.41 expressed as expected cell values, as given in Table 4.42, where an expected value is given by:

$$E_{ij} = \frac{n_{i.} n_{.j}}{N} \qquad \text{for } i = 1, \ldots, r \text{ and } j = 1, \ldots, c .$$

Table 4.42 Example expected values in a 3×3 contingency table with $N = 100$ observations

	x			
y	x_1	x_2	x_3	Total
y_1	6	8	6	20
y_2	15	20	15	50
y_3	9	12	9	30
Total	30	40	30	100

For example,

$$E_{11} = \frac{(20)(30)}{100} = 6 \quad \text{and} \quad E_{12} = \frac{(20)(40)}{100} = 8\,.$$

Following Leik and Gove, let a prime (′) indicate a sum of pairs calculated on the expected cell frequency values. Then, for the expected cell frequency values given in Table 4.42, consider all possible pairs of expected values partitioned into concordant pairs,

$$\begin{aligned} C' &= \sum_{i=1}^{r-1} \sum_{j=1}^{c-1} n_{ij} \left(\sum_{k=i+1}^{r} \sum_{l=j+1}^{c} n_{kl} \right) \\ &= (6)(20+15+12+9) + (8)(15+9) + (15)(12+9) \\ &\qquad + (20)(9) = 1{,}023\,, \end{aligned}$$

all discordant pairs of expected cell frequency values,

$$\begin{aligned} D' &= \sum_{i=1}^{r-1} \sum_{j=1}^{c-1} n_{i,c-j+1} \left(\sum_{k=i+1}^{r} \sum_{l=1}^{c-j} n_{kl} \right) \\ &= (6)(15+20+9+12) + (8)(15+9) + (15)(9+12) \\ &\qquad + (20)(9) = 1{,}023\,, \end{aligned}$$

all pairs of expected cell frequency values tied on variable x,

$$\begin{aligned} T_x' &= \sum_{j=1}^{c} \sum_{i=1}^{r-1} n_{ij} \left(\sum_{k=i+1}^{r} n_{kj} \right) \\ &= (6)(15+9) + (15)(9) + (8)(20+12) + (20)(12) \\ &\qquad + (6)(15+9) + (15)(9) = 1{,}054\,, \end{aligned}$$

all pairs of expected cell frequency values tied on variable y,

$$T'_y = \sum_{i=1}^{r} \sum_{j=1}^{c-1} n_{ij} \left(\sum_{k=j+1}^{c} n_{ik} \right)$$

$$(6)(8+6) + (8)(6) + (15)(20+15) + (20)(15)$$
$$+ (9)(12+9) + (12)(9) = 1{,}254 \; ,$$

and all pairs of expected cell frequency values tied on both variables x and y,

$$T'_{xy} = \frac{1}{2} \sum_{i=1}^{r} \sum_{j=1}^{c} n_{ij} \left(n_{ij} - 1 \right)$$
$$= \frac{1}{2} \big[(6)(6-1) + (8)(8-1) + (6)(6-1) + (15)(15-1)$$
$$+ (20)(20-1) + (15)(15-1) + (9)(9-1) + (12)(12-1)$$
$$+ (9)(9-1) \big] = 596 \; .$$

Then,

$$C' + D' + T'_x + T'_y + T'_{xy} = \frac{N(N-1)}{2}$$

and, for the expected frequency data given in Table 4.42,

$$1{,}023 + 1{,}023 + 1{,}054 + 1{,}254 + 596 = \frac{100(100-1)}{2} = 4{,}950 \; .$$

Fortunately, there is a more convenient way to calculate C', D', T'_x, T'_y, and T'_{xy} without first calculating the expected values. First, given the observed row and column marginal frequency distributions in Table 4.41, $\{20, 50, 30\}$ and $\{30, 40, 30\}$, respectively, calculate the number of pairs of expected cell frequency values tied on both variables x and y,

$$T'_{xy} = \frac{1}{2N^2} \left(\sum_{i=1}^{r} n_{i.}^2 \right) \left(\sum_{j=1}^{c} n_{.j}^2 \right) - \frac{N}{2}$$
$$= \frac{1}{2(100^2)} \left(20^2 + 50^2 + 30^2 \right) \left(30^2 + 40^2 + 30^2 \right) - \frac{100}{2} = 596 \; .$$

Next, calculate the number of pairs of expected cell frequency values tied on variable y,

$$T_y' = \frac{1}{2}\sum_{i=1}^{r} n_{i.}^2 - \frac{N}{2} - T_{xy}' = \frac{1}{2}\left(20^2 + 50^2 + 30^2\right) - \frac{100}{2} - 596 = 1{,}254 .$$

In like manner, calculate the number of pairs of expected cell frequency values tied on variable x,

$$T_x' = \frac{1}{2}\sum_{j=1}^{c} n_{.j}^2 - \frac{N}{2} - T_{xy}' = \frac{1}{2}\left(30^2 + 40^2 + 30^2\right) - \frac{100}{2} - 596 = 1{,}054 .$$

Finally, calculate the number of concordant and discordant pairs of expected cell frequency values,

$$C' = D' = \frac{1}{2}\left[\frac{N(N-1)}{2} - T_x' - T_y' - T_{xy}'\right]$$

$$= \frac{1}{2}\left[\frac{100(100-1)}{2} - 1054 - 1254 - 596\right] = 1{,}023 .$$

It should be noted that C', D', T_x', T_y', and T_{xy}' are all calculated on the observed marginal frequency totals of the observed contingency table, which are invariant under permutation.

4.9.3 Maximized Contingency Table

Test statistic d_N^c is based on three contingency tables: the table of observed values given in Table 4.41, the table of expected values given in Table 4.42, and a table of maximum values to be described next. A contingency table of maximum values is necessary for computing d_N^c. An algorithm for generating an arrangement of cell frequencies in an $r \times c$ contingency table that provides the maximum value of a test statistic was presented in Chap. 3, Sect. 3.2. The algorithm is reproduced here for convenience.

STEP 1: List the observed marginal frequency totals of an $r \times c$ contingency table with empty cell frequencies.

STEP 2: If any pair of marginal frequency totals, one from each set of marginals, are equal to each other, enter that value in the table as n_{ij} and subtract the value from the two marginal frequency totals. For example, if the marginal frequency total for Row 2 is equal to the marginal frequency total for Column 3, enter the marginal frequency total in the table as n_{23} and subtract the value of n_{23} from the marginal frequency totals of Row 2 and Column 3.

Repeat STEP 2 until no two marginal frequency totals are equal. If all marginal frequency totals have been reduced to zero, go to STEP 5; otherwise, go to STEP 3.

STEP 3: Find the largest remaining marginal frequency totals in each set and enter the smaller of the two values in n_{ij}. Then, subtract that (smaller) value from the two marginal frequency totals. Go to STEP 4.

STEP 4: If all marginal frequency totals have been reduced to zero, go to STEP 5; otherwise, go to STEP 2.

STEP 5: Set any remaining n_{ij} values to zero, $i = 1, \ldots, r$ and $j = 1, \ldots, c$.

To illustrate the algorithmic procedure, consider the 3×3 contingency table given in Table 4.41 on p. 192, replicated in Table 4.43 for convenience. Then, the procedure is:

STEP 1: List the observed row and column marginal frequency totals, leaving the cell frequencies empty, as in Table 4.44.

STEP 2: For the two sets of marginal frequency totals given in Table 4.44, three marginal frequency totals are equal to 30, one for Row 3, one for Column 1, and one for Column 3, i.e., $n_{3.} = n_{.1} = n_{.3} = 30$. Set $n_{31} = 30$ and subtract 30 from the two marginal frequency totals. The adjusted row and column marginal frequency totals are now {20, 50, 0} and {0, 40, 30}, respectively. No other two marginal frequency totals are identical, so go to STEP 3.

STEP 3: The two largest remaining marginal frequency totals are 50 in Row 2 and 50 in Column 2, i.e., $n_{2.} = 50$ and $n_{.2} = 40$. Set $n_{22} = 40$, the smaller of the two marginal frequency totals, and subtract 40 from the two adjusted marginal frequency totals. The adjusted row and column marginal frequency totals are now {20, 10, 0} and {0, 0, 30}, respectively. Go to STEP 4.

STEP 4: Not all marginal frequency totals have been reduced to zero, so go to STEP 2.

Table 4.43 Example observed values in a 3×3 contingency table with $N = 100$ observations

	x			
y	x_1	x_2	x_3	Total
y_1	15	5	0	20
y_2	15	25	10	50
y_3	0	10	20	30
Total	30	40	30	100

Table 4.44 Empty 3×3 contingency table with observed row marginal frequency distribution {20, 50, 30} and observed column marginal frequency distribution {30, 40, 30}

	x			
y	x_1	x_2	x_3	Total
y_1	–	–	–	20
y_2	–	–	–	50
y_3	–	–	–	30
Total	30	40	30	100

STEP 2: No two marginal frequency totals are identical, so go to STEP 3.

STEP 3: The two largest marginal frequency totals are 20 in Row 1 and 30 in Column 3, i.e., $n_{1.} = 20$ and $n_{.3} = 30$. Set $n_{13} = 20$, the smaller of the two marginal frequency totals and subtract 20 from the two adjusted marginal frequency totals. The adjusted row and column marginal frequency totals are now {0, 10, 0} and {0, 0, 10}. Go to STEP 4.

STEP 4: Not all marginal frequency totals have been reduced to zero, so go to STEP 2.

STEP 2: Two marginal frequency totals are equal to 10, one for Row 2 and one for Column 3, i.e., $n_{2.} = n_{.3} = 10$. Set $n_{23} = 10$ and subtract 10 from the two adjusted marginal frequency totals. The adjusted row and column marginals are now {0, 0, 0} and {0, 0, 0}. All adjusted marginal frequency totals are now zero, so go to STEP 5.

STEP 5: Set any remaining n_{ij} values to zero; in this case, $n_{11}, n_{12}, n_{21}, n_{32}$, and n_{33} are set to zero.

The completed contingency table is given in Table 4.45. When there are tied values in a marginal distribution, e.g., $n_{.1} = n_{.3} = 30$, there may be alternative cell locations for the non-zero entries, meaning that more than one arrangement of cell frequencies may satisfy the conditions, but the nine cell frequency values {0, 0, 20, 0, 40, 10, 30, 0, 0} must be included in the 3×3 maximized contingency table.

Let a double prime (″) indicate a sum of pairs calculated on the maximized cell frequency values. Then, for the maximized frequency data given in Table 4.45, the number of concordant pairs of maximized cell frequency values is

$$C'' = \sum_{i=1}^{r-1} \sum_{j=1}^{c-1} n_{ij} \left(\sum_{k=i+1}^{r} \sum_{l=j+1}^{c} n_{kl} \right)$$
$$= (0)(40 + 10 + 0 + 0) + (0)(10 + 0) + (0)(0 + 0) + (20)(0) = 0 \,,$$

Table 4.45 Completed 3×3 contingency table with row marginal frequency distribution {20, 50, 30} and column marginal frequency distribution {30, 40, 30}

	x			
y	x_1	x_2	x_3	Total
y_1	0	0	20	20
y_2	0	40	10	50
y_3	30	0	0	30
Total	30	40	30	100

the number of discordant pairs of maximized cell frequency values is

$$D'' = \sum_{i=1}^{r-1} \sum_{j=1}^{c-1} n_{i,c-j+1} \left(\sum_{k=i+1}^{r} \sum_{l=1}^{c-j} n_{kl} \right)$$
$$= (20)(0+40+30+0) + (0)(0+30) + (10)(30+0) + (40)(30) = 2{,}900 \; ,$$

the number of pairs of maximized cell frequency values tied on variable x is

$$T_x'' = \sum_{j=1}^{c} \sum_{i=1}^{r-1} n_{ij} \left(\sum_{k=i+1}^{r} n_{kj} \right)$$
$$= (0)(0+20) + (0)(20) + (0)(40+10) + (40)(10) + (30)(0+0) + (0)(0) = 400 \; ,$$

the number of pairs of maximized cell frequency values tied on variable y is

$$T_y'' = \sum_{i=1}^{r} \sum_{j=1}^{c-1} n_{ij} \left(\sum_{k=j+1}^{c} n_{ik} \right)$$
$$(0)(0+30) + (0)(30) + (0)(40+0) + (40)(0) + (20)(10+0) + (10)(0) = 200 \; ,$$

and the number of pairs of maximized cell frequency values tied on both variables x and y is

$$T_{xy}'' = \frac{1}{2} \sum_{i=1}^{r} \sum_{j=1}^{c} n_{ij} \left(n_{ij} - 1 \right)$$
$$= \frac{1}{2} \big[(20)(20-1) + (40)(40-1) + (10)(10-1) + (30)(30-1) \big] = 1{,}450 \; .$$

Then,

$$C'' + D'' + T_x'' + T_y'' + T_{xy}'' = \frac{N(N-1)}{2}$$

Table 4.46 Values for C, D, T_x, T_y, and T_{xy} obtained from the observed, expected, and maximized frequency tables

	Frequency table		
Pairs	Observed	Expected	Maximized
C	2,075	1,023	0
D	175	1,023	2,900
T_x	850	1,054	200
T_y	1,050	1,254	400
T_{xy}	800	596	1,450
Total	4,950	4,950	4,950

and for the maximized data given in Table 4.45,

$$C'' + D'' + T_x'' + T_y'' + T_{xy}''$$
$$= 0 + 2{,}900 + 200 + 400 + 1{,}450 = \frac{100(100-1)}{2} = 4{,}950\ .$$

Note that the maximized contingency table given in Table 4.45 occurs only when as few cells as possible contain non-zero entries. Thus, either C'' or D'' is maximized and the other is minimized; in this case, $C'' = 0$ is the minimum value of C possible, given the observed marginal frequency distributions, and $D'' = 2{,}900$ is the maximum value of D possible, given the observed marginal frequency distributions. Also, $T_x'' = 200$ and $T_y'' = 400$ are the minimum values of T_x and T_y possible, given the observed marginal frequency distributions. On the other hand, $T_{xy}'' = 1{,}450$ is the maximum value of T_{xy} possible, given the observed marginal frequency distributions.

Table 4.46 summarizes the C, D, T_x, T_y, and T_{xy} values obtained from the observed, expected, and maximized contingency tables.

4.9.4 Calculation of Leik and Gove's d_N^c

Given the observed, expected, and maximized values for C, D, T_x, T_y, and T_{xy} in Table 4.46, errors of the first kind (E_1)—the variation between independence and maximum association—are given by:

$$E_1 = T_y' - T_y'' = 1{,}254 - 400 = 854$$

and errors of the second kind (E_2)—the variation between the observed table and the table of maximum association—are given by:

$$E_2 = T_y - T_y'' = 1{,}050 - 400 = 650\ .$$

Then, in the manner of proportional-reduction-in-error measures of association,

$$d_N^c = \frac{E_1 - E_2}{E_1} = \frac{(T_y' - T_y'') - (T_y - T_y'')}{T_y' - T_y''} = \frac{T_y' - T_y}{T_y' - T_y''}$$

$$= \frac{1{,}254 - 1{,}050}{1{,}254 - 400} = 0.2389 \; .$$

Because d_N^c is a symmetrical measure, the number of tied values on variable x can be used in place of the number of tied values on variable y. Thus,

$$d_N^c = \frac{T_x' - T_x}{T_x' - T_x''} = \frac{1{,}054 - 850}{1{,}054 - 200} = 0.2389 \; .$$

Alternatively, d_N^c can be defined in terms of the number of values tied on both x and y. Thus,

$$d_N^c = \frac{T_{xy}' - T_{xy}}{T_{xy}' - T_{xy}''} = \frac{596 - 800}{596 - 1{,}450} = 0.2389 \; .$$

Because the data are categorical, C and D can be considered as grouped together. Thus,

$$d_N^c = \frac{(C' + D') - (C + D)}{(C' + D') - (C'' + D'')} = \frac{(1{,}023 + 1{,}023) - (2{,}075 + 175)}{(1{,}023 + 1{,}023) - (0 + 2{,}900)}$$

$$= 0.2389 \; .$$

Finally,

$$d_N^c = \frac{T_y' - T_y}{T_y' - T_y''} = \frac{T_x' - T_x}{T_x' - T_x''} = \frac{T_{xy}' - T_{xy}}{T_{xy}' - T_{xy}''} = \frac{(C' + D') - (C + D)}{(C' + D') - (C'' + D'')} \; .$$

As noted by Leik and Gove, for an aid in interpreting the relationship between variables x and y, it would be preferable to explicitly determine the number of pairs lost to the marginal requirements of the contingency table. Association can then be defined within those limits, enabling the index to reach unity if cell frequencies are as close to a perfect pattern as the marginal distributions allow [53, p. 286]. Thus, for the frequency data given in Table 4.41 on p. 192, the proportion of cases being considered is

$$1 - \frac{2\left(T_x'' + T_y''\right)}{N(N-1)} = 1 - \frac{2(200 + 600)}{100(100-1)} = 0.8384 \; .$$

4.9.5 A Permutation Test for d_N^c

Leik and Gove did not provide a standard error for test statistic d_N^c [52]. On the other hand, permutation tests neither assume nor require knowledge of standard errors. Consider the expression

$$d_N^c = \frac{T_y' - T_y}{T_y' - T_y''} .$$

It is readily apparent that T_y' and T_y'' are invariant under permutation. Therefore, the probability of d_N^c under the null hypothesis can be determined by the discrete permutation distribution of T_y alone, which is easily obtained from the observed contingency table. Exact permutation statistical methods are highly efficient when only the variable portion of the defined test statistic is calculated on each of the M possible arrangements of the observed data; in this case, T_y.

For the frequency data given in Table 4.41 on p. 192, there are only $M = 96{,}151$ possible, equally-likely arrangements in the reference set of all permutations of cell frequencies given the observed row and column marginal frequency distributions, $\{20, 50, 30\}$ and $\{30, 40, 30\}$, respectively, making an exact permutation analysis feasible. If all $M = 96{,}151$ arrangements occur with equal chance, the exact probability value of d_N^c under the null hypothesis is the sum of the hypergeometric point probability values associated with $d_N^c = 0.2389$ or greater. Based on the underlying hypergeometric probability distribution, the exact upper-tail probability value is $P = 0.1683 \times 10^{-11}$.

4.10 A Matrix Occupancy Problem

In many research situations, it is necessary to examine a sequence of observations on a small group of subjects, where each observation is classified in one of two ways. Suppose, for example, a Success (1) or Failure (0) is recorded for each of $N \geq 2$ subjects on each of $k \geq 2$ tasks. The standard test in such cases is Cochran's Q test, as described in Sect. 4.7.

However, when the number of subjects is small, e.g., $2 \leq N \leq 6$, and the number of treatments is large, e.g., $20 \leq k \leq 400$, an alternative test may be preferable to Cochran's Q test. Such research conditions arise for a number of reasons. First, a long-term panel study is proposed, but few subjects are willing to make a research commitment due to the extended time of the research, or the treatment is either distasteful or time-intensive for the subjects. Second, a longitudinal study begins with an adequate number of subjects, but there is a high drop-out rate and survival analysis cannot be justified. Third, very few subjects satisfy the research protocol. Fourth, the cost of each observation/treatment is expensive for the researcher. Fifth, subjects are very expensive, as in primate studies. Sixth, a pilot study with a small number of subjects may be implemented to establish the validity of the research prior to applying for funding for a larger study.

Consider an $N \times k$ occupancy matrix with N subjects (rows) and k treatment conditions (columns). Let x_{ij} denote the observation of the ith subject ($i = 1, \ldots, N$) in the jth treatment condition ($j = 1, \ldots, k$), where a success is coded 1 and a failure is coded 0. For any subject, a success might result from the treatment administered or it might result from some other cause or a random response, i.e., a false positive. Therefore, a successful treatment response is counted only when all N subjects score a success, i.e., a full column of 1 values. Clearly, this approach does not generalize well to a great number of subjects since it is unrealistic for a large number of subjects to respond in concert. The Q test of Cochran is preferable when N is large.

In 1965, Mielke and Siddiqui presented an exact permutation procedure for the matrix occupancy problem in *Journal of the American Statistical Association* that is appropriate for small samples (N) and a large number of treatments (k) [68]. Let

$$R_i = \sum_{j=1}^{k} x_{ij}$$

for $i = 1, \ldots, N$ denote subject (row) totals, let

$$M = \prod_{i=1}^{N} \binom{k}{R_i}$$

denote the number of equally-likely distinguishable $N \times k$ occupancy matrices in the reference set, under the null hypothesis, and let $v = \min(R_1, \ldots, R_N)$. The null hypothesis stipulates that each of the M distinguishable configurations of 1s and 0s within each of the N rows occurs with equal probability, given that the $R_1, \ldots, R_N$ values are fixed. If U_g is the number of distinct configurations where exactly k treatment conditions (columns) are filled with successes (1s), then

$$U_v = \binom{k}{v} \prod_{i=1}^{N} \binom{k-v}{R_i - v}$$

is the initial value of the recursive relation

$$U_g = \binom{k}{g} \left[\prod_{i=1}^{N} \binom{k-g}{R_i - g} - \sum_{j=g+1}^{v} \binom{k-g}{j-g} \frac{U_j}{\binom{k}{j}} \right] ,$$

where $0 \leq g \leq v - 1$. If $g = 0$, then

$$M = \sum_{g=0}^{v} U_g$$

and the exact probability of observing s or more treatment conditions (columns) completely filled with successes (1s) is given by:

$$P = \frac{1}{M} \sum_{g=s}^{v} U_g \; ,$$

where $0 \leq s \leq v$.

In 1972, Eicker, Siddiqui, and Mielke described extensions to the matrix occupancy problem [28]. In 1974, Mantel [58] observed that the solution to the matrix occupancy problem was also the solution to the "committee problem" considered by Mantel and Pasternack in 1968 [59], Gittelsohn in 1969 [36], Sprott in 1969 [81], and White in 1971 [85]. Whereas the matrix occupancy problem considers N subjects and k treatments, scoring a success by a subject for a specific treatment as a 1 and a failure as a 0, the committee problem considers N committees and k individuals, scoring a 1 if an individual is not a member of a specified committee and 0 otherwise. The committee problem is concerned with the number of individuals belonging to no committees, which is equivalent to the concern of the matrix occupancy problem with the number of treatments associated with successes among all subjects.

4.10.1 Example Analysis

Consider an experiment with $N = 6$ subjects and $k = 8$ treatment conditions, such as given in Table 4.47. For the binary data listed in Table 4.47, the R_i totals are $\{4, 6, 5, 7, 4, 6\}$, the minimum of R_i, $i = 1, \ldots, N$, is $v = 4$, the number of

Table 4.47 Successes (1s) and failures (0s) of $N = 6$ subjects on a series of $k = 8$ treatments

	Treatment								
Subject	1	2	3	4	5	6	7	8	R_i
1	0	1	1	1	0	0	1	0	4
2	1	1	1	0	0	1	1	1	6
3	0	1	0	1	1	0	1	1	5
4	1	1	1	1	0	1	1	1	7
5	0	1	1	0	0	0	1	1	4
6	1	1	1	1	0	1	1	0	6

treatment conditions filled with 1s is $s = 2$ (treatments 2 and 7),

$$\sum_{g=s}^{v} U_g = \sum_{g=2}^{4} U_g = 149{,}341{,}920 + 6{,}838{,}720 + 40{,}320 = 156{,}220{,}960 \;,$$

the number of $N{\times}k$ occupancy matrices in the reference set of all possible occupancy matrices, under the null hypothesis, is

$$M = \prod_{i=1}^{N} \binom{k}{R_i} = \binom{8}{4}\binom{8}{6}\binom{8}{5}\binom{8}{7}\binom{8}{4}\binom{8}{6}$$
$$= 70 \times 28 \times 56 \times 8 \times 70 \times 28 = 1{,}721{,}036{,}800 \;,$$

and the exact probability of observing $s = 2$ or more treatment conditions completely filled with 1s is

$$P = \frac{1}{M} \sum_{g=s}^{v} U_g = \frac{156{,}220{,}960}{1{,}721{,}036{,}800} = 0.0908 \;.$$

It is also possible to define a maximum-corrected measure of effect size as $R = s/k$ that varies between 0 when no treatments (columns) are completely filled with 1s, to a maximum of 1 when all k columns are filled with 1s; in this example,

$$R = \frac{s}{k} = \frac{2}{8} = 0.25.$$

4.11 Fisher's Exact Probability Test

While Fisher's exact probability (FEP) test is, strictly speaking, not a measure of association between two nominal-level variables, it has assumed such importance in the analysis of 2×2 contingency tables that excluding Fisher's exact test from consideration would be a serious omission. That said, however, Fisher's exact probability test provides the probability of association rather than a measure of the strength of association. The Fisher exact probability test was independently developed by R.A. Fisher, Frank Yates, and Joseph Irwin in the early 1930s [32, 47, 89]. Consequently, the test is often referred to as the Fisher–Yates or the Fisher–Irwin exact probability test.[5]

[5]In this research monograph "Fisher exact probability test" is used throughout.

Although the Fisher exact probability test was originally designed for 2×2 contingency tables and is used almost exclusively for this purpose, in this section the test is extended to apply to other contingency tables such as 2×3, 3×3, 3×4, 2×2×2, and other larger contingency tables. For ease of calculation and to avoid large factorial expressions, a recursion procedure with an arbitrary initial value provides an efficient method to obtain exact probability values; for a detailed description of recursion procedures, see Chap. 2, Sects. 2.6.1 and 2.6.2.

4.11.1 Fisher's Exact Analysis of a 2×2 Table

Consider a 2×2 contingency table with N cases, where x_o denotes the observed frequency of any cell and r and c represent the row and column marginal frequency totals, respectively, corresponding to x_o. Table 4.48 illustrates the notation for a 2×2 contingency table.

If $H(x|r, c, N)$ is a recursively defined positive function in which

$$H(x|r, c, N) = D \times \binom{r}{x}\binom{N-r}{c-x}\binom{N}{c}^{-1}$$

$$= D \times \frac{r!\; c!\; (N-r)!\; (N-c)!}{N!\; x!\; (r-x)!\; (c-x)!\; (N-r-c+x)!} ,$$

where $D > 0$ is an unknown constant, then solving the recursive relation

$$H(x+1|r, c, N) = H(x|r, c, N) \times g(x)$$

yields

$$g(x) = \frac{(r-x)(c-x)}{(x+1)(N-r-c+x+1)} .$$

The algorithm may then be employed to enumerate all values of

$$H(x|r, c, N) ,$$

Table 4.48 Example notation for a 2×2 contingency table

	A_1	A_2	Total
B_1	x	$r-x$	r
B_2	$c-x$	$N-r-c+x$	$N-r$
Total	c	$N-c$	N

where $a \leq x \leq b$, $a = \max(0, r + c - N)$, $b = \min(r, c)$, and $H(a|N, r, c)$ is initially set to some small positive value [14]. The total over the entire distribution may be found by:

$$T = \sum_{k=a}^{b} H(k|r, c, N) \ .$$

To calculate the probability value of x_o, given the observed marginal frequency distributions, the point probability of the observed table must be determined. This value, designated by $U_2 = H(x|r, c, N)$, is found recursively. Next, the tail of the probability distribution associated with U_2 must be identified. Let

$$U_1 = \begin{cases} H(x_o - 1|r, c, N) & \text{if } x_o > a \ , \\ 0 & \text{if } x_o = a \ , \end{cases}$$

and

$$U_3 = \begin{cases} H(x_o + 1|r, c, N) & \text{if } x_o < b \ , \\ 0 & \text{if } x_o = b \ . \end{cases}$$

If $U_1 > U_3$, U_2 is located in the right tail of the distribution; otherwise, U_2 is defined to be in the left tail of the distribution, and the one-tailed (S_1) and two-tailed (S_2) subtotals may be found by:

$$S_1(x_o|r, c, N) = \sum_{k=a}^{b} K_k H(k|r, c, N)$$

and

$$S_2(x_o|r, c, N) = \sum_{k=a}^{b} L_k H(k|r, c, N) \ ,$$

respectively, where

$$K_k = \begin{cases} 1 & \text{if } U_1 \leq U_3 \text{ and } k \leq x_o \text{ or if } U_1 > U_2 \text{ and } k \geq x_o \ , \\ 0 & \text{otherwise} \ , \end{cases}$$

and

$$L_k = \begin{cases} 1 & \text{if } H(k|r, c, N) \leq U_2 \, , \\ 0 & \text{otherwise} \, , \end{cases}$$

for $k = a, \ldots, b$. The one- and two-tailed exact probability values are then given by:

$$P_1 = \frac{S_1}{T} \quad \text{and} \quad P_2 = \frac{S_2}{T} \, ,$$

respectively.

A 2×2 Contingency Table Example

To illustrate the calculation of Fisher's exact probability test for a fourfold contingency table, consider the 2×2 contingency table given in Table 4.49 with $x_o = 6$, $r = 9$, $c = 8$, $N = 20$,

$$a = \max(0, r + c - N) = \max(0, 9 + 8 - 20) = \max(0, -3) = 0 \, ,$$

$$b = \min(r, c) = \min(9, 8) = 8 \, ,$$

and $b - a + 1 = 8 - 0 + 1 = 9$ possible table configurations in the reference set of all permutations of cell frequencies, given the observed row and column marginal frequency distributions, {9, 11} and {8, 12}, respectively.

Table 4.50 lists the nine possible values of x in the first column. The second column of Table 4.50 lists the exact point probability values for $x = 0, \ldots, 8$ calculated from the conventional hypergeometric probability expression given by:

$$p(x|r, c, N) = \binom{r}{x}\binom{N-r}{c-x}\binom{N}{c}^{-1}$$
$$= \frac{r! \, (N-r)! \, c! \, (N-c)!}{N! \, x! \, (r-x)! \, (c-x)! \, (N-r-c+x)!} \, .$$

Table 4.49 Example 2×2 contingency table

	A_1	A_2	Total
B_1	6	3	9
B_2	2	9	11
Total	8	12	20

Table 4.50 Example of statistical recursion with an arbitrary initial value

x	Probability	$H(x\|r, c, N)$	$H(x\|r, c, N)/T$
0	0.001310	1	0.001310
1	0.023577	18	0.023577
2	0.132032	100.80	0.132032
3	0.308073	235.20	0.308073
4	0.330079	252	0.330079
5	0.165039	126	0.165039
6	0.036675	28	0.036675
7	0.003144	2.40	0.003144
8	0.000071	0.054545	0.000071
Total	1.000000	763.454545	1.000000

The third column of Table 4.50 contains the recursion values where, for $x = 0$, the initial (starting) value is arbitrarily set to 1 for this example analysis. Then,

$$1\left[\frac{(9)(8)}{(1)(4)}\right] = 18\ ,$$

$$18\left[\frac{(8)(7)}{(2)(5)}\right] = 100.80\ ,$$

$$100.80\left[\frac{(7)(6)}{(3)(6)}\right] = 235.20\ ,$$

$$235.20\left[\frac{(6)(5)}{(4)(7)}\right] = 252\ ,$$

$$252\left[\frac{(5)(4)}{(5)(8)}\right] = 126\ ,$$

$$126\left[\frac{(4)(3)}{(6)(9)}\right] = 28\ ,$$

$$28\left[\frac{(3)(2)}{(7)(10)}\right] = 2.40\ ,$$

$$2.40\left[\frac{(2)(1)}{(8)(11)}\right] = 0.054545\ .$$

The total of $H(x|r, c, N)$ for $x = 0, \ldots, 8$ is

$$\begin{aligned} T &= 1 + 18 + 100.80 + 235.20 + 252 + 126 + 28 + 2.40 + 0.054545 \\ &= 763.454545\ . \end{aligned}$$

The fourth column of Table 4.50 corrects the entries of the third column by dividing each entry by T. For the frequency data given in Table 4.41 on p. 192,

$$U_2 = H(x_o|r, c, N) = H(6|9, 8, 20) = 28 .$$

Because $x_o > a$, i.e., $6 > 1$,

$$U_1 = H(x_o - 1|r, v, N) = H(5|9, 8, 20) = 126$$

and because $x_o < b$, i.e., $6 < 8$,

$$U_3 = H(x_o + 1|r, c, N) = H(7|9, 8, 20) = 2.40 .$$

Thus, $U_2 = 28$ is located in the right tail of the distribution since $U_1 > U_3$, i.e., $126 > 2.40$. Then, the one- and two-tailed subtotals are

$$S_1 = 28 + 2.40 + 0.054545 = 30.454545$$

and

$$S_2 = 1 + 18 + 28 + 2.40 + 0.054545 = 49.454545 ,$$

respectively, and the one- and two-tailed exact probability values are

$$P_1 = \frac{S_1}{T} = \frac{30.454545}{763.454545} = 0.039890$$

and

$$P_2 = \frac{S_2}{T} = \frac{49.454545}{763.454545} = 0.064777 ,$$

respectively.

4.11.2 Larger Contingency Tables

Although Fisher's exact probability test has largely been limited to the analysis of 2×2 contingency tables in the literature, it is not difficult to extend Fisher's exact test to larger contingency tables, although such extensions may be computationally intensive [71, pp. 127–130, 296–298]. Consider an example 2×3 contingency table with N cases, where x_o denotes the observed frequency of the cell in the first row and first column, y_o denotes the observed frequency of the cell in the second row and first column, and r_1, r_2, and c_1 are the observed marginal frequency totals in the first row, second row, and first column, respectively. If $H(x, y)$, given N, r_1,

r_2, and c_1, is a recursively defined positive function, then solving the recursive relation

$$H(x, y+1) = H(x, y) \times g_1(x, y)$$

yields

$$g_1(x, y) = \frac{(c_1 - x - y)(r_2 - y)}{(1 + y)(N - r_1 - r_2 - c_1 + 1 + x + y)} . \tag{4.14}$$

If $y = \min(r_2, c_1 - x)$, then $H(x + 1, y) = H(x, y) \times g_2(x, y)$, where

$$g_2(x, y) = \frac{(c_1 - x - y)(r_1 - x)}{(1 + x)(N - r_1 - r_2 - c_1 + 1 + x + y)} , \tag{4.15}$$

given that $\max(0, r_1 + r_2 + c_1 - N - x) = 0$. However, if $y = \min(r_2, c_1 - x)$ and $\max(0, r_1 + r_2 + c_1 - N - x) > 0$, then $H(x + 1, y - 1) = H(x, y) \times g_3(x, y)$, where

$$g_3(x, y) = \frac{y(r_1 - x)}{(1 + x)(r_2 + 1 - y)} . \tag{4.16}$$

The three recursive expressions given in Eqs. (4.14), (4.15), and (4.16) may be employed to completely enumerate the distribution of $H(x, y)$, where $a \leq x \leq b$, $a = \max(0, r_1 + c_1 - N)$, $b = \min(r_1, c_1)$, $c(x) \leq y \leq d(x)$, $c(x) = \max(0, r_1 + r_2 + c_1 - N + x)$, $d(x) = \min(r_2, c_1 - x)$, and $H[a, c(x)]$ is initially set to some small positive value [15]. The total over the completely enumerated distribution may be found by:

$$T = \sum_{x=a}^{b} \sum_{y=c(x)}^{d(x)} H(x, y) .$$

To calculate the probability value of (x_o, y_o), given the observed marginal frequency distributions, the hypergeometric point probability value of the observed 2×3 contingency table must be obtained; this value may also be found recursively. Next, the probability of a result this extreme or more extreme must be found. The subtotal is given by:

$$S = \sum_{x=a}^{b} \sum_{y=c(x)}^{d(x)} J_{x,y} H_{x,y} ,$$

Table 4.51 Example 2×3 contingency table

	A_1	A_2	A_3	Total
B_1	5	3	2	10
B_2	8	4	7	19
Total	13	7	9	29

where

$$J_{x,y} = \begin{cases} 1 & \text{if } H(x, y) \leq H(x_o, y_o) , \\ 0 & \text{otherwise} , \end{cases}$$

for $x = a, \ldots, b$ and $y = c(x), \ldots, d(x)$. The exact probability value for independence associated with the observed cell frequencies, x_o and y_o is given by $P = S/T$.

A 2×3 Contingency Table Example

To illustrate the calculation of Fisher's exact probability test for a 2×3 contingency table, consider the frequency data given in Table 4.51 where $x_o = 5$, $y_o = 3$, $r_1 = 10$, $c_1 = 13$, $c_2 = 7$, and $N = 29$. For the frequency data given in Table 4.51, there are only $M = 59$ arrangements[6] of cell frequencies that are consistent with the observed row and column marginal frequency distributions, $\{10, 19\}$ and $\{13, 7, 9\}$, respectively, and exactly 56 of the arrangements $M = 59$ have hypergeometric point probability values equal to or less than the point probability value of the observed table ($p = 0.8096 \times 10^{-1}$), yielding an exact probability value of $P = 0.6873$. Since the 2×3 table in Table 4.51 has only two degrees of freedom, Table 4.52 lists the $M = 59$ values for n_{11} and n_{12} for each possible arrangement of cell frequencies, given the observed marginal frequency totals, and the associated hypergeometric point probability values. Row 56 contains the observed values of $n_{11} = 5$ and $n_{12} = 3$ indicated by an asterisk.

A 2×6 Contingency Table Example

Fisher's exact probability test is easily extended to any $2 \times c$ contingency table. For example, consider the 2×6 contingency table given in Table 4.53 where $v_o = 1$, $w_o = 4$, $x_o = 3$, $y_o = 4$, $z_o = 8$, $r_1 = 6$, $r_2 = 5$, $r_3 = 10$, $r_4 = 9$, $r_5 = 10$,

[6] Although it is relatively simple to calculate the number of possible arrangements of cell frequencies (M) for a 2×2 contingency tables prior to analysis, it is considerably more difficult to calculate M for larger contingency tables; thus, M is usually determined at the conclusion of the analysis. For an algorithm to approximate the number of possible arrangements of cell frequencies, see a 1977 article in *Journal of the American Statistical Association* by Gail and Mantel [35].

Table 4.52 Listing of the $M = 59$ possible cell arrangements for the data given in Table 4.51 with cell frequencies n_{11}, n_{12}, and associated exact hypergeometric point probability values

Table	n_{11}	n_{12}	Probability	Table	n_{11}	n_{12}	Probability
1	0	1	0.3495×10^{-6}	31	6	4	0.2999×10^{-2}
2	1	0	0.6490×10^{-6}	32	7	3	0.2999×10^{-2}
3	0	7	0.4194×10^{-5}	33	8	1	0.4048×10^{-2}
4	0	2	0.9436×10^{-5}	34	4	5	0.6747×10^{-2}
5	10	0	0.1428×10^{-4}	35	2	2	0.6869×10^{-2}
6	3	7	0.1428×10^{-4}	36	2	5	0.6869×10^{-2}
7	1	7	0.2336×10^{-4}	37	7	0	0.7196×10^{-2}
8	2	0	0.3505×10^{-4}	38	5	0	0.8096×10^{-2}
9	2	7	0.3505×10^{-4}	39	3	1	0.8396×10^{-2}
10	1	1	0.4089×10^{-4}	40	3	5	0.1079×10^{-1}
11	0	6	0.4404×10^{-4}	41	6	0	0.1079×10^{-1}
12	0	3	0.6291×10^{-4}	42	7	2	0.1619×10^{-1}
13	0	5	0.1321×10^{-3}	43	2	3	0.1717×10^{-1}
14	0	4	0.1468×10^{-3}	44	2	4	0.1717×10^{-1}
15	4	6	0.2499×10^{-3}	45	5	4	0.2024×10^{-1}
16	9	1	0.2499×10^{-3}	46	7	1	0.2159×10^{-1}
17	9	0	0.3213×10^{-3}	47	6	3	0.2699×10^{-1}
18	1	6	0.3816×10^{-3}	48	4	1	0.3148×10^{-1}
19	1	2	0.4907×10^{-3}	49	3	2	0.3778×10^{-1}
20	3	0	0.5140×10^{-3}	50	3	4	0.4198×10^{-1}
21	3	6	0.8996×10^{-3}	51	4	4	0.4498×10^{-1}
22	2	6	0.9813×10^{-3}	52	6	1	0.5037×10^{-1}
23	2	1	0.9813×10^{-3}	53	5	1	0.5667×10^{-1}
24	5	5	0.1349×10^{-2}	54	3	3	0.6297×10^{-1}
25	8	2	0.1349×10^{-2}	55	6	2	0.6447×10^{-1}
26	1	5	0.1717×10^{-2}	56*	5	3	0.8096×10^{-1}
27	1	3	0.1908×10^{-2}	57	4	2	0.9445×10^{-1}
28	8	0	0.2313×10^{-2}	58	4	3	0.1049
29	1	4	0.2862×10^{-2}	59	5	2	0.1133
30	4	0	0.2999×10^{-2}				

Table 4.53 Example 2×6 contingency table

	A_1	A_2	A_3	A_4	A_5	A_6	Total
B_1	1	4	3	4	8	9	29
B_2	5	1	7	5	2	3	23
Total	6	5	10	9	10	12	52

$c_1 = 29$, and $N = 52$. For the frequency data given in Table 4.53, $M = 33{,}565$ arrangements of cell frequencies are consistent with the observed row and column marginal frequency distributions, $\{29, 23\}$ and $\{6, 5, 10, 9, 10, 12\}$, respectively, and exactly 27,735 of the $M = 33{,}565$ arrangements have hypergeometric point probability values equal to or less than the point probability value of the observed table ($p = 0.1159\times10^{-3}$), yielding an exact probability value of $P = 0.0338$.

A 3×3 Contingency Table Example

Fisher's exact probability test can also be applied to larger contingency tables, although calculation time increases substantially as the number of rows and columns increase. In this section, Fisher's exact probability test is applied to a 3×3 contingency table. Consider the 3×3 contingency table given in Table 4.54 where $w_o = 3$, $x_o = 5$, $y_o = 2$, $z_o = 9$, $r_1 = 10$, $r_2 = 14$, $c_1 = 13$, $c_2 = 16$, and $N = 40$. For the frequency data given in Table 4.54, $M = 4{,}818$ arrangements of cell frequencies are consistent with the observed row and column marginal frequency distributions, $\{10, 14, 16\}$ and $\{13, 16, 11\}$, respectively, and exactly 3,935 of the $M = 4{,}818$ arrangements have hypergeometric point probability values equal to or less than the point probability value of the observed table ($p = 0.1273\times10^{-4}$), yielding an exact probability value of $P = 0.0475$.

A 3×4 Contingency Table Example

Finally, consider the sparse 3×4 contingency table given in Table 4.55. For the frequency data given in Table 4.55, only $M = 706$ arrangements of cell frequencies are consistent with the observed row and column marginal frequency distributions, $\{5, 5, 4\}$ and $\{4, 3, 4, 3\}$, respectively, and 168 of the $M = 706$ arrangements have hypergeometric point probability values equal to or less than the point probability value of the observed table ($p = 0.1903\times10^{-3}$), yielding an exact probability value of $P = 0.0187$.

Table 4.54 Example 3×3 contingency table

	A_1	A_2	A_3	Total
B_1	3	5	2	10
B_2	2	9	3	14
B_3	8	2	6	16
Total	13	16	11	40

Table 4.55 Example 3×4 contingency table

	A_1	A_2	A_3	A_4	Total
B_1	3	0	0	2	5
B_2	0	3	1	1	5
B_3	1	0	3	0	4
Total	4	3	4	3	14

4.12 Analyses of 2×2×2 Tables

Fisher's exact probability test is not limited to two-way contingency tables. Consider a 2×2×2 contingency table, such as depicted in Fig. 4.1, where n_{ijk} denotes the cell frequency of the ith row, jth column, and kth slice for $i, j, k = 1, 2$. Denote by a dot $(\cdot)$ the partial sum of all rows, all columns, or all slices, depending on the position of the $(\cdot)$ in the subscript list. If the $(\cdot)$ is in the first subscript position, the sum is over all rows, if the $(\cdot)$ is in the second subscript position, the sum is over all columns, and if the $(\cdot)$ is in the third subscript position, the sum is over all slices. Thus, $n_{i..}$ denotes the marginal frequency total of the ith row, $i = 1, \ldots, r$, summed over all columns and slices; $n_{.j.}$ denotes the marginal frequency total of the jth column, $j = 1, \ldots, c$, summed over all rows and slices; and $n_{..k}$ denotes the marginal frequency total of the kth slice, $k = 1, \ldots, s$, summed over all rows and columns. Therefore, $A = n_{1..}$, $B = n_{.1.}$, $C = n_{..1}$, and $N = n_{...}$ denote the observed marginal frequency totals of the first row, first column, first slice, and entire table, respectively, such that $1 \leq A \leq B \leq C \leq N/2$. Also, let $w = n_{111}$, $x = n_{112}$, $y = n_{121}$, and $z = n_{211}$ denote cell frequencies of the 2×2×2 contingency table. Then, the probability for any w, x, y, and z is given by:

$$
\begin{aligned}
P(w, x, y, z|A, B, C, N) = \\
&\big[A!(N-A)!\, B!\,(N-B)!\, C!(N-C)!\big] \\
&\times \big[(N!)^2\, w!\, x!\, y!\, z!\,(A-w-x-y)!\,(B-w-x-z)! \\
&\quad (C-w-y-z)!\,(N-A-B-C+2w+x+y+z)!\big]^{-1}
\end{aligned}
$$

[67]. An algorithm to compute Fisher's exact probability test involves a nested looping structure and requires two distinct passes. The first pass yields the exact

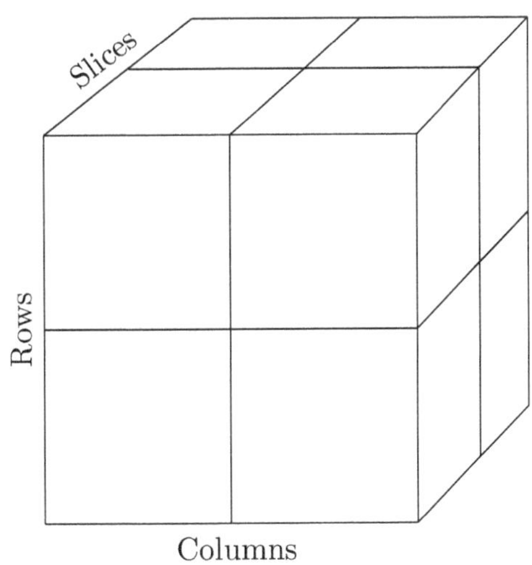

Fig. 4.1 Graphic depiction of a 2×2×2 contingency table

probability, U, of the observed 2×2×2 contingency table and is terminated when U is obtained. The second pass yields the exact probability value of all tables with hypergeometric point probability values equal to or less than the point probability of the observed contingency table. The four nested loops within each pass are over the cell frequency indices w, x, y, and z, respectively. The bounds for w, x, y, and z are

$$0 \leq w \leq M_w \;,$$
$$0 \leq x \leq M_x \;,$$
$$0 \leq y \leq M_y \;,$$

and

$$L_x \leq z \leq M_z \;,$$

respectively, where $M_w = A$, $M_x = A - w$, $M_y = A - w - x$, $M_z = \min(B - w - x, C - w - y)$, and $L_z = \max(0, A + B + C - N - 2w - x - y)$.

The recursion method can be illustrated with the fourth (inner) loop over z, given w, x, y, A, B, C, and N because the inner loop yields both U on the first pass and the exact probability value on the second pass. Let $H(w, x, y, z)$ be a recursively defined positive function given A, B, C, and N, satisfying

$$H(w, x, y, z + 1) = H(w, x, y, z) \times g(w, x, y, z) \;,$$

where

$$g(w, x, y, z) = \frac{(B - w - x - z)(C - w - z)}{(z + 1)(N - A - B - C + 2w + x + y + z + 1)} \;.$$

The remaining three loops of each pass initialize $H(w, x, y, z)$ for continued enumerations. Let $I_x = \max(0, A + B + C - N)$ and set the initial value of $H(0, 0, 0, I_z)$ to an arbitrary small positive constant. Then, the total over the completely enumerated distribution is found by:

$$T = \sum_{w=0}^{M_w} \sum_{x=0}^{M_x} \sum_{y=0}^{M_y} \sum_{z=L_x}^{M_x} H(w, x, y, z) \;.$$

If w_o, x_o, y_o, and z_o are the values of w, x, y, and z in the observed 2×2×2 contingency table, then U and the exact probability value (P) are given by:

$$U = H(w_o, x_o, y_o, z_o)/T$$

and

$$P = \sum_{w=0}^{M_w} \sum_{x=0}^{M_x} \sum_{y=0}^{M_y} \sum_{z=L_x}^{M_x} H(w, x, y, z)\, \psi(w, x, y, z,)/T \; .$$

respectively, where

$$\psi(w, x, y, z) = \begin{cases} 1 & \text{if } H(w, x, y, z) \leq H(w_o, x_o, y_o, z_o) \; , \\ 0 & \text{otherwise} \; . \end{cases}$$

4.12.1 A 2×2×2 Contingency Table Example

Consider a scenario in which $N = 1{,}663$ respondents were asked if they agreed with the statement that women should have equal pay for the same job as men (No, Yes). The respondents were then classified by region of the country (North, South) and by year of the survey (2000, 2010). For the frequency data given in Table 4.56, $M = 3{,}683{,}159{,}504$ arrangements of cell frequencies are consistent with the observed row, column, and slice marginal frequency distributions, {623, 1040}, $\{1{,}279, 384\}$, and $\{1{,}039, 624\}$, respectively. Exactly 2,761,590,498 of the arrangements have hypergeometric point probability values equal to or less than the point probability value of the observed table ($p = 0.1684 \times 10^{-72}$), yielding an exact probability value of $P = 0.1684 \times 10^{-65}$.

4.12.2 A 3×4×2 Contingency Table Example

Fisher's exact probability test is not limited to multi-way contingency tables with only two categories in each dimension. Consider the $r \times c \times s$ contingency table given in Table 4.57 with $r = 3$ rows, $c = 4$ columns, and $s = 2$ slices. In general, it is not efficient to analyze complex multi-way tables with exact permutation procedures, as there are usually too many arrangements of cell frequencies in the reference set of all possible arrangements of cell frequencies. For the frequency data given in Table 4.57 with row, column, and slice marginal frequency distributions, $\{71, 31\}$,

Table 4.56 Cross-classification of responses (No, Yes), categorized by year and region

	Region			
	North		South	
Year	No	Yes	No	Yes
2000	410	56	126	31
2010	439	374	64	163

Table 4.57 Three-way contingency table with $r = 3$ rows, $c = 4$ columns, and $s = 2$ slices

		C_1	C_2	C_3	C_4
S_1	R_1	3	4	1	6
	R_2	7	8	4	9
	R_3	7	8	9	5
S_2	R_1	2	6	5	2
	R_2	0	2	6	1
	R_3	2	4	0	1

$\{21, 32, 25, 24\}$, and $\{29, 37, 36\}$, respectively, the approximate resampling probability value based on $L = 1{,}000{,}000$ random arrangements of cell frequencies is

$$P = \frac{29{,}600}{1{,}000{,}000} = 0.0296 .$$

4.13 Coda

Chapter 3 applied permutation statistical methods to measures of association for two nominal-level variables that are based on Pearson's chi-squared test statistic. Chapter 4 applied exact and resampling permutation statistical methods to measures of association for two nominal-level variables that are not based on Pearson's chi-squared test statistic. Included in Chap. 4 were Goodman and Kruskal's asymmetric λ_a, λ_b, t_a, and t_b measures, Cohen's unweighted chance-corrected κ coefficient, McNemar's and Cochran's Q measures of change, Leik and Gove's d_N^c measure, Mielke and Siddiqui's exact probability for the matrix occupancy problem, and Fisher's exact probability test, extended to cover a variety of contingency tables. For each test, examples illustrated the measures and either exact or resampling probability values based on the appropriate permutation analysis were provided.

Chapter 5 applies permutation statistical methods to a variety of measures of association designed for ordinal-level variables that are based on all possible paired comparisons. Included in Chap. 5 are Kendall's τ_a and τ_b and Stuart's τ_c measures of ordinal association, Somers' asymmetric d_{yx} and d_{xy} measures, Kim's $d_{y.x}$ and $d_{x.y}$ measures, Wilson's e measure, and Cureton's rank-biserial correlation coefficient.

References

1. Acock, A.C., Stavig, G.R.: A measure of association for nonparametric statistics. Social Forces **57**, 1381–1386 (1979)
2. Agresti, A., Finlay, B.: Statistical Methods for the Social Sciences. Prentice–Hall, Upper Saddle River, NJ (1997)
3. Armitage, P., Blendis, L.M., Smyllie, H.C.: The measurement of observer disagreement in the recording of signs. J. R. Stat. Soc. A Gen. **129**, 98–109 (1966)

4. Bartko, J.J.: The intraclass correlation coefficient as a measure of reliability. Psychol. Rep. **19**, 3–11 (1966)
5. Bartko, J.J., Carpenter, W.T.: On the methods and theory of reliability. J. Nerv. Ment. Dis. **163**, 307–317 (1976)
6. Berkson, J.: Some difficulties of interpretation encountered in the application of the chi-square test. J. Am. Stat. Assoc. **33**, 526–536 (1938)
7. Berry, K.J., Jacobsen, R.B., Martin, T.W.: Clarifying the use of chi-square: Testing the significance of Goodman and Kruskal's gamma. Soc. Sci. Quart. **57**, 687–690 (1976)
8. Berry, K.J., Johnston, J.E., Mielke, P.W.: Exact and resampling probability values for measures associated with ordered R by C contingency tables. Psychol. Rep. **99**, 231–238 (2006)
9. Berry, K.J., Johnston, J.E., Mielke, P.W.: An alternative measure of effect size for Cochran's Q test for related proportions. Percept. Motor Skill **104**, 1236–1242 (2007)
10. Berry, K.J., Martin, T.W., Olson, K.F.: A note on fourfold point correlation. Educ. Psychol. Meas. **34**, 53–56 (1974)
11. Berry, K.J., Martin, T.W., Olson, K.F.: A note on fourfold point correlation. Educ. Psychol. Meas. **34**, 53–56 (1974)
12. Berry, K.J., Martin, T.W., Olson, K.F.: Testing theoretical hypotheses: A PRE statistic. Social Forces **53**, 190–196 (1974)
13. Berry, K.J., Mielke, P.W.: Goodman and Kruskal's tau-b statistic: A nonasymptotic test of significance. Sociol Method Res. **13**, 543–550 (1985)
14. Berry, K.J., Mielke, P.W.: Subroutines for computing exact chi-square and Fisher's exact probability tests. Educ. Psychol. Meas. **45**, 153–159 (1985)
15. Berry, K.J., Mielke, P.W.: Exact chi-square and Fisher's exact probability test for 3 by 2 cross-classification tables. Educ. Psychol. Meas. **47**, 631–636 (1987)
16. Berry, K.J., Mielke, P.W.: A generalization of Cohen's kappa agreement measure to interval measurement and multiple raters. Educ. Psychol. Meas. **48**, 921–933 (1988)
17. Blalock, H.M.: Probabilistic interpretations for the mean square contingency. J. Am. Stat. Assoc. **53**, 102–105 (1958)
18. Blalock, H.M.: Social Statistics, 2nd edn. McGraw–Hill, New York (1979)
19. Böhning, D., Holling, H.: A Monte Carlo study on minimizing chi-square distances under the hypothesis of homogeneity or independence for a two-way contingency table. Statistics **20**, 55–70 (1989)
20. Brennan, R.L., Prediger, D.J.: Coefficient kappa: Some uses, misuses, and alternatives. Educ. Psychol. Meas. **41**, 687–699 (1981)
21. Cicchetti, D.V., Showalter, D., Tyrer, P.J.: The effect of number of rating scale categories on levels of interrater reliability. Appl. Psychol. Meas. **9**, 31–36 (1985)
22. Cochran, W.G.: The comparison of percentages in matched samples. Biometrika **37**, 256–266 (1950)
23. Cohen, J.: A coefficient of agreement for nominal scales. Educ. Psychol. Meas. **20**, 37–46 (1960)
24. Cohen, J.: Weighted kappa: Nominal scale agreement with provision for scaled disagreement or partial credit. Psychol. Bull. **70**, 213–220 (1968)
25. Conger, A.J.: Integration and generalization of kappas for multiple raters. Psychol. Bull. **88**, 322–328 (1980)
26. Conger, A.J.: Kappa reliabilities for continuous behaviors and events. Educ. Psychol. Meas. **45**, 861–868 (1985)
27. Costner, H.L.: Criteria for measures of association. Am. Sociol. Rev. **30**, 341–353 (1965)
28. Eicker, P.J., Siddiqui, M.M., Mielke, P.W.: A matrix occupancy problem. Ann. Math. Stat. **43**, 988–996 (1972)
29. Feinstein, A.R.: Clinical Biostatistics XXIII: The role of randomization in sampling, testing, allocation, and credulous idolatry (Part 2). Clin. Pharmacol. Ther. **14**, 898–915 (1973)
30. Ferguson, G.A.: Statistical Analysis in Psychology and Education, 5th edn. McGraw–Hill, New York (1981)

31. Fisher, R.A.: Statistical Methods for Research Workers, 5th edn. Oliver and Boyd, Edinburgh (1934)
32. Fisher, R.A.: The logic of inductive inference (with discussion). J. R. Stat. Soc. **98**, 39–82 (1935)
33. Fleiss, J.L.: Measuring nominal scale agreement among many raters. Psych. Bull. **76**, 378–382 (1971)
34. Fleiss, J.L., J, C.: The equivalence of weighted kappa and the intraclass coefficient as measures of reliability. Educ. Psychol. Meas. **33**, 613–619 (1973)
35. Gail, M., Mantel, N.: Counting the number of $r \times c$ contingency tables with fixed margins. J. Am. Stat. Assoc. **72**, 859–862 (1977)
36. Gittelsohn, A.M.: An occupancy problem. Am. Stat. **23**, 11–12 (1969)
37. Goodman, L.A., Kruskal, W.H.: Measures of association for cross classifications. J. Am. Stat. Assoc. **49**, 732–764 (1954)
38. Goodman, L.A., Kruskal, W.H.: Measures of association for cross classifications, II: Further discussion and references. J. Am. Stat. Assoc. **54**, 123–163 (1959)
39. Goodman, L.A., Kruskal, W.H.: Measures of association for cross classifications, III: Approximate sampling theory. J. Am. Stat. Assoc. **58**, 310–364 (1963)
40. Goodman, L.A., Kruskal, W.H.: Measures of association for cross classifications, IV: Simplification of asymptotic variances. J. Am. Stat. Assoc. **67**, 415–421 (1972)
41. Graham, P., Jackson, R.: The analysis of ordinal agreement data: Beyond weighted kappa. J. Clin. Epidemiol. **46**, 1055–1062 (1993)
42. Guilford, J.P.: Fundamental Statistics in Psychology and Education. McGraw–Hill, New York (1950)
43. Guttman, L.: An outline of the statistical theory of prediction. In: Horst, P., Wallin, P., Guttman, L., et al. (eds.) The Prediction of Personal Adjustment, pp. 253–318. Social Science Research Council, New York (1941)
44. Hubert, L.J.: Kappa revisited. Psychol. Bull. **84**, 289–297 (1977)
45. Hunter, A.A.: On the validity of measures of association: The nominal-nominal two-by-two case. Am. J. Sociol. **79**, 99–109 (1973)
46. Iachan, R.: Measures of agreement for incompletely ranked data. Educ. Psychol. Meas. **44**, 823–830 (1984)
47. Irwin, J.O.: Tests of significance for differences between percentages based on small numbers. Metron **12**, 83–94 (1935)
48. Kendall, M.G., Babington Smith, B.: On the method of paired comparisons. Biometrika **31**, 324–345 (1940)
49. Kramer, M., Schmidhammer, J.: The chi-squared statistic in ethology: Use and misuse. Animal. Beh. **44**, 833–841 (1992)
50. Krippendorff, K.: Bivariate agreement coefficients for reliability of data. In: Borgatta, E.F. (ed.) Sociological Methodology, pp. 139–150. Jossey–Bass, San Francisco (1970)
51. Landis, J.R., Koch, G.G.: An application of hierarchical kappa-type statistics in the assessment of majority agreement among multiple observers. Biometrics **33**, 363–374 (1977)
52. Leik, R.K., Gove, W.R.: The conception and measurement of asymmetric monotonic relationships in sociology. Am. J. Sociol. **74**, 696–709 (1969)
53. Leik, R.K., Gove, W.R.: Integrated approach to measuring association. In: Costner, H.L. (ed.) Sociological Methodology, pp. 279–301. Jossey Bass, San Francisco, CA (1971)
54. Light, R.J.: Measures of response agreement for qualitative data: Some generalizations and alternatives. Psychol. Bull. **76**, 365–377 (1971)
55. Light, R.J., Margolin, B.H.: An analysis of variance for categorical data. J. Am. Stat. Assoc. **66**, 534–544 (1971)
56. Lunney, G.H.: Using analysis of variance with a dichotomous dependent variable: An empirical study. J. Educ. Meas. **7**, 263–269 (1970)
57. Maclure, M., Willett, W.C.: Misinterpretation and misuse of the kappa statistic. Am. J. Epidemiol. **126**, 161–169 (1987)

58. Mantel, N.: 361: Approaches to a health research occupancy problem. Biometrics **30**, 355–362 (1974)
59. Mantel, N., Pasternack, B.S.: A class of occupancy problems. Am. Stat. **22**, 23–24 (1968)
60. Marascuilo, L.A., McSweeney: Nonparametric and Distribution-free methods in the Social Sciences. Brooks–Cole, Monterey, CA (1977)
61. Margolin, B.H., Light, R.J.: An analysis of variance for categorical data, II: Small sample comparisons with chi square and other competitors. J. Am. Stat. Assoc. **69**, 755–764 (1974)
62. May, R.B., Masson, M.E., Hunter, M.A.: Applications of Statistics in Behavioral Research. Harper & Row, New York (1990)
63. McNemar, Q.: Note on the sampling error of the differences between correlated proportions and percentages. Psychometrika **12**, 153–157 (1947)
64. Mielke, P.W., Berry, K.J.: Cumulant methods for analyzing independence of r-way contingency tables and goodness-of-fit frequency data. Biometrika **75**, 790–793 (1988)
65. Mielke, P.W., Berry, K.J.: Nonasymptotic inferences based on Cochran's Q test. Percept. Motor Skill **81**, 319–322 (1995)
66. Mielke, P.W., Berry, K.J., Johnston, J.E.: Resampling programs for multiway contingency tables with fixed marginal frequency totals. Psychol. Rep. **101**, 18–24 (2007)
67. Mielke, P.W., Berry, K.J., Zelterman, D.: Fisher's exact test of mutual independence for $2 \times 2 \times 2$ cross-classification tables. Educ. Psychol. Meas. **54**, 110–114 (1994)
68. Mielke, P.W., Siddiqui, M.M.: A combinatorial test for independence of dichotomous responses. J. Am. Stat. Assoc. **60**, 437–441 (1965)
69. Pearson, K.: On the criterion that a given system of deviations from the probable in the case of a correlated system of variables is such that it can be reasonably supposed to have arisen from random sampling. Philos. Mag. 5 **50**, 157–175 (1900)
70. Pearson, K.: On the laws of inheritance in man: II. On the inheritance of the mental and moral characters in man, and its comparison with the inheritance of the physical characters. Biometrika **3**, 131–190 (1904)
71. Pierce, A.: Fundamentals of Nonparametric Statistics. Dickenson, Belmont, CA (1970)
72. Robinson, W.S.: Ecological correlations and the behavior of individuals. Am. Soc. Rev. **15**, 351–357 (1950). [Reprinted in Int J Epidem **38**, 337–341 (2009)]
73. Robinson, W.S.: The statistical measurement of agreement. Am. Sociol. Rev. **22**, 17–25 (1957)
74. Robinson, W.S.: The geometric interpretation of agreement. Am. Sociol. Rev. **24**, 338–345 (1959)
75. Särndal, C.E.: A comparative study of association measures. Psychometrika **39**, 165–187 (1974)
76. Scott, W.A.: Reliability of content analysis: The case of nominal scale coding. Public Opin. Quart. **19**, 321–325 (1955)
77. Serlin, R.C., Carr, J., Marascuilo, L.A.: A measure of association for selected non-parametric procedures. Psychol. Bull. **92**, 786–790 (1982)
78. Somers, R.H.: A new asymmetric measure of association for ordinal variables. Am. Sociol. Rev. **27**, 799–811 (1962)
79. Spearman, C.E.: The proof and measurement of association between two things. Am. J. Psychol. **15**, 72–101 (1904)
80. Spearman, C.E.: 'Footrule' for measuring correlation. Brit. J. Psychol. **2**, 89–108 (1906)
81. Sprott, D.A.: A note on a class of occupancy problems. Am. Stat. **23**, 12–13 (1969)
82. Tschuprov, A.A.: Principles of the Mathematical Theory of Correlation. Hodge, London (1939). [Translated by M. Kantorowitsch]
83. Vanbelle, S., Albert, A.: A note on the linearly weighted kappa coefficient for ordinal scales. Stat. Methodol. **6**, 157–163 (2008)
84. Wasserstein, R., Lazar, N.A.: The ASA's statement on p-values: Context, process, and purpose. Am. Stat. **70**, 129–133 (2016)
85. White, C.: The committee problem. Am. Stat. **25**, 25–26 (1971)
86. Wickens, T.D.: Multiway Contingency Tables Analysis for the Social Sciences. Erlbaum, Hillsdale, NJ (1989)

87. Wilkinson, L.: Statistical methods in psychology journals: Guidelines and explanations. Am. Psychol. **54**, 594–604 (1999)
88. Williams, G.W.: Comparing the joint agreement of several raters with another rater. Biometrics **32**, 619–627 (1976)
89. Yates, F.: Contingency tables involving small numbers and the χ^2 test. Suppl. J. R. Stat. Soc. **1**, 217–235 (1934)
90. Yule, G.U.: On the methods of measuring association between two attributes. J. R. Stat. Soc. **75**, 579–652 (1912). [Originally a paper read before the Royal Statistical Society on 23 April 1912]

Chapter 5
Ordinal-Level Variables, I

Measures of relationships between two ordinal-level (ranked) variables are typically more informative than measures of relationships between simple nominal-level (categorical) variables, as disjoint, ordered categories usually contain more information than disjoint, unordered categories. Examples of ordinal-level variables are: Race Finishes (Win, Place, Show), Birth Order (1st, 2nd, 3rd, etc.), Academic Rank (Assistant Professor, Associate Professor, Professor), and Likert Scales (Strongly Agree, Agree, Neutral, Disagree, Strongly Disagree). Measures of association for two ordinal-level variables are typically of two types: those based on pairwise differences, such as Kendall's τ_a and τ_b measures and Goodman and Kruskal's γ measure, and those based on criteria other than pairwise differences, such as Cohen's weighted kappa measure of inter-rater agreement and Bross's ridit analysis.

Chapter 5 of *The Measurement of Association* provides exact and Monte Carlo permutation statistical methods for a variety of measures of association designed for ordinal-level variables that are based on all possible pairwise comparisons between ranked scores. Included in this chapter are exact and Monte Carlo permutation statistical methods for Kendall's τ_a and τ_b measures of ordinal association, Stuart's τ_c measure, Goodman and Kruskal's γ measure, Somers' d_{yx} and d_{xy} measures, Kim's $d_{y \cdot x}$ and $d_{x \cdot y}$ measures, Wilson's e measure, Whitfield's S measure of ordinal association between one ordinal-level variable and one binary variable, and Cureton's rank-biserial correlation coefficient. Measures of association for two ordinal-level variables that are not based on pairwise comparisons are considered in Chap. 6 and include Spearman's rank-order correlation coefficient, Spearman's footrule measure of agreement, Kendall's coefficient of concordance, Kendall's u measure of inter-rater agreement, Cohen's weighted kappa measure of agreement, and Bross's ridit analysis.

The measurement of objects by ordering or ranking them has an early and distinguished beginning. It is not widely recognized that Francis Galton was an early advocate of ranked data. In 1922, on the centenary of Francis Galton's birth, Sir Henry Rew attributed Galton's first contribution to statistics to an 1875 article in

K. J. Berry et al., *The Measurement of Association*,
https://doi.org/10.1007/978-3-319-98926-6_5

Philosophical Magazine, Series 4 on "Statistics by intercomparison, with remarks on the law of frequency of error" [41]. Galton's method of intercomparison was expressly designed to bring attributes that could be ordered or ranked, but not measured, within the purview of statistical analysis [39, p. 144]. Galton's objective was to describe a method for obtaining simple statistical results that was "applicable to a multitude of objects lying outside the present limits of statistical enquiry" [13, p. 33]. Galton contended that the objects needed only to be ranked in order as regards the characteristic considered—the middlemost (median) indicating the average and those objects one-quarter distant from either end (quartiles) indicating the divergence of the series, i.e., the probable or median error. Galton argued that these three values, median and two quartiles, were sufficient to characterize or compare populations [39, p. 144].[1]

5.1 Pairwise Measures of Ordinal Association

A number of measures of association for two ordinal-level variables are based on pairwise comparisons of differences between rank scores. The test statistic S, as defined by Maurice Kendall in 1938 [21] and more extensively in 1948 [23], plays an important role in a variety of statistical measures where Kendall's test statistic is often expressed as $S = C - D$, where C and D indicate the number of concordant pairs and discordant pairs, respectively, *vide infra*.[2] Consider two ordinal variables that have been cross-classified into an $r \times c$ contingency table, where r and c denote the number of rows and columns, respectively. Let $n_{i.}$, $n_{.j}$, and n_{ij} denote the row marginal frequency totals, column marginal frequency totals, and number of objects in the ijth cell, respectively, for $i = 1, \ldots, r$ and $j = 1, \ldots, c$, and let N denote the total number of objects in the $r \times c$ contingency table, i.e.,

$$n_{i.} = \sum_{j=1}^{c} n_{ij} \, , \quad n_{.j} = \sum_{i=1}^{r} n_{ij} \, , \quad \text{and} \quad N = \sum_{i=1}^{r} \sum_{j=1}^{c} n_{ij} \, .$$

Table 5.1 depicts a conventional notation for a typical $r \times c$ contingency table for two categorical variables, x_i for $i = 1, \ldots, r$ and y_j for $j = 1, \ldots, c$.

If x and y represent the row and column variables, respectively, there are $N(N-1)/2$ pairs of objects in the table that can be partitioned into five mutually exclusive, exhaustive types of pairs: concordant pairs, discordant pairs, pairs tied on variable

[1] For an alternative, more mathematical, approach to measuring the variation among disjoint, ordered categories, see three articles by Berry and Mielke [5, 6, 7].

[2] Some authors prefer to indicate the number of concordant pairs by P and the number of discordant pairs by Q. Still others indicate the number of concordant pairs by N^+ and the number of discordant pairs by N^-.

Table 5.1 Notation for the cross-classification of two categorical variables, x_i for $i = 1, \ldots, r$ and y_j for $j = 1, \ldots, c$

x	y 1	2	$\cdots$	c	Total
1	n_{11}	n_{12}	$\cdots$	n_{1c}	$n_{1.}$
2	n_{21}	n_{22}	$\cdots$	n_{2c}	$n_{2.}$
$\vdots$	$\vdots$	$\vdots$	$\ddots$	$\vdots$	$\vdots$
r	n_{r1}	n_{r2}	$\cdots$	n_{rc}	$n_{r.}$
Total	$n_{.1}$	$n_{.2}$	$\cdots$	$n_{.c}$	N

x but not tied on variable y, pairs tied on variable y but not tied on variable x, and pairs tied on both variables x and y.

For an $r \times c$ contingency table, concordant pairs (pairs of objects that are ranked in the same order on both variable x and variable y) are given by

$$C = \sum_{i=1}^{r-1} \sum_{j=1}^{c-1} n_{ij} \left(\sum_{k=i+1}^{r} \sum_{l=j+1}^{c} n_{kl} \right) , \tag{5.1}$$

discordant pairs (pairs of objects that are ranked in one order on variable x and the reverse order on variable y) are given by

$$D = \sum_{i=1}^{r-1} \sum_{j=1}^{c-1} n_{i,c-j+1} \left(\sum_{k=i+1}^{r} \sum_{l=1}^{c-j} n_{kl} \right) , \tag{5.2}$$

pairs of objects tied on variable x but not tied on variable y are given by

$$T_x = \sum_{i=1}^{r} \sum_{j=1}^{c-1} n_{ij} \left(\sum_{k=j+1}^{c} n_{ik} \right) , \tag{5.3}$$

pairs of objects tied on variable y but not tied on variable x are given by

$$T_y = \sum_{j=1}^{c} \sum_{i=1}^{r-1} n_{ij} \left(\sum_{k=i+1}^{r} n_{kj} \right) , \tag{5.4}$$

and pairs of objects tied on both variable x and variable y are given by

$$T_{xy} = \frac{1}{2} \sum_{i=1}^{r} \sum_{j=1}^{c} n_{ij} \left(n_{ij} - 1 \right) = \frac{1}{2} \left(\sum_{i=1}^{r} \sum_{j=1}^{c} n_{ij}^2 - N \right) . \tag{5.5}$$

Then,

$$C + D + T_x + T_y + T_{xy} = \frac{N(N-1)}{2} \,.$$

Given C, D, T_x, T_y, and N, six measures of ordinal association are commonly defined, each having the same numerator, $S = C - D$, but different denominators [2].[3] [4] The earliest of these pairwise measures was Kendall's τ_a [23].[5] Kendall's τ_a is a symmetrical measure of ordinal association that is most suitable when there are no tied pairs and is defined as the simple difference between the proportions of concordant and discordant pairs given by

$$\tau_a = \frac{C}{\dfrac{N(N-1)}{2}} - \frac{D}{\dfrac{N(N-1)}{2}} = \frac{C-D}{\dfrac{N(N-1)}{2}} = \frac{2S}{N(N-1)} \,. \tag{5.6}$$

Kendall's τ_b [23] extends τ_a to measure strong monotonicity in contingency tables and is most appropriate when $r = c$. The denominator for τ_b is adjusted for the number of tied pairs for both variable x and variable y. Kendall's τ_b is given by

$$\tau_b = \frac{S}{\sqrt{(C+D+T_x)(C+D+T_y)}} \,. \tag{5.7}$$

Stuart's τ_c [46] modifies Kendall's τ_b for contingency tables where $r \neq c$ and is given by

$$\tau_c = \frac{2mS}{N^2(m-1)} \,, \tag{5.8}$$

where $m = \min(r, c)$. Goodman and Kruskal's γ [15] is a symmetrical measure of weak monotonicity in which tied pairs of all types are ignored and is given by

$$\gamma = \frac{C-D}{C+D} = \frac{S}{C+D} \,. \tag{5.9}$$

Somers' d_{yx} and d_{xy} [44] are asymmetric measures of ordinal association. Unlike the four symmetrical measures, τ_a, τ_b, τ_c, and γ, Somers' d_{yx} and d_{xy} measures

[3] The number of pairs tied on both variables x and y (T_{xy}) is not used in any of the six measures.

[4] There are actually many more than six measures of ordinal association based on pairwise comparisons; only the most common six measures are discussed here.

[5] Yule's Q for 2×2 contingency tables also has S in the numerator and preceded Kendall's τ_a by some 40 years [51, 52]. While Yule's Q is occasionally prescribed for rank-score data [29, p. 255–256], it was originally designed for categorical data and 2×2 contingency tables; it is therefore described more appropriately in Chap. 9.

depend on which variable, y or x, is considered to be the dependent variable. If variable y is the dependent variable, then

$$d_{yx} = \frac{S}{C + D + T_y} , \quad (5.10)$$

and if variable x is the dependent variable, then

$$d_{xy} = \frac{S}{C + D + T_x} . \quad (5.11)$$

Thus, for both d_{yx} and d_{xy}, when a difference between paired values on the independent variable (i.e., untied pair) is not reflected as a difference between the corresponding paired values on the dependent variable (i.e., tied pair) the denominators of Eqs. (5.10) and (5.11) are increased by T_y or T_x, respectively, and the values of d_{yx} and d_{xy} are diminished accordingly. Finally, it is readily apparent that Kendall's τ_b measure of ordinal association given in Eq. (5.7) is simply the geometric mean of Somers' d_{yx} and d_{xy} measures given by

$$\tau_b = \sqrt{d_{yx}\, d_{xy}} .$$

5.2 Permutation Statistical Methods

For an exact permutation analysis of an $r \times c$ contingency table, it is necessary to calculate the selected measure of ordinal association for the observed cell frequencies and exhaustively enumerate all M possible, equally-likely arrangements of the N objects in the rc cells, given the observed marginal frequency distributions. For each arrangement in the reference set of all permutations of cell frequencies a measure of ordinal association, say T, and the exact hypergeometric point probability value under the null hypothesis, $p(n_{ij}|n_{i.}, n_{.j}, N)$, are calculated, where

$$p(n_{ij}|n_{i.}, n_{.j}, N) = \frac{\left(\prod_{i=1}^{r} n_{i.}!\right)\left(\prod_{j=1}^{c} n_{.j}!\right)}{N! \prod_{i=1}^{r}\prod_{j=1}^{c} n_{ij}!} ,$$

n_{ij} is an observed cell frequency for $i = 1, \ldots r$ and $j = 1, \ldots, c$, $n_{i.}$ is the ith of r row marginal frequency totals summed over all columns, $n_{.j}$ is the jth of c column marginal frequency totals summed over all rows, and N is the total of all n_{ij} values for $i = 1, \ldots, r$ and $j = 1, \ldots, c$ [8, 33, p. 258]. If T_{o} denotes the value of the observed test statistic, the exact one-sided upper- and lower-tail probability

(P) values of T_o are the sums of the $p(n_{ij}|n_{i.}, n_{.j}, N)$ values associated with the T values computed on all possible, equally-likely arrangements of cell frequencies that are equal to or greater than T_o when T_o is positive and equal to or less than T_o when T_o is negative, respectively. Thus, the exact hypergeometric probability value of T_o when T is positive is given by

$$P = \sum_{k=1}^{M} \Psi(T_k)\, p(n_{ij}|n_{i.}, n_{.j}, N) \ ,$$

where

$$\Psi(T_k) = \begin{cases} 1 & \text{if } T_k \geq T_o \ , \\ 0 & \text{otherwise} \ , \end{cases}$$

and the exact hypergeometric probability value of T_o when T is negative is given by

$$P = \sum_{k=1}^{M} \Psi(T_k)\, p(n_{ij}|n_{i.}, n_{.j}, N) \ ,$$

where

$$\Psi(T_k) = \begin{cases} 1 & \text{if } T_k \leq T_o \ , \\ 0 & \text{otherwise} \ . \end{cases}$$

When the number of possible arrangements of cell frequencies is very large, exact tests are impractical and Monte Carlo methods become necessary. Monte Carlo resampling permutation statistical methods generate a random sample of all possible arrangements of cell frequencies, drawn with replacement, given the observed marginal frequency distributions. The resampling one-sided upper- and lower-tail probability values of statistic T are simply the proportions of the T values computed on the randomly selected arrangements of cell frequencies that are equal to or greater than T_o when T_o is positive and equal to or less than T_o when T_o is negative, respectively. Thus, the Monte Carlo resampling probability value of T_o when T is positive is given by

$$P(T \geq T_o|H_0) = \frac{\text{number of } T \text{ values } \geq T_o}{L} \ ,$$

where L denotes the number of random arrangements of the observed data.[6]

[6]In general, setting $L = 1{,}000{,}000$ ensures a probability value with three decimal places of accuracy [19].

5.3 Kendall's τ_a Measure of Ordinal Association

Kendall's τ_a measure of ordinal association [21], given by

$$\tau_a = \frac{2S}{N(N-1)} ,$$

was originally designed to measure the association between two sets of untied rank scores, where the two sets of rank scores are customarily labeled as x and y, although the rank scores can also be represented in an $r \times c$ contingency table where $n_{i.} = n_{.j} = 1$ for $i = 1, \ldots, r$ and $j = 1, \ldots, c$. Kendall's τ_a is occasionally touted as an alternative to Spearman's rank-order correlation coefficient [26, p. 179]. Note also that because it is assumed that there are no ties in the data, τ_a may also be given by

$$\tau_a = \frac{2S}{N(N-1)} = \frac{C-D}{C+D} .$$

Finally, a method based on systematic reversals of observed values advocated by Henry Mann in 1945 may be employed to calculate Kendall's τ_a [30].[7] Table 5.2 illustrates the counting of reversal arrangements in a sequence of ranks from 1 to 5. The first set of paired columns in Table 5.2 lists the observed ranks for two groups, and subsequent sets of paired columns illustrate the number of reversals necessary to produce the first column from the second. In this case, seven reversal sequences are required with one reversal arrangement per sequence. For example, reversal sequence 1 in Table 5.2 exchanges ranks 2 and 1 in the observed column, reversal sequence 2 exchanges ranks 5 and 1 in reversal sequence 1, reversal sequence 3 exchanges ranks 4 and 1 in reversal sequence 2, and so on until reversal sequence 7 exchanges ranks 3 and 2 in reversal sequence 6 to achieve the ordered sequence in reversal sequence 7. The technique that Mann described is similar to a graphic computation of disarray first constructed by S.D. Holmes and published in an appendix to a book on *Educational Psychology* by P. Sandiford in 1928 with application to Pearson's product-moment correlation coefficient, r_{xy} [43, pp. 391–394], and in a later publication by H.D. Griffin in 1958 with application to Kendall's rank-order correlation coefficient, τ_a [16].

A proof that the number of interchanges of nearest neighbors required to reduce one ranking to the other was provided by P.A.P. Moran in 1947 [34] and was, according to Moran, first proved by Olinde Rodrigues in 1839 [42].[8] In 1948

[7] James Durbin and Alan Stuart introduced an inversion procedure for rank-correlation coefficients in 1951 [11]. Alan Stuart also developed a method to calculate Kendall's τ_a based on inversions of ranks in 1977 [47].

[8] A summary in English of the Rodrigues 1839 article is available in *Mathematics and Social Utopias in France: Olinde Rodrigues and His Times* [1, pp. 110–112].

Table 5.2 Reversal sequences for $N = 5$ ranks to obtain no reversals from an observed data set

Observed	Reversal sequence 1	2	3	4	5	6	7
1 3	1 3	1 3	1 3	1 1	1 1	1 1	1 1
2 4	2 4	2 4	2 1	2 3	2 3	2 3	2 2
3 5	3 5	3 1	3 4	3 4	3 4	3 2	3 3
4 2	4 1	4 5	4 5	4 5	4 2	4 4	4 4
5 1	5 2	5 2	5 2	5 2	5 5	5 5	5 5

Moran mathematically established the relationship between rank-order correlation and permutation distributions [35].[9] Consider N objects denoted by $1, \ldots, N$ and let s be the least number of interchanges of adjacent objects required to restore the permutations to the normal order. Utilizing a theorem by Haden [17], Moran proved that $s = N(N-1)/4 - S/2$ so that

$$\tau_a = 1 - \frac{4s}{N(N-1)} = -\frac{4t}{N(N-1)} ,$$

where $t = s - N(N-1)/4$. Thus, Moran showed that Kendall's τ_a rank-order correlation coefficient could be defined in terms of s and, therefore, the theory of rank-order correlation could be mathematically linked with the theory of permutations.

A graphic that depicts the number of reversals consists of lines that are drawn between like values in the two columns and the number of reversals is represented by the number of times the lines cross [16]. For example, consider the two sets of ranks given in Fig. 5.1.[10]

There are five crosses ($\times$s) among the $N = 5$ lines, i.e., both diagonal lines cross two horizontal lines and each other, indicating the five reversals required to produce the distribution of ranks on the left from the distribution of ranks on the right. Thus, beginning with the right column of {4, 2, 3, 1, 5} and for the first reversal, exchange ranks 3 and 1, yielding {4, 2, 1, 3, 5}; for the second reversal, exchange ranks 2 and 1, yielding {4, 1, 2, 3, 5}; for the third reversal, exchange ranks 4 and 1, yielding {1, 4, 2, 3, 5}; for the fourth reversal, exchange ranks 4 and 2, yielding {1, 2, 4, 3, 5}; and for the fifth reversal, exchange ranks 4 and 3, yielding {1, 2, 3, 4, 5}.

[9]This paper was cited by Moran in 1947 as "Rank correlation and a paper by H.G. Haden," [36, p. 162] but apparently the title was changed at some point to "Rank correlation and permutation distributions" when it was published in *Proceedings of the Cambridge Philosophical Society* in 1948.

[10]Technically, Fig. 5.1 is a permutation graph of a family of line segments that connect two parallel lines in the Euclidean plane. Given a permutation {4, 2, 3, 1, 5} of the positive integers {1, 2, 3, 4, 5}, there exists a vertex for each number {1, 2, 3, 4, 5} and an edge between two numbers where the segments cross in the permutation diagram.

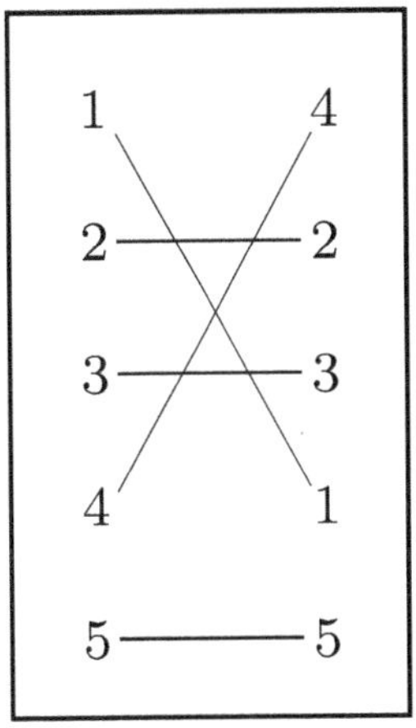

Fig. 5.1 Graphic depiction of the number of reversals for two sets of ranks, from 1 to 5

For the $N = 5$ rank scores in Fig. 5.1, $C = 5$, $D = 5$, $S = C - D = 5 - 5 = 0$ and $s = 5$ crosses; thus,

$$\tau_a = 1 - \frac{4s}{N(N-1)} = 1 - \frac{4(5)}{5(5-1)} = 0.00$$

and

$$\tau_a = \frac{2S}{N(N-1)} = \frac{2(0)}{5(5-1)} = 0.00\ .$$

5.3.1 *Example 1*

To illustrate the calculation of Kendall's τ_a measure of ordinal association, consider the two sets of rankings with no tied values listed in Table 5.3, where there are

$$\binom{N}{2} = \frac{N(N-1)}{2} = \frac{8(8-1)}{2} = 28$$

possible pairs and N denotes the number of paired rankings; in this case, $N = 8$. The 28 paired differences are listed in Table 5.4 for convenience.

Because there are no tied rank scores in Table 5.3, the $N(N-1)/2$ pairs can be exhaustively divided into just two types: concordant (C) and discordant (D) pairs. To clarify the calculation of Kendall's S, consider the x and y rank scores for the first pair of objects in Table 5.3: Objects 1 and 2. For variable x calculate $1-3 = -2$ and for variable y calculate $3 - 4 = -1$. When the signs agree, either both negative or both positive, as in this case with both signs negative, the pair is considered a concordant (C) pair. Now consider the x and y rank scores for the second pair:

Table 5.3 Two sets of $N = 8$ rank scores for Kendall's τ_a measure of ordinal association

Object	Variable	
	x	y
1	1	3
2	3	4
3	2	1
4	4	2
5	5	5
6	7	8
7	8	6
8	6	7

Table 5.4 Paired differences, r_{ij}, s_{ij}, $r_{ij}s_{ij}$, and $|r_{ij} - s_{ij}|$ values for the rank scores listed in Table 5.3

Pair	$x_i - x_j$	$y_i - y_j$	r_{ij}	s_{ij}	$r_{ij}s_{ij}$	$\|r_{ij} - s_{ij}\|$
1	1 − 3	3 − 4	−1	−1	+1	0
2	1 − 2	3 − 1	−1	+1	−1	2
3	1 − 4	3 − 2	−1	+1	−1	2
4	1 − 5	3 − 5	−1	−1	+1	0
5	1 − 7	3 − 8	−1	−1	+1	0
6	1 − 8	3 − 6	−1	−1	+1	0
7	1 − 6	3 − 7	−1	−1	+1	0
8	3 − 2	4 − 1	+1	+1	+1	0
9	3 − 4	4 − 2	−1	+1	−1	2
10	3 − 5	4 − 5	−1	−1	+1	0
11	3 − 7	4 − 8	−1	−1	+1	0
12	3 − 8	4 − 6	−1	−1	+1	0
13	3 − 6	4 − 7	−1	−1	+1	0
14	2 − 4	1 − 2	−1	−1	+1	0
15	2 − 5	1 − 5	−1	−1	+1	0
16	2 − 7	1 − 8	−1	−1	+1	0
17	2 − 8	1 − 6	−1	−1	+1	0
18	2 − 6	1 − 7	−1	−1	+1	0
19	4 − 5	2 − 5	−1	−1	+1	0
20	4 − 7	2 − 8	−1	−1	+1	0
21	4 − 8	2 − 6	−1	−1	+1	0
22	4 − 6	2 − 7	−1	−1	+1	0
23	5 − 7	5 − 8	−1	−1	+1	0
24	5 − 8	5 − 6	−1	−1	+1	0
25	5 − 6	5 − 7	−1	−1	+1	0
26	7 − 8	8 − 6	−1	+1	−1	2
27	7 − 6	8 − 7	+1	+1	+1	0
28	8 − 6	6 − 7	+1	−1	−1	2
Total					+18	10

Objects 1 and 3. For variable x calculate $1 - 2 = -1$ and for variable y calculate $3 - 1 = +2$. When the signs disagree, as in this case with one negative sign and one positive sign, the pair is considered a discordant (D) pair.

Given the $N = 8$ bivariate rank scores listed in Table 5.3, for $i < j$ define

$$r_{ij} = \begin{cases} +1 & \text{if } x_i > x_j \,, \\ 0 & \text{if } x_i = x_j \,, \\ -1 & \text{if } x_i < x_j \,, \end{cases} \qquad \text{and} \qquad s_{ij} = \begin{cases} +1 & \text{if } y_i > y_j \,, \\ 0 & \text{if } y_i = y_j \,, \\ -1 & \text{if } y_i < y_j \,. \end{cases}$$

Then, following Kendall [23],

$$S = \sum_{i=1}^{N-1} \sum_{j=i+1}^{N} r_{ij} s_{ij}$$

as given in the sixth column of Table 5.4, where there are 23 concordant pairs, each indicated by $+1$ ($C = 23$) and 5 discordant pairs, each indicated by -1 ($D = 5$); therefore, the observed value of Kendall's test statistic is $S = C - D = 23 - 5 = +18$. For the rank scores with no tied values listed in Table 5.3, the observed value of Kendall's τ_a test statistic is

$$\tau_a = \frac{2S}{N(N-1)} = \frac{2(+18)}{8(8-1)} = +0.6429$$

and, because there are no tied rank scores for the data listed in Table 5.3, $\tau_a = \tau_b = \tau_c = \gamma = d_{yx} = d_{xy} = +0.6429$.

As Kendall pointed out in his 1948 book on *Rank Correlation Methods*, there is one rather disappointing feature of rank-correlation coefficients, such as τ_a; namely, the comparatively large standard errors that they usually possess [24, p. 65]. Kendall noted that, whatever the value of τ_a might be, the standard error is of the order of $\sqrt{2N}$ and cautioned:

> It is clearly impossible to locate the parent correlation very closely unless the ranking contains 30 or 40 members. This provides a useful caution against attributing reality to correlation coefficients calculated from rankings of small extent, unless several sample values are available [24, p. 65].

Permutation statistical methods, being exact, are ideally suited for small sample sizes as they do not assume a specific sampling distribution nor do they depend on a theoretical approximating function.

Let $N = 8$ denote the number of bivariate scores listed in Table 5.3 and $b = 2$ denote the number of variables, in this case variables x and y. Then, for the rank scores listed in Table 5.3 there are

$$M = \left(N!\right)^b = \left(8!\right)^2 = 1{,}625{,}702{,}400$$

possible, equally-likely arrangements in the reference set of all permutations of the observed rank scores. However, considering variable x fixed, relative to variable y, M can be reduced to

$$M = (N!)^{b-1} = (8!)^{2-1} = 40{,}320$$

and an exact permutation analysis is easily accomplished. Since $N(N-1)/2$ is invariant under permutation, it is sufficient to find the probability of S [8].

If all $M = 40{,}320$ possible arrangements of the observed rank scores listed in Table 5.3 occur with equal chance, the exact probability value of Kendall's S under the null hypothesis is the sum of the hypergeometric point probability values associated with $S = +18$ or greater. Based on the hypergeometric probability distribution, the exact upper-tail probability value is $P = 0.0310$.

5.3.2 *Example 2*

For a second example of Kendall's τ_a measure of ordinal association, consider the small set of rank scores listed in Table 5.5 in which tied rank scores on variables x and y (T_x and T_y, respectively) are introduced.

Table 5.6 lists the 10 paired differences, r_{ij}, s_{ij}, $r_{ij}s_{ij}$, and $|r_{ij} - s_{ij}|$ values for the rank scores listed in Table 5.5. Following Kendall,

$$S = \sum_{i=1}^{N-1} \sum_{j=i+1}^{N} r_{ij}s_{ij}$$

as given in the sixth column of Table 5.6, where there are $C = 5$ concordant pairs, each indicated by $+1$ and $D = 3$ discordant pairs, each indicated by -1; therefore, $S = C - D$ implies that the observed value of S is $S = 5 - 3 = +2$. Also, there is $T_x = 1$ pair of rank scores tied on variable x but not tied on variable y, indicated by a 0 in row 5 of the sixth column and $T_y = 1$ pair of rank scores tied on variable y but not tied on variable x, indicated by a 0 in row 8 of the sixth column. Then, the observed value of Kendall's τ_a test statistic based on $S = +2$ is

$$\tau_a = \frac{2S}{N(N-1)} = \frac{2(+2)}{5(5-1)} = +0.20\,.$$

Table 5.5 Two sets of $N = 5$ rank scores with ties for Kendall's τ_a measure of ordinal association

	Variable	
Object	x	y
1	1	2
2	2.5	1
3	2.5	4.5
4	4	4.5
5	5	3

Table 5.6 Paired differences, r_{ij}, s_{ij}, $r_{ij}s_{ij}$, and $|r_{ij} - s_{ij}|$ values for the rank scores listed in Table 5.5

Pair	$x_i - x_j$	$y_i - y_j$	r_{ij}	s_{ij}	$r_{ij}s_{ij}$	$\lvert r_{ij} - s_{ij}\rvert$
1	1.0 − 2.5	2.0 − 1.0	−1	+1	−1	2
2	1.0 − 2.5	2.0 − 4.5	−1	−1	+1	0
3	1.0 − 4.0	2.0 − 4.5	−1	−1	+1	0
4	1.0 − 5.0	2.0 − 3.0	−1	−1	+1	0
5	2.5 − 2.5	1.0 − 4.5	0	−1	0	1
6	2.5 − 4.0	1.0 − 4.5	−1	−1	+1	0
7	2.5 − 5.0	1.0 − 3.0	−1	−1	+1	0
8	2.5 − 4.0	4.5 − 4.5	−1	0	0	1
9	2.5 − 5.0	4.5 − 3.0	−1	+1	−1	2
10	4.0 − 5.0	4.5 − 3.0	−1	+1	−1	2
Total					+2	8

For the rank scores listed in Table 5.5, there are only

$$M = (N!)^b = (5!)^2 = 14{,}400$$

possible, equally-likely arrangements in the reference set of all permutations of the observed rank scores, making an exact permutation analysis feasible. If all $M = 14{,}400$ possible arrangements of the observed rank scores listed in Table 5.5 occur with equal chance, the exact probability value of Kendall's S under the null hypothesis is the sum of the hypergeometric point probability values associated with $S = +2$ or greater. Based on the hypergeometric probability distribution, the exact upper-tail probability value is $P = 0.7660$.

5.3.3 Example 3

For a third example of Kendall's τ_a measure of ordinal association, consider the two sets of rank scores listed in Table 5.7, where there are multiple tied rank scores on both variable x and variable y (T_x and T_y, respectively). For the rank scores listed in Table 5.7, $N = 6$, the number of concordant pairs is $C = 8$, the number of discordant pairs is $D = 2$, the number of pairs tied on variable x is $T_x = 1$, the number of pairs tied on variable y is $T_y = 2$, and the number of pairs tied on both variable x and variable y is $T_{xy} = 2$. Table 5.8 lists the

$$\frac{N(N-1)}{2} = \frac{6(6-1)}{2} = 15$$

paired differences, r_{ij}, s_{ij}, $r_{ij}s_{ij}$, and $|r_{ij} - s_{ij}|$ values for the rank scores given in Table 5.7.

Table 5.7 Two sets of rank scores with ties for Kendall's τ_a measure of ordinal association

	Variable	
Object	x	y
1	1.5	2
2	1.5	2
3	3.5	4.5
4	5.5	2
5	3.5	4.5
6	5.5	6

Table 5.8 Paired differences, r_{ij}, s_{ij}, $r_{ij}s_{ij}$, and $|r_{ij} - s_{ij}|$ values for the rank scores listed in Table 5.7

Pair	$x_i - x_j$	$y_i - y_j$	r_{ij}	s_{ij}	$r_{ij}s_{ij}$	$\|r_{ij} - s_{ij}\|$	Type
1	1.5 − 1.5	2.0 − 2.0	0	0	0	0	T_{xy}
2	1.5 − 3.5	2.0 − 4.5	−1	−1	+1	0	C
3	1.5 − 5.5	2.0 − 2.0	−1	0	0	1	T_y
4	1.5 − 3.5	2.0 − 4.5	−1	−1	+1	0	C
5	1.5 − 5.5	2.0 − 6.0	−1	−1	+1	0	C
6	1.5 − 3.5	2.0 − 4.5	−1	−1	+1	0	C
7	1.5 − 5.5	2.0 − 2.0	−1	0	0	1	T_y
8	1.5 − 3.5	2.0 − 4.5	−1	−1	+1	0	C
9	1.5 − 5.5	2.0 − 6.0	−1	−1	+1	0	C
10	3.5 − 5.5	4.5 − 2.0	−1	+1	−1	2	D
11	3.5 − 3.5	4.5 − 4.5	0	0	0	0	T_{xy}
12	3.5 − 5.5	4.5 − 6.0	−1	−1	+1	0	C
13	5.5 − 3.5	2.0 − 4.5	+1	−1	−1	2	D
14	5.5 − 5.5	2.0 − 6.0	0	−1	0	1	T_x
15	3.5 − 5.5	4.5 − 6.0	−1	−1	+1	0	C
Total					+6	7	

Following Kendall,

$$S = \sum_{i=1}^{N-1} \sum_{j=i+1}^{N} r_{ij}s_{ij}$$

as given in the sixth column of Table 5.8, where there are $C = 8$ concordant pairs in rows 2, 4, 5, 6, 8, 9, 12, and 15, indicated by $+1$ values, and $D = 2$ discordant pairs in rows 10 and 13, indicated by -1 values. Values of T_x, T_y, and T_{xy} receive values of 0. Thus, the observed value of S is

$$S = \sum_{i=1}^{N-1} \sum_{j=i+1}^{N} r_{ij}s_{ij} = C - D = 8 - 2 = +6$$

and, following Eq. (5.6) on p. 226, the observed value of Kendall's τ_a test statistic is

$$\tau_a = \frac{2S}{N(N-1)} = \frac{2(+6)}{6(6-1)} = +0.40 \ .$$

For the rank scores listed in Table 5.7, there are only

$$M = (N!)^b = (6!)^2 = 518{,}400$$

possible, equally-likely arrangements in the reference set of all permutations of the observed rank scores, making an exact permutation analysis possible. If all $M = 518{,}400$ possible arrangements of the observed rank scores listed in Table 5.7 occur with equal chance, the exact probability value of Kendall's S under the null hypothesis is the sum of the hypergeometric point probability values associated with $S = +6$ or greater. Based on the hypergeometric probability distribution, the exact upper-tail probability value is $P = 0.1333$.

5.3.4 *Example 4*

For a fourth example of Kendall's τ_a measure of ordinal association, consider the frequency data given in Table 5.9, where $N = 20$ bivariate observations have been cross-classified into a 3×3 ordered contingency table, which is a more typical application of measures of ordinal association, such as τ_a. For the frequency data given in Table 5.9, the number of concordant pairs is

$$C = \sum_{i=1}^{r-1}\sum_{j=1}^{c-1} n_{ij} \left(\sum_{k=i+1}^{r} \sum_{l=j+1}^{c} n_{kl} \right)$$
$$= (6)(2+1+1+5) + (2)(1+5) + (2)(1+5) + (2)(5) = 88 \ ,$$

Table 5.9 Example rank-score data for $N = 20$ bivariate observations cross-classified on ordinal variables x and y into a 3×3 contingency table

	y			
x	1	2	3	Total
1	6	2	0	8
2	2	2	1	5
3	1	1	5	7
Total	9	5	6	20

the number of discordant pairs is

$$D = \sum_{i=1}^{r-1} \sum_{j=1}^{c-1} n_{i,c-j+1} \left(\sum_{k=i+1}^{r} \sum_{l=1}^{c-j} n_{kl} \right)$$

$$= (0)(2+2+1+1) + (2)(2+1) + (1)(1+1) + (2)(1) = 10 ,$$

the number of pairs tied on variable x but not tied on variable y is

$$T_x = \sum_{i=1}^{r} \sum_{j=1}^{c-1} n_{ij} \left(\sum_{k=j+1}^{c} n_{ik} \right)$$

$$= (6)(2+0) + (2)(0) + (2)(2+1) + (2)(1) + (1)(1+5) + (1)(5) = 31 ,$$

the number of pairs tied on variable y but not tied on variable x is

$$T_y = \sum_{j=1}^{c} \sum_{i=1}^{r-1} n_{ij} \left(\sum_{k=i+1}^{r} n_{kj} \right)$$

$$= (6)(2+1) + (2)(1) + (2)(2+1) + (2)(1) + (0)(1+5) + (1)(5) = 33 ,$$

and the number of pairs tied on both variable x and variable y is

$$T_{xy} = \frac{1}{2} \sum_{i=1}^{r} \sum_{j=1}^{c} n_{ij} \left(n_{ij} - 1 \right)$$

$$= \frac{1}{2} \big[(6)(6-1) + (2)(2-1) + (0)(0-1) + (2)(2-1) + (2)(2-1)$$

$$+ (1)(1-1) + (1)(1-1) + (1)(1-1) + (5)(5-1) \big] = 28 .$$

Alternatively,

$$T_{xy} = \frac{1}{2} \left(\sum_{i=1}^{r} \sum_{j=1}^{c} n_{ij}^2 - N \right)$$

$$= \frac{1}{2} \left(6^2 + 2^2 + 0^2 + 2^2 + 2^2 + 1^2 + 1^2 + 1^2 + 5^2 - 20 \right) = 28 .$$

Then, the observed value of Kendall's S is $S = C - D = 88 - 10 = +78$ and the observed value of Kendall's τ_a test statistic is

$$\tau_a = \frac{2S}{N(N-1)} = \frac{2(+78)}{20(20-1)} = +0.4105 \ .$$

For the frequency data given in Table 5.9, there are only $M = 412$ possible, equally-likely arrangements in the reference set of all permutations of cell frequencies given the observed row and column marginal frequency distributions, $\{8, 5, 7\}$ and $\{9, 5, 6\}$, respectively, making an exact permutation analysis feasible. If all $M = 412$ possible arrangements of the observed data given in Table 5.9 occur with equal chance, the exact probability value of Kendall's S under the null hypothesis is the sum of the hypergeometric point probability values associated with $S = +78$ or greater. Based on the hypergeometric probability distribution, the exact upper-tail probability value is $P = 0.0026$.

5.4 Kendall's τ_b Measure of Ordinal Association

Because tied values occur in the data sets in Examples 2, 3, and 4 (Tables 5.5, 5.7, and 5.9), Kendall's τ_a measure of ordinal association is less than satisfactory, as it ignores the two sets of tied values, T_x and T_y. For this reason Kendall developed τ_b, an alternative to τ_a, given by

$$\tau_b = \frac{S}{\sqrt{(C + D + T_x)(C + D + T_y)}} \ ,$$

which incorporated tied values on variables x and y (T_x and T_y, respectively).

5.4.1 *Example 1*

Consider the frequency data given in Table 5.10, where $N = 41$ bivariate observations have been cross-classified into a 3×3 ordered contingency table. For

Table 5.10 Example rank-score data for $N = 41$ bivariate observations cross-classified on ordinal variables x and y into a 3×3 contingency table

	y			
x	1	2	3	Total
1	7	6	3	16
2	5	2	7	14
3	3	2	6	11
Total	15	10	16	41

the frequency data given in Table 5.10, the number of concordant pairs is

$$C = \sum_{i=1}^{r-1} \sum_{j=1}^{c-1} n_{ij} \left(\sum_{k=i+1}^{r} \sum_{l=j+1}^{c} n_{kl} \right)$$

$$= (7)(2+7+2+6) + (6)(7+6) + (5)(2+6) + (2)(6) = 249 ,$$

the number of discordant pairs is

$$D = \sum_{i=1}^{r-1} \sum_{j=1}^{c-1} n_{i,c-j+1} \left(\sum_{k=i+1}^{r} \sum_{l=1}^{c-j} n_{kl} \right)$$

$$= (3)(5+2+3+2) + (6)(5+3) + (7)(3+2) + (2)(3) = 125 ,$$

the number of pairs tied on variable x is

$$T_x = \sum_{i=1}^{r} \sum_{j=1}^{c-1} n_{ij} \left(\sum_{k=j+1}^{c} n_{ik} \right)$$

$$= (7)(6+3) + (6)(3) + (5)(2+7) + (2)(7) + (3)(2+6) + (2)(6) = 176 ,$$

the number of pairs tied on variable y is

$$T_y = \sum_{j=1}^{c} \sum_{i=1}^{r-1} n_{ij} \left(\sum_{k=i+1}^{r} n_{kj} \right)$$

$$= (7)(5+3) + (5)(3) + (6)(2+2) + (2)(2) + (3)(7+6) + (7)(6) = 180 ,$$

$S = C - D = 249 - 125 = +124$, and the observed value of Kendall's τ_b test statistic is

$$\tau_b = \frac{S}{\sqrt{(C+D+T_x)(C+D+T_y)}}$$

$$= \frac{+124}{\sqrt{(249+125+176)(249+125+180)}} = +0.2246 .$$

For the frequency data given in Table 5.10, there are only $M = 5{,}225$ possible, equally-likely arrangements in the reference set of all permutations of cell frequencies given the observed row and column marginal frequency distributions, $\{16, 14, 11\}$ and $\{15, 10, 16\}$, respectively, making an exact permutation analysis possible. The exact probability value of Kendall's τ_b under the null hypothesis is the sum of the hypergeometric point probability values associated with the values of $\tau_b = +0.2246$ or greater. Based on the hypergeometric probability distribution, the exact upper-tail probability value is $P = 0.0555$.

5.4.2 Example 2

For a second example analysis of Kendall's τ_b measure of ordinal association, consider the frequency data given in Table 5.11 where $N = 72$ bivariate observations have been cross-classified into a 3×5 ordered contingency table. For the frequency data given in Table 5.11, the number of concordant pairs is

$$C = \sum_{i=1}^{r-1} \sum_{j=1}^{c-1} n_{ij} \left(\sum_{k=i+1}^{r} \sum_{l=j+1}^{c} n_{kl} \right)$$
$$= (8)(2+8+5+5+5+3+7+7) + (4)(8+5+5+3+7+7)$$
$$+ \cdots + (8)(7+7) + (5)(7) = 855 ,$$

the number of discordant pairs is

$$D = \sum_{i=1}^{r-1} \sum_{j=1}^{c-1} n_{i,c-j+1} \left(\sum_{k=i+1}^{r} \sum_{l=1}^{c-j} n_{kl} \right)$$
$$= (3)(3+2+8+5+4+5+3+7) + (5)(3=2+8+4+5+3)$$
$$+ \cdots + (8)(4+5) + (2)(4) = 541 ,$$

Table 5.11 Example rank-score data for $N = 72$ bivariate observations cross-classified on ordinal variables x and y into a 3×5 contingency table

	y					
x	1	2	3	4	5	Total
1	8	4	3	5	3	23
2	3	2	8	5	5	23
3	4	5	3	7	7	26
Total	15	11	14	17	15	72

the number of pairs tied on variable x is

$$T_x = \sum_{i=1}^{r} \sum_{j=1}^{c-1} n_{ij} \left(\sum_{k=j+1}^{c} n_{ik} \right)$$

$$= (8)(4+3+5+3) + (4)(3+5+3)$$

$$+ \cdots + (3)(7+7) + (7)(7) = 668 ,$$

the number of pairs tied on variable y is

$$T_y = \sum_{j=1}^{c} \sum_{i=1}^{r-1} n_{ij} \left(\sum_{k=i+1}^{r} n_{kj} \right)$$

$$= (8)(3+4) + (3)(4) + (4)(2+5) + (2)(5)$$

$$+ \cdots + (3)(5+7) + (5)(7) = 329 ,$$

$S = C - D = 866 - 541 = +314$, and the observed value of Kendall's τ_b test statistic is

$$\tau_b = \frac{S}{\sqrt{(C+D+T_x)(C+D+T_y)}}$$

$$= \frac{+314}{\sqrt{(855+541+668)(855+541+329)}} = +0.1664 .$$

For the data listed in Table 5.11, there are $M = 70{,}148{,}145$ possible, equally-likely arrangements in the reference set of all permutations of cell frequencies given the observed row and column marginal frequency distributions, $\{23, 23, 26\}$ and $\{15, 11, 14, 17, 15\}$, respectively. Therefore, an exact test is not practical and a Monte Carlo resampling probability analysis based on $L = 1{,}000{,}000$ random arrangements of cell frequencies is utilized. The resampling probability value of τ_b under the null hypothesis is the proportion of τ_b values equal to or greater than $\tau_b = +0.1664$; in this case there are 48,600 τ_b values that are equal to greater than the observed value of $\tau_b = +0.1664$. Thus, the Monte Carlo resampling approximate upper-tail probability value is

$$P(\tau_b \geq \tau_o) = \frac{\text{number of } \tau_b \text{ values } \geq \tau_o}{L} = \frac{48{,}600}{1{,}000{,}000} = 0.0486 ,$$

where τ_o denotes the observed value of τ_b.

While an exact permutation analysis is not practical for the frequency data given in Table 5.11, it is not impossible. The exact probability value of Kendall's τ_b under the null hypothesis is the sum of the hypergeometric point probability values

Table 5.12 Example rank data (y values) for three time periods: t_1, t_2, and t_3

Time		
t_1	t_2	t_3
1	2	5
3	4	6
	7	8
		9

associated with the values of $\tau_b = +0.1664$ or greater. Based on the hypergeometric probability distribution, the exact upper-tail probability value conditioned on the reference set of all $M = 70{,}148{,}145$ arrangements of cell frequencies is $P = 0.0488$.[11]

5.4.3 Kendall's τ_b and Wilcoxon's W Measures

Kendall's τ_b measure of ordinal association can be shown to be a function of the Wilcoxon two-sample rank-sum test and, consequently, of the Mann–Whitney two-sample rank-sum test. Kraft and van Eeden [26, pp. 179-181] showed that Kendall's τ_b can be computed as a sum of Wilcoxon test statistics as follows. Suppose that N rank observations have been taken at k times periods. Let S_1 be the sum of the ranks among all the y values at t_1; let S_2 be the sum of the ranks among all the y values at t_2; and let $S_3, \ldots, S_{k-1}$ be defined analogously. S_{k-1} is the sum of the ranks among the y values for t_{k-1} and t_k of the y values at t_{k-1}. Then Wilcoxon's $W = S_1 + S_2 + \cdots + S_{k-1}$ is a linear function of Kendall's τ_b. This relationship between Wilcoxon's W and Kendall's τ_b was noted by Whitfield in 1947 [48] and by Kendall in 1948 [23, p. 165], but it was Kraft and van Eeden who made it explicit.

To illustrate the Kraft and van Eeden procedure, consider the rank data given in Table 5.12 where nine observations (y values) have been taken at three time periods, indicated by t_1, t_2, and t_3. For the rank data given in Table 5.12, the number of concordant pairs is $C = 23$, the number of discordant pairs is $D = 3$, the number of pairs tied on variable t is $T_t = 10$, the number of pairs tied on variable y is $T_y = 0$, the number of pairs tied on both variables t and y is $T_{ty} = 0$, and $S = C - D = 23 - 3 = +20$. Then Kendall's τ_b test statistic is

$$\tau_b = \frac{S}{\sqrt{(C + D + T_y)(C + D + T_t)}}$$

$$= \frac{+20}{\sqrt{(23 + 3 + 0)(23 + 3 + 10)}} = +0.6537\ .$$

[11] In general, $L = 1{,}000{,}000$ randomly selected values ensure a probability value with three decimal places of accuracy [19].

Table 5.13 Example rank data (y values) for two time periods: t_2 and t_3

Time	
t_2	t_3
1	3
2	4
5	6
	7

For the rank-score data given in Table 5.12, S_1 is the sum of the ranks in t_1; thus, $S_1 = 1 + 3 = 4$. Then re-ranking the seven y values in t_2 and t_3 in Table 5.12 as given in Table 5.13, S_2 is the sum of the ranks in t_2; thus, $S_2 = 1+2+5 = 8$. Then, Wilcoxon's W is $W = S_1 + S_2 = 4+8 = 12$. Proceeding in this manner, Kraft and van Eeden demonstrated that Wilcoxon's W is simply a linear function of Kendall's τ_b test statistic.

5.5 Stuart's τ_c Measure of Ordinal Association

Kendall's τ_b is a strongly monotonic measure of ordinal association, i.e., for every ordered category increase in variable x, there is expected to be an ordered category increase in variable y. Consequently, τ_b can only achieve limits of ± 1 for contingency tables where $r = c$ and the row and column marginal frequency distributions are identical, e.g., $\{20, 40, 60\}$ and $\{20, 40, 60\}$. More specifically, τ_b cannot generally attain values of ± 1 because of the Cauchy inequality:

> The square of the sum of the products of two sets will be equal to or less than the product of the squared sums of two sets.

More formally, for variables x and y,

$$\left(\sum_{i=1}^{N} x_i y_i \right)^2 \leq \sum_{i=1}^{N} x_i^2 \sum_{i=1}^{N} y_i^2 \; .$$

Consequently, the numerator of τ_b will be equal to or less than the denominator, permitting τ_b to attain ± 1 only when all the observations are concentrated on one of the two principal diagonals of the contingency table. If no marginal frequency is to be zero, this means that τ_b can attain ± 1 only for a square contingency table with identical marginal frequency distributions. It is important to note that, because the categories are ordered, the marginal frequency distributions must be identical, not merely equivalent. Thus, marginal frequency distributions for rows and columns of $\{50, 30, 20\}$ and $\{50, 30, 20\}$, respectively, are identical, providing the possibility that t_b will be equal to $+1$, and marginal frequency distributions for rows and columns of $\{50, 30, 20\}$ and $\{20, 30, 50\}$, respectively, are identical, providing the possibility that τ_b will be equal to -1, but row and column marginal frequency distributions of $\{50, 30, 20\}$ and $\{30, 20, 50\}$, respectively, are equivalent but not identical, and therefore constrain Kendall's t_b to be less than $+1$ or greater than -1.

Thus, Kendall's τ_b is not the most appropriate measure of ordinal association for the 3×5 contingency table given in Table 5.11 on p. 241. To correct for this limitation, Alan Stuart proposed τ_c for contingency tables where $r \neq c$, given by

$$\tau_c = \frac{2mS}{N^2(m-1)} , \tag{5.12}$$

where $m = \min(r, c)$ [46], which in a classic case of Stigler's [45] law of eponymy, is often erroneously labeled as Kendall's τ_c. Stuart showed that if N is a multiple of m and $r = c$ with identical marginal frequency distributions such that all observations fall on the diagonal of the contingency table and all cell frequencies are equal, the maximum value of Kendall's S is given by

$$S_{\max} = \frac{N^2(m-1)}{2m} . \tag{5.13}$$

Then, if $N = m$,

$$\frac{N^2(m-1)}{2m} = \frac{N^2(N-1)}{2N} = \frac{N(N-1)}{2} .$$

However, if N is not a multiple of m, the expression in Eq. (5.13) remains an upper bound that cannot be attained. It follows that Stuart's τ_c can sometimes attain, and for large N, can generally almost always attain ± 1.

5.5.1 *Example 1*

Consider the frequency data given in Table 5.14, where $N = 40$ bivariate observations have been cross-classified into a 3×3 ordered contingency table. For the frequency data given in Table 5.14, the number of concordant pairs is

$$C = \sum_{i=1}^{r-1} \sum_{j=1}^{c-1} n_{ij} \left(\sum_{k=i+1}^{r} \sum_{l=j+1}^{c} n_{kl} \right)$$
$$= (8)(6+2+4+7) + (5)(2+7) + (3)(4+7) + (6)(7) = 272 ,$$

Table 5.14 Example rank-score data for Stuart's τ_c with $N = 40$ bivariate observations cross-classified on ordinal variables x and y into a 3×3 contingency table

	y			
x	1	2	3	Total
1	8	5	3	16
2	3	6	2	11
3	2	4	7	13
Total	13	15	12	40

the number of discordant pairs is

$$D = \sum_{i=1}^{r-1} \sum_{j=1}^{c-1} n_{i,c-j+1} \left(\sum_{k=i+1}^{r} \sum_{l=1}^{c-j} n_{kl} \right)$$

$$= (3)(3+6+2+4) + (5)(3+2) + (2)(2+4) + (6)(2) = 94 \;,$$

$S = C - D = 272 - 94 = +178$, $m = \min(3, 3) = 3$, and the observed value of Stuart's τ_c test statistic is

$$\tau_c = \frac{2mS}{N^2(m-1)} = \frac{2(3)(+178)}{40^2(3-1)} = +0.3338 \;.$$

For the frequency data given in Table 5.14 with $N = 40$ observations, there are only $M = 5{,}329$ possible, equally-likely arrangements in the reference set of all permutations of cell frequencies given the observed row and column marginal frequency distributions, {16, 11, 13} and {13, 15, 12}, respectively, making an exact permutation analysis possible. The exact probability value of Stuart's τ_c under the null hypothesis is the sum of the hypergeometric point probability values associated with the values of $\tau_c = +0.3338$ or greater. Based on the hypergeometric probability distribution, the exact upper-tail probability value is $P = 0.0088$.

5.5.2 Example 2

For a second example of Stuart's τ_c measure of ordinal association, consider the frequency data given in Table 5.11 on p. 241, replicated for convenience in Table 5.15, where $N = 72$ bivariate observations have been cross-classified into a 3×5 ordered contingency table. For the frequency data given in Table 5.15, the number of concordant pairs is

$$C = \sum_{i=1}^{r-1} \sum_{j=1}^{c-1} n_{ij} \left(\sum_{k=i+1}^{r} \sum_{l=j+1}^{c} n_{kl} \right)$$

$$= (8)(2+8+5+5+5+3+7+7) + (4)(8+5+5+3+7+7)$$
$$+ \cdots + (8)(7+7) + (5)(7) = 855 \;,$$

Table 5.15 Example rank-score data for Stuart's τ_c with $N = 72$ bivariate observations cross-classified on ordinal variables x and y into a 3×5 contingency table

	y					
x	1	2	3	4	5	Total
1	8	4	3	5	3	23
2	3	2	8	5	5	23
3	4	5	3	7	7	26
Total	15	11	14	17	15	72

the number of discordant pairs is

$$D = \sum_{i=1}^{r-1} \sum_{j=1}^{c-1} n_{i,c-j+1} \left(\sum_{k=i+1}^{r} \sum_{l=1}^{c-j} n_{kl} \right)$$

$$= (3)(3+2+8+5+4+5+3+7) + (5)(3+2+8+4+5+3)$$
$$+ \cdots + (8)(4+5) + (2)(4) = 541 ,$$

$S = C - D = 855 - 541 = +314$, and the observed value of Stuart's τ_c test statistic is

$$\tau_c = \frac{2mS}{N^2(m-1)} = \frac{2(3)(+314)}{72^2(3-1)} = +0.1817 .$$

Note that Stuart's test statistic $\tau_c = +0.1817$ is slightly larger than Kendall's test statistic $\tau_b = +0.1664$, calculated on the same set of frequency data.

For the frequency data given in Table 5.15, there are $M = 70{,}148{,}145$ possible, equally-likely arrangements in the reference set of all permutations of cell frequencies given the observed row and column marginal frequency distributions, $\{23, 23, 26\}$ and $\{15, 11, 14, 17, 15\}$, respectively, making an exact permutation analysis possible. The exact probability value of Stuart's τ_c under the null hypothesis is the sum of the hypergeometric point probability values associated with the values of $\tau_c = +0.1817$ or greater. Based on the hypergeometric probability distribution, the exact upper-tail probability value is $P = 0.0600$.

5.5.3 *Measures of Effect Size*

A measure of effect size for Stuart's τ_c that norms properly between ± 1 would be useful. Consider Table 5.16 with the same marginals as Table 5.15, but with the cell frequencies constructed to produce the maximum value of τ_c. Note that because two row marginal frequency totals are identical ($n_{1.} = n_{2.} = 23$) and two column marginal frequency totals are identical ($n_{.1} = n_{.5} = 15$), the cell frequencies in Table 5.16 constitute only one possible arrangement of cell frequencies yielding

Table 5.16 Example maximized rank-score data for $N = 72$ bivariate observations cross-classified on ordinal variables x and y into a 3×5 contingency table

	y					
x	1	2	3	4	5	Total
1	15	8	0	0	0	23
2	0	3	5	0	15	23
3	0	0	9	17	0	26
Total	15	11	14	17	15	72

the maximum value of τ_c, given the observed row and column marginal frequency distributions, {23, 23, 26} and {15, 11, 14, 17, 15}, respectively.

For the frequency data given in Table 5.16, the number of concordant pairs is

$$C = \sum_{i=1}^{r-1}\sum_{j=1}^{c-1} n_{ij} \left(\sum_{k=i+1}^{r} \sum_{l=j+1}^{c} n_{kl} \right)$$

$$= (15)(3+5+0+15+0+9+17+0) + (8)(5+0+15+9+17+0) + \cdots + (5)(17+0) + (0)(0) = 1{,}266\ ,$$

the number of discordant pairs is

$$D = \sum_{i=1}^{r-1}\sum_{j=1}^{c-1} n_{i,c-j+1} \left(\sum_{k=i+1}^{r} \sum_{l=1}^{c-j} n_{kl} \right)$$

$$= (0)(0+3+5+0+0+0+9+17) + (0)(0+3+5+0+0+9) + \cdots + (5)(0+0) + (3)(0) = 390\ ,$$

the maximum value of S is $S_{\max} = C - D = 1{,}266 - 390 = 876$, and the maximum value of Stuart's τ_c is

$$\tau_{\max} = \frac{2mS_{\max}}{N^2(m-1)} = \frac{2(3)(876)}{72^2(3-1)} = +0.5069\ .$$

Then, a maximum-corrected measure of effect size is given by

$$ES = \frac{\tau_c}{\tau_{\max}} = \frac{+0.1817}{+0.5069} = +0.3584\ ,$$

indicating that $\tau_c = +0.1817$ is approximately 36% of the maximum possible value of τ_c, given the observed row and column marginal frequency distributions, {23, 23, 26} and {15, 11, 14, 17, 15}, respectively.

5.5.4 Sharper Bounds

There is an alternative, more general method for standardizing measures of ordinal association [4]. The "sharper-bounds" approach applies to a variety of measures of association and is illustrated here with Stuart's τ_c measure. Stuart's τ_c is based on the unstandardized measure of effect size, S. Several possibilities exist to bound S between -1 and $+1$, representing complete dissociation and complete association of variables x and y, respectively. As noted in Eq. (5.12) on p. 245, Stuart proposed that the maximum value of S be defined as

$$S_{\max} = \frac{N^2(m-1)}{2m} ,$$

where $m = \min(r, c)$ and provided $N \bmod m = 0$.

In order for S to equal $N^2(m-1)/(2m)$ and, thus, for τ_c to attain the maximum value when $-1 \leq \tau_c \leq +1$, two conditions must be met. For simplicity, consider an $r \times c$ contingency table with $r \leq c$, then $r = \min(r, c)$ and $c = \max(r, c)$. First, each row marginal frequency total must equal N/m, implying $N \bmod m = 0$ [46]. Second, some sum of 1 to c column marginal frequency totals must equal N/m, summing sequentially either from left to right, beginning with the first column, or from right to left, beginning with column c. Thus, the problem with the τ_c measure of ordinal association lies in the definition for the maximum value for S provided by Stuart. The denominator, $N^2(m-1)/(2m)$, provides only an upper bound for S computed on an idealized $r \times c$ contingency table. The solution is to find a sharper bound for the maximum value of τ_c based on the observed data than Stuart's $N^2(m-1)/(2m)$ can provide.

An alternative to Stuart's proposed maximum value of S, $N^2(m-s)/(2m)$, is provided by a Monte Carlo resampling algorithm. Given two integral marginal vectors, the set of all $r \times c$ contingency tables with row marginal frequency distribution $\{n_{1.}, \ldots, n_{r.}\}$ and column marginal frequency distribution $\{n_{.1}, \ldots, n_{.c}\}$ is a Fréchet class of matrices of nonnegative integer elements given fixed marginal frequency distributions and denoted by $F(r, c)$. Enumerating all M members of $F(r, c)$ to find an exact solution is computationally prohibitive and impractical, since the reference set of all possible permutations of cell frequencies is usually very large, even for modest values of r and c. The alternative is a Monte Carlo resampling algorithm that enumerates a random sample of size L from all M members of $F(r, c)$. If T denotes the statistic of interest, a nine-step Monte Carlo resampling algorithm is constructed as follows.

STEP 1: Let L denote a random sample with replacement of a large number of the M possible arrangements of the n_{ij} cell frequencies for $i = 1, \ldots, r$ and $j = 1, \ldots, c$ with fixed marginal frequency distributions $\{n_{1.}, \ldots, n_{r.}\}$ and $\{n_{.1}, \ldots, n_{.c}\}$.

STEP 2: Set counter k and the maximum value of statistic T ($T_{\max}$) to zero.

STEP 3: If each $\{n_{1.}, \ldots, n_{r.}\}$ or $\{n_{.1}, \ldots, n_{.c}\}$ marginal frequency distribution corresponding to $m = \min(r, c)$ equals N/m, go to STEP 4; otherwise, go to STEP 5.

STEP 4: Set $w = \max(r, c)$. If $w = c$ and any sequence of marginal frequency totals beginning with Column 1 or Column w sums to N/m, or if $w = r$ and any sequence of marginal frequency totals beginning with Row 1 or Row w sums to N/m, then set $T_{\max} = N^2(m-1)/(2m)$ and go to STEP 9; otherwise, go to STEP 5.

STEP 5: Generate a random arrangement of the n_{ij} cell frequencies for $i = 1, \ldots, r$ and $j = 1, \ldots, c$, satisfying the fixed marginal frequency distributions $\{n_{1.}, \ldots, n_{r.}\}$ and $\{n_{.1}, \ldots, n_{.c}\}$.

STEP 6: Compute statistic T on the random arrangement of the n_{ij} values and set counter $k = k + 1$.

STEP 7: If $T > T_{\max}$, $T_{\max}$ is replaced by T.

STEP 8: If $k = L$, the maximum randomly selected value of T is $T_{\max}$, go to STEP 9; otherwise, go to STEP 5.

STEP 9: Exit.

Determination of the exact maximum value of S is impractical for many $r \times c$ contingency tables. However, generation of all M arrangements of $F(r, c)$ is possible when r and c are small [32]. Table 5.17 contains maximum values of Kendall's S utilizing exact, Monte Carlo resampling, and Stuart's procedures for

Table 5.17 Maximum values of S based on exact, resampling, and Stuart's procedures for 2×2, 2×3, 2×4, 2×5, 3×3, 3×4, and 4×4 contingency tables with uniform and skewed row and column marginal frequency distributions

		Marginal		Procedure		
Table	Size	Row	Column	Exact	Resampling	Stuart's
1	2×2	{9, 9}	{9, 9}	81	81	81
2		{9, 9}	{6, 12}	54	54	81
3		{6, 12}	{6, 12}	72	72	81
4	2×3	{18, 18}	{12, 12, 12}	288	288	324
5		{18, 18}	{6, 12, 18}	324	324	324
6		{12, 24}	{12, 12, 12}	288	288	324
7		{12, 24}	{6, 12, 18}	252	252	324
8	2×4	{30, 30}	{15, 15, 15, 15}	900	900	900
9		{30, 30}	{6, 12, 18, 24}	828	828	900
10		{20, 40}	{15, 15, 15, 15}	750	750	900
11		{20, 40}	{6, 12, 18, 24}	768	708	900
12	2×5	{45, 45}	{18, 18, 18, 18, 18}	1,944	1,944	2,025
13		{45, 45}	{6, 12, 18, 24, 30}	1,890	1,764	2,025
14		{30, 60}	{18, 18, 18, 18, 18}	1,728	1,728	2,025
15		{30, 60}	{6, 12, 18, 24, 30}	1,728	1,728	2,025
16		{12, 12, 12}	{6, 12, 18}	324	324	432
17		{6, 12, 18}	{6, 12, 18}	396	396	432
18	3×4	{20, 20, 20}	{15, 15, 15, 15}	1,100	1,100	1,200
19		{20, 20, 20}	{6, 12, 18, 24}	1,088	876	1,200
20		{10, 20, 30}	{15, 15, 15, 15}	1,050	1,050	1,200
21		{10, 20, 30}	{6, 12, 18, 24}	996	996	1,200
22	4×4	{15, 15, 15, 15}	{15, 15, 15, 15}	1,350	1,350	1,350
23		{15, 15, 15, 15}	{6, 12, 18, 24}	1,116	1,035	1,350
24		{6, 12, 18, 24}	{6, 12, 18, 24}	1,260	1,260	1,350

2×2, 2×3, 2×4, 2×5, 3×3, 3×4, and 4×4 contingency tables. Because the true maximum value of S is dependent on the observed marginal frequency distributions, a variety of uniform and skewed marginal frequency distributions are utilized in Table 5.17.

Uniform marginal frequency distributions imply that the probability of an observation falling into Row i is given by $1/r$ and the probability of an observation falling into Column j is given by $1/c$. On the other hand, the skewed marginal frequency distributions in Table 5.17 imply that the probability of an observation falling into Row i is given by $(2i)/[r(r+1)]$ and the probability of an observation falling into Column j is given by $(2j)/[c(c+1)]$. The various values of $N = 18$ for the 2×2 tables; $N = 36$ for the 2×3 and 3×3 tables; $N = 60$ for the 2×4, 3×4 and 4×4 tables; and $N = 90$ for the 2×5 tables were obtained from $N = 3\max[r(r+1), c(c+1)]$, ensuring integral values for the $r = 2, 3, 4$ and $c = 2, 3, 4, 5$ marginal frequency totals. The column in Table 5.17 headed "Exact" lists maximum values of S based on all M members of $F(r, c)$; the column headed "Resampling" lists maximum values of S based on $L =$ 1,000,000 random arrangements of cell frequencies; and the column headed "Stuart's" lists maximum values of S based on Stuart's proposed $S_{\max} = N^2(m-1)/(2m)$.

It is evident in Table 5.17 that the maximum values of Kendall's S based on resampling are always less than the obtained by the maximum proposed by Stuart, except in five cases: the 2×2 table (Table 1) with row and column marginal frequency distributions, $\{9, 9\}$ and $\{9, 9\}$, respectively; the 2×3 table (Table 5) with row and column marginal frequency distributions, $\{18, 18\}$ and $\{6, 12, 18\}$, respectively; the 2×4 table (Table 8) with row and column marginal frequency distributions, $\{30, 30\}$ and $\{15, 15, 15, 15\}$, respectively; the 3×3 table (Table 20) with row and column marginal frequency distributions, $\{12, 12, 12\}$ and $\{12, 12, 12\}$, respectively; and the 4×4 table (Table 27) with row and column marginal frequency distributions, $\{15, 15, 15, 15\}$ and $\{15, 15, 15, 15\}$, respectively. All five cases satisfy the two conditions for Stuart's $N^2(m-1)/(2m)$—row marginals are either equal to N/m or some sequential sum of column marginals are equal to N/m.

Proper comparisons in Table 5.17 are between the randomly selected maximum values of S and Stuart's maximum values of S. The purpose of these analyses is to obtain sharper bounds on $S_{\max}$ through Monte Carlo resampling; the exact values of $S_{\max}$ are listed in Table 5.17 only to demonstrate optimal results and, for the example analyses in Table 5.17, constitute a gold standard for purposes of comparison.

Stuart's procedure matches the exact maximum value of S for only 5 of the 25 marginal conditions specified in Table 5.17, i.e., Tables 1, 5, 8, 16, and 23. Thus, Stuart's suggested procedure often overestimates the maximum value of S and, consequently, underestimates effect size. As is evident in Table 5.17, there are four tables where the Monte Carlo resampling and exact procedures differ on the maximum value of S: Tables 11, 13, 24, and 28. Note that all four tables have similar skewed column marginal frequency distributions of either $\{6, 12, 18, 24\}$ or $\{6, 12, 18, 24, 30\}$. Consequently, the number of possible cell frequency configurations yielding the maximum value of S is severely circumscribed, other

Table 5.18 Tables 11, 13, 20, and 24 from Table 5.17 with total number of possible cell frequency configurations, maximum S values, hypergeometric point probability values, and cell frequency configurations corresponding to the maximum value of S

Table number	Number of configurations	Maximum S value	Point probability	Cell frequencies
11	1,088	768	0.3650×10^{-13}	6 12 2 0 0 0 16 24
13	37,775	1,890	0.1259×10^{-19}	6 12 18 9 0 0 0 0 15 30 0 0 0 15 30 6 12 18 9 0
24	358,267	1,088	0.2814×10^{-20}	6 12 2 0 0 0 16 4 0 0 0 20
28	28,904,292	1,116	0.1877×10^{-20}	6 9 0 0 0 3 12 0 0 0 6 9 0 0 0 15

factors being equal. Table 5.18 lists the table numbers from Table 5.17 for the tables where the resampling and exact maximum values of S do not agree, the exact number of possible cell frequency configurations given the fixed marginal frequency distributions, the exact maximum value of S, the point probability value of each table yielding the maximum value of S, and a listing of the cell frequency configurations yielding the maximum value of S.

To illustrate, consider Table 11 in Table 5.18 for which there are $M = 1{,}088$ cell frequency configurations in the reference set of all permutations of cell frequencies given the observed row and column marginal frequency distributions, $\{20, 40\}$ and $\{6, 12, 18, 24\}$, respectively. The maximum value of S is $S_{\max} = 768$, the hypergeometric point probability value is only 0.3650×10^{-13}, and only one of the $M = 1{,}088$ possible cell configurations yields a maximum value of $S_{\max} = 768$. Note that for Table 13 in Table 5.18, there are two cell frequency configurations yielding a maximum value of $S_{\max} = 1{,}890$, because the row marginal frequency totals are both equal to $N/m = 90/2$, i.e., $\{45, 45\}$. For the four tables listed in Table 5.18, it is not surprising that the exact and resampling values of $S_{\max}$ differ, given $L = 1{,}000{,}000$, the large number of possible cell frequency configurations, the skewed marginal frequency distributions, the limited number(s) of cell frequency configurations yielding the maximum value of S, and the very small hypergeometric point probability values of the cell frequency configuration(s) yielding the maximum value of S.

Although Table 5.17 documents the possible limitations of Stuart's proposed maximum value of S, the question remains as to the effect of the maximum value on the standardized measure of effect size, τ_c. It is obvious that different maximum values of S obtained by the resampling and Stuart's procedures have little effect on

Table 5.19 Example 2×2, 2×3, and 2×4 contingency tables with $N = 60$, row marginal frequency totals of {30, 30}, and observed cell frequencies chosen to maximize the observed value of S

Table size	Column marginals	Observed cell frequencies	Resampling τ_c value	Stuart's τ_c value
2×2	{30, 30}	30 0 0 30	+1.0000	+1.0000
	{20, 40}	20 10 0 30	+1.0000	+0.6667
	{10, 50}	10 20 0 30	+1.0000	+0.3333
	{5, 55}	5 25 0 30	+1.0000	+0.1667
2×3	{10, 20, 30}	10 20 0 0 0 30	+1.0000	+1.0000
	{20, 20, 20}	20 10 0 0 10 20	+1.0000	+0.8889
	{5, 20, 35}	5 20 5 0 0 30	+1.0000	+0.8333
	{5, 15, 40}	5 15 10 0 0 30	+1.0000	+0.6667
2×4	{15, 15, 15, 15}	15 15 0 0 0 0 15 15	+1.0000	+1.0000
	{10, 15, 15, 20}	10 15 5 0 10 15 5 0	+1.0000	+0.9444
	{5, 15, 15, 25}	5 15 10 0 0 0 5 25	+1.0000	+0.9444
	{5, 10, 10, 35}	5 10 10 5 0 0 0 30	+1.0000	+0.8333

the value of τ_c when the observed value of S is zero or close to zero. Moreover, researchers typically care little about very small effect sizes. Table 5.19 lists four 2×2, four 2×3, and four 2×4 contingency tables, with the column marginal frequency distributions, observed cell frequencies, maximum values of S based on Monte Carlo resampling, maximum values of S based on Stuart's $N^2(m-1)/(2m)$, observed values of τ_c based on the randomly selected maximum value of S, and observed values of τ_c based on Stuart's maximum value of S for each of the 12 tables.

In order to isolate the effect of skewed marginals on the value of τ_c, each of the 12 tables in Table 5.19 has $N = 60$, $r = 2$ rows, identical uniform row marginals of $N/m = 60/2 = \{30, 30\}$, and observed cell frequencies designed to ensure a maximum value of S, thus controlling for N, r, $n_{i.}$ for $i = 1, 2$, and S. The fourth and fifth columns in Table 5.19 list the maximum values of Kendall's S obtained from the resampling and Stuart procedures. It should be noted that the Monte Carlo resampling and exact maximum values of S are identical in these examples. Since Stuart's procedure is based solely on $N = 60$ and $m = 2$, the maximum value is identical for all 12 tables listed in Table 5.19. The last two columns of Table 5.19 list the observed values of τ_c on the basis of the resampling and Stuart procedures. Comparison of the last two columns reveals that, whereas differences between the two procedures are at times nonexistent or very small, at other times the differences are quite large, due to skewed column marginal frequency distributions that neither equal N/m nor sum sequentially to one of the row marginals, the most extreme example being the 2×2 contingency table with highly skewed column marginals totals of $\{5, 55\}$, where τ_c is = +1.00 under the Monte Carlo resampling procedure and only +0.1667 under Stuart's procedure.

The Monte Carlo resampling method for calculating sharper bounds, illustrated with Stuart's τ_c, is an example of a relatively new technique, applied to an existing statistic that enables improvement in measurement accuracy. The Monte Carlo resampling permutation procedure provided sharper bounds for the maximum value of S, permitting better estimation of effect sizes than can be accomplished with Stuart's maximum value of S based on $N^2(m-1)/(2m)$. Table 5.17 demonstrates the effectiveness of resampling in providing sharper bounds for S_{max} than Stuart's $N^2(m-1)/(2m)$ over a variety of table sizes, sample sizes, and marginal distributions. Stuart's procedure systematically deflates effect sizes by overestimating S_{max} in 20 of the 25 marginal conditions specified. Table 5.18 provides some rationale for those instances when the exact and resampling maximum values of S do not agree.

Establishing S_{max} with Monte Carlo resampling is not a simple matter of identifying one out of M possible cell frequency arrangements, since the probabilities of different configurations vary considerably. In general, the success of the resampling procedure depends on the size of M, the skewness of the marginal frequency distributions, the number of cell frequency configurations yielding S_{max}, and the point probability value of the cell frequency configuration(s) yielding S_{max}. Table 5.19 explores the impact of the wrong maximum value of S on the value of Stuart's τ_c, while controlling for N, r, $n_{i.}$ for $i = 1, \ldots, r$, and S. Inspection of Table 5.19 reveals that skewed marginal frequency distributions often lead to inflated values of S_{max} and generate τ_c values that are too small, sometimes by a substantial amount.

5.6 Goodman and Kruskal's γ Measure

In 1954 Goodman and Kruskal developed a new measure of association for two ordinal-level variables that they called gamma (γ) [15].[12] Gamma is a proportional-reduction-in-error measure of ordinal association that is based solely on the untied

[12] A number of authors prefer to reserve the symbol gamma (γ) for the population parameter and indicate the sample statistic by the letter G.

pairs, C and D, and is given by

$$\gamma = \frac{S}{C+D} = \frac{C-D}{C+D} = \frac{C}{C+D} - \frac{D}{C+D} \,. \tag{5.14}$$

It is clear from the expression on the right side of Eq. (5.14) that γ is simply the difference between the proportions of like and unlike pairs, ignoring all tied pairs, i.e., T_x, T_y, and T_{xy}.

There is a potential problem with γ that was immediately recognized by Goodman and Kruskal. Gamma is unstable over various "cutting points." That is to say, γ tends to increase as the categories of a contingency table are collapsed because γ gives no consideration to tied pairs and the number of tied pairs increases as the table is collapsed. Gamma also usually yields greater association values than other measures of ordinal association as it does not consider any of the tied pairs. Finally, γ is a weakly monotonic measure of ordinal association, i.e., for every ordered category increase (decrease) in variable x, variable y either increases (decreases) or stays the same.

5.6.1 *Monotonicity*

Strongly monotonic and weakly monotonic relationships can be illustrated with some simple graphics. A strongly monotonic relationship, such as measured by Kendall's τ_b, is illustrated in Fig. 5.2 with an **X** denoting a non-zero cell frequency and a blank cell denoting a zero cell frequency. In a strongly monotonic relationship, for every increase (decrease) in one variable there is an increase (decrease) in the other variable. In this case, if the **X**s were replaced with actual cell frequencies, Kendall's τ_b would equal $+1.00$, C would be a positive integer, D, T_x, and T_y would be zero, and Goodman and Kruskal's γ would equal $+1.00$.

Compare the strongly monotonic graphic illustrated in Fig. 5.2 with the graphic in Fig. 5.3 in which a typical weakly monotonic relationship is illustrated. For a weakly monotonic relationship, for every increase (decrease) in one variable, the other variable either increases (decreases) or stays the same. In this case, with actual cell frequencies, Goodman and Kruskal's γ would equal $+1.00$ and Kendall's τ_b would be less than $+1.00$.

Fig. 5.2 Graphic for a simulated strongly monotonic relationship

	1	2	3	4	5	6
1	X					
2		X				
3			X			
4				X		
5					X	
6						X

Fig. 5.3 Graphic for a simulated weakly monotonic relationship

	1	2	3	4	5	6
1	X	X				
2		X	X			
3			X	X		
4				X	X	
5					X	X
6						X

Fig. 5.4 Graphic for a simulated weakly monotonic relationship

	1	2	3	4	5	6
1	X	X	X	X	X	X
2						X
3						X
4						X
5						X
6						X

Table 5.20 Example rank-score data for Goodman and Kruskal's γ with $N = 60$ bivariate observations cross-classified on ordinal variables x and y into a 3×3 contingency table

	y			
x	1	2	3	Total
1	15	3	2	20
2	7	12	1	20
3	8	5	7	20
Total	30	20	10	60

Finally, compare the strongly monotonic graphic illustrated in Fig. 5.2 with the weakly monotonic graphic illustrated in Fig. 5.4, where with actual cell frequencies, Goodman and Kruskal's γ would again be $+1.00$ and Kendall's τ_b would be less than $+1.00$.

5.6.2 *Example 1*

To illustrate the calculation of Goodman and Kruskal's γ measure of ordinal association, consider the frequency data given in Table 5.20, where $N = 60$ bivariate observations have been cross-classified into a 3×3 ordered contingency table. For the frequency data given in Table 5.20, the number of concordant pairs is

$$C = \sum_{i=1}^{r-1} \sum_{j=1}^{c-1} n_{ij} \left(\sum_{k=i+1}^{r} \sum_{l=j+1}^{c} n_{kl} \right)$$

$$= (15)(12+1+5+7) + (3)(1+7) + (7)(5+7) + (12)(7) = 567 ,$$

the number of discordant pairs is

$$D = \sum_{i=1}^{r-1} \sum_{j=1}^{c-1} n_{i,c-j+1} \left(\sum_{k=i+1}^{r} \sum_{l=1}^{c-j} n_{kl} \right)$$

$$= (2)(7+12+8+5) + (3)(7+8) + (1)(8+5) + (12)(8) = 218 ,$$

$S = C - D = 567 - 218 = +349$, and the observed value of Goodman and Kruskal's γ test statistic is

$$\gamma = \frac{C-D}{C+D} = \frac{S}{C+D} = \frac{567-218}{567+218} = \frac{+349}{785} = +0.4446 .$$

For the ordered frequency data given in Table 5.20, there are only $M = 13{,}101$ possible, equally-likely arrangements in the reference set of all permutations of cell frequencies given the observed row and column marginal frequency distributions, $\{20, 20, 20\}$ and $\{30, 20, 10\}$, respectively, making an exact permutation analysis possible. The exact probability value of Goodman and Kruskal's γ under the null hypothesis is the sum of the hypergeometric point probability values associated with the values of $\gamma = +0.4446$ or greater. Based on the hypergeometric probability distribution, the exact upper-tail probability value is $P = 0.0055$.

5.6.3 Example 2

For a second example of Goodman and Kruskal's γ measure of ordinal association, consider the frequency data given in Table 5.21, where $N = 75$ bivariate observations have been cross-classified into a 3×5 ordered contingency table. For the frequency data given in Table 5.21, the number of concordant pairs is

$$C = \sum_{i=1}^{r-1} \sum_{j=1}^{c-1} n_{ij} \left(\sum_{k=i+1}^{r} \sum_{l=j+1}^{c} n_{kl} \right)$$

$$= (9)(7+8+3+2+4+8+8+10) + (5)(8+3+2+8+8+10)$$
$$+ \cdots + (8)(8+10) + (3)(10) = 1{,}202 ,$$

Table 5.21 Example rank-score data for Goodman and Kruskal's γ with $N = 75$ bivariate observations cross-classified on ordinal variables x and y into a 3×5 contingency table

	y					
x	1	2	3	4	5	Total
1	9	5	3	1	1	19
2	4	7	8	3	2	24
3	2	4	8	8	10	32
Total	15	16	19	12	13	75

the number of discordant pairs is

$$D = \sum_{i=1}^{r-1} \sum_{j=1}^{c-1} n_{i,c-j+1} \left(\sum_{k=i+1}^{r} \sum_{l=1}^{c-j} n_{kl} \right)$$
$$= (1)(4+7+8+3+2+4+8+8) + (1)(4+7+8+2+4+8)$$
$$+ \cdots + (8)(2+4) + (7)(2) = 306 ,$$

$S = C - D = 1{,}202 - 306 = +896$, and the observed value of Goodman and Kruskal's γ test statistic is

$$\gamma = \frac{C-D}{C+D} = \frac{S}{C+D} = \frac{+896}{1{,}202+306} = +0.5942 .$$

For the ordered frequency data given in Table 5.21, there are only $M = 68{,}161{,}105$ possible, equally-likely arrangements in the reference set of all permutations of cell frequencies given the observed row and column marginal frequency distributions, {19, 24, 32} and {15, 16, 19, 12, 13}, respectively, making an exact permutation analysis feasible. The exact probability value of Goodman and Kruskal's γ under the null hypothesis is the sum of the hypergeometric point probability values associated with the values of $\gamma = +0.5942$ or greater. Based on the hypergeometric probability distribution, the exact upper-tail probability value is only $P = 0.1518 \times 10^{-5}$.

5.7 Somers' d_{yx} and d_{xy} Measures of Association

In 1962 sociologist Robert Somers took exception to Goodman and Kruskal's symmetric measure of ordinal association, γ, and proposed two asymmetric alternatives given by

$$d_{yx} = \frac{C-D}{C+D+T_y} = \frac{S}{C+D+T_y} , \tag{5.15}$$

where T_y denotes the number of pairs tied on variable y but not tied on variable x, and

$$d_{xy} = \frac{C-D}{C+D+T_x} = \frac{S}{C+D+T_x} , \tag{5.16}$$

where T_x denotes the number of pairs tied on variable x but not tied on variable y.

Table 5.22 Example rank-score data for Somers' d_{yx} with $N = 18$ bivariate observations cross-classified on ordinal variables x and y into a 3×3 contingency table

	y			
x	1	2	3	Total
1	3	2	1	6
2	2	2	2	6
3	1	2	3	6
Total	6	6	6	18

As is evident in Eqs. (5.15) and (5.16), Somers included in the denominators of d_{yx} and d_{xy} the number of tied values on the dependent variable: T_y for d_{yx} and T_x for d_{xy}. The rationale for including tied values is simply that when variable y is the dependent variable (d_{yx}), then if two values of the independent variable, x, differ but the corresponding two values of the dependent variable, y, do not differ (are tied), there is evidence of a lack of association and the ties on variable y (T_y) should be included in the denominator where they act to decrease the value of d_{yx}. The same rationale holds for Somers' d_{xy} where the ties on variable x (T_x) are included in the denominator.

5.7.1 *Example 1*

To illustrate Somers' d_{yx} measure of ordinal association with y the dependent variable, consider the frequency data given in Table 5.22 where $N = 18$ bivariate observations have been cross-classified into a 3×3 ordered contingency table. For the frequency data given in Table 5.22, the number of concordant pairs is

$$C = \sum_{i=1}^{r-1}\sum_{j=1}^{c-1} n_{ij}\left(\sum_{k=i+1}^{r}\sum_{l=j+1}^{c} n_{kl}\right)$$
$$= (3)(2+2+2+3)+(2)(2+3)+(2)(2+3)+(2)(3) = 53\ ,$$

the number of discordant pairs is

$$D = \sum_{i=1}^{r-1}\sum_{j=1}^{c-1} n_{i,c-j+1}\left(\sum_{k=i+1}^{r}\sum_{l=1}^{c-j} n_{kl}\right)$$
$$= (1)(2+2+1+2)+(2)(2+1)+(2)(1+2)+(2)(1) = 21\ ,$$

the number of pairs tied on variable y but not tied on variable x is

$$T_y = \sum_{j=1}^{c} \sum_{i=1}^{r-1} n_{ij} \left(\sum_{k=i+1}^{r} n_{kj} \right)$$

$$= (3)(2+1) + (2)(1) + (2)(2+2) + (2)(2)$$

$$+ (1)(2+3) + (2)(3) = 34 \,,$$

$S = C - D = 53 - 21 = +32$, and the observed value of Somers' d_{yx} test statistic is

$$d_{yx} = \frac{C - D}{C + D + T_y} = \frac{S}{C + D + T_y} = \frac{+32}{53 + 21 + 34} = +0.2963 \,.$$

For the ordered frequency data given in Table 5.22, there are only $M = 406$ possible, equally-likely arrangements in the reference set of all permutations of cell frequencies given the observed row and column marginal frequency distributions, $\{6, 6, 6\}$ and $\{6, 6, 6\}$, respectively, making an exact permutation analysis possible. The exact probability value of d_{yx} under the null hypothesis is the sum of the hypergeometric point probability values associated with the values of $d_{yx} = +0.2963$ or greater. Based on the hypergeometric probability distribution, the exact upper-tail probability value is $P = 0.0994$.

5.7.2 Example 2

To illustrate Somers' d_{xy} measure of ordinal association with x the dependent variable, consider the ordered frequency data given in Table 5.23 where $N = 42$

Table 5.23 Example rank-score data for Somers' d_{xy} with $N = 42$ bivariate observations cross-classified on ordinal variables x and y into a 3×4 contingency table

	y				
x	1	2	3	4	Total
1	6	5	6	1	18
2	4	3	5	2	14
3	2	1	4	3	10
Total	12	9	15	6	42

bivariate observations have been cross-classified into a 3×4 ordered contingency table. For the frequency data given in Table 5.23, the number of concordant pairs is

$$C = \sum_{i=1}^{r-1} \sum_{j=1}^{c-1} n_{ij} \left(\sum_{k=i+1}^{r} \sum_{l=j+1}^{c} n_{kl} \right)$$
$$= (6)(3+5+2+1+4+3) + (5)(5+2+4+3) + (6)(2+3)$$
$$+ (4)(1+4+3) + (3)(4+3) + (5)(3) = 276 ,$$

the number of discordant pairs is

$$D = \sum_{i=1}^{r-1} \sum_{j=1}^{c-1} n_{i,c-j+1} \left(\sum_{k=i+1}^{r} \sum_{l=1}^{c-j} n_{kl} \right)$$
$$= (1)(4+3+5+2+1+4) + (6)(4+3+2+1) + (5)(4+2)$$
$$+ (2)(2+1+4) + (5)(2+1) + (3)(2) = 144 ,$$

the number of pairs tied on variable x but not tied on variable y is

$$T_x = \sum_{i=1}^{r} \sum_{j=1}^{c-1} n_{ij} \left(\sum_{k=j+1}^{c} n_{ik} \right)$$
$$= (6)(5+6+1) + (5)(6+1) + (6)(1) + (4)(3+5+2)$$
$$+ (3)(5+2) + (5)(2) + (2)(1+4+3) + (1)(4+3) + (4)(3) = 219 ,$$

$S = C - D = 276 - 144 = +132$, and the observed value of Somers' d_{xy} test statistic is

$$d_{xy} = \frac{C - D}{C + D + T_x} = \frac{S}{C + D + T_x} = \frac{+132}{276 + 144 + 219} = +0.2066 .$$

For the ordered frequency data given in Table 5.23, there are only $M = 72{,}143$ possible, equally-likely arrangements in the reference set of all permutations of cell frequencies given the observed row and column marginal frequency distributions, {18, 14, 10} and {12, 9, 15, 6}, respectively, making an exact permutation analysis feasible. However, in this case consider over-sampling via Monte Carlo resampling. Over-sampling occurs quite often in the permutation literature as commercial resampling programs often do not have an exact probability option. In addition, resampling can be much more efficient than an exact procedure as the hypergeometric point probability values need not be calculated for each arrangement of the data. Conversely, exact procedures can sometimes be more efficient than resampling procedures because repeated calls to a pseudorandom number generator can be expensive in terms of execution time.

The Monte Carlo resampling probability value of d_{xy} is simply the proportion of randomly selected d_{xy} values that are equal to or greater than $d_{xy} = +0.2066$. If d_o denotes the observed value of d_{xy}, the approximate resampling probability value based on $L = 1{,}000{,}000$ random arrangements of the cell frequencies, given the observed row and column marginal frequency distributions, $\{18, 14, 10\}$ and $\{12, 9, 15, 6\}$, respectively, is

$$P(d_{xy} \geq d_o|H_0) = \frac{\text{number of } d_{xy} \text{ values } \geq d_o}{L} = \frac{55{,}581}{1{,}000{,}000} = 0.0556\,.$$

5.8 Kim's $d_{y \cdot x}$ and $d_{x \cdot y}$ Measures of Association

In 1971 Jae-On Kim proposed alternative asymmetric proportional-reduction-in-error measures of ordinal association given by

$$d_{y \cdot x} = \frac{C - D}{C + D + T_x} \quad \text{and} \quad d_{x \cdot y} = \frac{C - D}{C + D + T_y}$$

[25]. In contrast to Somers' d_{yx} and d_{xy} measures of ordinal association, which adjust for ties on the dependent variable—paired differences on the independent variable that do not result in paired differences on the dependent variable—Kim's $d_{y \cdot x}$ and $d_{x \cdot y}$ measures adjust for ties on the independent variable—pairs with no differences on the independent variable that correspond to pairs with differences on the dependent variable. It is immediately apparent that Kim's $d_{y \cdot x}$ and $d_{x \cdot y}$ measures are equivalent to Somers' d_{xy} and d_{yx} measures, respectively [25, p. 899].

5.8.1 *Example 1*

To illustrate Kim's $d_{y \cdot x}$ asymmetric measure of ordinal association, consider the frequency data given in Table 5.24 with $N = 8$ observations cross-classified into

Table 5.24 Example frequency data for Kim's $d_{y \cdot x}$ with $N = 8$ observations cross-classified on ordinal variables x and y into a 3×2 contingency table

	y		
x	Correct	Wrong	Total
High	2	1	3
Medium	1	2	3
Low	0	2	2
Total	3	5	8

a 3×2 ordered contingency table. For the frequency data given in Table 5.24, the number of concordant pairs is

$$C = \sum_{i=1}^{r-1} \sum_{j=1}^{c-1} n_{ij} \left(\sum_{k=i+1}^{r} \sum_{l=j+1}^{c} n_{kl} \right) = (2)(2+2) + (1)(2) = 10 \ ,$$

the number of discordant pairs is

$$D = \sum_{i=1}^{r-1} \sum_{j=1}^{c-1} n_{i,c-j+1} \left(\sum_{k=i+1}^{r} \sum_{l=1}^{c-j} n_{kl} \right) = (1)(1+0) + (2)(0) = 1 \ ,$$

the number of pairs tied on variable x but not tied on variable y is

$$T_x = \sum_{i=1}^{r} \sum_{j=1}^{c-1} n_{ij} \left(\sum_{k=j+1}^{c} n_{ik} \right) = (2)(1) + (1)(2) + (0)(2) = 4 \ ,$$

the number of pairs tied on variable y but not tied on variable x is

$$T_y = \sum_{j=1}^{c} \sum_{i=1}^{r-1} n_{ij} \left(\sum_{k=i+1}^{r} n_{kj} \right) = (2)(1+0) + (1)(0) + (1)(2+2) + (2)(2) = 10 \ ,$$

and the observed value of Kim's $d_{y\cdot x}$ test statistic is

$$d_{y\cdot x} = \frac{C - D}{C + D + T_x} = \frac{10 - 1}{10 + 1 + 4} = +0.60 \ .$$

Because Kim did not provide a standard error for $d_{y\cdot x}$, an asymptotic solution is not defined. However, for the ordered frequency data given in Table 5.24, there are only $M = 9$ possible, equally-likely arrangements in the reference set of all permutations of cell frequencies given the observed row and column marginal frequency distributions, {3, 3, 2} and {3, 5}, respectively, making an exact permutation analysis feasible. Since $M = 9$ is a very small number of arrangements, it will be illustrative to list the nine sets of cell frequencies, the $d_{y\cdot x}$ values, and the associated hypergeometric point probability values in Table 5.25, where the rows with hypergeometric point probability values associated with $d_{y\cdot x}$ values equal to or greater than the observed $d_{y\cdot x}$ value are indicated with asterisks.

If all $M = 9$ possible arrangements of cell frequencies in Table 5.24 occur with equal chance, the exact probability value of $d_{y\cdot x}$ under the null hypothesis is the

Table 5.25 Cell frequencies, $d_{y \cdot x}$ values, and exact hypergeometric point probability values for $M = 9$ possible arrangements of the observed data in Table 5.24

	Cell frequency							
Table	n_{11}	n_{12}	n_{21}	n_{22}	n_{31}	n_{32}	$d_{y \cdot x}$	Probability
1	0	3	1	2	2	0	−0.8667	0.0536
2	0	3	2	1	1	1	−0.5333	0.1071
3	1	2	0	3	2	0	−0.4667	0.0536
4	0	3	3	0	0	2	−0.2000	0.0179
5	1	2	1	2	1	1	−0.1333	0.3215
6	1	2	2	1	0	2	+0.2000	0.1607
7	2	1	0	3	1	1	+0.4667	0.1071
8*	2	1	1	2	0	2	+0.6000	0.1607
9*	3	0	0	3	0	2	+1.0000	0.0179
Sum								1.0000

sum of the hypergeometric point probability values in Table 5.25 associated with the values of $d_{y \cdot x} = +0.60$ or greater; in this case

$$P = 0.1607 + 0.0179 = 0.1786 \ .$$

It is not widely recognized that the numerator of $d_{y \cdot x}$, $C + D + T_x$, can be defined strictly in terms of the marginal frequency totals, i.e.,

$$C + D + T_x = \frac{1}{2}\left(N^2 - \sum_{j=1}^{c} n_{.j}^2\right) ,$$

where $n_{.j}$ denotes the column marginal frequency totals for $j = 1, \ldots, c$ columns and N denotes the total number of observations. Thus, for the frequency data given in Table 5.24 on p. 262,

$$C + D + T_x = 10 + 1 + 4 = 15$$

and

$$\frac{1}{2}\left(N^2 - \sum_{j=1}^{c} n_{.j}^2\right) = \frac{1}{2}\left[8^2 - (3^2 + 5^2)\right] = 15 \ .$$

Since the marginal frequency totals are invariant under permutation, the exact probability value depends solely on the distribution of $S = C - D$. Table 5.26 lists the $M = 9$ sets of cell frequencies, the S values, and the associated hypergeometric point probability values, where the rows with hypergeometric point probability values associated with S values that are equal to or greater than the observed value of $S = +9$ are indicated with asterisks.

Table 5.26 Cell frequencies, S values, and exact hypergeometric point probability values for $M = 9$ possible arrangements of the observed data in Table 5.24

	Cell frequency							
Table	n_{11}	n_{12}	n_{21}	n_{22}	n_{31}	n_{32}	S	Probability
1	0	3	1	2	2	0	−13	0.0536
2	0	3	2	1	1	1	−8	0.1071
3	1	2	0	3	2	0	−7	0.0536
4	0	3	3	0	0	2	−5	0.0179
5	1	2	1	2	1	1	−2	0.3215
6	1	2	2	1	0	2	+3	0.1607
7	2	1	0	3	1	1	+4	0.1071
8*	2	1	1	2	0	2	+9	0.1607
9*	3	0	0	3	0	2	+15	0.0179
Sum								1.0000

If the $M = 9$ possible arrangements of the cell frequencies in Table 5.24 occur with equal chance, the exact probability value of S under the null hypothesis is the sum of the hypergeometric point probability values in Table 5.26 associated with the values of $S = C - D = 10 - 1 = +9$ or greater; in this case, the exact upper-tail probability value is

$$P = 0.1607 + 0.0179 = 0.1786 \; .$$

5.8.2 Example 2

Similarly, for Kim's $d_{x \cdot y}$ test statistic,

$$d_{x \cdot y} = \frac{C - D}{C + D + T_y} = \frac{10 - 1}{10 + 1 + 10} = +0.4286 \; .$$

For the frequency data given in Table 5.24 on p. 262, there are only $M = 9$ possible, equally-likely arrangements in the reference set of all permutations of cell frequencies given the observed row and column marginal frequency distributions, $\{3, 3, 2\}$ and $\{3, 5\}$, respectively, making an exact permutation analysis feasible. Since $M = 9$ is a very small number, it will be illustrative to list the nine sets of cell frequencies, the $d_{x \cdot y}$ values, and the associated hypergeometric point probability values in Table 5.27, where the rows with hypergeometric point probability values associated with $d_{x \cdot y}$ values equal to or greater than the observed $d_{y \cdot x}$ value are indicated with asterisks.

If all $M = 9$ possible arrangements of cell frequencies in Table 5.27 occur with equal chance, the exact probability value of $d_{x \cdot y}$ under the null hypothesis is the

Table 5.27 Cell frequencies, $d_{x \cdot y}$ values, and exact hypergeometric point probability values for $M = 9$ possible arrangements of the observed data in Table 5.24

Table	Cell frequency						$d_{x \cdot y}$	Probability
	n_{11}	n_{12}	n_{21}	n_{22}	n_{31}	n_{32}		
1	0	3	1	2	2	0	−0.6190	0.0536
2	0	3	2	1	1	1	−0.3810	0.1071
3	1	2	0	3	2	0	−0.3333	0.0536
4	0	3	3	0	0	2	−0.1429	0.0179
5	1	2	1	2	1	1	−0.0952	0.3215
6	1	2	2	1	0	2	+0.1429	0.1607
7	2	1	0	3	1	1	+0.3333	0.1071
8*	2	1	1	2	0	2	+0.4286	0.1607
9*	3	0	0	3	0	2	+0.7143	0.0179
Sum								1.0000

sum of the hypergeometric point probability values associated with the values of $d_{x \cdot y} = +0.4286$ or greater; in this case

$$P = 0.1607 + 0.0179 = 0.1786\ .$$

Also,

$$C + D + T_y = \frac{1}{2}\left(N^2 - \sum_{i=1}^{r} n_{i.}^2\right)\ ,$$

where $n_{i.}$ denotes the row marginal frequency totals for $i = 1, \ldots, r$ rows and N denotes the total number of observations. Thus, for the frequency data given in Table 5.24 on p. 262,

$$C + D + T_y = 10 + 1 + 10 = 21$$

and

$$\frac{1}{2}\left(N^2 - \sum_{i=1}^{r} n_{i.}^2\right) = \frac{1}{2}\left[8^2 - (3^2 + 3^2 + 2^2)\right] = 21\ .$$

Since the marginal frequency totals are invariant under permutation, the exact probability value depends solely on the distribution of $S = C - D$. If the $M = 9$ possible arrangements of the cell frequencies in Table 5.24 occur with equal chance, the exact probability value of S under the null hypothesis is the sum of the hypergeometric probability values associated with the values of $S = C - D = 10 - 1 = +9$ or greater. Based on the hypergeometric probability distribution, the exact upper-tail probability value is

$$P = 0.1607 + 0.0179 = 0.1786\ .$$

5.9 Wilson's *e* Measure of Ordinal Association

In 1974 Thomas Wilson proposed yet another measure of ordinal association that he called e [50]. Arguing that a measure of association should be adjusted for tied values on both variable x and variable y, Wilson suggested a symmetric measure of ordinal association given by

$$e = \frac{C - D}{C + D + T_x + T_y} = \frac{S}{C + D + T_x + T_y} \, . \tag{5.17}$$

As Wilson noted, e takes the values of ± 1 if and only if the data exhibit a perfect positive or a perfect negative strongly monotonic relationship [50, p. 334].

It is obvious from Eq. (5.17) that Wilson's e is equivalent to Somers' d_{yx} when $T_x = 0$ and is equivalent to Somers' d_{xy} when $T_y = 0$. Moreover, if both $T_x = 0$ and $T_y = 0$, then $e = d_{yx} = d_{xy} = \gamma = \tau_a = \tau_b$.

5.9.1 Example 1

To illustrate Wilson's symmetric measure of ordinal association, consider the frequency data given in Table 5.28 with $N = 70$ observations on variables, Education and Responsibility, cross-classified into a 3×3 ordered contingency table.

For the frequency data given in Table 5.28, the number of concordant pairs is

$$C = \sum_{i=1}^{r-1} \sum_{j=1}^{c-1} n_{ij} \left(\sum_{k=i+1}^{r} \sum_{l=j+1}^{c} n_{kl} \right)$$
$$= (15)(20 + 5 + 0 + 5) + (5)(5 + 5) + (10)(0 + 5) + (20)(5) = 650 \, ,$$

Table 5.28 Example frequency data for Wilson's e with $N = 70$ observations cross-classified by Responsibility and Educational level into a 3×3 ordered contingency table

	Education			
Responsibility	B.S.	M.A.	Ph.D.	Total
High	15	5	5	25
Medium	10	20	5	35
Low	5	0	5	10
Total	30	25	15	70

the number of discordant pairs is

$$D = \sum_{i=1}^{r-1} \sum_{j=1}^{c-1} n_{i,c-j+1} \left(\sum_{k=i+1}^{r} \sum_{l=1}^{c-j} n_{kl} \right)$$

$$= (5)(10+20+5+0) + (5)(10+5) + (5)(5+0) + (20)(5) = 375 ,$$

the number of pairs tied on Responsibility (variable x) but not tied on Education (variable y) is

$$T_x = \sum_{i=1}^{r} \sum_{j=1}^{c-1} n_{ij} \left(\sum_{k=j+1}^{c} n_{ik} \right)$$

$$= (15)(5+5) + (5)(5) + (10)(20+5) + (20)(5)$$

$$+ (5)(0+5) + (0)(5) = 550 ,$$

the number of pairs tied on Education (variable y) but not tied on Responsibility (variable x) is

$$T_y = \sum_{j=1}^{c} \sum_{i=1}^{r-1} n_{ij} \left(\sum_{k=i+1}^{r} n_{kj} \right)$$

$$= (15)(10+5) + (10)(5) + (5)(20+0) + (20)(0)$$

$$+ (5)(5+5) + (5)(5) = 450 ,$$

and the observed value of Wilson's e test statistic is

$$e = \frac{C - D}{C + D + T_x + T_y} = \frac{S}{C + D + T_x + T_y}$$

$$= \frac{650 - 375}{650 + 375 + 550 + 450} = \frac{275}{2{,}025} = +0.1358 .$$

Because Wilson did not provide a standard error for e, an asymptotic solution is not defined. However, for the frequency data given in Table 5.28, there are only $M = 15{,}836$ possible, equally-likely arrangements in the reference set of all permutations of cell frequencies given the observed row and column marginal frequency distributions, {25, 35, 10} and {30, 25, 15}, respectively, making an exact permutation analysis feasible. If the $M = 15{,}836$ possible arrangements of cell frequencies given in Table 5.28 occur with equal chance, the exact probability value of Wilson's e under the null hypothesis is the sum of the hypergeometric point probability values associated with the values of $e = +0.1358$ or greater. Based on

Table 5.29 Example frequency data for Wilson's e with $N = 49$ observations cross-classified into a 4×4 ordered contingency table

	y				
x	1	2	3	4	Total
1	5	4	1	2	12
2	1	5	4	3	13
3	3	3	6	2	14
4	3	2	1	4	10
Total	12	14	12	11	49

the hypergeometric probability distribution, the exact upper-tail probability value is $P = 0.0501$.

5.9.2 Example 2

For a second example of Wilson's e measure of ordinal association, consider the frequency data given in Table 5.29 where $N = 49$ objects have been cross-classified into a 4×4 ordered contingency table. For the frequency data given in Table 5.29, the number of concordant pairs is

$$C = \sum_{i=1}^{r-1} \sum_{j=1}^{c-1} n_{ij} \left(\sum_{k=i+1}^{r} \sum_{l=j+1}^{c} n_{kl} \right)$$
$$= (5)(5+4+3+3+6+2+2+1+4) + (4)(4+3+6+2+1+4)$$
$$+ (3)(1+4) + (6)(4) = 406 \; ,$$

the number of discordant pairs is

$$D = \sum_{i=1}^{r-1} \sum_{j=1}^{c-1} n_{i,c-j+1} \left(\sum_{k=i+1}^{r} \sum_{l=1}^{c-j} n_{kl} \right)$$
$$= (2)(1+5+4+3+3+6+3+2+1) + (1)(1+5+3+3+3+2)$$
$$+ (6)(3+2) + (3)(3) = 280 \; ,$$

the number of pairs tied on variable x but not tied on variable y is

$$T_x = \sum_{i=1}^{r} \sum_{j=1}^{c-1} n_{ij} \left(\sum_{k=j+1}^{c} n_{ik} \right)$$
$$= (5)(4+1+2) + (4)(1+2) + (1)(2)$$
$$+ \cdots + (3)(2+1+4) + (2)(1+4) + (4)(1) = 212 \; ,$$

the number of pairs tied on variable y but not tied on variable x is

$$T_y = \sum_{j=1}^{c} \sum_{i=1}^{r-1} n_{ij} \left(\sum_{k=i+1}^{r} n_{kj} \right)$$

$$= (5)(1+3+3) + (1)(3+3) + (3)(3)$$

$$+ \cdots + (2)(3+2+4) + (3)(2+4) + (2)(4) = 210 \,,$$

and the observed value of Wilson's e test statistic is

$$e = \frac{C-D}{C+D+T_x+T_y} = \frac{S}{C+D+T_x+T_y}$$

$$= \frac{406-280}{406+280+212+210} = \frac{126}{1{,}108} = +0.1137 \,.$$

There are only $M = 20{,}597{,}720$ possible, equally-likely arrangements in the reference set of all permutations of cell frequencies given the observed row and column marginal frequency distributions, {12, 13, 14, 10} and {12, 14, 12, 11}, respectively, making an exact permutation analysis possible. If the $M = 20{,}597{,}720$ possible arrangements of cell frequencies given in Table 5.29 occur with equal chance, the exact probability value of Wilson's e under the null hypothesis is the sum of the hypergeometric point probability values associated with the values of $e = +0.1137$ or greater. Based on the hypergeometric probability distribution, the exact upper-tail probability value is $P = 0.1236$.

5.10 Comparisons of Pairwise Measures

Using a common set of cell frequencies, a comparison of the six most common measures based on Kendall's S demonstrates the differences among the measures. Consider the sparse frequency data given in Table 5.30 where $N = 55$ bivariate observations have been cross-classified into a 3×5 ordered contingency table.

Table 5.30 Example rank-score data for $N = 55$ bivariate observations cross-classified on ordinal variables x and y into a 3×5 contingency table

	y					
x	1	2	3	4	5	Total
1	5	3	2	1	0	11
2	2	8	7	6	2	25
3	0	2	4	4	9	19
Total	7	13	13	11	11	55

For the frequency data given in Table 5.30, the number of concordant pairs is

$$C = \sum_{i=1}^{r-1} \sum_{j=1}^{c-1} n_{ij} \left(\sum_{k=i+1}^{r} \sum_{l=j+1}^{c} n_{kl} \right)$$
$$= (5)(8+7+6+2+2+4+4+9) + (3)(7+6+2+4+4+9)$$
$$+ \cdots + (7)(4+9) + (6)(9) = 678 \; ,$$

the number of discordant pairs is

$$D = \sum_{i=1}^{r-1} \sum_{j=1}^{c-1} n_{i,c-j+1} \left(\sum_{k=i+1}^{r} \sum_{l=1}^{c-j} n_{kl} \right)$$
$$= (0)(2+8+7+6+0+2+4+4) + (1)(2+8+7+0+2+4)$$
$$+ \cdots + (7)(0+2) + (8)(0) = 123 \; ,$$

the number of pairs tied on variable x but not tied on variable y is

$$T_x = \sum_{i=1}^{r} \sum_{j=1}^{c-1} n_{ij} \left(\sum_{k=j+1}^{c} n_{ik} \right)$$
$$= (5)(3+2+1+0) + (3)(2+1+0) + (2)(1+0) + (1)(0)$$
$$+ \cdots + (0)(2+4+4+9) + (2)(4+4+9) + (4)(4+9)$$
$$+ (4)(9) = 397 \; ,$$

the number of pairs tied on variable y but not tied on variable x is

$$T_y = \sum_{j=1}^{c} \sum_{i=1}^{r-1} n_{ij} \left(\sum_{k=i+1}^{r} n_{kj} \right)$$
$$= (5)(2+0) + (2)(0) + (3)(8+2) + (8)(2)$$
$$+ \cdots + (0)(2+9) + (2)(9) = 158 \; ,$$

$S = C - D = 678 - 123 = +555$, and the observed value of Kendall's τ_a is

$$\tau_a = \frac{2S}{N(N-1)} = \frac{2(+555)}{55(55-1)} = +0.3737 \; ,$$

the observed value of Kendall's τ_b test statistic is

$$\tau_b = \frac{S}{\sqrt{(C+D+T_x)(C+D+T_y)}}$$

$$= \frac{+555}{\sqrt{(678+123+397)(678+123+158)}} = +0.5178\,,$$

with $m = \min(r, c) = \min(3, 5) = 3$, the observed value of Stuart's τ_c test statistic is

$$\tau_c = \frac{2mS}{N^2(m-1)} = \frac{2(3)(+555)}{55^2(3-1)} = +0.5504\,,$$

the observed value of Goodman and Kruskal's γ test statistic is

$$\gamma = \frac{S}{C+D} = \frac{+555}{678+123} = +0.6929\,,$$

the observed value of Somers' d_{yx} test statistic is

$$d_{yx} = \frac{S}{C+D+T_y} = \frac{+555}{678+123+158} = +0.5787\,,$$

and the observed value of Somers' d_{xy} test statistic is

$$d_{xy} = \frac{S}{C+D+T_x} = \frac{+555}{678+123+397} = +0.4633\,.$$

For the frequency data given in Table 5.30, there are only $M = 4{,}788{,}153$ possible, equally-likely arrangements in the reference set of all permutations of cell frequencies, given the observed row and column marginal frequency distributions, $\{11, 25, 19\}$ and $\{7, 13, 13, 11, 11\}$, respectively, making an exact permutation analysis possible. The exact probability value of τ_a, τ_b, τ_c, d_{yx}, and d_{xy} under the null hypothesis is the sum of the hypergeometric point probability values associated with the values of the observed statistics or greater; in this case the exact upper-tail probability value for the five measures is $P = 0.1550{\times}10^{-5}$; on the other hand, the exact upper-tail probability value for Goodman and Kruskal's γ is $P = 0.1416{\times}10^{-5}$. The results are summarized in Table 5.31.

It is, perhaps, curious that the five measures of ordinal association, τ_a, τ_b, τ_c, d_{yx}, and d_{xy}, yield identical probability values. It follows from the fact that $C + D + T_y$ and $C + D + T_x$ can be computed from just the marginal frequency distributions, which are fixed for all possible arrangements of cell frequencies. Thus, the denominators of Kendall's τ_a, Kendall's τ_b, Stuart's τ_c, Somers' d_{yx}, and Somers' d_{xy} can all be calculated from the marginals of the observed contingency table,

Table 5.31 Summary of computed values and probability values for Kendall's τ_a, Kendall's τ_b, Stuart's τ_c, Goodman and Kruskal's γ, Somers' d_{yx}, and Somers' d_{xy}

Measure	Statistic	Probability
Kendall's τ_a	+0.3737	0.1550×10^{-5}
Kendall's τ_b	+0.5178	0.1550×10^{-5}
Stuart's τ_c	+0.5504	0.1550×10^{-5}
G/K's γ	+0.6929	0.1416×10^{-5}
Somers' d_{yx}	+0.5787	0.1550×10^{-5}
Somers' d_{xy}	+0.4633	0.1550×10^{-5}

which are invariant under permutation. However, the denominator of Goodman and Kruskal's γ is $C + D$, cannot be obtained from the marginals alone, and is not invariant under permutation.

For the observed cell frequencies given in Table 5.30, the number of concordant pairs is

$$C = \sum_{i=1}^{r-1} \sum_{j=1}^{c-1} n_{ij} \left(\sum_{k=i+1}^{r} \sum_{l=j+1}^{c} n_{kl} \right)$$

$$= 5(8+7+6+2+2+4+4+9) + 3(7+6+2+4+4+9)$$

$$+ 2(6+2+4+9) + 1(2+9) + 2(2+4+4+9) + 8(4+4+9)$$

$$+ 7(4+9) + 6(9) = 678 \ ,$$

the number of discordant pairs is

$$D = \sum_{i=1}^{r-1} \sum_{j=1}^{c-1} n_{i,c-j+1} \left(\sum_{k=i+1}^{r} \sum_{l=1}^{c-j} n_{kl} \right)$$

$$= 0(2+8+7+6+0+2+4+4) + 1(2+8+7+0+2+4)$$

$$+ 2(2+8+0+2) + 3(2+0) + 2(0+2+4+4) + 6(0+2+4)$$

$$+ 7(0+2) + 8(0) = 123 \ ,$$

the number of pairs tied on variable x but not tied on variable y is

$$T_x = \sum_{i=1}^{r} \sum_{j=1}^{c-1} n_{ij} \left(\sum_{k=j+1}^{c} n_{ik} \right)$$

$$= 5(3+2+1+0) + 3(2+1+0) + 2(1+0) + 1(0)$$

$$+ 2(8+7+6+2) + 8(7+6+2) + 7(6+2) + 6(2)$$

$$+ 0(2+4+4+9) + 2(4+4+9) + 4(4+9) + 4(9) = 397 \ ,$$

and the number of pairs tied on variable y but not tied on variable x is

$$\begin{aligned} T_y = \sum_{j=1}^{c} \sum_{i=1}^{r-1} n_{ij} \left(\sum_{k=i+1}^{r} n_{kj} \right) \\ &= 5(2+0) + 2(0) + 3(8+2) + 8(2) + 2(7+4) + 7(4) \\ &\quad + 1(6+4) + 6(4) + 0(2+9) + 2(9) = 158 \; . \end{aligned}$$

Thus,

$$C + D + T_y = 678 + 123 + 158 = 959$$

and

$$C + D + T_x = 678 + 123 + 397 = 1{,}198 \; .$$

It is easily shown that $C + D + T_y$ can be obtained from N and the row marginal frequency distribution; accordingly,

$$C + D + T_y = \frac{1}{2}\left(N^2 - \sum_{i=1}^{r} n_{i.}^2 \right) = \frac{1}{2}\left[55^2 - \left(11^2 + 25^2 + 19^2 \right) \right] = 959 \; ,$$

and $C + D + T_x$ can be obtained from N and the column marginal frequency distribution; accordingly,

$$\begin{aligned} C + D + T_x &= \frac{1}{2}\left(N^2 - \sum_{j=1}^{c} n_{.j}^2 \right) \\ &= \frac{1}{2}\left[55^2 - \left(7^2 + 13^2 + 13^2 + 11^2 + 11^2 \right) \right] = 1{,}198 \; . \end{aligned}$$

5.10.1 Marginal Frequency Distributions

In this section, it is demonstrated that all pairwise components can be obtained from the observed marginal frequency totals. Let C denote the number of concordant pairs, D denote the number of discordant pairs, T_x denote the number of pairs tied on variable x but not tied on variable y, T_y denote the number of pairs tied on variable y but not tied on variable x, and T_{xy} denote the number of pairs tied on both variable x and variable y. Then the total number of pairs can be partitioned as

$$\binom{N}{2} = \frac{N(N-1)}{2} = C + D + T_x + T_y + T_{xy} \; .$$

Note that

$$\frac{1}{2}\left(N^2 - \sum_{j=1}^{c} n_{.j}^2\right) = C + D + T_x$$

and

$$\frac{1}{2}\left[\sum_{j=1}^{c} n_{.j}(n_{.j} - 1)\right] = T_y + T_{xy} ,$$

where $n_{.j}$ denotes the jth column marginal frequency total, $j = 1, \ldots, c$.

Then, all possible pairs can be partitioned in terms of the marginal frequency totals as

$$\begin{aligned}\binom{N}{2} &= \frac{1}{2}\left(N^2 - \sum_{j=1}^{c} n_{.j}^2\right) + \frac{1}{2}\left[\sum_{j=1}^{c} n_{.j}(n_{.j} - 1)\right] \\ &= \frac{1}{2}\left[N^2 - \sum_{j=1}^{c} n_{.j}^2 + \sum_{j=1}^{c} n_{.j}(n_{.j} - 1)\right] \\ &= \frac{1}{2}\left(N^2 - \sum_{j=1}^{c} n_{.j}\right) = \frac{N(N-1)}{2} .\end{aligned} \tag{5.18}$$

While the relationship given in Eq. (5.18) is in terms of the column marginal frequency totals, the same results can be obtained from the row marginal frequency totals, i.e.,

$$\binom{N}{2} = \frac{1}{2}\left[N^2 - \sum_{i=1}^{r} n_{i.}^2 + \sum_{i=1}^{r} n_{i.}(n_{i.} - 1)\right] , \tag{5.19}$$

where $n_{i.}$ denotes the ith row marginal frequency total, $i = 1, \ldots, r$.

For the frequency data given in Table 5.30 on p. 270 and following the first expression in Eq. (5.18),

$$\begin{aligned}\binom{N}{2} &= \frac{1}{2}\left[N^2 - \sum_{j=1}^{c} n_{.j}^2 + \sum_{j=1}^{c} n_{.j}(n_{.j} - 1)\right] \\ &= \frac{1}{2}\Big[55^2 - (7^2 + 13^2 + 13^2 + 11^2 + 11^2) + (7)(7-1)\end{aligned}$$

$$+ (13)(13-1) + (13)(13-1) + (11)(11-1) + (11)(11-1)\Big]$$

$$= \frac{1}{2}\big(3{,}025 - 629 + 574\big) = 1{,}485\ ,$$

and following Eq. (5.19)

$$\binom{N}{2} = \frac{1}{2}\left[N^2 - \sum_{i=1}^{r} n_{i.}^2 + \sum_{i=1}^{r} n_{i.}(n_{i.}-1)\right]$$

$$= \frac{1}{2}\Big[55^2 - \big(11^2 + 25^2 + 19^2\big)$$

$$+ (11)(11-1) + (25)(25-1) + (19)(19-1)\Big]$$

$$= \frac{1}{2}\big(3{,}025 - 1{,}107 + 1{,}052\big) = 1{,}485\ .$$

Thus, since the marginal frequency distributions are fixed under permutation, the exact probability values of Kendall's τ_a, Kendall's τ_b, Somers' d_{yx}, and Somers' d_{xy} are based entirely on the permutation distribution of the common numerator, S [8]. In the case of Stuart's measure of ordinal association, the formula for τ_c does not include either $C + D + T_x$ or $C + D + T_y$, but utilizes $m = \min(r, c)$, which is based on the number of rows or columns that are fixed under permutation. Consequently, the probability value for Stuart's τ_c is also based solely on the permutation distribution of statistic S. In the case of Goodman and Kruskal's measure of ordinal association, γ does not consider either T_x or T_y as providing any usable information; therefore, its probability value differs slightly from the common probability value for Kendall's τ_a and τ_b, Stuart's τ_c, and Somers' d_{yx} and d_{xy}.

5.11 Whitfield's *S* Measure

In 1947 John Whitfield, an experimental psychologist at the University of Cambridge, proposed a measure of correlation between two variables in which one variable was composed of N rank scores and the other variable was dichotomous [48]. An example analysis will serve to illustrate Whitfield's procedure. Consider the rank scores listed in Table 5.32 where the dichotomous variable categories are two samples indicated by the letters A and B and the rank scores

Table 5.32 Ranking of a dichotomous variable with $n_1 = 4$, $n_2 = 2$, and $N = n_1 + n_2 = 6$

Rank	1	2	3	4	5	6
Sample	*A*	*B*	*A*	*A*	*A*	*B*

are from 1 to 6. Let $n_1 = 4$ denote the number of rank scores in the A category, let $n_2 = 2$ denote the number of rank scores in the B category, and let $N = n_1 + n_2$.

Whitfield designed a procedure to calculate a statistic that he labeled S, following Kendall's notation in a 1945 *Biometrika* article on "The treatment of ties in ranking problems" [22]. Given the $N = 6$ rank scores listed in Table 5.32, consider the $n_1 = 4$ rank scores in the category identified by the letter A: $1, 3, 4$, and 5. Beginning with rank score 1 with the letter A, there are no rank scores with the letter B to the left of $A = 1$ and two rank scores with the letter B to the right of $A = 1$ (ranks 2 and 6); so Whitfield calculated $0 - 2 = -2$. For rank score 3 with the letter A, there is one rank score to the left of $A = 3$ with the letter B (rank 2) and one rank score to the right of $A = 3$ with the letter B (rank 6); so $1 - 1 = 0$. For rank score 4 with the letter A, there is one rank score to the left of $A = 4$ with the letter B (rank 2) and one rank score to the right of $A = 4$ with the letter B (rank 6); so $1 - 1 = 0$. Finally, for rank score 5 with the letter A, there is one rank score to the left of $A = 5$ with the letter B (rank 2) and one rank score to the right of $A = 5$ with the letter B (rank 6); so $1 - 1 = 0$. The sum of the differences between variables A and B is $S = -2 + 0 + 0 + 0 = -2$. In this manner, Whitfield's approach accommodated samples with $n_1 \neq n_2$ as well as any number of tied rank scores.

Since the number of possible pairs of N consecutive integers is given by

$$\frac{N(N-1)}{2} ,$$

Whitfield defined and calculated a measure of rank-order association between variables A and B as

$$\tau = \frac{2S}{N(N-1)} = \frac{2(-2)}{6(6-1)} = -0.1333 .$$

Whitfield's S is identical to Kendall's S [22] and is directly related to the two-sample rank-sum U statistic of Mann and Whitney [31] and to the two-sample rank-sum W statistic of Wilcoxon [49]. This can be demonstrated with a simple comparison. For the rank scores listed in Table 5.32, there are $n_1 = 4$ A rank scores and $n_2 = 2$ B rank scores, so considering the smaller of the two sample sizes (the $n_2 = 2$ B rank scores), the first letter B (rank 2) precedes three letter A rank scores (ranks 3, 4, and 5) and the second letter B (rank 6) precedes no letter A, so $U = 3 + 0 = 3$. The relationships between Whitfield's S and Mann and Whitney's U statistics are given by

$$S = 2U - n_1 n_2 \quad \text{and} \quad U = \frac{S + n_1 n_2}{2} .$$

Thus, for the rank scores listed in Table 5.32 the observed values of S and U are

$$S = (2)(3) - (4)(2) = -2 \quad \text{and} \quad U = \frac{-2 + (4)(2)}{2} = 3 ,$$

respectively [8, 27]. Also, for the example rank scores listed in Table 5.32, the observed Wilcoxon W statistic for the smaller of the two sums (the $n_2 = 2$ B rank scores) is $W = 2 + 6 = 8$ and the relationships between Whitfield's S and Wilcoxon's W are given by

$$S = n_2(N + 1) - 2W \quad \text{and} \quad W = \frac{n_2(N + 1) - S}{2} .$$

Thus, the observed values of S and W are

$$S = (2)(6 + 1) - (2)(8) = -2 \quad \text{and} \quad W = \frac{(2)(6 + 1) - (-2)}{2} = 8 ,$$

respectively [8, 27].

As Whitfield noted, the calculation of S was fashioned after a procedure introduced by Maurice Kendall in 1945 and Whitfield might have been unaware of the two-sample rank-sum tests previously published by Wilcoxon in 1945 [49], Festinger in 1946 [12], and Mann and Whitney in 1947 [31], as they are not referenced in the 1947 Whitfield article. Kendall considered the number of concordant (C) and discordant (D) pairs, of which there is a total of $N(N - 1)/2$ pairs when there are no tied values among the N integers [22]. For the example rank scores listed in Table 5.32 there are

$$\frac{N(N - 1)}{2} = \frac{6(6 - 1)}{2} = 15$$

pairs of rank scores. Table 5.33 lists and numbers the 15 rank pairs, the concordant/discordant classification of rank pairs, and the rank-pair values, where concordant pairs ($-, -$ and $+, +$) are given a value of 0, and discordant pairs ($+, -$ and $-, +$) are given values of $+1$ and -1, respectively. The observed sum of the pair values listed in Table 5.33 for the 15 pairs is $S = -5 + 3 = -2$.

Today it is well-known, although poorly documented, that when one classification is a dichotomy and the other classification is rank ordered, with or without tied

Table 5.33 Fifteen pairs of observations with concordant/discordant (C/D) pairs and associated rank-pair values

Number	Pair	C/D	Value	Number	Pair	C/D	Value
1	1–2	$-, +$	-1	9	2–6	$+, +$	0
2	1–3	$-, -$	0	10	3–4	$-, -$	0
3	1–4	$-, -$	0	11	3–5	$-, -$	0
4	1–5	$-, -$	0	12	3–6	$-, +$	-1
5	1–6	$-, +$	-1	13	4–5	$-, -$	0
6	2–3	$+, -$	$+1$	14	4–6	$-, +$	-1
7	2–4	$+, -$	$+1$	15	5–6	$-, +$	-1
8	2–5	$+, -$	$+1$				

Table 5.34 Listing of the $n_1 = 9$ and $n_2 = 6$ rank scores from Samples A and B, respectively

Rank	1	2	3	4	5	6	7	8	9	10	11	12	13	14	15
Sample	A	A	B	A	A	A	B	B	A	A	A	A	B	B	B

values, the S statistic of Kendall is equivalent to the Mann–Whitney U statistic; see articles on this topic by Lincoln Moses in 1956 [37] and Edmund John Burr in 1960 [8]. Whitfield apparently was the first to uncover the relationship between S, the statistic underlying Kendall's τ_a and τ_b rank-order correlation coefficients, and U, the Mann–Whitney two-sample rank-sum statistic for two independent samples.

However, it was Hemelrijk in 1952 [18] and Jonckheere in 1954 [20] who made the relationship between S and U explicit; see also a discussion by Leach in 1979 [28, p. 183]. Because the Jonckheere–Terpstra test, when restricted to two independent samples, is mathematically identical in reverse application to the Wilcoxon and Mann–Whitney tests, see references [20, p. 138] and [40, p. 396], the two-sample rank-sum test is sometimes referred to as the Kendall–Wilcoxon–Mann–Whitney–Jonckheere–Festinger test [37, p. 246].

5.11.1 Example 1

Consider the rank scores listed in Table 5.34 consisting of $n_1 = 9$ rank scores from Sample A and $n_2 = 6$ rank scores from Sample B. Calculating Mann and Whitney's U statistic for the data listed in Table 5.34, the number of A rank scores to the left of (less than) the first B rank score (rank 3) is 2; the number of A rank scores to the left of the second and third B rank scores (ranks 7 and 8) is 5 each; and the number of A rank scores to the left of the last three B rank scores (ranks 13, 14, and 15) is 9 each. Then $U = 2 + 5 + 5 + 9 + 9 + 9 = 39$. To calculate Wilcoxon's W statistic for the rank data listed in Table 5.34, the sum of the rank scores in Sample A is $W = 1 + 2 + 4 + 5 + 6 + 9 + 10 + 11 + 12 = 60$.[13]

To calculate Whitfield's S statistic for the data listed in Table 5.34, there are two A rank scores to the left of $B = 3$ (ranks 1 and 2) and seven A rank scores to the right of $B = 3$ (ranks 4, 5, 6, 9, 10 11, and 12), so $2 - 7 = -5$. There are five A rank scores to the left of $B = 7$ and $B = 8$ (ranks 1, 2, 4, 5, and 6) and four A rank scores to the right of $B = 7$ and $B = 8$ (ranks 9, 10, 11, and 12), so $(5 - 4) + (5 - 4) = 2$. There are nine A rank scores to the left of $B = 13$, 14, and 15 (ranks 1, 2, 4, 5, 6, 9, 10, 11, and 12) and zero A rank scores to the right of $B = 13$, 14, and 15, so $(9 - 0) + (9 - 0) + (9 - 0) = 27$. Then $S = -5 + 2 + 27 = +24$. Note that the

[13]Coincidentally, in this example analysis the sum of the $n_1 = 9$ rank scores in Sample B is also 60.

relationships among Whitfield's S, Mann and Whitney's U, and Wilcoxon's W are given by

$$S = 2U - n_1 n_2 = 2(39) - (9)(6) = 78 - 54 = +24 \;,$$

$$U = \frac{S + n_1 n_2}{2} = \frac{24 + (9)(6)}{2} = \frac{78}{2} = 39 \;,$$

$$S = n_1(N+1) - 2W = 9(15+1) - (2)(60) = 144 - 120 = +24 \;,$$

and

$$W = \frac{n_1(N+1) - S}{2} = \frac{9(15+1) - 24}{2} = \frac{120}{2} = 60 \;.$$

Alternatively, as Whitfield suggested, arrange the two samples into a contingency table with two rows and columns equal to the frequency distribution of the combined samples, as depicted in Table 5.35. Here the first row of frequencies in Table 5.35 represents the runs in the list of rank scores in Table 5.34 labeled as A, i.e., there are two occurrences of A in ranks 1 and 2; no occurrence of A in rank 3; three occurrences of A in ranks 4, 5, and 6; no occurrence of A in ranks 7 and 8; four occurrences of A in ranks 10, 11, and 12; and no occurrence of A in ranks 13, 14, and 15. The second row of frequencies in Table 5.35 represents the runs in the list of rank scores in Table 5.34 labeled as B, i.e., there are no occurrences of B in ranks 1 and 2; one occurrence of B in rank 3; no occurrences of B in ranks 4, 5, and 6; two occurrences of B in ranks 7 and 8; no occurrences of B in ranks 9, 10, 11, and 12; and three occurrences of B in ranks 13, 14, and 15.

Given the $r \times c$ contingency table in Table 5.35 with $r = 2$ rows and $c = 6$ columns, let n_{ij} indicate a cell frequency for $i = 1, \ldots, r$ and $j = 1, \ldots, c$. Then, as Kendall showed in 1948 [23], the number of concordant pairs is given by

$$C = \sum_{i=1}^{r-1} \sum_{j=1}^{c-1} n_{ij} \left(\sum_{k=i+1}^{r} \sum_{l=j+1}^{c} n_{kl} \right) \tag{5.20}$$

and the number of discordant pairs is given by

$$D = \sum_{i=1}^{r-1} \sum_{j=1}^{c-1} n_{i,c-j+1} \left(\sum_{k=i+1}^{r} \sum_{l=1}^{c-j} n_{kl} \right) . \tag{5.21}$$

Table 5.35 Contingency table of the frequencies of rank scores in Table 5.34

A	2	0	3	0	4	0
B	0	1	0	2	0	3

Thus, for the cell frequencies given in Table 5.35, C is calculated by proceeding from the upper-left cell with frequency $n_{11} = 2$ downward and to the right, multiplying each cell frequency by the sum of all cell frequencies below and to the right, and summing the products. Thus, following Eq. (5.20), the number of concordant pairs in Table 5.35 is

$$C = \sum_{i=1}^{r-1} \sum_{j=1}^{c-1} n_{ij} \left(\sum_{k=i+1}^{r} \sum_{l=j+1}^{c} n_{kl} \right)$$
$$= (2)(1+0+2+0+3) + (0)(0+2+0+3)$$
$$+ (3)(2+0+3) + (0)(0+3) + (4)(3) = 39 ,$$

and D is calculated by proceeding from the upper-right cell with frequency $n_{16} = 0$ downward and to the left, multiplying each cell frequency by the sum of all cell frequencies below and to the left, and summing the products. Thus, following Eq. (5.21), the number of discordant pairs in Table 5.35 is

$$D = \sum_{i=1}^{r-1} \sum_{j=1}^{c-1} n_{i,c-j+1} \left(\sum_{k=i+1}^{r} \sum_{l=1}^{c-j} n_{kl} \right)$$
$$= (0)(0+1+0+2+0) + (4)(0+1+0+2)$$
$$+ (0)(0+1+0) + (3)(0+1) + (0)(0) = 15 .$$

Then, the observed value of S is $C - D = 39 - 15 = +24$.

For the rank scores listed in Table 5.34 on p. 279, there are only

$$M = \frac{N!}{n_1!\, n_2!} = \frac{15!}{9!\, 6!} = 5{,}005$$

possible, equally-likely arrangements in the reference set of all permutations of the observed rank scores, making an exact permutation analysis feasible. If all arrangements of the $N = 15$ observed rank scores listed in Table 5.34 occur with equal chance, the exact probability value under the null hypothesis of S computed on the $M = 5{,}005$ possible, equally-likely arrangements of the observed data with $n_1 = 9$ A rank scores and $n_2 = 6$ B rank scores preserved for each arrangement is the sum of the hypergeometric point probability values associated with the values of $S = +24$ or greater. Based on the hypergeometric probability distribution, the exact upper-tail probability value is $P = 0.0905$.

Table 5.36 Listing of the $n_1 = 8$ and $n_2 = 4$ rank scores from Samples A and B, respectively

Rank	1	2	3	4	5	6	7	8	9	10	11	12
Sample	A	A	A	A	A	A	B	A	B	B	A	B

Table 5.37 Contingency table of the frequencies of rank scores in Table 5.36

A	6	0	1	0	1	0
B	0	1	0	2	0	1

5.11.2 Example 2

For a second example of Whitfield's S statistic, consider the rank scores listed in Table 5.36 consisting of $n_1 = 8$ rank scores from Sample A and $n_2 = 4$ rank scores from Sample B. To calculate Whitfield's S statistic for the data listed in Table 5.36, there are six A rank scores to the left of $B = 7$ (ranks, 1, 2, 3, 4, 5, 6) and two A ranks to the right of $B = 7$ (ranks 8 and 11), so $6 - 2 = 4$. There are seven A ranks to the left of $B = 9$ and $B = 10$ (ranks 1, 2, 3, 4, 5, 6, 8) and one A rank to the right of $B = 9$ and $B = 10$ (rank 11), so $(7 - 1) + (7 - 1) = 12$. There are eight A ranks to the left of $B = 12$ (ranks 1, 2, 3, 4, 5, 6, 8, 11) and no A ranks to the right of $B = 12$, so $8 - 0 = 8$. Then, $S = 4 + 12 + 8 = +24$.

Alternatively, arrange the two samples into a contingency table with two rows and columns equal to the frequency distribution of the combined samples, as depicted in Table 5.37. Here the first row of frequencies in Table 5.37 represents the runs in the list of rank scores in Table 5.36 labeled as A, i.e., there are six occurrences of A in ranks 1, 2, 3, 4, 5, and 6; no occurrence of A in rank 7; one occurrence of A in rank 8; no occurrences of A in ranks 9 and 10; one occurrence of A in rank 11; and no occurrence of A in rank 12. The second row of frequencies in Table 5.37 represents the runs in the list of rank scores in Table 5.36 labeled as B, i.e., there are no occurrences of B in ranks 1, 2, 3, 4, 5, and 6; one occurrence of B in rank 7; no occurrence of B in rank 8; two occurrences of B in ranks 9 and 10; no occurrence of B in rank 11; and one occurrence of B in rank 12.

Given the $r \times c$ contingency table in Table 5.37 with $r = 2$ rows and $c = 6$ columns, let n_{ij} indicate a cell frequency for $i = 1, \ldots, r$ and $j = 1, \ldots, c$. For the cell frequencies given in Table 5.37, C is calculated by proceeding from the upper-left cell with frequency $n_{11} = 2$ downward and to the right, multiplying each cell frequency by the sum of all cell frequencies below and to the right, and summing the products. Thus, following Eq. (5.20) on p. 280, the number of concordant pairs in Table 5.37 is

$$C = \sum_{i=1}^{r-1} \sum_{j=1}^{c-1} n_{ij} \left(\sum_{k=i+1}^{r} \sum_{l=j+1}^{c} n_{kl} \right)$$

$$= (6)(1 + 0 + 2 + 0 + 1) + (0)(0 + 2 + 0 + 1)$$

$$+ (1)(2 + 0 + 1) + (0)(0 + 1) + (1)(1) = 28 ,$$

and D is calculated by proceeding from the upper-right cell with frequency $n_{16} = 0$ downward and to the left, multiplying each cell frequency by the sum of all cell frequencies below and to the left, and summing the products. Thus, following Eq. (5.21) on p. 280, the number of discordant pairs in Table 5.37 is

$$D = \sum_{i=1}^{r-1} \sum_{j=1}^{c-1} n_{i,c-j+1} \left(\sum_{k=i+1}^{r} \sum_{l=1}^{c-j} n_{kl} \right)$$

$$= (0)(0 + 1 + 0 + 2 + 0) + (1)(0 + 1 + 0 + 2)$$

$$+ (0)(0 + 1 + 0) + (1)(0 + 1) + (0)(0) = 4 .$$

Then, the observed value of S is $C - D = 28 - 4 = +24$.

For the rank scores listed in Table 5.36, there are only

$$M = \frac{N!}{n_1!\, n_2!} = \frac{12!}{8!\, 4!} = \frac{479{,}001{,}600}{(40{,}320)(24)} = 495$$

possible, equally-likely arrangements in the reference set of all permutations of the observed rank scores, making an exact permutation analysis feasible.

If all arrangements of the $N = 12$ observed rank scores listed in Table 5.36 occur with equal chance, the exact probability value under the null hypothesis of S computed on the $M = 495$ possible, equally-likely arrangements of the observed data with $n_1 = 8$ and $n_2 = 4$ preserved for each arrangement is the sum of the hypergeometric point probability values associated with the values of $S = +24$ or greater. Based on the hypergeometric probability distribution, the exact upper-tail probability value is $P = 0.0242$.

5.12 Cureton's Rank-Biserial Correlation Coefficient

Consider two correlated variables, one represented by a ranking and the other by a dichotomy, similar to Whitfield's data in Table 5.34 on p. 279. In 1956 psychologist Edward Cureton proposed a new measure of correlation for a ranking

Table 5.38 Example (0, 1) coded data for Cureton's rank-biserial correlation coefficient with $n_0 = 6$ and $n_1 = 4$

	Variable	
Object	x	y
1	0	1
2	1	2
3	0	3
4	0	4
5	0	5
6	0	6
7	1	7
8	0	8
9	1	9
10	1	10

and a dichotomous variable called r_{rb} for rank-biserial correlation [9].[14] The rank-biserial correlation coefficient was introduced by Cureton as a measure of effect size for the Wilcoxon–Mann–Whitney two-sample rank-sum test. Twelve years later, in 1968, Cureton extended r_{rb} to include tied rank scores [10]. Cureton stated that the new correlation coefficient should norm properly between ± 1 and should be strictly non-parametric, defined solely in terms of inversions and agreements between rank pairs, without the use of means, variances, covariances, or regression [9, p. 287]. Consequently, as Cureton stated, "clearly r_{rb} is a Kendall-type coefficient" [9, p. 289]. However, Cureton also stated that r_{rb} "is also a Spearman-type coefficient" [9, p. 289]. It is clear that r_{rb} is, indeed, a Kendall-type coefficient as Kendall's tau-like family of measures and Cureton's r_{rb} are both based on $S = C - D$, where C and D denote the number of concordant and discordant pairs of x, y values, respectively. It is less clear that Cureton's r_{rb} belongs to the Spearman family of correlation measures [3, pp. 302–303].

5.12.1 *Example 1*

Consider an example data set such as listed in Table 5.38 in which $N = 10$ objects are ranked (variable y) and simultaneously classified into two groups coded 0 and 1 (variable x). Cureton defined r_{rb} as

$$r_{rb} = \frac{S}{S_{\max}} ,$$

[14] Technically, Cureton's r_{rb} is not considered a measure of correlation [14, p. 629].

where C is the number of concordant pairs, D is the number of discordant pairs, $S = C - D$ is the test statistic of Kendall [21] and Whitfield [48], and $S_{\max} = n_0 n_1$, where n_0 is the number of objects coded 0 and n_1 is the number of objects coded 1.

Table 5.39 lists the

$$\binom{N}{2} = \frac{N(N-1)}{2} = \frac{10(10-1)}{2} = 45$$

possible paired comparisons of x_i and x_j with y_i and y_j, where $i < j$ and n_0 and n_1 are the number of objects coded 0 and 1, respectively. Each paired difference is labeled as concordant (C) or discordant (D). Paired differences not labeled as C or D are not relevant in the present context as they are tied by either $x_i = x_j = 0$ or $x_i = x_j = 1$. In Table 5.39 there are $C = 18$ concordant and $D = 6$ discordant paired differences; thus, for the $N = 10$ paired differences listed in Table 5.39, the observed value of S is $C - D = 18 - 6 = +12$.

Alternatively, as suggested by Whitfield [48], the rank scores listed in Table 5.38 can be rearranged into a contingency table to make calculation of C and D much

Table 5.39 Paired differences and concordant (C) and discordant (D) values for the univariate rank scores listed in Table 5.38

Pair	$x_i - x_j$	$y_i - y_j$	Type	Pair	$x_i - x_j$	$y_i - y_j$	Type
1	$1 - 0$	$1 - 2$	C	24	$0 - 1$	$3 - 10$	C
2	$0 - 0$	$1 - 3$		25	$0 - 0$	$4 - 5$	
3	$0 - 0$	$1 - 4$		26	$0 - 0$	$4 - 6$	
4	$0 - 0$	$1 - 5$		27	$0 - 1$	$4 - 7$	C
5	$0 - 0$	$1 - 6$		28	$0 - 0$	$4 - 8$	
6	$0 - 1$	$1 - 7$	C	29	$0 - 1$	$4 - 9$	C
7	$0 - 0$	$1 - 8$		30	$0 - 1$	$4 - 10$	C
8	$0 - 1$	$1 - 9$	C	31	$0 - 0$	$5 - 6$	
9	$0 - 1$	$1 - 10$	C	32	$0 - 1$	$5 - 7$	C
10	$1 - 0$	$2 - 3$	D	33	$0 - 0$	$5 - 8$	
11	$1 - 0$	$2 - 4$	D	34	$0 - 1$	$5 - 9$	C
12	$1 - 0$	$2 - 5$	D	35	$0 - 1$	$5 - 10$	C
13	$1 - 0$	$2 - 6$	D	36	$0 - 1$	$6 - 7$	C
14	$1 - 1$	$2 - 7$		37	$0 - 0$	$6 - 8$	
15	$1 - 0$	$2 - 8$	D	38	$0 - 1$	$6 - 9$	C
16	$1 - 1$	$2 - 9$		39	$0 - 1$	$6 - 10$	C
17	$1 - 1$	$2 - 10$		40	$1 - 0$	$7 - 8$	D
18	$0 - 0$	$3 - 4$		41	$1 - 1$	$7 - 9$	
19	$0 - 0$	$3 - 5$		42	$1 - 1$	$7 - 10$	
20	$0 - 0$	$3 - 6$		43	$0 - 1$	$8 - 9$	C
21	$0 - 1$	$3 - 7$	C	44	$0 - 1$	$8 - 10$	C
22	$0 - 0$	$3 - 8$		45	$1 - 1$	$9 - 10$	
23	$0 - 1$	$3 - 9$	C				

Table 5.40 Contingency table of the frequencies of rank scores in Table 5.38

0	1	0	4	0	1	0
1	0	1	0	1	0	2

more convenient [48]. Consider the data listed in Table 5.38 arranged into a 2×6 contingency table, such as given in Table 5.40. The top row of frequencies given in Table 5.40 represents the runs in the list of rank scores given in Table 5.38 coded 0, i.e., there is one occurrence of a 0 in rank 1, no occurrence of a 0 in rank 2, four occurrences of a 0 in ranks 3, 4, 5, and 6, no occurrence of a 0 in rank 7, one occurrence of a 0 in rank 8, and two occurrences of a 0 in ranks 9 and 10. The bottom row of frequencies given in Table 5.40 represents the runs in the list of rank scores given in Table 5.38 coded 1, i.e., there is no occurrence of a 1 in rank 1, one occurrence of a 1 in rank 2, no occurrence of a 1 in ranks 3, 4, 5, and 6, one occurrence of a 1 in rank 7, no occurrence of a 1 in rank 8, and two occurrences of a 1 in ranks 9 and 10.

Given the $r \times c$ contingency table in Table 5.40 with $r = 2$ rows and $c = 6$ columns, let x_{ij} indicate a cell frequency for $i = 1, \ldots, r$ and $j = 1, \ldots, c$. Then, as Kendall showed in 1948 [23], the number of concordant and discordant pairs is given by

$$C = \sum_{i=1}^{r-1} \sum_{j=1}^{c-1} x_{ij} \left(\sum_{k=i+1}^{r} \sum_{l=j+1}^{c} x_{kl} \right)$$

and

$$D = \sum_{i=1}^{r-1} \sum_{j=1}^{c-1} x_{i,c-j+1} \left(\sum_{k=i+1}^{r} \sum_{l=1}^{c-j} x_{kl} \right) ,$$

respectively. Thus, the observed values of C and D are

$$C = (1)(1+0+1+0+2) + (0)(0+1+0+2) + (4)(1+0+2) + (0)(0+2) + (1)(2) = 18$$

and

$$D = (0)(0+1+0+1+0) + (1)(0+1+0+1) + (0)(0+1+0) + (4)(0+1) + (1)(0) = 6 ,$$

respectively, and the observed value of S is $C - D = 18 - 6 = +12$. It is easily shown that the maximum value of Cureton's S, $S_{\max}$, is given by $n_0 n_1$, where n_0

is the number of objects coded 0 and n_1 is the number of objects coded 1. Then, Cureton's rank-biserial coefficient is given by

$$r_{rb} = \frac{S}{S_{\max}} = \frac{S}{n_0 n_1} = \frac{+12}{(6)(4)} = +0.50 \; .$$

In 1966 Glass derived a simplified formula for r_{rb}, assuming no tied rank scores [14], given by

$$r_{rb} = \frac{2}{N} \left(\bar{y}_1 - \bar{y}_0 \right) \; ,$$

where $\bar{y}_0$ and $\bar{y}_1$ are the arithmetic averages of the y values coded 0 and 1, respectively. In this case, $\bar{y}_0 = 4.50$ and $\bar{y}_1 = 7.00$. Note that under (0, 1) binary coding, $\bar{y}_0$ and $\bar{y}_1 - \bar{y}_0$ are the intercept (a_{yx}) and slope (b_{yx}), respectively, of a regression line passing through the two points ($x = 0, \bar{y}_0 = 4.40$) and ($x = 1, \bar{y}_1 = 7.00$), as illustrated in Fig. 5.5.

Glass provided two alternative calculating formulæ given by

$$r_{rb} = \frac{2}{n_0} \left(\bar{y}_1 - \frac{N+1}{2} \right) \quad \text{or} \quad r_{rb} = \frac{2}{n_1} \left(\frac{N+1}{2} - \bar{y}_0 \right) \; .$$

Thus, for the data listed in Table 5.38 on p. 284 where

$$\bar{y}_0 = \frac{1}{n_0} \sum_{i=1}^{n_0} = \frac{1}{6}(1 + 3 + 4 + 5 + 6 + 8) = \frac{1}{6}(27) = 4.50$$

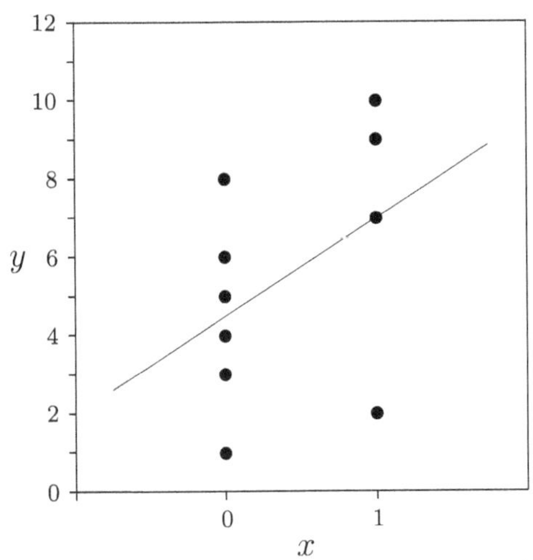

Fig. 5.5 Graphic depicting the regression line for the data listed in Table 5.38 with intercept equal to $\bar{y}_0 = 4.50$ and slope equal to $\bar{y}_1 - \bar{y}_0 = 7.00 - 4.50 = 2.50$

and

$$\bar{y}_1 = \frac{1}{n_1} \sum_{i=1}^{n_1} = \frac{1}{4}(2+7+9+10) = 7.00 \, ,$$

Cureton's rank-biserial correlation coefficient is given by either

$$r_{rb} = \frac{2}{n_0}\left(\bar{y}_1 - \frac{N+1}{2}\right) = \frac{2}{6}\left(7.00 - \frac{10+1}{2}\right) = +0.50$$

or

$$r_{rb} = \frac{2}{n_1}\left(\frac{N+1}{2} - \bar{y}_0\right) = \frac{2}{4}\left(\frac{10+1}{2} - 4.50\right) = +0.50 \, .$$

Since n_0 and n_1 are constants under permutation,

$$P(r_{rb} \geq r_o | H_0) = P(S \geq S_o | H_0) = \frac{\text{number of } S \text{ values} \geq S_o}{M} \, ,$$

where r_o and S_o denote the observed values of r_{rb} and S, respectively.

For the rank scores listed in Table 5.38, there are only

$$M = \frac{N!}{n_0!\, n_1!} = \frac{10!}{6!\, 4!} = 210$$

possible, equally-likely arrangements in the reference set of all permutations of the observed rank scores, making an exact permutation analysis feasible. If all arrangements of the $N = 10$ observed rank scores listed in Table 5.38 occur with equal chance, the exact upper-tail probability value of $S = +12$ computed on the $M = 210$ possible arrangements of the observed data with $n_0 = 6$ and $n_1 = 4$ rank scores preserved for each arrangement is

$$P(S \geq S_o | H_0) = \frac{\text{number of } S \text{ values } \geq S_o}{M} = \frac{54}{210} = 0.2571 \, .$$

5.12.2 Example 2

For a second example of Cureton's rank-biserial correlation coefficient, consider the rank-score data given in Table 5.41 in which $N = 12$ objects are ranked (variable y) and also classified into two groups coded 0 and 1 (variable x).

For the rank-score data given in Table 5.41, $N = 12$, $n_0 = 5$, $n_1 = 7$, the number of concordant pairs is $C = 18$, the number of discordant pairs is $D = 14$, the number of pairs with tied values on variable x is $T_x = 30$, the number of pairs

Table 5.41 Example (0, 1) coded data for Cureton's rank-biserial correlation coefficient with $n_0 = 5$ and $n_1 = 7$

	Variable	
Object	x	y
1	0	1
2	1	2.5
3	0	2.5
4	1	4
5	0	5
6	1	6
7	1	7
8	1	8
9	1	9
10	0	11
11	1	11
12	0	11

with tied values on variable y is $T_y = 3$, the number of pairs with tied values on both variable x and variable y is $T_{xy} = 1$, and Kendall's test statistic is $S = C - D = 18 - 14 = +4$. Then Cureton's rank-biserial correlation coefficient is

$$r_{rb} = \frac{S}{n_0 n_1} = \frac{+4}{(5)(7)} = +0.1143 \; .$$

As in Example 1, n_0 and n_1 are constants under permutation, therefore

$$P(r_{rb} \geq r_o | H_0) = P(S \geq S_o | H_0) = \frac{\text{number of } S \text{ values } \geq S_o}{M} \; ,$$

where r_o and S_o denote the observed values of r_{rb} and S, respectively. For the rank scores listed in Table 5.41 there are only

$$M = \frac{N!}{n_0!\, n_1!} = \frac{12!}{5!\; 7!} = \frac{479{,}001{,}600}{(120)(5{,}040)} = 792$$

possible, equally-likely arrangements in the reference set of all permutations of the observed rank scores, making an exact permutation analysis feasible. If all arrangements of the $N = 12$ observed rank scores listed in Table 5.41 occur with equal chance, the exact upper-tail probability value of $S = +4$ computed on the $M = 792$ possible arrangements of the observed data with $n_0 = 5$ and $n_1 = 7$ rank scores preserved for each arrangement is

$$P(S \geq S_o | H_0) = \frac{\text{number of } S \text{ values } \geq S_o}{M} = \frac{614}{792} = 0.7753 \; .$$

Table 5.42 Example (0, 1) coded data for Cureton's rank-biserial correlation coefficient with $n_0 = 6$ and $n_1 = 4$

	Variable	
Object	x	y
1	0	1
2	1	2
3	0	3
4	0	4
5	0	5
6	0	6
7	1	7
8	0	8
9	1	9
10	1	10

5.13 Relationships Among Measures

It is sometimes of interest to examine the relationships among seemingly unrelated statistical tests and measures. Since Cureton originally proposed r_{rb} as a measure of effect size for the Wilcoxon–Mann–Whitney two-sample rank-sum test, it is expected that Cureton's r_{rb} and the Wilcoxon–Mann–Whitney test would be related. In addition, since Cureton's rank-biserial measure is based on Kendall's S, it is to be expected that Cureton's r_{rb} and Kendall's τ_a would be related. Finally, in 2008 Roger Newson established the identity between Cureton's r_{rb} statistic and Somers' d_{yx} statistic [38].

For the rank-score data listed in Table 5.38 on p. 284, replicated in Table 5.42 for convenience, Cureton's rank-biserial test statistic is $r_{rb} = +0.50$. Wilcoxon's two-sample rank-sum test, W, is simply the smaller of the sums of the rank scores of the two samples, i.e.,

$$W = \sum_{i=1}^{n_0} = 1 + 3 + 4 + 5 + 6 + 8 = 27 \, .$$

When there are no tied rank values, the relationships between Wilcoxon's W and Cureton's r_{rb} are given by

$$W = \frac{n_0(N+1) - n_0 n_1 r_{rb}}{2} \quad \text{and} \quad r_{rb} = \frac{n_0(N+1) - 2W}{n_0 n_1} \, , \tag{5.22}$$

where n_0 is the number of objects in the group with the smaller of the two sums; in this case, $W = 27$. Thus, following the expressions in Eq. (5.22), the observed value of Wilcoxon's W is

$$W = \frac{6(10+1) - (6)(4)(0.50)}{2} = 27$$

and the observed value of Cureton's r_{rb} test statistic is

$$r_{rb} = \frac{6(10+1) - 2(27)}{(6)(4)} = +0.50\ .$$

For the rank-score data listed in Table 5.42, Mann and Whitney's two-sample rank-sum test, U, is the sum of the number of values in one group, preceded by the number of values in the other group. Thus, for the rank-score data listed in Table 5.42, the value of 1 in Group 0 is less than values 2, 7, 9, and 10 in Group 1, yielding $U = 4$. Then, the value of 3 in Group 0 is less than values 7, 9, and 10 in Group 1, yielding $U = 3+4 = 7$. Next, the value of 4 in Group 0 is less than values 7, 9, and 10 in Group 1, yielding $U = 3+3+4 = 10$. Next, the value of 5 in Group 0 is less than values 7, 9, and 10 in Group 1, yielding $U = 3+3+3+4 = 13$. Next, the value of 6 in Group 0 is less than values 7, 9, and 10 in Group 1, yielding $U = 3+3+3+3+4 = 16$. Finally, the value of 8 in Group 0 is less than values 9 and 10 in Group 1, yielding $U = 3+3+3+3+4+2 = 18$. Alternatively,

$$U = n_0 n_1 + \frac{n_0(n_0+1)}{2} - W = (6)(4) + \frac{6(6+1)}{2} - 27 = 18\ .$$

When there are no tied rank values, the relationships between Mann and Whitney's U and Cureton's r_{rb} are given by

$$U = \frac{n_0 n_1 (1 + r_{rb})}{2} \quad \text{and} \quad r_{rb} = \frac{2U}{n_0 n_1} - 1\ . \tag{5.23}$$

Thus, following the expressions in Eq. (5.23), the observed value of Mann and Whitney's U is

$$U = \frac{(6)(4)(1+0.50)}{2} = 18$$

and the observed value of Cureton's r_{rb} test statistic is

$$r_{rb} = \frac{2(18)}{(6)(4)} - 1 = +0.50\ .$$

For the rank scores listed in Table 5.42, Kendall's τ_a test statistic is

$$\tau_a = \frac{2S}{N(N-1)} = \frac{2(12)}{10(10-1)} = 0.2667\ .$$

The relationships between Kendall's τ_a and Cureton's r_{rb} are given by

$$\tau_a = \frac{2 n_0 n_1 r_{rb}}{N(N-1)} \quad \text{and} \quad r_{rb} = \frac{\tau_a N(N-1)}{2 n_0 n_1}\ . \tag{5.24}$$

Thus, following the expressions in Eq. (5.24), the observed value of Kendall's τ_a test statistic is

$$\tau_a = \frac{2(6)(4)(0.50)}{10(10-1)} = 0.2667$$

and the observed value of Cureton's r_{rb} test statistic is

$$r_{rb} = \frac{(0.2667)(10)(10-1)}{(2)(6)(4)} = +0.50 \; .$$

In a clever piece of mathematics, Roger Newson established the identity between Cureton's rank-biserial coefficient and Somers' d_{yx} measure of ordinal relationship [38]. The identity is complicated to prove, but easy to demonstrate. For the rank scores listed in Table 5.42, there are no tied rank scores in variable y, so the number of values tied on y but not tied on x is $T_y = 0$; consequently, the number of values tied on both x and y is also $T_{xy} = 0$. There are six 0 values in variable x, yielding $n_0(n_0 - 1)/2 = 6(6-1)/2 = 15$ tied values, and there are four 1 values in variable x, yielding $n_1(n_1 - 1)/2 = 4(4-1)/2 = 6$ tied values. Thus, there are $T_x = 15 + 6 = 21$ values tied on variable x, but not tied on variable y. Finally, for the rank scores listed in Table 5.42, the number of concordant pairs is $C = 18$, the number of discordant pairs is $D = 6$, and $S = C - D = 18 - 6 = +12$.

Somers' asymmetric measure of ordinal relationship is

$$d_{yx} = \frac{C-D}{C+D+T_y} = \frac{S}{C+D+T_y} = \frac{18-6}{18+6+0} = \frac{+12}{24} = +0.50$$

and Cureton's rank-biserial correlation coefficient is

$$r_{rb} = \frac{S}{S_{\max}} = \frac{S}{n_0 n_1} = \frac{+12}{(6)(4)} = +0.50 \; .$$

Because there are tied values on variable y, the relationships between Cureton's r_{rb}, Wilcoxon's W, and Mann and Whitney's U given in Eqs. (5.23) and (5.24) do not hold. However, Kendall's τ_a test statistic is

$$\tau_a = \frac{2S}{N(N-1)} = \frac{2(+4)}{12(12-1)} = +0.0606$$

and the relationships between Cureton's r_{rb} and Kendall's τ_a are

$$\tau_a = \frac{2n_0 n_1 r_{rb}}{N(N-1)} = \frac{2(5)(7)(0.1143)}{12(12-1)} = 0.0606$$

and

$$r_{rb} = \frac{\tau_a N(N-1)}{2n_0 n_1} = \frac{(0.0606)(12)(12-1)}{(2)(5)(7)} = 0.1143 .$$

Similarly, Somers' d_{yx} test statistic is

$$d_{yx} = \frac{C-D}{C+D+T_y} = \frac{S}{C+D+T_y} = \frac{18-14}{18+14+3} = \frac{+4}{35} = 0.1143$$

and, as expected, Somers' d_{yx} and Cureton's r_{rb} yield identical values.

5.14 Coda

Chapter 5 applied exact and Monte Carlo permutation statistical methods to measures of association for two ordinal-level variables based on pairwise differences between rank scores. Included in Chap. 5 were Kendall's τ_a and τ_b measures, Stuart's τ_c measure, Somers' asymmetric d_{yx} and d_{xy} measures, Kim's $d_{y \cdot x}$ and $d_{x \cdot y}$ measures, Wilson's e measure, and Cureton's rank-biserial correlation coefficient. For each test, examples illustrated the measures and either exact or resampling probability values based on the appropriate permutation analysis were provided.

Chapter 6 continues the examination of measures of association for two ordinal-level variables, but concentrates on permutation statistical methods for measures of association that are not based on pairwise differences of rank scores. Included in Chap. 6 are Spearman's rank-order correlation coefficient, Spearman's footrule measure of agreement, Kendall's coefficient of concordance, Kendall's u measure of inter-rater agreement, Cohen's weighted kappa measure of agreement, and Bross's ridit analysis.

References

1. Askey, R.: The 1839 paper on permutations: Its relation to the Rodrigues formula and further developments. In: Altman, S., Ortiz, E.L. (eds.) Mathematics and Social Utopias in France: Olinde Rodrigues and His Times, Vol. 28. History of Mathematics, pp. 105–118. American Mathematical Society, Providence, RI (2005)
2. Berry, K.J., Johnston, J.E., Mielke, P.W.: Exact and resampling probability values for measures associated with ordered R by C contingency tables. Psychol. Rep. **99**, 231–238 (2006)
3. Berry, K.J., Johnston, J.E., Mielke, P.W.: A Chronicle of Permutation Statistical Methods: 1920–2000 and Beyond. Springer–Verlag, Cham, CH (2014)
4. Berry, K.J., Johnston, J.E., Zahran, S., Mielke, P.W.: Stuart's tau measure of effect size for ordinal variables: Some methodological considerations. Beh. Res. Meth. **41**, 1144–1148 (2009)
5. Berry, K.J., Mielke, P.W.: Assessment of variation in ordinal data. Percept. Motor Skill **74**, 63–66 (1992)

6. Berry, K.J., Mielke, P.W.: Indices of ordinal variation. Percept. Motor Skill **74**, 576–578 (1992)
7. Berry, K.J., Mielke, P.W.: A test of significance for the index of ordinal variation. Percept. Motor Skill **79**, 1291–1295 (1994)
8. Burr, E.J.: The distribution of Kendall's score S for a pair of tied rankings. Biometrika **47**, 151–171 (1960)
9. Cureton, E.E.: Rank-biserial correlation. Psychometrika **21**, 287–290 (1956)
10. Cureton, E.E.: Rank-biserial correlation when ties are present. Educ. Psychol. Meas. **28**, 77–79 (1968)
11. Durbin, J., Stuart, A.: Inversions and rank correlation coefficients. J. R. Stat. Soc. B Meth. **13**, 303–309 (1951)
12. Festinger, L.: The significance of differences between means without reference to the frequency distribution function. Psychometrika **11**, 97–105 (1946)
13. Galton, F.: Statistics by intercomparison, with remarks on the law of frequency of error. Philos. Mag. 4 **49**(322), 33–46 (1875)
14. Glass, G.V.: Note on rank-biserial correlation. Educ. Psychol. Meas. **26**, 623–631 (1966)
15. Goodman, L.A., Kruskal, W.H.: Measures of association for cross classifications. J. Am. Stat. Assoc. **49**, 732–764 (1954)
16. Griffin, H.D.: Graphic computation of tau as a coefficient of disarray. J. Am. Stat. Assoc. **53**, 441–447 (1958)
17. Haden, H.G.: A note on the distribution of the different orderings of n objects. Math. Proc. Cambridge **43**, 1–9 (1947)
18. Hemelrijk, J.: Note on Wilcoxon's two-sample test when ties are present. Ann. Math. Stat. **23**, 133–135 (1952)
19. Johnston, J.E., Berry, K.J., Mielke, P.W.: Permutation tests: Precision in estimating probability values. Percept. Motor Skill **105**, 915–920 (2007)
20. Jonckheere, A.R.: A distribution-free k-sample test against ordered alternatives. Biometrika **41**, 133–145 (1954)
21. Kendall, M.G.: A new measure of rank correlation. Biometrika **30**, 81–93 (1938)
22. Kendall, M.G.: The treatment of ties in ranking problems. Biometrika **33**, 239–251 (1945)
23. Kendall, M.G.: Rank Correlation Methods. Griffin, London (1948)
24. Kendall, M.G.: Rank Correlation Methods, 3rd edn. Griffin, London (1962)
25. Kim, J.-O.: Predictive measures of ordinal association. Am. J. Soc. **76**, 891–907 (1971)
26. Kraft, C.A., van Eeden, C.: A Nonparametric Introduction to Statistics. Macmillan, New York (1968)
27. Kruskal, W.H.: Historical notes on the Wilcoxon unpaired two-sample test. J. Am. Stat. Assoc. **52**, 356–360 (1957)
28. Leach, C.: Introduction to Statistics: A Nonparametric Approach for the Social Sciences. Wiley, New York (1979)
29. Loether, H.J., McTavish, D.G.: Descriptive and Inferential Statistics: An Introduction, 4th edn. Allyn and Bacon, Boston (1993)
30. Mann, H.B.: Nonparametric tests against trend. Econometrica **13**, 245–259 (1945)
31. Mann, H.B., Whitney, D.R.: On a test of whether one of two random variables is stochastically larger than the other. Ann. Math. Stat. **18**, 50–60 (1947)
32. Mielke, P.W., Berry, K.J.: Fisher's exact probability test for cross-classification tables. Educ. Psychol. Meas. **52**, 97–101 (1992)
33. Mielke, P.W., Berry, K.J.: Permutation Methods: A Distance Function Approach. Springer–Verlag, New York (2001)
34. Moran, P.A.P.: On the method of paired comparisons. Biometrika **34**, 363–365 (1947)
35. Moran, P.A.P.: Rank correlation and permutation distributions. Math. Proc. Cambridge **44**, 142–144 (1948)
36. Moran, P.A.P.: Recent developments in ranking theory. J. R. Stat. Soc. B Meth. **12**, 152–162 (1950)
37. Moses, L.E.: Statistical theory and research design. Annu. Rev. Psychol. **7**, 233–258 (1956)

38. Newson, R.: Identity of Somers' D and the rank biserial correlation coefficient (2008). http://www.imperial.ac.uk/nhli/r.newson/miscdocs/ransum1.pdf (2008). Accessed 19 Jan 2016
39. Porter, T.M.: The Rise of Statistical Thinking, 1820–1900. Princeton University Press, Princeton, NJ (1986)
40. Randles, R.H., Wolfe, D.A.: Introduction to the Theory of Nonparametric Statistics. Wiley, New York (1979)
41. Rew, H.: Francis Galton. J. R. Stat. Soc. **85**, 293–298 (1922)
42. Rodrigues, O.: Note sur les inversions, ou dérangements produits dans les permutations (Note on inversions, or products of derangements in permutations). J. Math. Pure. Appl. **4**, 236–240 (1839). [The Journal de Mathématiques Pures et Appliquées is also known as the Journal de Liouville]
43. Sandiford, P.: Educational Psychology. Longmans, Green & Company, New York (1928). [The graphical method appears in an Appendix by S.D. Holmes, 'A graphical method of estimating *R* for small groups', pp. 391–394]
44. Somers, R.H.: A new asymmetric measure of association for ordinal variables. Am. Sociol. Rev. **27**, 799–811 (1962)
45. Stigler, S.M.: Stigler's law of eponymy. In: Gieryn, T.F. (ed.) Science and Social Structure: A Festschrift for Robert K. Merton, pp. 147–157. New York Academy of Sciences, New York (1980)
46. Stuart, A.: The estimation and comparison of strengths of association in contingency tables. Biometrika **40**, 105–110 (1953)
47. Stuart, A.: Spearman-like computation of Kendall's tau. Brit. J. Math. Stat. Psy. **30**, 104–112 (1977)
48. Whitfield, J.W.: Rank correlation between two variables, one of which is ranked, the other dichotomous. Biometrika **34**, 292–296 (1947)
49. Wilcoxon, F.: Individual comparisons by ranking methods. Biometrics Bull. **1**, 80–83 (1945)
50. Wilson, T.P.: Measures of association for bivariate ordinal hypotheses. In: Blalock, H.M. (ed.) Measurement in the Social Sciences: Theories and Strategies, pp. 327–342. Aldine, Chicago (1974)
51. Yule, G.U.: On the association of attributes in statistics: With illustrations from the material childhood society. Philos. T. R. Soc. Lond. **194**, 257–319 (1900)
52. Yule, G.U.: On the methods of measuring association between two attributes. J. R. Stat. Soc. **75**, 579–652 (1912). [Originally a paper read before the Royal Statistical Society on 23 April 1912]

Chapter 6
Ordinal-Level Variables, II

Chapter 5 applied exact and Monte Carlo permutation statistical methods to measures of association designed for two ordinal-level (ranked) variables that are based on pairwise comparisons between rank scores. This sixth chapter of *The Measurement of Association* continues the examination of measures of association designed for two ordinal-level variables initiated in Chap. 5, but concentrates on measures of association that are based on criteria other than pairwise comparisons between rank scores, although some overlap is unavoidable. Included in Chap. 6 are exact and Monte Carlo permutation statistical methods for Spearman's rank-order correlation coefficient, Spearman's footrule measure of agreement, Kendall and Babington Smith's coefficient of concordance, Kendall's and Babington Smith's u measure of inter-rater agreement, Cohen's weighted kappa measure of chance-corrected agreement, and Bross's ridit analysis.

6.1 Spearman's Rank-Order Correlation Coefficient

Consider two rankings of N objects consisting of the first N integers and let x_i and y_i for $i = 1, \ldots, N$ denote the first and second rankings, respectively. Rank-order correlation is not without its critics, as the squaring of ranks is quite controversial. S.S. Stevens relates that Frederick Mosteller convinced him that:

> [R]ank order correlation does not apply to ordinal scales because the derivation of the formula for this correlation involves the assumption that the differences between successive ranks are equal.[1]

[1]Quoted in Cowles [16, p. 206].

K. J. Berry et al., *The Measurement of Association*,
https://doi.org/10.1007/978-3-319-98926-6_6

A popular measure of correlation between the two rankings is Spearman's rank-order correlation coefficient given by

$$\rho = 1 - \frac{\displaystyle\sum_{i=1}^{N} d_i^2}{\dfrac{N(N^2-1)}{6}} = 1 - \frac{6\displaystyle\sum_{i=1}^{N} d_i^2}{N(N^2-1)} \,, \tag{6.1}$$

where $d_i = x_i - y_i$ for $i = 1, \ldots, N$. Charles Spearman developed ρ in the first of two articles on the measurement of association and correlation in 1904 and 1906 that appeared in *American Journal of Psychology* and *British Journal of Psychology*, respectively [82, 83].[2] Recognizing that with two sets of untied rank scores, x_i and y_i for $i = 1, \ldots, N$,

$$\sum_{i=1}^{N} x_i = \sum_{i=1}^{N} y_i = \frac{N(N+1)}{2}$$

and

$$\sum_{i=1}^{N} x_i^2 = \sum_{i=1}^{N} y_i^2 = \frac{N(N+1)(2N+1)}{6} \,,$$

Spearman simply substituted into Pearson's formula for the product-moment correlation coefficient given by

$$r_{xy} = \frac{N\displaystyle\sum_{i=1}^{N} x_i y_i - \sum_{i=1}^{N} x_i \sum_{i=1}^{N} y_i}{\sqrt{N\displaystyle\sum_{i=1}^{N} x_i^2 - \left(\sum_{i=1}^{N} x_i\right)^2}\sqrt{N\displaystyle\sum_{i=1}^{N} y_i^2 - \left(\sum_{i=1}^{N} y_i\right)^2}}$$

and simplified the equation, yielding Eq. (6.1).

Note that the denominator of Spearman's rank-order correlation coefficient, $N(N^2 - 1)/6$, as given in Eq. (6.1), represents one-half of the maximum value of $\sum_{i=1}^{N} d_i^2$ when x_i and y_i, $i = 1, \ldots, N$, both consist of untied rank scores and the y_i rank scores are the exact inverse of the x_i rank scores, i.e., $y_i = N - x_i + 1$ for $i = 1, \ldots, N$. Thus, Spearman's ρ is a maximum-corrected measure of rank-order

[2] Spearman published a second article in *American Journal of Psychology* in 1904 on general intelligence that was not related to the measurement of association [81].

correlation and norms properly between ± 1, where $+1$ indicates perfect positive association and -1 indicates perfect negative association.

It is easily confirmed that the denominator of Eq. (6.1), $N(N^2-1)/6$, is one-half of the maximum value of $\sum_{i=1}^{N} d_i^2$ when x_i and y_i for $i = 1, \ldots, N$ are both untied rank scores and the y_i rank scores are the inverse of the x_i rank scores. For the maximum value of $\sum_{i=1}^{N} d_i^2$, define

$$\sum_{i=1}^{N} d_i^2 = \sum_{i=1}^{N} (x_i - y_i)^2 = \sum_{i=1}^{N} x_i^2 + \sum_{i=1}^{N} y_i^2 - 2\sum_{i=1}^{N} x_i y_i \ .$$

Since, for N untied rank scores,

$$\sum_{i=1}^{N} x_i^2 = \sum_{i=1}^{N} y_i^2 = \frac{N(N+1)(2N+1)}{6}$$

and, for $x_i = 1, \ldots, N$ and $y_i = N - x_i + 1, i = 1, \ldots, N$,

$$\sum_{i=1}^{N} x_i y_i = \frac{N(N+1)(N+2)}{6} \ ,$$

then substituting into Eq. (6.1) yields

$$\sum_{i=1}^{N} d_i^2 = \frac{2N(N+1)(2N+1)}{6} - \frac{2N(N+1)(N+2)}{6}$$
$$= \frac{2N(N+1)(N-1)}{6} = \frac{N(N^2-1)}{3} \ ,$$

which is twice the value of $N(N^2-1)/6$.

Kendall, Kendall, and Babington Smith observed that to judge the significance of a value of ρ, it is necessary to consider only the distribution of values obtained from the observed rankings with all other possible permutations of the integers from 1 to N, and further noted that in practice it is generally more convenient to consider only the distribution of $\sum_{i=1}^{N} d_i^2$ as $N(N^2-1)/6$ is invariant under permutation [45, p. 25]. Kendall et al. provided tables of explicit values up to and including $N = 8$ with some experimental distributions for $N = 10$ and $N = 20$. The distributions for $N = 2, \ldots, 8$ were exact, but the distributions for $N = 10$ and $N = 20$ were based on a sample of 2,000 randomly selected permutations of the rank scores, making this an early example of Monte Carlo resampling permutation statistical methods [45, pp. 261–267].

6.1.1 Example 1

Consider the rank-correlation data listed in Table 6.1 with $N = 8$ objects and two sets of rank scores, x and y. For the rank-correlation data listed in Table 6.1, the columns headed x and y contain the observed raw scores, the columns headed r_x and r_y contain the corresponding rank scores, the column headed d contains the signed differences between r_x and r_y, and the column headed d^2 contains the squared rank differences. Let ρ_o denote the observed value of Spearman's rank-order correlation coefficient, then following Eq. (6.1) on p. 298,

$$\rho_o = 1 - \frac{6\sum_{i=1}^{N} d_i^2}{N(N^2-1)} = 1 - \frac{6(18)}{8(8^2-1)} = +0.7857\,.$$

Because there are only $M = N! = 8! = 40{,}320$ possible, equally-likely arrangements in the reference set of all permutations of the observed r_x and r_y rank scores listed in Table 6.1, an exact permutation analysis is easily accomplished. If all $M = 40{,}320$ arrangements of the observed rank scores listed in Table 6.1 occur with equal chance, the exact upper-tail probability of the observed value of $\rho = +0.7857$ under the null hypothesis is

$$P(\rho \geq \rho_o|H_0) = \frac{\text{number of } \rho \text{ values } \geq \rho_o}{M} = \frac{563}{40{,}320} = 0.0140\,,$$

where ρ_o denotes the observed value of ρ. The exact upper-tail probability value of $P = 0.0140$ agrees with the value provided by Kendall, Kendall, and Babington Smith [45, p. 255].

Table 6.1 Example rank-order correlation data for Spearman's rank-order correlation coefficient with $N = 8$ objects and two sets of scores, x and y

Pair	x	y	r_x	r_y	d	d^2
1	72	63	8	7	+1	1
2	46	49	6	6	0	0
3	13	35	2	4	−2	4
4	27	17	4	2	+2	4
5	53	81	7	8	−1	1
6	34	41	5	5	0	0
7	11	26	1	3	−2	4
8	22	15	3	1	+2	4
Total						18

6.1.2 Example 2

For a second example of Spearman's rank-order correlation coefficient, consider the rank data listed in Table 6.2 with $N = 13$ objects and two sets of scores, x and y. For the rank-correlation data listed in Table 6.2, the columns headed x and y contain the observed raw scores, the columns headed r_x and r_y contain the corresponding rank scores, the column headed d contains the signed differences between r_x and r_y, and the column headed d^2 contains the squared rank differences. Following Eq. (6.1) on p. 298, the observed value of Spearman's rank-order correlation coefficient is

$$\rho = 1 - \frac{6\sum_{i=1}^{N} d_i^2}{N(N^2-1)} = 1 - \frac{6(42)}{13(13^2-1)} = +0.8846 \ .$$

Because there are $M = N! = 13! = 6{,}227{,}020{,}800$ possible, equally-likely arrangements of the observed data listed in Table 6.2, an exact permutation test is not practical and a Monte Carlo resampling permutation procedure based on $L = 1{,}000{,}000$ random arrangements of the rank scores is utilized. If the M arrangements in the reference set of all permutations of the observed rank scores listed in Table 6.2 occur with equal chance, the approximate resampling probability of the observed value of $\rho = +0.8846$ under the null hypothesis is

$$P(\rho \geq \rho_{\text{o}}|H_0) = \frac{\text{number of } \rho \text{ values} \geq \rho_{\text{o}}}{L} = \frac{138}{1{,}000{,}000} = 0.1380\times10^{-3} \ ,$$

where ρ_{o} denotes the observed value of ρ.

Table 6.2 Example rank-order correlation data for Spearman's rank-order correlation coefficient with $N = 13$ objects and two sets of scores, x and y

Pair	x	y	r_x	r_y	d	d^2
1	21	26	3	1	+2	4
2	39	41	7	5	+2	4
3	57	81	11	10	+1	1
4	27	39	4	4	0	0
5	45	94	9	12	−3	9
6	73	72	13	9	+4	16
7	32	59	5	7	−2	4
8	41	64	8	8	0	0
9	69	99	12	13	−1	1
10	36	43	6	6	0	0
11	13	29	1	2	−1	1
12	53	88	10	11	−1	1
13	17	33	2	3	−1	1
Total						42

While $M = N! = 13! = 6{,}227{,}020{,}800$ possible arrangements makes an exact permutation analysis impractical, it is not impossible. If the reference set of all possible permutations of the rank scores in Table 6.2 occur with equal chance, the exact probability of $\rho = +0.8846$ under the null hypothesis is

$$P(\rho \geq \rho_{\text{o}}|H_0) = \frac{\text{number of } \rho \text{ values } \geq \rho_{\text{o}}}{M} = \frac{868{,}215}{6{,}227{,}020{,}800} = 0.1394\times 10^{-3}\ .$$

6.2 Spearman's Footrule Agreement Measure

The oft-cited 1904 and 1906 articles by Charles Spearman contained two new measures of rank-order correlation: the well-known Spearman rank-order correlation coefficient, ρ, and a second, lesser-known, correlation coefficient that Spearman named "the footrule" [82, 83].[3,4] Consider two rankings of N objects consisting of the first N integers and let x_i and y_i for $i = 1, \ldots, N$ denote the first and second rankings, respectively. Then, Spearman's footrule is given by

$$\mathcal{R} = 1 - \frac{\displaystyle\sum_{i=1}^{N} |x_i - y_i|}{\dfrac{N^2-1}{3}} = 1 - \frac{3\displaystyle\sum_{i=1}^{N} |x_i - y_i|}{N^2-1}\ . \tag{6.2}$$

Unlike Spearman's rank-order correlation coefficient, the denominator of Spearman's footrule coefficient, $(N^2 - 1)/3$, as given in Eq. (6.2), does not represent one-half of the maximum value of $\sum_{i=1}^{N} |x_i - y_i|$ when x_i and y_i for $i = 1, \ldots, N$ are both untied rank scores and the y_i rank scores are the exact inverse of the x_i rank scores, i.e., $y_i = N - x_i + 1$ for $i = 1, \ldots, N$. Thus, Spearman's $\mathcal{R}$ is not a maximum-corrected measure of rank-order correlation and is, instead, a chance-corrected measure of agreement.

It can easily be shown that Spearman's $\mathcal{R}$ is a chance-corrected measure of agreement and is not, in fact, a conventional measure of correlation, which explains why $\mathcal{R}$ can, on occasion, yield negative values and can only attain a value of -1 when $N = 2$. To show that the expected value of $\sum_{i=1}^{N} |d_i|$ is given by $(N^2 - 1)/3$,

[3] The "footrule" coefficient, under another name, had been proposed a few years earlier by Alfred Binet and his collaborators in France [85].

[4] Presented in these two articles were a number of other measures of ordinal association for comparison that were not new, e.g., Yule's Q and Y measures.

let

$$\begin{aligned}\sum_{i=1}^{N} |d_i| &= \frac{1}{N}\sum_{i=1}^{N}\sum_{j=1}^{N} |i-j| \\ &= \frac{2}{N}\sum_{i=1}^{N-1}\sum_{j=i+1}^{N} (j-i) \\ &= \frac{1}{N}\sum_{i=1}^{N-1}\left[N(N+1)+i^2-i(2N+1)\right] \\ &= \frac{N(N+1)}{6N}\left[6(N+1)+(2N-1)-3(2N+1)\right] \\ &= \frac{N^2-1}{3}\ .\end{aligned}$$

Therefore, Spearman's footrule coefficient given by

$$\mathcal{R} = 1 - \frac{\displaystyle\sum_{i=1}^{N} |d_i|}{\dfrac{N^2-1}{3}}$$

is a chance-corrected measure of agreement when the expected value of $\sum_{i=1}^{N} |d_i|$ is given by $(N^2-1)/3$, as it takes the classic form of chance-corrected measures of agreement given by

$$\text{agreement} = 1 - \frac{\text{observed disagreement}}{\text{expected disagreement}}$$

[48, p. 140].[5]

Three limitations of Spearman's footrule contribute to its lack of use in contemporary research, where it is rarely encountered [85, p. 104]. First, unlike other measures of rank correlation, $\mathcal{R}$ does not norm properly between the limits of ± 1; second, like Spearman's ρ, $\mathcal{R}$ is limited to fully ranked data and does not accommodate tied rank scores; and third, because of the summation of absolute differences between the rank scores, it has traditionally been somewhat cumbersome

[5] Spearman offered a somewhat different, more elegant, derivation of $(N^2-1)/3$ in the Appendix to his 1906 paper on the footrule [83, p. 105].

to establish the probability value of an observed value of $\mathcal{R}$, especially when N is small.

Spearman's $\mathcal{R}$ attains a maximum value of $+1$ when x_i is identical to y_i for $i = 1, \ldots, N$ and no tied values are present. However, if $y_i = N - x_i + 1$ for $i = 1, \ldots, N$, then $\mathcal{R} = -0.5$ when N is odd and

$$\mathcal{R} = -0.5\left(1 + \frac{3}{N^2 - 1}\right)$$

when N is even [42]. Consequently, $\mathcal{R}$ cannot attain a minimum value of -1, except when $N = 2$. Spearman, apparently unaware that $\mathcal{R}$ was a chance-corrected measure and recognizing that negative values of $\mathcal{R}$ did not represent inverse correlation, naïvely suggested that "it is better to treat every correlation as positive" [82, pp. 87–88]. Maurice Kendall explicitly pointed to this apparent lack of proper norming as a defect in the footrule and suggested a correction given by

$$\mathcal{R}' = 1 - \frac{4\sum_{i=1}^{N} |x_i - y_i|}{N^2}$$

that ensured a proper limit of $+1$ when the two rankings were in complete agreement and -1 when the two rankings were inverse to each other [42, p. 33]. However, the correction, while well intended, completely destroyed the chance-corrected interpretation of Spearman's footrule, an important and valuable attribute that was neither understood nor appreciated at the time.

6.2.1 *Probability of Spearman's Footrule*

When both variables x and y consist entirely of untied rank scores from 1 to N and variable y is a permutation of the rank observations in variable x, then methods exist to determine the probability of an observed $\mathcal{R}$ under the null hypothesis that any of the $N!$ orderings of either the x or y values is equally likely. If

$$D = \sum_{i=1}^{N} |x_i - y_i|$$

then, since $\mathcal{R}$ is simply a linear transformation of D, the probability of an observed value of D is the probability of an observed value of $\mathcal{R}$. Tables of the exact cumulative distribution function of D for $2 \leq N \leq 10$ and approximate probability values based on Monte Carlo methods for $11 \leq N \leq 15$ were published by Ury and Kleinecke in 1979 [88]. In 1988 Franklin extended the work of Ury and Kleinecke, reported the exact cumulative distribution function of D for $11 \leq N \leq 18$, and discussed the rate of convergence to an approximating normal distribution [31]. In 1990 Salama and Quade used Markov-chain properties to obtain the exact cumulative distribution function of D for $4 \leq N \leq 40$ and further investigated approximations to the discrete distribution of D [71]. If either variable x or variable y contains tied values, then the calculation of an exact probability value is more complex.

6.2.2 Example 1

Consider the paired-rank data listed in Table 6.3 where there are $N = 8$ paired observations and there are no tied rank scores. If $\mathcal{R}_{\text{o}}$ denotes the observed value of Spearman's footrule, then following Eq. (6.2) on p. 302,

$$\mathcal{R}_{\text{o}} = 1 - \frac{3\sum_{i=1}^{N} |x_i - y_i|}{N^2 - 1} = 1 - \frac{3(10)}{8^2 - 1} = +0.5238 ,$$

indicating approximately 52% agreement above that expected by chance.

Since there are only $M = N! = 8! = 40{,}320$ possible, equally-likely arrangements in the reference set of all permutations of the observed x and y rank scores listed in Table 6.3, an exact permutation analysis is feasible. If all $M = 40{,}320$ arrangements of the observed rank scores listed in Table 6.3 occur with equal chance, the exact probability of the observed value of $\mathcal{R} = +0.5238$ under the null hypothesis is

$$P(\mathcal{R} \geq \mathcal{R}_{\text{o}}|H_0) = \frac{\text{number of } \mathcal{R} \text{ values } \geq \mathcal{R}_{\text{o}}}{M} = \frac{1{,}248}{40{,}320} = 0.0310 ,$$

where $\mathcal{R}_{\text{o}}$ denotes the observed value of $\mathcal{R}$. The probability value $P = 0.0310$ is in agreement with the exact tabled probability value provided by Ury and Kleinecke [88, p. 272].

Table 6.3 Example data for Spearman's footrule rank-correlation coefficient with $N = 8$ objects and two sets of rankings, x and y

Pair	x	y	$x - y$	$\lvert x - y\rvert$
1	8	7	+1	1
2	6	6	0	0
3	2	4	−2	2
4	4	2	+2	2
5	7	8	−1	1
6	5	5	0	0
7	1	3	−2	2
8	3	1	+2	2
Total				10

6.2.3 Example 2

For a second example of Spearman's footrule measure, consider the paired-rank data listed in Table 6.4 where there are $N = 12$ paired observations and there are no tied rank scores. Following Eq. (6.2) on p. 302, the observed value of Spearman's footrule is

$$\mathcal{R}_o = 1 - \frac{3\sum_{i=1}^{N}|x_i - y_i|}{N^2 - 1} = 1 - \frac{3(26)}{12^2 - 1} = +0.4545 ,$$

indicating approximately 45% agreement above that expected by chance.

Because there are $M = N! = 12! = 479{,}001{,}600$ possible, equally-likely arrangements in the reference set of all permutations of the observed x and y rank scores listed in Table 6.4, an exact permutation analysis is not practical and a Monte Carlo resampling probability procedure based on $L = 1{,}000{,}000$ random arrangements of cell frequencies is utilized. If all M arrangements of the observed rank scores listed in Table 6.4 occur with equal chance, the approximate resampling upper-tail probability of the observed value of $\mathcal{R} = +0.4545$ under the null hypothesis is

$$P(\mathcal{R} \geq \mathcal{R}_o | H_0) = \frac{\text{number of } \mathcal{R} \text{ values } \geq \mathcal{R}_o}{L} = \frac{19{,}115}{1{,}000{,}000} = 0.0191 ,$$

where $\mathcal{R}_o$ denotes the observed value of $\mathcal{R}$.

While $M = 479{,}001{,}600$ possible arrangements makes an exact permutation analysis impractical, it is not impossible. If the reference set of all M arrangements of the observed rank scores listed in Table 6.4 occur with equal chance, the exact

Table 6.4 Example data for Spearman's footrule rank-correlation coefficient with $N = 12$ objects and two rankings, x and y

Pair	x	y	$x - y$	$\lvert x - y\rvert$
1	7	5	+2	2
2	3	1	+2	2
3	4	2	+2	2
4	11	10	+1	1
5	9	12	−3	3
6	8	9	−1	1
7	5	8	−3	3
8	6	7	−1	1
9	12	6	+6	6
10	10	11	−1	1
11	1	3	−2	2
12	2	4	−2	2
Total				26

probability of $\mathcal{R} = +0.4545$ under the null hypothesis is

$$P(\mathcal{R} \geq \mathcal{R}_{o}|H_0) = \frac{\text{number of } \mathcal{R} \text{ values } \geq \mathcal{R}_{o}}{M} = \frac{9{,}226{,}950}{479{,}001{,}600} = 0.0193 ,$$

where $\mathcal{R}_{o}$ denotes the observed value of $\mathcal{R}$.

6.2.4 Example 3

For a third example of Spearman's footrule measure, consider the paired-rank data listed in Table 6.5 where $N = 10$ paired observations and there are several tied scores. Following Eq. (6.2) on p. 302, the observed value of Spearman's footrule is

$$\mathcal{R} = 1 - \frac{3\sum_{i=1}^{N} |x_i - y_i|}{N^2 - 1} = 1 - \frac{3(19)}{10^2 - 1} = +0.5758 ,$$

indicating approximately 58% agreement above that expected by chance.

Since there are only $M = N! = 10! = 3{,}628{,}800$ possible, equally-likely arrangements in the reference set of all permutations of the observed x and y rank scores listed in Table 6.5, an exact permutation analysis is feasible. If all M arrangements of the observed rank scores listed in Table 6.5 occur with equal chance, the exact probability of $\mathcal{R} = +0.5758$ under the null hypothesis is

$$P(\mathcal{R} \geq \mathcal{R}_{o}|H_0) = \frac{\text{number of } \mathcal{R} \text{ values } \geq \mathcal{R}_{o}}{M} = \frac{117{,}216}{3{,}628{,}800} = 0.0323 ,$$

where $\mathcal{R}_{o}$ denotes the observed value of $\mathcal{R}$.

Table 6.5 Example data for Spearman's footrule rank-correlation coefficient with $N = 10$ objects and two rankings, x and y

Pair	x	y	$x - y$	$\|x - y\|$
1	4	1	−3	3
2	5.5	2	−3.5	3.5
3	1	4	+3	3
4	5.5	4	−1.5	1.5
5	2	4	+2	2
6	3	6	+3	3
7	7	7	0	0
8	8.5	8	−0.5	0.5
9	10	9	−1	1
10	8.5	10	+1.5	1.5
Total				19

6.2.5 *Multiple Rankings*

Spearman's footrule, as originally presented in his 1904 and 1906 articles in *American Journal of Psychology* and *British Journal of Psychology*, respectively, was limited to $N \geq 2$ untied rank scores and $b = 2$ judges/raters [82, 83]. However, as Berry and Mielke showed in 1998, Spearman's footrule can be generalized to include both tied or untied rank scores and $b \geq 2$ sets of rankings [5]. Let

$$\delta = \left[N \binom{b}{2} \right]^{-1} \sum_{i=1}^{N} \sum_{r<s} \left| x_{ri} - x_{si} \right| \tag{6.3}$$

denote an average distance function based on all $\binom{b}{2}$ possible paired absolute differences among values of the rankings by b judges and let

$$\mu_\delta = \left[N^2 \binom{b}{2} \right]^{-1} \sum_{i=1}^{N} \sum_{j=1}^{N} \sum_{r<s} \left| x_{ri} - x_{sj} \right| \tag{6.4}$$

denote the expected value of δ where b is the number of judges, N is the number of objects, and $\sum_{r<s}$ is the sum over all r and s such that $1 \leq r < s \leq N$. Then, the generalization of Spearman's footrule measure is given by

$$\Re = 1 - \frac{\delta}{\mu_\delta} \, , \tag{6.5}$$

where $\Re$ is a chance-corrected measure of the agreement among the b judges that is not limited to untied rank scores. Note that in the case of $b = 2$ judges, Eq. (6.5) reduces to Spearman's 1906 footrule for $b = 2$ judges as given in Eq. (6.2) on p. 302.

Illustration with $b = 2$ Independent Judges

The calculation of test statistics δ, μ_δ, and $\Re$, as given in Eqs. (6.3), (6.4), and (6.5), respectively, can be described and compared with Spearman's equation for the footrule given in Eq. (6.2) on p. 302 using an example data set with $b = 2$ independent judges. To illustrate the calculation of Spearman's footrule, consider the small set of rank data listed in Table 6.6 with $N = 5$ objects and $b = 2$ independent judges. Table 6.7 illustrates the calculation of Spearman's footrule for the rank data given in Table 6.6. Given the calculations in Table 6.7, Spearman's footrule is

$$\mathcal{R} = \frac{3 \displaystyle\sum_{i=1}^{N} |x_i - y_i|}{N^2 - 1} = \frac{3(4)}{5^2 - 1} = +0.50 \, .$$

Table 6.6 Rank scores assigned to $N = 5$ objects by $b = 2$ independent judges

	Judge	
Object	1	2
1	5	4
2	2	1
3	1	2
4	3	3
5	4	5

Table 6.7 Calculations for Spearman's footrule coefficient with $N = 5$ objects and $b = 2$ independent judges

Pair	x	y	$x - y$	$\lvert x - y\rvert$
1	5	4	−1	1
2	2	1	+1	1
3	1	2	−1	1
4	3	3	0	0
5	4	5	−1	1
Total				4

Table 6.8 Calculation of $\lvert x_{ri} - x_{si}\rvert$ for $r < s$ and $i = 1, \ldots, N$ for δ

i	$\lvert x_{ri} - x_{si}\rvert$, $r < s$	Sum
1	$\lvert 5 - 4\rvert$	1
2	$\lvert 2 - 1\rvert$	1
3	$\lvert 1 - 2\rvert$	1
4	$\lvert 3 - 3\rvert$	0
5	$\lvert 4 - 5\rvert$	1

Table 6.8 illustrates the calculation of δ for the rank data given in Table 6.6. Given the calculations in Table 6.8, the observed value of δ is

$$\delta_o = \left[N\binom{b}{2}\right]^{-1} \sum_{i=1}^{N} \sum_{r<s} \lvert x_{ri} - x_{si}\rvert$$
$$= \left[5\binom{2}{2}\right]^{-1} (1+1+1+0+1) = \frac{4}{5} = 0.80\,.$$

Table 6.9 illustrates the calculation of μ_δ for the rank data given in Table 6.6. Given the calculations in Table 6.9, the exact expected value of the M δ values is

$$\mu_\delta = \left[N^2\binom{b}{2}\right]^{-1} \sum_{i=1}^{N} \sum_{j=1}^{N} \sum_{r<s} \lvert x_{ri} - x_{sj}\rvert$$
$$= \left[5^2\binom{2}{2}\right]^{-1} (1+0+2+\cdots+2+0+1) = \frac{40}{25} = 1.60\,.$$

Table 6.9 Calculation of $|x_{ri} - x_{si}|$ for $r < s$, $i = 1, \ldots, N$, and $j = 1, \ldots, N$

Pair	i	j	$\lvert x_{ri} - x_{sj}\rvert$, $r < s$	Sum	Pair	i	j	$\lvert x_{ri} - x_{sj}\rvert$, $r < s$	Sum
1	1	2	$\lvert 1-2\rvert$	1	14	3	5	$\lvert 3-5\rvert$	2
2	1	1	$\lvert 1-1\rvert$	0	15	3	4	$\lvert 3-4\rvert$	1
3	1	3	$\lvert 1-3\rvert$	2	16	4	2	$\lvert 4-2\rvert$	2
4	1	5	$\lvert 1-5\rvert$	4	17	4	1	$\lvert 4-1\rvert$	3
5	1	4	$\lvert 1-4\rvert$	3	18	4	3	$\lvert 4-3\rvert$	1
6	2	2	$\lvert 2-2\rvert$	0	19	4	5	$\lvert 4-5\rvert$	1
7	2	1	$\lvert 2-1\rvert$	1	20	4	4	$\lvert 4-4\rvert$	0
8	2	3	$\lvert 2-3\rvert$	1	21	5	2	$\lvert 5-2\rvert$	3
9	2	5	$\lvert 2-5\rvert$	3	22	5	1	$\lvert 5-1\rvert$	4
10	2	4	$\lvert 2-4\rvert$	2	23	5	3	$\lvert 5-3\rvert$	2
11	3	2	$\lvert 3-2\rvert$	1	24	5	5	$\lvert 5-5\rvert$	0
12	3	1	$\lvert 3-1\rvert$	2	25	5	4	$\lvert 5-4\rvert$	1
13	3	3	$\lvert 2-5\rvert$	0					

Table 6.10 Rank scores assigned to $N = 8$ objects by $b = 3$ independent judges

	Judge		
Object	1	2	3
1	1	1	1
2	2	2	3
3	3	3	2

Then, the chance-corrected measure of agreement between the $b = 2$ independent judges is

$$\mathfrak{R} = 1 - \frac{\delta_o}{\mu_\delta} = 1 - \frac{0.80}{1.60} = +0.50\,,$$

indicating 50% agreement above that expected by chance. Thus, the equivalence between

$$\mathcal{R} = 1 - \frac{3\sum_{i=1}^{N} |x_i - y_i|}{N^2 - 1} \quad \text{and} \quad \mathfrak{R} = 1 - \frac{\delta}{\mu_\delta}$$

is established for $b = 2$ independent judges.

Illustration with $b = 3$ Independent Judges

To illustrate the calculation of Spearman's footrule with $b > 2$ independent judges, consider the small set of rank data listed in Table 6.10 with $N = 3$ objects and $b = 3$ judges. The example is deliberately kept small to clarify the calculations.

Table 6.11 Calculation of $|x_{ri} - x_{si}|$ for $r < s$ and $i = 1, \ldots, N$ for δ

i	$\lvert x_{ri} - x_{si}\rvert$, $r < s$	Sum
1	$\lvert 1-1\rvert + \lvert 1-1\rvert + \lvert 1-1\rvert$	0
2	$\lvert 2-2\rvert + \lvert 2-3\rvert + \lvert 2-3\rvert$	2
3	$\lvert 3-3\rvert + \lvert 3-2\rvert + \lvert 3-2\rvert$	2

Table 6.12 Calculation of $|x_{ri} - x_{si}|$ for $r < s$, $i = 1, \ldots, N$, and $j = 1, \ldots, N$ for μ_δ

Pair	i	j	$\lvert x_{ri} - x_{sj}\rvert$, $r < s$	Sum
1	1	1	$\lvert 1-1\rvert + \lvert 1-1\rvert + \lvert 1-1\rvert$	0
2	1	2	$\lvert 1-2\rvert + \lvert 1-3\rvert + \lvert 1-3\rvert$	5
3	1	3	$\lvert 1-3\rvert + \lvert 1-2\rvert + \lvert 1-2\rvert$	4
4	2	1	$\lvert 2-1\rvert + \lvert 2-1\rvert + \lvert 2-1\rvert$	3
5	2	2	$\lvert 2-2\rvert + \lvert 2-3\rvert + \lvert 2-3\rvert$	2
6	2	3	$\lvert 2-3\rvert + \lvert 2-2\rvert + \lvert 2-2\rvert$	1
7	3	1	$\lvert 3-1\rvert + \lvert 3-1\rvert + \lvert 3-1\rvert$	6
8	3	2	$\lvert 3-2\rvert + \lvert 3-3\rvert + \lvert 3-3\rvert$	1
9	3	3	$\lvert 3-3\rvert + \lvert 3-2\rvert + \lvert 3-2\rvert$	2

Table 6.11 illustrates the calculation of δ for the rank data given in Table 6.10. Given the calculations in Table 6.11, the observed value of δ is

$$\delta_o = \left[N\binom{b}{2}\right]^{-1} \sum_{i=1}^{N} \sum_{r<s} |x_{ri} - x_{si}| = \left[3\binom{3}{2}\right]^{-1} (0+2+2)$$

$$= \frac{4}{9} = 0.4444 \; .$$

Table 6.12 illustrates the calculation of μ_δ for the rank data given in Table 6.10. Given the calculations in Table 6.12, the exact expected value of the M δ values is

$$\mu_\delta = \left[N^2\binom{b}{2}\right]^{-1} \sum_{i=1}^{N} \sum_{j=1}^{N} \sum_{r<s} |x_{ri} - x_{sj}|$$

$$= \left[3^2\binom{3}{2}\right]^{-1} (0+5+4+3+2+1+6+1+2) = \frac{24}{27} = 0.8889 \; .$$

Then, the observed chance-corrected measure of agreement among the $b = 3$ independent judges is

$$\Re_o = 1 - \frac{\delta_o}{\mu_\delta} = 1 - \frac{0.4444}{0.8889} = +0.50 \; ,$$

indicating 50% agreement above that expected by chance.

6.2.6 Example Analysis

Consider a generalized footrule analysis where rankings by $b = 4$ independent judges contain untied rank scores for $N = 8$ objects. The data are listed in Table 6.13. Following Eq. (6.3) on p. 308, the observed value of δ is

$$\delta_o = \left[N \binom{b}{2} \right]^{-1} \sum_{i=1}^{N} \sum_{r<s} |x_{ri} - x_{si}| = \left[8 \binom{4}{2} \right]^{-1} (68.00) = \frac{68}{48} = 1.4167 \,,$$

and following Eq. (6.4) on p. 308, the exact expected value of the M δ values is

$$\mu_\delta = \left[N^2 \binom{b}{2} \right]^{-1} \sum_{i=1}^{N} \sum_{j=1}^{N} \sum_{r<s} |x_{ri} - x_{sj}|$$

$$= \left[8^2 \binom{4}{2} \right]^{-1} (1{,}008) = \frac{1{,}008}{384} = 2.6250 \,.$$

Then, following Eq. (6.5) on p. 308, the observed chance-corrected measure of effect size is

$$\Re_o = 1 - \frac{\delta_o}{\mu_\delta} = 1 - \frac{1.4167}{2.6250} = +0.4603 \,,$$

indicating approximately 46% agreement above that expected by chance.

An exact permutation analysis is not possible for the data listed in Table 6.13 since there are

$$M = (N!)^b = (8!)^4 = 2{,}642{,}908{,}293{,}365{,}760{,}000$$

possible, equally-likely arrangements in the reference set of all permutations of the observed rank scores. Therefore, a Monte Carlo resampling permutation analysis

Table 6.13 Rank scores assigned to $N = 8$ objects by $b = 4$ independent judges

	Judge			
Object	1	2	3	4
1	6	7	8	8
2	8	5	4	7
3	1	3	6	4
4	2	1	2	2
5	3	2	1	1
6	5	6	7	5
7	4	4	3	3
8	7	8	5	6

is mandated. If all M possible, equally-likely arrangements of the observed rank scores listed in Table 6.13 occur with equal chance, the approximate resampling upper-tail probability value of $\Re = +0.4603$ computed on $L = 1{,}000{,}000$ random arrangements of the observed rank scores is

$$P(\Re \geq \Re_{\text{o}}|H_0) = \frac{\text{number of } \Re \text{ values } \geq \Re_{\text{o}}}{L} = \frac{195}{1{,}000{,}000} = 0.1950 \times 10^{-3} ,$$

where $\Re_{\text{o}}$ denotes the observed value of $\Re$.

6.3 The Coefficient of Concordance

The measurement of the degree of association among multiple sets of rank scores is useful in studies of inter-test reliability. Whereas Spearman's rank-order correlation coefficient and Kendall's τ_a and τ_b measures express the degree of association between two variables measured in, or transformed to, rank scores, the coefficient of concordance expresses the degree of association among multiple sets of rank scores.

In 1939 Maurice Kendall and Bernard Babington Smith published an article in *The Annals of Mathematical Statistics* on "The problem of m rankings" in which they developed the well-known coefficient of concordance [43].[6] Let N and m denote the number of rank scores and the number of judges, respectively, then Kendall and Babington Smith defined the coefficient of concordance as

$$W = \frac{12S}{m^2(N^3 - N)} , \tag{6.6}$$

where S is the observed sum of squares of the deviations of sums of ranks from the mean value $m(N + 1)/2$.[7]

Since $m^2(N^3 - N)$ in the denominator of Eq. (6.6) is invariant over all permutations of the observed data, Kendall and Babington Smith showed that in order to test whether an observed value of W is statistically significant it is only necessary to consider the distribution of S by permuting the N ranks in all possible, equally-likely ways. Letting one of the rankings be fixed, there are $(N!)^{m-1}$ possible values of S. Based on this permutation procedure, Kendall and Babington Smith created four tables that provided exact probability values for $N = 3$ and $m = 2, \ldots, 10$, $N = 4$ and $m = 2, \ldots, 6$, and $N = 5$ and $m = 3$.

---

[6] The coefficient of concordance was independently developed by W. Allen Wallis in 1939, which he termed the "correlation ratio for ranked data" [91].

[7] The squaring of rank scores and calculating the mean of ranks are, to say the least, controversial mathematical operations.

In a form more conducive to calculation, W can be defined as

$$W = \frac{12 \sum_{i=1}^{N} R_i^2 - 3m^2 N(N+1)}{m^2 N(N^2 - 1)} ,$$

where R_i for $i = 1, \ldots, N$ is the sum of the rank scores for the ith of N objects and there are no tied rank scores. It is also well known that W can be defined as a function of the average value of all pairwise Spearman rank-order correlation coefficients given by

$$\bar{\rho} = \frac{2}{m(m-1)} \sum_{i=1}^{m-1} \sum_{j=i+1}^{m} \rho_{ij} .$$

In this regard, Kendall and Babington Smith showed that $\bar{\rho}$ is simply the intraclass coefficient, r_{I}, for the m sets of rankings, and also observed that the coefficient of concordance is equivalent to Friedman's two-way analysis of variance for ranks, as noted by I.R. Savage [72, p. 335]. The relationships between W and $\bar{\rho}$ are given by

$$\bar{\rho} = \frac{mW - 1}{m - 1} \quad \text{and} \quad W = \frac{\bar{\rho}(m-1) + 1}{m} .$$

If all arrangements of the m sets of observed rank scores occur with equal chance, the exact probability value of the observed value of W computed on M possible, equally-likely arrangements of the observed rank scores under the null hypothesis is

$$P(W \geq W_{\mathrm{o}} | H_0) = \frac{\text{number of } W \text{ values } \geq W_{\mathrm{o}}}{M} ,$$

where W_{o} denotes the observed value of W.

6.3.1 Example 1

To illustrate Kendall and Babington Smith's coefficient of concordance, consider the rank data listed in Table 6.14 with $N = 6$ objects and $m = 3$ sets of rankings. For the rank scores listed in Table 6.14, the sum of the squared rank scores is

$$\sum_{i=1}^{N} R_i^2 = 4^2 + 14^2 + 15^2 + 13^2 + 11^2 + 6^2 = 763 ,$$

the observed value of Kendall and Babington Smith's coefficient of concordance is

$$W = \frac{12\sum_{i=1}^{N} R_i^2 - 3m^2N(N+1)}{m^2N(N^2-1)}$$

$$= \frac{12(763) - 3(3^2)(6)(6+1)^2}{3^2(6)(6^2-1)} = 0.6444\ ,$$

and the observed value of the pairwise average Spearman rank-order correlation with

$$\rho_{12} = 1 - \frac{6\sum_{i=1}^{N} d_i^2}{N(N^2-1)} = 1 - \frac{6(20)}{6(6^2-1)} = +0.4286\ ,$$

$$\rho_{13} = 1 - \frac{6\sum_{i=1}^{N} d_i^2}{N(N^2-1)} = 1 - \frac{6(22)}{6(6^2-1)} = +0.3714\ ,$$

and

$$\rho_{23} = 1 - \frac{6\sum_{i=1}^{N} d_i^2}{N(N^2-1)} = 1 - \frac{6(14)}{6(6^2-1)} = +0.60$$

is

$$\bar{\rho} = \frac{2}{m(m-1)} \sum_{i=1}^{m-1} \sum_{j=i+1}^{m} \rho_{ij} = \frac{2(0.4286 + 0.3714 + 0.60)}{3(3-1)} = 0.4667\ .$$

Finally, the observed relationships between $\bar{\rho}$ and Kendall and Babington Smith's W are

$$\bar{\rho} = \frac{mW - 1}{m-1} = \frac{3(0.6444) - 1}{3-1} = 0.4667$$

and

$$W = \frac{\bar{\rho}(m-1) + 1}{m} = \frac{(0.4667)(3-1) + 1}{3} = 0.6444\ .$$

For the $m = 3$ sets of rank scores listed in Table 6.14 there are only

$$M = \left(N!\right)^{m-1} = \left(6!\right)^{3-1} = 518{,}400$$

Table 6.14 Example data for Kendall and Babington Smith's coefficient of concordance with $m = 3$ rankings and $N = 6$ objects

	Ranking			
Object	1	2	3	R_i
1	1	1	2	4
2	6	5	3	14
3	3	6	6	15
4	4	4	5	13
5	5	2	4	11
6	2	3	1	6

Table 6.15 Example data for Kendall and Babington Smith's coefficient of concordance with $m = 3$ sets of rankings and $N = 8$ objects

	Ranking			
Object	1	2	3	R_i
1	4	2	5	11
2	6	6	3	15
3	2	1	1	4
4	1	3	2	6
5	3	5	8	16
6	5	4	4	13
7	7	8	7	22
8	8	7	6	21

possible, equally-likely arrangements in the reference set of all permutations of the observed data, making an exact permutation analysis practical. If all M arrangements of the observed rank scores listed in Table 6.14 occur with equal chance, the exact probability of $W = 0.6444$ under the null hypothesis is

$$P(W \geq W_{\text{o}}|H_0) = \frac{\text{number of } W \text{ values } \geq W_{\text{o}}}{M} = \frac{29{,}030}{518{,}400} = 0.0560\,,$$

where W_{o} denotes the observed value of W.

6.3.2 Example 2

For a second example of Kendall and Babington's Smith's coefficient of concordance, consider the rank data listed in Table 6.15 with $N = 8$ objects and $m = 3$ sets of rankings.

For the rank scores listed in Table 6.15, the sum of the squared rank scores is

$$\sum_{i=1}^{N} R_i^2 = 11^2 + 15^2 + 4^2 + 6^2 + 16^2 + 132 + 22^2 + 21^2 = 1{,}748\,,$$

the observed value of Kendall and Babington Smith's coefficient of concordance is

$$W = \frac{12\sum_{i=1}^{N} R_i^2 - 3m^2N(N+1)}{m^2N(N^2-1)}$$
$$= \frac{12(1{,}748) - (3)(3^2)(8)(8+1)^2}{3^2(8)(8^2-1)} = 0.7672\,,$$

and the observed value of the pairwise average Spearman rank-order correlation with

$$\rho_{12} = 1 - \frac{6\sum_{i=1}^{N} d_i^2}{N(N^2-1)} = 1 - \frac{6(16)}{8(8^2-1)} = +0.8095\,,$$

$$\rho_{13} = 1 - \frac{6\sum_{i=1}^{N} d_i^2}{N(N^2-1)} = 1 - \frac{6(42)}{8(8^2-1)} = +0.50\,,$$

and

$$\rho_{23} = 1 - \frac{6\sum_{i=1}^{N} d_i^2}{N(N^2-1)} = 1 - \frac{6(30)}{8(8^2-1)} = +0.6429$$

is

$$\bar{\rho} = \frac{2}{m(m-1)} \sum_{i=1}^{m-1} \sum_{j=i+1}^{m} \rho_{ij} = \frac{2(0.8095 + 0.50 + 0.6429)}{3(3-1)} = 0.6508\,.$$

Finally, the observed relationships between $\bar{\rho}$ and Kendall and Babington Smith's W are

$$\bar{\rho} = \frac{mW - 1}{m-1} = \frac{3(0.7672) - 1}{3-1} = 0.6508$$

and

$$W = \frac{\bar{\rho}(m-1) + 1}{m} = \frac{(0.6508)(3-1) + 1}{3} = 0.7672\,.$$

For the $m = 3$ sets of rank scores listed in Table 6.15 there are

$$M = \left(N!\right)^m = \left(8!\right)^3 = 65{,}548{,}320{,}768{,}000$$

possible arrangements of the observed data—too many for an exact permutation analysis. However, holding one set of rank scores constant relative to the other two sets of rank scores reduces the number of possible arrangements to

$$M = (N!)^{m-1} = (8!)^{3-1} = 1{,}625{,}702{,}400 \, .$$

While even this number of possible arrangements makes an exact permutation analysis impractical, it is not impossible given modern computing operating speeds. If the reference set of all M arrangements of the observed rank scores listed in Table 6.15 occur with equal chance, the exact probability of $W = 0.7672$ under the null hypothesis is

$$P(W \geq W_{\text{o}}|H_0) = \frac{\text{number of } W \text{ values } \geq W_{\text{o}}}{M} = \frac{5{,}125{,}594}{1{,}625{,}702{,}400} = 0.3153\times10^{-2} \, ,$$

where W_{o} denotes the observed value of W.

6.3.3 A Related Procedure

It has long been recognized that the data structure for Kendall and Babington Smith's coefficient of concordance [43] is the same as the Friedman two-way analysis of variance for ranks [32] and the same as the Wallis correlation ratio for rank-score data [91]. While the Friedman test, for example, provides a global probability value of overall differences among ranks, there is a related procedure that provides an exact probability value for the sum of ranks of just a single object, answering the question: when is single object total not due to chance under the null hypothesis of random assignment?

Suppose that each of N judges independently assigns K distinct untied ranks to $K \geq 2$ objects [6]. If S denotes the sum of the N ranks for a specified object under the null hypothesis that each of the N judges assigns the K ranks to the K objects at random, i.e., each object occurs with probability $1/K$, then the exact point probability of S is given by

$$p_S = K^{-N} C_{S-N} \tag{6.7}$$

for $S = N,\ N+1,\ \ldots,\ NK$. Let $m = S - N$, then

$$C_m = \sum_{j=0}^{v} (-1)^j \binom{N}{j} \binom{m - jK + N - 1}{N - 1} \tag{6.8}$$

and $v = \min(N, m/K)$, i.e., the largest nonnegative integer less than or equal to N or m/K. The exact one-sided probability value for S is given by

$$P_1 = \sum_{j=N}^{w} p_j \; ,$$

where $w = \min(S, NK + N - S)$ and the exact two-sided probability value for S is given by

$$P_2 = \min(2P_1, 1) \; ,$$

since the distribution of S is symmetric about $N(K+1)/2$ under the null hypothesis.

The mean and variance of S are given by

$$\mu_S = \frac{N(K+1)}{2} \quad \text{and} \quad \sigma_S^2 = \frac{N(K^2-1)}{12} \; ,$$

respectively, and the limiting distribution of

$$z = \frac{S - \mu_S}{\sigma_S}$$

under the null hypothesis is $N(0, 1)$ as $N \to \infty$.

Example Analysis

A panel of $N = 3$ reviewers evaluates $K = 15$ submitted manuscripts for inclusion in a special issue of a journal. Each reviewer independently ranks the 15 manuscripts from 15 (highest) to 1 (lowest). The manuscript with the largest total receives $S = 13 + 11 + 10 = 34$. Table 6.16 lists the values of j from N to w, where

$$w = \min(SN, NK + N - S) = \min[34, (3)(15) + 3 - 34] = 14 \; .$$

The exact point probability values of $S = 34$ under the null hypothesis is $p_S = 0.2311{\times}10^{-1}$, indicated with an asterisk in Table 6.16. The exact one-sided probability value of $S = 34$ under the null hypothesis is

$$P_1 = \sum_{j=N}^{w} p_j = 0.2963{\times}10^{-3} + 0.8889{\times}10^{-3} + \cdots + 0.2311{\times}10^{-1} = 0.1079 \; ,$$

Table 6.16 Listing of values of j from N to w and p_j probability values for $j = N, \ldots, NK + N - S$

j	p_j
3	0.2963×10^{-3}
4	0.8889×10^{-3}
5	0.1778×10^{-2}
6	0.2963×10^{-2}
7	0.4444×10^{-2}
8	0.6222×10^{-2}
9	0.8296×10^{-2}
10	0.1067×10^{-1}
11	0.1333×10^{-1}
12	0.1630×10^{-1}
13	0.1956×10^{-1}
14*	0.2311×10^{-1}
Sum	0.1079

and the exact two-sided probability value of $S = 34$ under the null hypothesis is

$$P_2 = \min(2P_1, 1) = \min[2(0.1079), 1] = 0.2158 .$$

For comparison, the mean of S is

$$\mu_S = \frac{N(K+1)}{2} = \frac{3(15+1)}{2} = 24 ,$$

the variance of S is

$$\sigma_S^2 = \frac{N(K^2-1)}{12} = \frac{3(15^2-1)}{12} = 56 ,$$

the standard score of S is

$$z = \frac{S - \mu_S}{\sigma_S} = \frac{34 - 24}{\sqrt{56}} = +1.3363 ,$$

the approximate one-sided $N(0, 1)$ probability value of $S = 34$ under the null hypothesis is $P = 0.0907$, and the approximate two-sided $N(0, 1)$ probability value of $S = 34$ under the null hypothesis is $P = 0.1815$. If the value of S is corrected for continuity, then

$$z = \frac{(S - 0.5) - \mu_S}{\sigma_S} = \frac{33.5 - 24}{\sqrt{56}} = +1.2695 ,$$

the approximate one-sided $N(0, 1)$ probability value of $S = 33.5$ under the null hypothesis is $P = 0.1021$, and the approximate two-sided $N(0, 1)$ probability value of $S = 33.5$ under the null hypothesis is $P = 0.2043$.

History of the Problem

The solution to the problem given in Eqs. (6.7) and (6.8) is not new. On the other hand, it is not well known. Historically, the problem has been associated with gaming where it is desired to know the probability of the various sums of N fair dice. The number of ways any given total can be obtained from a throw of $N = 3$ common dice appears to be first given in the late Medieval Latin poem *De Vetula*, and is ascribed to Richard de Fournival (A.D. 1200–1250), Chancellor of Amiens Cathedral [7, 18, 41]. Girolamo Cardano wrote *Liber de Ludo Aleae* about 1526, although it was not published until 1663 [41, p. 7]. Cardano delineated the number of cases favorable for each throw that can be made with $N = 3$ common dice.

Galileo Galilei also examined the problem of three dice, which was posed to him when he was First Philosopher and Mathematician to Cosimo II, Duke of Tuscany. Although Galileo died in 1642, *Sopra le Scoperte dei Dadi* was not published until 1718 [18, pp. 64–66] and is translated in David [18, pp. 192–195]. Galileo solved the problem of why three dice yield sums of 10 and 11 more frequently than sums of 9 and 12 by exhaustively enumerating all 216 permutations and showing that there are 27 permutations yielding sums of 10 and 11, but only 25 permutations yielding sums of 9 and 12 [7, 17, 34, p. 52].

Thomas Strode (1693) first generalized the rules of enumeration to any number of dice, but limited the rules to those die shapes corresponding to the five Platonic solids, i.e., tetrahedron (4-sided), hexahedron (6-sided), octahedron (8-sided), dodecahedron (12-sided), and icosahedron (20-sided), using tables of the figurate numbers [84]. The problem of two-sided dice is less interesting as it follows the symmetric binomial distribution, i.e., N tosses of a fair coin. The general solution for the sum of any number of dice with any number of faces, corresponding to Eqs. (6.7) and (6.8), was first given by Abraham de Moivre [87]. The result is presented without demonstration by de Moivre in *De Mensura Sortis*, published in 1711 [19], which is translated in Hald [35], and presented with demonstration in *Miscellanea Analytica*, published in 1730 [20]. The result also appears as a lemma in *The Doctrine of Chances*, published in 1738 [21, pp. 35–39].

6.4 Kendall's *u* Measure of Agreement

Oftentimes, rather than ask a group of judges to rank a set of objects, the judges might be presented with a series of pairs of objects and asked to indicate a preference for one of the two objects in each pairing. Such a procedure in which judges are asked to indicate a preference for one of a pair of objects is called *paired comparisons*. A classic example of paired comparisons is presenting all possible pairs of N brands of dry dog food to k individual dogs and recording the choices. When data are gathered by the method of paired comparisons, it is possible to calculate the degree of agreement among the judges. In 1940 Kendall and Babington Smith [44] proposed a coefficient of agreement to evaluate paired comparisons among k judges for N rankings, given by

$$u = \frac{2S}{\binom{k}{2}\binom{N}{2}} - 1 ,$$

where

$$S = \sum_{i=1}^{N} \sum_{j=1}^{N} \binom{a_{ij}}{2} = \sum_{i=1}^{N} \sum_{j=1}^{N} a_{ij}^2 - k \sum_{i=1}^{N} \sum_{j=1}^{N} a_{ij} + \binom{k}{2}\binom{N}{2} ,$$

a_{ij} is the number of times that an object associated with row i of a preference matrix is preferred to the object associated with row j, and $a_{ij} \geq 2$ for $i, j = 1, \ldots, N$. The maximum number of agreements, occurring when $\binom{N}{2}$ cells of the preference matrix each contain k, is $\binom{N}{2}\binom{k}{2}$ and thus, in the case of complete agreement and only in this case, $u = +1$ [44, p. 334].

While the maximum value of u is +1 when there is complete agreement among all k judges, the minimum number of agreements occurs when each cell of the preference matrix contains $k/2$ if k is even or $(k \pm 1)/2$ if k is odd. Thus, when k is even the minimum value of u is $-1/(k-1)$ and when k is odd the minimum value of u is $-1/k$. Since the expected value of u is zero [44, p. 339] and the minimum values of u are $-1/(k-1)$ when k is even and $-1/k$ when k is odd, u is clearly a chance-corrected measure of agreement, although this was apparently not recognized by Kendall and Babington Smith, when u was developed in 1940.

6.4.1 Example 1

To illustrate the method of paired comparisons, consider the rank-score data listed in Table 6.17, where $k = 3$ judges have ranked $N = 6$ objects, labeled a to f. Now transform the rank data in Table 6.17 into a preference matrix as given in Table 6.18. The preference matrix is composed from the $k = 3$ rankings given in Table 6.17 by looking at all possible pairs of objects. Consider first Objects a and b. Judge 1

Table 6.17 Rankings of $N = 6$ objects by $k = 3$ independent judges, where 1 denotes the highest ranking

	Judge		
Object	1	2	3
a	1	1	1
b	6	5	6
c	3	6	5
d	2	4	2
e	5	2	4
f	4	3	3

preferred Object a to b, assigning rank 1 to Object A and rank 6 to Object b; Judge 2 preferred Object a to Object b, assigning rank 1 to Object a and rank 5 to Object b; and Judge 3 also preferred Object a to Object b, assigning rank 1 to Object a and rank 6 to Object b. Thus, since Object a was preferred to Object b three times, cell (a, b) of the preference matrix is 3, and since Object b was preferred to Object a zero times, cell (b, a) of the preference matrix is 0.

Now consider Objects e and f. Judge 1 preferred Object f to Object e, assigning rank 4 to Object f and rank 5 to Object e; Judge 2 preferred Object e to Object f, assigning rank 2 to Object e and rank 3 to Object f; and Judge 3 preferred Object f to Object e, assigning rank 3 to Object f and rank 4 to Object e. Thus, since Object e was preferred to Object f one time, cell (e, f) of the preference matrix is 1, and since Object f was preferred to Object e two times, cell (f, e) of the preference matrix is 2.

For the preference matrix given in Table 6.18,

$$S = \sum_{i=1}^{N} \sum_{j=1}^{N} \binom{a_{ij}}{2} = 9\binom{3}{2} + 6\binom{2}{2} = 33$$

and

$$u = \frac{2S}{\binom{k}{2}\binom{N}{2}} - 1 = \frac{2(33)}{\binom{3}{2}\binom{6}{2}} - 1 = +0.4667\ ,$$

indicating approximately 47% agreement above that expected by chance. There is another, more convenient, way to calculate u given by

$$u = \frac{8\left(\sum_{i=1}^{N} \sum_{j=1}^{N} a_{ij}^2 - k \sum_{i=1}^{N} \sum_{j=1}^{N} a_{ij}\right)}{k(k-1)N(N-1)} + 1\ ,$$

where the summation may be taken over the a_{ij} values either below or above the principal diagonal; in this case, the preference values below the principal diagonal are summed. For the preference matrix given in Table 6.18, consider the lower

Table 6.18 Preference matrix of $N = 6$ objects by $k = 3$ independent judges

	a	b	c	d	e	f
a	–	3	3	3	3	3
b	0	–	1	0	0	0
c	0	2	–	0	1	1
d	0	3	3	–	2	2
e	0	3	2	1	–	1
f	0	3	2	1	2	–

triangle of a_{ij} values where

$$\sum_{i=2}^{N}\sum_{j=1}^{N-1} a_{ij} = 0+0+2+0+3+3+0+3+2+1$$

$$+0+3+2+1+2 = 22$$

and

$$\sum_{i=2}^{N}\sum_{j=1}^{N-1} a_{ij}^2 = 0^2+0^2+2^2+0^2+3^2+3^2+0^2+3^2+2^2+1^2$$

$$+0^2+3^2+2^2+1^2+2^2 = 54\,.$$

Then, with the two lower-triangle summations,

$$u = \frac{8\left(\displaystyle\sum_{i=2}^{N}\sum_{j=1}^{N-1} a_{ij}^2 - k\sum_{i=2}^{N}\sum_{j=1}^{N-1} a_{ij}\right)}{k(k-1)N(N-1)} + 1$$

$$= \frac{8\big[54-(3)(22)\big]}{3(3-1)(6)(6-1)} + 1 = +0.4667\,.$$

If the upper triangle of a_{ij} values of the preference matrix is chosen instead of the lower-triangle values,

$$\sum_{i=1}^{N-1}\sum_{j=2}^{N} a_{ij} = 3+3+3+3+3+1+0+0+0+0$$

$$+1+1+2+2+1 = 23\,,$$

$$\sum_{i=1}^{N-1}\sum_{j=2}^{N} a_{ij}^2 = 3^2+3^2+3^2+3^2+3^2+1^2+0^2+0^2+0^2+0^2$$

$$+1^2+1^2+2^2+2^2+1^2 = 57\,,$$

and

$$u = \frac{8\left(\sum_{i=1}^{N-1}\sum_{j=2}^{N} a_{ij}^2 - k\sum_{i=1}^{N-1}\sum_{j=2}^{N} a_{ij}\right)}{k(k-1)N(N-1)} + 1$$

$$= \frac{8\big[57 - (3)(23)\big]}{3(3-1)(6)(6-1)} + 1 = +0.4667 \; .$$

In the same manner that Kendall and Babington Smith's coefficient of concordance, W, is a function of the average Spearman rank-order correlation coefficient, ρ, Kendall and Babington Smith's coefficient of agreement may be thought of as a generalization of Kendall's τ_a statistic, published two years prior in 1938, as u is the average value of the $k(k-1)/2$ τ_a statistics calculated on all possible paired rankings of the k judges. Given the rank-score data for Judges 1 and 2, the number of objects is $N = 6$, the number of concordant pairs is $C = 9$, the number of discordant pairs is $D = 6$, and $S = C - D = 9 - 6 = +3$. Then, Kendall's τ_a for Judges 1 and 2 is

$$\tau_{12} = \frac{2S}{N(N-1)} = \frac{2(+3)}{6(6-1)} = +0.20 \; .$$

Given the rank-score data for Judges 1 and 3, the number of objects is $N = 6$, the number of concordant pairs is $C = 13$, the number of discordant pairs is $D = 2$, and $S = C - D = 13 - 2 = +11$. Then, Kendall's τ_a for Judges 1 and 3 is

$$\tau_{13} = \frac{2S}{N(N-1)} = \frac{2(+11)}{6(6-1)} = +0.7333 \; .$$

Finally, given the rank-score data for Judges 2 and 3, the number of objects is $N = 6$, the number of concordant pairs is $C = 11$, the number of discordant pairs is $D = 4$, and $S = C - D = 11 - 4 = +7$. Then, Kendall's τ_a for Judges 2 and 3 is

$$\tau_{23} = \frac{2S}{N(N-1)} = \frac{2(+7)}{6(6-1)} = +0.4667 \; .$$

The arithmetic average of the three τ_a values is equal to u; thus,

$$u = \frac{2}{k(k-1)}\sum_{i=1}^{k-1}\sum_{j=i+1}^{k} \tau_{ij} = \frac{2(0.20 + 0.7333 + 0.4667)}{3(3-1)} = +0.4667 \; .$$

Because the lower limits of u are $-1/(k-1)$ when k is even and $-1/k$ when k is odd, Siegel and Castellan [80, p. 275] proposed an index of agreement similar to

Table 6.19 Upper-tail probability values for the Kendall and Babington Smith coefficient of agreement, u, with $k = 3$ judges

N	S	u	Probability
2	1	−0.3333	1.0000
	3	+1.0000	0.2500
3	3	−0.3333	1.0000
	5	+0.1111	0.5781
	7	+0.5556	0.1563
	9	+1.0000	0.0156

the Kendall coefficient of concordance, where

$$W = \frac{u(k-1)+1}{k} \qquad \text{if } k \text{ is even}$$

and

$$W = \frac{ku+1}{k+1} \qquad \text{if } k \text{ is odd} .$$

Thus, $0 \leq W \leq 1$ and is interpretable as a percentage of agreement among the k judges. For the example data in Table 6.18 where k is odd,

$$W = \frac{ku+1}{k+1} = \frac{(3)(0.4667)+1}{3+1} = 0.60 ,$$

indicating 60% agreement among the three judges. It should be noted, however, that the transformation of u to W as suggested by Siegel and Castellan destroys the chance-corrected interpretation of Kendall and Babington Smith's u measure of agreement.[8]

Exact Probability Values

Kendall and Babington Smith provided tables of exact probability values in terms of S for $k = 3$ and $N = 2, \ldots, 8$; $k = 4$ and $N = 2, \ldots, 6$; $k = 5$ and $N = 2, \ldots, 5$; and $k = 6$ and $N = 2, \ldots, 4$ [44, pp. 336–337]. Given the range of values for k and N, the tabled values are suitable for most applications of u. Table 6.19 illustrates the upper-tail probability values of Kendall and Babington Smith's u statistic for $k = 3$ and $N = 2, \ldots, 3$. Since k and N are invariant under permutation, the permutation distribution of S is sufficient to establish an exact upper-tail probability value.

[8]The introduction of W was apparently the work of N. John Castellan as it appears for the first time in the second edition of Siegel and Castellan *Nonparametric Statistics for the Behavioral Sciences* which was published in 1988 and Sidney Siegel had passed away much earlier in 1961, just five years after *Nonparametric Statistics for the Behavioral Sciences* was published. Coincidentally, N. John Castellan passed away in 1993, five years after the second edition was published.

Table 6.20 Rankings by $k = 3$ independent judges for $N = 2$ objects and associated preference matrices

		Judge			Preference		
Table 1	Object	1	2	3		a	b
	a	1	1	1	a	–	3
	b	2	2	2	b	0	–
		Judge			Preference		
Table 2	Object	1	2	3		a	b
	a	1	1	2	a	–	2
	b	2	2	1	b	1	–
		Judge			Preference		
Table 3	Object	1	2	3		a	b
	a	1	2	1	a	–	2
	b	2	1	2	b	1	–
		Judge			Preference		
Table 4	Object	1	2	3		a	b
	a	2	1	1	a	–	2
	b	1	2	2	b	1	–
		Judge			Preference		
Table 5	Object	1	2	3		a	b
	a	1	2	2	a	–	2
	b	2	1	1	b	1	–
		Judge			Preference		
Table 6	Object	1	2	3		a	b
	a	2	1	2	a	–	2
	b	1	2	1	b	1	–
		Judge			Preference		
Table 7	Object	1	2	3		a	b
	a	2	2	1	a	–	2
	b	1	1	2	b	1	–
		Judge			Preference		
Table 8	Object	1	2	3		a	b
	a	2	2	2	a	–	3
	b	1	2	1	b	0	–

To illustrate how the probability values in Table 6.19 were calculated, consider $k = 3$ and $N = 2$ in Table 6.19. There are only

$$M = 2^{k\binom{N}{2}} = 2^{3\binom{2}{2}} = 8$$

possible arrangements of the $k = 3$ rankings with $N = 2$ objects, making an exact permutation analysis easily accomplished. The $M = 8$ arrangements and associated preference matrices are listed in Table 6.20.

For Table 1 in Table 6.20,

$$S = \sum_{i=1}^{N} \sum_{j=1}^{N} a_{ij}^2 - k \sum_{i=1}^{N} \sum_{j=1}^{N} a_{ij} + \binom{k}{2}\binom{N}{2}$$

$$= 3^2 + 0^2 - (3)(3+0) + \binom{3}{2}\binom{2}{2} = +3 \,,$$

for Tables 2 through 7, $S = +1$, and for Table 8, $S = +3$. Thus, for $S = +3$ there are two occurrences (Tables 1 and 8) out of a possible $M = 8$ tables and the probability for $S = +3$ is $2/8 = 0.25$. For $S = +1$ there are six occurrences (Tables 8 through 7) and the cumulative upper-tail probability is $(2 + 6)/8 = 1.00$. Table 6.21 illustrates the calculation with a frequency distribution where the column headed f denotes the frequency of occurrence for values of S and the column headed F denotes the cumulative frequency distribution.

Now consider the upper-tail probability values for $k = 3$ and $N = 3$. There are

$$M = 2^{k\binom{N}{2}} = 2^{3\binom{3}{2}} = 512$$

possible arrangements of the $k = 3$ rankings with $N = 3$ objects. The frequency distribution of the $M = 512$ arrangements is given in Table 6.22, illustrating how the probability values were calculated by Kendall and Babington Smith.

For the example data in Table 6.17 on p. 322 with $k = 3$ judges and $N = 6$ objects, there are

$$M = 2^{k\binom{N}{2}} = 2^{3\binom{6}{2}} = 0.3518 \times 10^{14}$$

possible arrangements of the preference matrix. For $k = 3$, $N = 6$, $S = +33$, and $u = +0.4667$, the upper-tail probability value as given in Table 6.19 is $P = 0.0042$.

Table 6.21 Upper-tail probability values for S with $k = 3$ and $N = 2$ where f denotes the frequency of occurrence and F denotes the cumulative frequency

u	S	f	F	Probability
−0.3333	1	6	8	1.0000
+1.0000	3	2	2	0.2500

Table 6.22 Upper-tail probability values for S with $k = 3$ and $N = 3$ where f denotes the frequency of occurrence and F denotes the cumulative frequency of occurrence

u	S	f	F	Probability
−0.3333	3	216	512	1.0000
+0.1111	5	216	296	0.5781
+0.5556	7	72	80	0.1563
+1.0000	9	8	8	0.0156

6.4.2 Example 2

For a second example of Kendall's u measure of agreement, consider a situation where $k = 4$ members of a selection committee are asked to rank the final $N = 3$ applicants for a new position. The data are given in Table 6.23. The question is: to what degree do the $k = 4$ judges agree on the ranking of the $N = 3$ candidates? Table 6.24 shows the rank data given in Table 6.23 rearranged into a preference matrix.

For the preference matrix given in Table 6.24,

$$S = \sum_{i=1}^{N} \sum_{j=1}^{N} \binom{a_{ij}}{2} = 2\binom{3}{2} + 2\binom{2}{2} = +8$$

and

$$u = \frac{2S}{\binom{k}{2}\binom{N}{2}} - 1 = \frac{2(+8)}{\binom{4}{2}\binom{3}{2}} - 1 = -0.1111 ,$$

indicating less than chance agreement among the $k = 4$ judges.

Alternatively, using the upper triangle of a_{ij} values in the preference matrix in Table 6.24,

$$\sum_{i=1}^{N-1} \sum_{j=2}^{N} a_{ij} = 1 + 1 + 2 = 4 ,$$

$$\sum_{i=1}^{N-1} \sum_{j=2}^{N} a_{ij}^2 = 1^2 + 1^2 + 2^2 = 6$$

Table 6.23 Rank scores for $N = 3$ candidates by $k = 4$ judges

	Judge			
Candidate	1	2	3	4
a	1	2	2	1
b	2	1	3	3
c	3	3	1	2

Table 6.24 Preference matrix of $N = 3$ candidates by $k = 4$ judges

	a	b	c
a	–	1	1
b	3	–	2
c	3	2	–

and

$$u = \frac{8\left(\sum_{i=1}^{N-1}\sum_{j=2}^{N} a_{ij}^2 - k\sum_{i=1}^{N-1}\sum_{j=2}^{N} a_{ij}\right)}{k(k-1)N(N-1)} + 1$$

$$= \frac{8[6-(4)(4)]}{4(4-1)(3)(3-1)} + 1 = -0.1111 \; .$$

Since $k = 4$ is even, u can be normed between 0 and 1 as

$$W = \frac{u(k-1)+1}{k} = \frac{(-0.1111)(4-1)+1}{4} = 0.1667 \; ,$$

indicating approximately 17% agreement among the $k = 4$ judges.

As previously, *vide supra*, Kendall's u measure of agreement may also be thought of as a generalization of Kendall's τ_a measure of ordinal association, as u is the average of the $k(k-1)/2$ τ_a statistics calculated on the paired rankings of the $k = 4$ judges. Given the rank-score data for Judges 1 and 2, the number of objects is $N = 3$, the number of concordant pairs is $C = 2$, the number of discordant pairs is $D = 1$, $S = C - D = 2 - 1 = +1$, and Kendall's τ_a for Judges 1 and 2 is

$$\tau_{12} = \frac{2S}{N(N-1)} = \frac{2(+1)}{3(3-1)} = +0.3333 \; .$$

For Judges 1 and 3, the number of objects is $N = 3$, the number of concordant pairs is $C = 1$, the number of discordant pairs is $D = 2$, $S = C - D = 1 - 2 = -1$, and Kendall's τ_a for Judges 1 and 3 is

$$\tau_{13} = \frac{2S}{N(N-1)} = \frac{2(-1)}{3(3-1)} = -0.3333 \; .$$

For Judges 1 and 4, the number of objects is $N = 3$, the number of concordant pairs is $C = 2$, the number of discordant pairs is $D = 1$, $S = C - D = 2 - 1 = +1$, and Kendall's τ_a for Judges 1 and 4 is

$$\tau_{14} = \frac{2S}{N(N-1)} = \frac{2(+1)}{3(3-1)} = +0.3333 \; .$$

For Judges 2 and 3, the number of objects is $N = 3$, the number of concordant pairs is $C = 0$, the number of discordant pairs is $D = 3$, $S = C - D = 0 - 3 = -3$, and Kendall's τ_a for Judges 2 and 3 is

$$\tau_{23} = \frac{2S}{N(N-1)} = \frac{2(-3)}{3(3-1)} = -1.00 \; .$$

For Judges 2 and 4, the number of objects is $N = 3$, the number of concordant pairs is $C = 1$, the number of discordant pairs is $D = 2$, $S = C - D = 1 - 2 = -1$, and Kendall's τ_a for Judges 2 and 4 is

$$\tau_{24} = \frac{2S}{N(N-1)} = \frac{2(-1)}{3(3-1)} = -0.3333 \, .$$

And for Judges 3 and 4, the number of objects is $N = 3$, the number of concordant pairs is $C = 2$, the number of discordant pairs is $D = 1$, $S = C - D = 2 - 1 = +1$, and Kendall's τ_a for Judges 3 and 4 is

$$\tau_{34} = \frac{2S}{N(N-1)} = \frac{2(+1)}{3(3-1)} = +0.3333 \, .$$

The arithmetic average of the six τ_a values is equal to u; thus,

$$u = \frac{2}{k(k-1)} \sum_{i=1}^{k-1} \sum_{j=i+1}^{k} \tau_{ij}$$
$$= \frac{2(0.3333 - 0.3333 + 0.3333 - 1.00 - 0.3333 + 0.3333)}{4(4-1)} = -0.1111 \, .$$

Exact Probability Values

Kendall and Babington Smith provided tables of exact probability values for a variety of combinations of k and N. The permutation distribution for $k = 4$ and $N = 3$ given in Table 6.25 illustrates the exact probability values provided by Kendall and Babington Smith.

Table 6.25 Upper-tail probability values for S with $k = 4$ and $N = 3$ where f denotes the frequency of occurrence and F denotes the cumulative frequency

u	S	f	F	Probability
−0.3333	6	217	4,096	1.0000
−0.2222	7	864	3,879	0.9470
−0.1111	8	1,151	3,015	0.7361
+0.0000	9	512	1,864	0.4551
+0.1111	10	216	1,352	0.3301
+0.2222	11	576	1,136	0.2773
+0.3333	12	384	560	0.1367
+0.5556	14	72	176	0.0430
+0.6667	15	96	104	0.0254
+1.0000	18	8	8	0.0020

For the example data given in Table 6.25 with $k = 4$ judges and $N = 3$ candidates, there are only

$$M = 2^{k\binom{N}{2}} = 2^{4\binom{3}{2}} = 2^{12} = 4{,}096$$

possible arrangements of the preference matrix, making an exact permutation analysis practical. For $u = -0.1111$ and $S = 8$, the exact upper-tail probability value under the null hypothesis as given in Table 6.25 is

$$P(S \geq S_{\text{o}}|H_0) = \frac{\text{number of } S \text{ values} \geq S_{\text{o}}}{M} = \frac{3{,}015}{4{,}096} = 0.7361 ,$$

where S_{o} denotes the observed value of S.

6.5 Cohen's Weighted Kappa

In 1960 Jacob Cohen developed statistic kappa, a chance-corrected measure of inter-rater agreement between two judges for a set of c disjoint, unordered categories [13]. In 1968 Cohen extended kappa to measure the agreement between two judges for a set of c disjoint, ordered categories [14]. The original kappa for c disjoint, unordered categories became known as "unweighted" kappa, or κ, and kappa for c disjoint, ordered categories became known as "weighted" kappa, or κ_w. Whereas unweighted kappa did not distinguish among magnitudes of disagreement, weighted kappa incorporated the magnitude of each disagreement and provided partial credit for disagreements when agreement was not complete [52]. The usual approach is to assign weights to each disagreement pair with larger weights indicating greater disagreement.[9] Unweighted kappa for c disjoint, unordered categories is discussed in Chap. 4; weighted kappa for c disjoint, ordered categories is discussed in this chapter.

The measurement of agreement is a special case of measuring association between two ordinal-level variables. A number of statistical research problems require the measurement of agreement, rather than association or correlation. Agreement indices measure the extent to which a set of response measurements are identical to another set, i.e., agree, rather than the extent to which one set of response measurements is a linear function of another set of response measurements, i.e., correlated. Like Spearman's footrule, Cohen's weighted kappa measure of inter-rater agreement is a chance-corrected measure, reflecting the amount of agreement in excess of what would be expected by chance. Thus, weighted kappa is equal to one when perfect agreement occurs, is equal to zero under independence, and can be slightly negative when agreement is less than expected by chance [30, p. 434].

[9] Some authors prefer to define weighted kappa in terms of agreement weights, instead of disagreement weights [11, 89].

Table 6.26 Notation for the cross-classification of N objects by $b = 2$ judges into c disjoint, ordered categories denoted by $a_1, \ldots, a_c$

	Judge 2				
Judge 1	a_1	a_2	$\cdots$	a_c	Total
a_1	n_{11}	n_{12}	$\cdots$	n_{1c}	$n_{1.}$
a_2	n_{21}	n_{22}	$\cdots$	n_{2c}	$n_{2.}$
$\vdots$	$\vdots$	$\vdots$	$\ddots$	$\vdots$	$\vdots$
a_c	n_{c1}	n_{c2}	$\cdots$	n_{cc}	$n_{c.}$
Total	$n_{.1}$	$n_{.2}$	$\cdots$	$n_{.c}$	N

For simplicity, consider $N \geq 2$ objects cross-classified by $b = 2$ independent judges into a $c \times c$ contingency table with c disjoint, ordered categories denoted by $a_1, \ldots, a_c$, such as in Table 6.26. Denote by a dot $(\cdot)$ the partial sum of all rows or all columns, depending on the position of the $(\cdot)$ in the subscript list. If the $(\cdot)$ is in the first subscript position, the sum is over all rows, and if the $(\cdot)$ is in the second subscript position, the sum is over all columns. Thus, $n_{i.}$ denotes the marginal frequency total of the ith row, $i = 1, \ldots, c$, summed over all columns, and $n_{.j}$ denotes the marginal frequency total of the jth column, $j = 1, \ldots, c$, summed over all rows. Then, n_{ij}, w_{ij}, $n_{i.}$, and $n_{.j}$ denote the cell frequencies, cell weights, row marginal frequency totals, and column marginal frequency totals, respectively, where

$$n_{i.} = \sum_{j=1}^{c} n_{ij} \; , \quad n_{.j} = \sum_{i=1}^{c} n_{ij} \; , \quad \text{and} \quad N = \sum_{i=1}^{c} \sum_{j=1}^{c} n_{ij} \; .$$

When the c categories for the $b = 2$ judges are similarly arranged, then n_{ii}, $i = 1, \ldots, c$, and n_{ij}, $i \neq j$, denote the agreement and disagreement cell frequencies, respectively.

Although a variety of weighting schemes have been proposed for Cohen's weighted kappa, the most popular is quadratic weighting given by $w_{ij} = (i - j)^2$ for $i, j = 1, \ldots, c$, where category disagreement weights progress geometrically outward from the agreement diagonal, i.e., 0^2, 1^2, 2^2, 3^2, and so on. However, linear weighting in which $w_{ij} = |i - j|$ for $i, j = 1, \ldots, c$, where category disagreement weights progress linearly outward from the agreement diagonal, i.e., 0, 1, 2, 3, and so on, is perhaps more intuitive.

A simple calculation formula for Cohen's weighted kappa test statistic with $b = 2$ judges is given by

$$\kappa_w = 1 - \frac{\dfrac{1}{N} \displaystyle\sum_{i=1}^{c} \sum_{j=1}^{c} w_{ij} n_{ij}}{\dfrac{1}{N^2} \displaystyle\sum_{i=1}^{c} \sum_{j=1}^{c} w_{ij} n_{i.} n_{.j}} \; . \tag{6.9}$$

Given a $c \times c$ agreement table with N objects classified by the ratings of two independent judges into c disjoint, ordered categories, an exact permutation test generates a reference set of all M possible, equally-likely arrangements of the N objects in the c^2 cells, while preserving the total number of objects in each category, i.e., the marginal frequency distributions. For each arrangement of cell frequencies with fixed marginal frequency distributions, the weighted kappa statistic, κ_w, and the exact probability value, $p(n_{ij}|n_{i.}, n_{.j}, N)$, are calculated, where

$$p(n_{ij}|n_{i.}, n_{.j}, N) = \frac{\left(\prod_{i=1}^{c} n_{i.}!\right)\left(\prod_{j=1}^{c} n_{.j}!\right)}{N! \prod_{i=1}^{c} \prod_{j=1}^{c} n_{ij}!}$$

is the conventional hypergeometric probability value of a $c \times c$ contingency (agreement) table.

Let κ_o denote the value of the observed weighted kappa statistic and M denote the total number of distinct cell frequency arrangements of the N objects in the $c \times c$ classification table, given fixed marginal frequency totals. Then the exact probability value of κ_o under the null hypothesis is given by

$$P(\kappa_o|H_0) = \sum_{k=1}^{M} \Psi(\kappa_k)\, p(n_{ij}|n_{i.}, n_{.j}, N) \;,$$

where

$$\Psi(\kappa_k) = \begin{cases} 1 & \text{if } \kappa_k \geq \kappa_o \;, \\ 0 & \text{otherwise} \;. \end{cases}$$

When the reference set of all M possible arrangements is very large, exact permutation analyses are impractical and Monte Carlo resampling approximations become necessary. Let L denote a random sample of all M possible values of κ_w. Then, under the null hypothesis, the resampling approximate probability value for the observed value of κ_w, κ_o, is given by

$$P(\kappa_o) = \frac{1}{L} \sum_{l=1}^{L} \Psi_l(\kappa_w)$$

where

$$\Psi_l(\kappa_w) = \begin{cases} 1 & \text{if } \kappa_w \geq \kappa_o \;, \\ 0 & \text{otherwise} \;. \end{cases}$$

6.5.1 Example 1

Consider a small example data set of $N = 5$ objects classified into $c = 3$ disjoint, ordered categories by $b = 2$ independent judges. Table 6.27 contains the $c^2 = 9$ cell frequencies. The corresponding linear and quadratic disagreement cell weights are given in parentheses and brackets, respectively. The number of objects and the number of categories are deliberately kept small to simplify the example analysis.

Linear Weighting

Utilizing linear disagreement weights, given in parentheses in Table 6.27, and following the numerator of Eq. (6.9) on p. 333 with $N = 5$ objects, $c = 3$ disjoint, ordered categories, and $b = 2$ judges,

$$\frac{1}{N}\sum_{i=1}^{c}\sum_{j=1}^{c} w_{ij}n_{ij} = \frac{1}{5}\big[(0)(0) + (1)(1) + (2)(0) + (1)(0) + (0)(2) + (1)(0) + (2)(1) + (1)(0) + (0)(1)\big] = 0.60\ ,$$

and for the denominator of Eq. (6.9),

$$\frac{1}{N^2}\sum_{i=1}^{c}\sum_{j=1}^{c} w_{ij}n_{i.}n_{.j} = \frac{1}{5^2}\big[(0)(1)(1) + (1)(1)(3) + (2)(1)(1) + (1)(2)(1) + (0)(2)(3) + (1)(2)(1) + (2)(2)(1) + (1)(2)(3) + (0)(2)(1)\big] = 0.76\ .$$

Table 6.27 Example data for a weighted kappa analysis with $N = 5$ observations, $c = 3$ disjoint, ordered categories, and $b = 2$ judges

	Judge 2			
Judge 1	Category A	Category B	Category C	Total
Category A	0 (0) [0]	1 (1) [1]	0 (2) [4]	1
Category B	0 (1) [1]	2 (0) [0]	0 (1) [1]	2
Category C	1 (2) [4]	0 (1) [1]	1 (0) [0]	2
Total	1	3	1	5

Note—Linear cell weights are in parentheses and quadratic cell weights are in brackets

Then the observed value of Cohen's weighted kappa with linear weighting is

$$\kappa_w = 1 - \frac{\dfrac{1}{N} \displaystyle\sum_{i=1}^{c} \sum_{j=1}^{c} w_{ij} n_{ij}}{\dfrac{1}{N^2} \displaystyle\sum_{i=1}^{c} \sum_{j=1}^{c} w_{ij} n_{i.} n_{.j}} = 1 - \frac{0.60}{0.76} = +0.2105 \,,$$

indicating approximately 21% agreement above that expected by chance.

There are only $M = 8$ possible, equally-likely arrangements of cell frequencies given the observed row and column marginal frequency distributions, $\{1, 2, 2\}$ and $\{1, 3, 1\}$, respectively, in Table 6.27. The eight arrangements of cell frequencies are listed in Table 6.28, where Table 1 of Table 6.28 contains the observed cell frequencies.

Table 6.29 lists the computed kappa values and associated hypergeometric point probability values for the $M = 8$ classification tables in Table 6.28, ordered from high to low by the κ_w values. As is evident from the κ_w test statistics and associated probability values listed in Table 6.29, the observed value of $\kappa_w = +0.2105$ is not unusual as four κ_w values are less than $\kappa_w = +0.2105$ (-0.3158, -0.3158, -0.3158, and -0.3158) and four values are equal to or greater than $\kappa_w = +0.2105$ ($+0.2105$, $+0.2105$, $+0.2105$, and $+0.7368$). Thus, the exact probability value of the observed cell configuration under the null hypothesis is the sum of the hypergeometric point probability values associated with the values of $\kappa_w = +0.2105$ or greater. Based on the hypergeometric probability distribution,

Table 6.28 Eight possible arrangements of the cell frequencies in Table 6.27, given fixed marginal frequency distributions

Table 1			Table 2			Table 3			Table 4		
0	1	0	1	0	0	1	0	0	0	1	0
0	2	0	0	1	1	0	2	0	1	0	1
1	0	1	0	2	0	0	1	1	0	2	0
Table 5			Table 6			Table 7			Table 8		
0	1	0	0	0	1	0	0	1	0	1	0
1	1	0	0	2	0	1	1	0	0	1	1
0	1	1	1	1	0	0	2	0	1	1	0

Table 6.29 Weighted kappa and hypergeometric probability values for the eight 3×3 classification tables given in Table 6.28 with linear weighting

Table	κ_w	Probability
3	+0.7368	0.1000
1	+0.2105	0.1000
2	+0.2105	0.1000
5	+0.2105	0.2000
4	−0.3158	0.1000
6	−0.3158	0.1000
7	−0.3158	0.1000
8	−0.3158	0.2000

Table 6.30 Example data for a weighted kappa analysis with $N = 5$ observations, $c = 3$ ordered categories, $b = 2$ judges and quadratic weights in brackets

	Judge 2			
Judge 1	A	B	C	Total
A	0 [0]	1 [1]	0 [4]	1
B	0 [1]	2 [0]	0 [1]	2
C	1 [4]	0 [1]	1 [0]	2
Total	1	3	1	5

the exact upper-tail probability value is $P = 0.1000 + 0.1000 + 0.1000 + 0.2000 = 0.5000$.

Quadratic Weighting

Consider again the frequency data listed in Table 6.27 on p. 335, replicated for convenience in Table 6.30, absent the linear weights, with $N = 5$ objects classified into $c = 3$ disjoint, ordered categories by $b = 2$ independent judges.

Utilizing quadratic cell disagreement weights, given in brackets in Table 6.30, and following the numerator of Eq. (6.9) on p. 333 with $N = 5$ objects, $c = 3$ disjoint, ordered categories, and $b = 2$ judges,

$$\frac{1}{N}\sum_{i=1}^{c}\sum_{j=1}^{c} w_{ij}n_{ij} = \frac{1}{5}\big[(0)(0) + (1)(1) + (4)(0) + (1)(0) + (0)(2) + (1)(0) + (4)(1) + (1)(0) + (0)(1)\big] = 1.00\,,$$

and for the denominator of Eq. (6.9),

$$\frac{1}{N^2}\sum_{i=1}^{c}\sum_{j=1}^{c} w_{ij}n_{i.}n_{.j} = \frac{1}{5^2}\big[(0)(1)(1) + (1)(1)(3) + (4)(1)(1) + (1)(2)(1) + (0)(2)(3) + (1)(2)(1) + (4)(2)(1) + (1)(2)(3) + (0)(2)(1)\big] = 1.00\,.$$

Then, the observed value of Cohen's weighted kappa with quadratic weighting is

$$\kappa_w = 1 - \frac{\dfrac{1}{N}\displaystyle\sum_{i=1}^{c}\sum_{j=1}^{c} w_{ij}n_{ij}}{\dfrac{1}{N^2}\displaystyle\sum_{i=1}^{c}\sum_{j=1}^{c} w_{ij}n_{i.}n_{.j}} = 1 - \frac{1.00}{1.00} = 0.00\,,$$

indicating only chance agreement between the two judges.

As noted in the linear weighted analysis, there are only $M = 8$ possible, equally-likely arrangements of cell frequencies given the observed row and column marginal frequency distributions, $\{1, 2, 2\}$ and $\{1, 3, 1\}$, respectively, in Table 6.30. The eight arrangements of cell frequencies are listed in Table 6.28, where Table 6.1 of Table 6.28 contains the observed cell frequencies.

Table 6.31 lists the computed kappa values and associated hypergeometric point probability values for the $M = 8$ classification tables in Table 6.28, ordered from high to low by the κ_w values. As is evident from the κ_w test statistics and associated probability values listed in Table 6.31, for the observed value of $\kappa_w = 0.00$ three of the κ_w values are less than $\kappa_w = 0.00$ (−0.40, −0.40, and −0.80) and five values are equal to or greater than $\kappa_w = 0.00$ (0.00, 0.00, +0.40, +0.40, and +0.80). Thus, the exact probability value of the observed cell configuration under the null hypothesis is the sum of the hypergeometric point probability values associated with the values of $\kappa_w = 0.00$ or greater. Based on the hypergeometric probability distribution, the exact upper-tail probability value is $P = 0.1000 + 0.1000 + 0.2000 + 0.1000 + 0.1000 = 0.6000$.

6.5.2 Example 2

While the first example with $N = 5$ objects and only $M = 8$ possible arrangements of cell frequencies illustrates an exact permutation statistical procedure, it does not reflect a typical agreement analysis. A second example with $N = 71$ objects provides a more realistic assessment of agreement data. Consider the frequency data listed in Table 6.32 with $N = 71$ objects classified into $c = 3$ disjoint, ordered categories by $b = 2$ independent judges.

Table 6.31 Weighted kappa and hypergeometric probability values for the eight 3×3 classification tables given in Table 6.28 with quadratic weighting

Table	κ_w	Probability
3	+0.80	0.1000
2	+0.40	0.1000
5	+0.40	0.2000
4	0.00	0.1000
1	0.00	0.1000
7	−0.40	0.1000
8	−0.40	0.2000
6	−0.80	0.1000

Table 6.32 Example data for a weighted kappa analysis with $N = 71$ observations, $c = 3$ disjoint, ordered categories, $b = 2$ judges, and linear weights in parentheses

	Judge 2			
Judge 1	A	B	C	Total
A	12 (0)	9 (1)	8 (2)	29
B	7 (1)	10 (0)	6 (1)	23
C	5 (2)	6 (1)	8 (0)	19
Total	24	25	22	71

Linear Weighting

For the frequency data given in Table 6.32, utilizing linear cell disagreement weights given in parentheses, and following the numerator of Eq. (6.9) on p. 333 with $N = 71$ objects, $c = 3$ disjoint, ordered categories, and $b = 2$ judges,

$$\frac{1}{N}\sum_{i=1}^{c}\sum_{j=1}^{c} w_{ij}n_{ij} = \frac{1}{71}\big[(0)(12) + (1)(9) + (2)(8) + (1)(7) + (0)(10) + (1)(6) + (2)(5) + (1)(6) + (0)(8)\big] = 0.7606\ ,$$

and for the denominator of Eq. (6.9) on p. 333,

$$\frac{1}{N^2}\sum_{i=1}^{c}\sum_{j=1}^{c} w_{ij}n_{i.}n_{.j} = \frac{1}{71^2}\big[(0)(29)(24) + (1)(29)(25) + (2)(29)(22) + (1)(23)(24) + (0)(23(25) + (1)(23)(22) + (2)(19)(24) + (1)(19)(25 + (0)(19)(22)\big] = 0.8820\ .$$

Then, the observed value of Cohen's weighted kappa with linear weighting is

$$\kappa_w = 1 - \frac{\dfrac{1}{N}\displaystyle\sum_{i=1}^{c}\sum_{j=1}^{c} w_{ij}n_{ij}}{\dfrac{1}{N^2}\displaystyle\sum_{i=1}^{c}\sum_{j=1}^{c} w_{ij}n_{i.}n_{.j}} = 1 - \frac{0.7606}{0.8820} = +0.1377\ ,$$

indicating approximately 14% agreement above that expected by chance.

Since there are only $M = 43{,}315$ arrangements in the reference set of all permutations of cell frequencies consistent with the observed row and column marginal frequency distributions, $\{29, 23, 19\}$ and $\{24, 25, 22\}$, respectively, an exact permutation analysis is feasible. The exact probability value of the observed cell configuration under the null hypothesis is the sum of the hypergeometric point probability values associated with the values of $\kappa_w = +0.1377$ or greater. Based on the hypergeometric probability distribution, the exact upper-tail probability value is $P = 0.0970$.

Quadratic Weighting

For comparison, contrast linear cell weighting with quadratic cell weighting, utilizing the common data set given in Table 6.32, replicated in Table 6.33 for convenience, with $N = 71$ objects classified into $c = 3$ disjoint, ordered categories

Table 6.33 Example data for a weighted kappa analysis with $N = 71$ observations, $c = 3$ disjoint, ordered categories, $b = 2$ judges, and quadratic weights in brackets

	Judge 2			
Judge 1	A	B	C	Total
A	12 [0]	9 [1]	8 [4]	29
B	7 [1]	10 [0]	6 [1]	23
C	5 [4]	6 [1]	8 [0]	19
Total	24	25	22	71

by $b = 2$ independent judges. For the frequency data given in Table 6.33, utilizing quadratic cell disagreement weights given in brackets, and following the numerator of Eq. (6.9) on p. 333 with $N = 71$, $c = 3$ disjoint, ordered categories, and $b = 2$ judges,

$$\frac{1}{N}\sum_{i=1}^{c}\sum_{j=1}^{c} w_{ij}n_{ij} = \frac{1}{71}\big[(0)(12) + (1)(9) + (4)(8) + (1)(7) + (0)(10)$$

$$+ (1)(6) + (4)(5) + (1)(6) + (0)(8)\big] = 1.1268\ ,$$

and for the denominator of Eq. (6.9) on p. 333,

$$\frac{1}{N^2}\sum_{i=1}^{c}\sum_{j=1}^{c} w_{ij}n_{i.}n_{.j} = \frac{1}{71^2}\big[(0)(29)(24) + (1)(29)(25) + (4)(29)(22)$$

$$+ (1)(23)(24) + (0)(23(25) + (1)(23)(22) + (4)(19)(24)$$

$$+ (1)(19)(25 + (0)(19)(22)\big] = 1.3160\ .$$

Then the observed value of Cohen's weighted kappa with quadratic weighting is

$$\kappa_w = 1 - \frac{\dfrac{1}{N}\displaystyle\sum_{i=1}^{c}\sum_{j=1}^{c} w_{ij}n_{ij}}{\dfrac{1}{N^2}\displaystyle\sum_{i=1}^{c}\sum_{j=1}^{c} w_{ij}n_{i.}n_{.j}} = 1 - \frac{1.1268}{1.3160} = +0.1438\ ,$$

indicating approximately 14% agreement above that expected by chance.

Since there are only $M = 43{,}315$ arrangements in the reference set of all permutations of cell frequencies consistent with the observed row and column marginal frequency distributions, $\{29, 23, 19\}$ and $\{24, 25, 22\}$, respectively, an exact permutation analysis is feasible. The exact probability value of the observed cell configuration under the null hypothesis is the sum of the hypergeometric point probability values associated with the values of $\kappa_w = +0.1438$ or greater. Based on the hypergeometric probability distribution, the exact upper-tail probability value is $P = 0.1311$.

6.5.3 Linear and Quadratic Weighting Compared

There exists considerable controversy over exactly which cell disagreement weights should be used with Cohen's weighted kappa statistic, κ_w. On the one hand, the choice of weights is completely arbitrary and any disagreement cell weights may be utilized [89, p. 157]. On the other hand, linear and quadratic cell weights are observed almost exclusively in the literature. Linear weighting is perhaps the more useful of the two approaches in which $w_{ij} = |i - j|$ for $i, j = 1, \ldots, c$, where disagreement cell weights progress linearly outward from the agreement diagonal. In addition, linear weighting has been shown to have some interesting and valuable properties. In 2008 Vanbelle and Albert demonstrated that linear-weighted kappa for $b = 2$ independent judges and $c \geq 3$ disjoint, ordered categories is equivalent to deriving the weighted kappa agreement coefficient from unweighted kappa values computed on $c - 1$ embedded 2×2 classification tables [89]. In 2009 Mielke and Berry generalized the results of Vanbelle and Albert to $b \geq 2$ independent judges [63].

It is patently obvious that linear weighting and quadratic weighting yield the same results for 2×2 contingency tables. It is also abundantly clear that linear weighted and quadratic weighted kappa values often differ very little for 3×3 contingency tables. For example, for the frequency data in Tables 6.32 and 6.33, the observed value of weighted kappa with linear weighting was $\kappa_w = +0.1377$ and the observed value of weighted kappa with quadratic weighting was $\kappa_w = +0.1438$, a difference of only 0.0061. Linear and quadratic weighting generally yield greater differences with larger contingency tables. Consider the 5×5 contingency table given in Table 6.34 with $N = 10$ objects, $c = 5$ disjoint, ordered categories, and $b = 2$ judges. For the frequency data given in Table 6.34 with linear weights given in parentheses and quadratic weights given in brackets, the observed value of weighted kappa with linear weighting is $\kappa_w = +0.7222$ and the observed value of weighted kappa with quadratic weighting is $\kappa_w = +0.5122$, for a difference of 0.2100. The single frequency in the first row (A) and fifth column (E) of Table 6.34 has a linear weight of $w_{15} = 4$, a quadratic weight of $w_{15} = 16$, and accounts for the entire difference in the two κ_w values. As demonstrated by Brenner and Kliebsch,

Table 6.34 Example data for a weighted kappa analysis with $N = 10$ observations, $c = 5$ ordered categories, $b = 2$ judges, linear weights in parentheses, and quadratic weights in brackets

	Judge 2					
Judge 1	A	B	C	D	E	Total
A	1 (0) [0]	0 (1) [1]	0 (2) [4]	0 (3) [9]	1 (4) [16]	2
B	0 (1) [1]	2 (0) [0]	0 (1) [1]	0 (2) [4]	0 (3) [9]	2
C	0 (2) [4]	0 (1) [1]	3 (0) [0]	0 (1) [1]	0 (2) [4]	3
D	0 (3) [9]	0 (2) [4]	0 (1) [1]	2 (0) [0]	0 (1) [1]	2
E	0 (4) [16]	0 (3) [9]	0 (2) [4]	0 (1) [1]	1 (0) [0]	1
Total	1	2	3	2	2	10

the linear form of the weighted kappa coefficient is less sensitive to the number of categories than the quadratic form; consequently, they recommended that the linear form be used whenever the number of categories of the ordinal scale is large [9].

6.5.4 Weighted Kappa with Multiple Judges

While Cohen's weighted kappa was originally designed for and is limited to $b = 2$ independent judges, weighted kappa can be generalized and extended to measure agreement among multiple judges [4]. The generalization of Cohen's kappa to multiple judges has long been controversial, with many missteps and dead-ends along the way; see Sect. 4.5 in Chap. 4. In 1988 Berry and Mielke generalized Cohen's kappa agreement measure to accommodate multiple judges [4] and in 2008 Mielke, Berry, and Johnston provided an efficient Monte Carlo resampling algorithm to analyze agreement data with multiple judges [60].

In this section, an algorithmic procedure to compute unweighted and weighted kappa with multiple raters is presented [60]. Although the procedure is appropriate for any number of $c \geq 2$ disjoint, ordered categories and $b \geq 2$ judges, the description of the procedure and the examples are limited to $b = 3$ independent judges to simplify presentation, with no loss of generality.

Consider $b = 3$ judges who independently classify N objects into c disjoint, ordered categories. The classification may be conceptualized as a $c \times c \times c$ contingency table with c rows, c columns, and c slices. Let n_{ijk}, R_i, C_j, and S_k denote the cell frequencies and row, column, and slice marginal frequency totals for $i, j, k = 1, \ldots, c$ and let the frequency total be given by

$$N = \sum_{i=1}^{c} \sum_{j=1}^{c} \sum_{k=1}^{c} n_{ijk} .$$

Cohen's weighted kappa test statistic for a three-way contingency table is given by

$$\kappa_w = \frac{N^2 \displaystyle\sum_{i=1}^{c} \sum_{i=1}^{c} \sum_{i=1}^{c} w_{ijk} n_{ijk}}{\displaystyle\sum_{i=1}^{c} \sum_{i=1}^{c} \sum_{i=1}^{c} w_{ijk} R_i C_j S_k} , \tag{6.10}$$

where w_{ijk} are disagreement weights assigned to each cell for $i, j, k = 1, \ldots, c$. Under the null hypothesis that the judges classify the N objects independently with fixed marginal frequency totals, $\mathrm{E}[\kappa_w] = 0$.

As discussed previously, *vide supra*, a variety of weighting functions have been proposed for weighted kappa for two judges, where the arbitrary cell weights are denoted as w_{ij} and i and j designate the c categories for each judge, $i, j = 1, \ldots, c$ [77, p. 246]. Typically, the cell weights are defined such that $w_{ii} = 0$ for $i = 1, \ldots, c$ and the weights are symmetrical, i.e., $w_{ij} = w_{ji}$ for $i, j = 1, \ldots, c$. Examples of weighting systems for two judges include linear weighting where $w_{ij} = |i - j|$, quadratic weighting where $w_{ij} = (i - j)^2$, and unweighted kappa where

$$w_{ij} = \begin{cases} 0 & \text{if } i = j \,, \\ 1 & \text{otherwise} \,. \end{cases}$$

For three judges, the cell disagreement weights are given by w_{ijk}, where i, j, and k designate the c categories for each judge. Analogously to w_{ij}, w_{ijk} may be defined such that $w_{iii} = 0$ for $i = 1, \ldots, c$ and the weights are symmetrical, i.e., $w_{ijk} = w_{ikj} = w_{jik} = w_{jki} = w_{kij} = w_{kji}$ for $i, j, k = 1, \ldots, c$. Examples of weighting systems for three judges include linear weighting where

$$w_{ijk} = |i - j| + |i - k| + |j - k|$$

and quadratic weighting where

$$w_{ijk} = (i - j)^2 + (i - k)^2 + (j - k)^2$$

for $i, j, k = 1, \ldots, c$.

Weighted kappa for three judges reduces to unweighted kappa when

$$w_{ijk} = \begin{cases} 0 & \text{if } i = j = k \,, \\ 1 & \text{otherwise} \,. \end{cases}$$

Given a $c{\times}c{\times}c$ contingency table with N objects cross-classified by three independent judges, an exact permutation test involves generating all possible, equally-likely arrangements of the N objects to the c^3 cells, while preserving the observed marginal frequency distributions. For each arrangement in the reference set of all permutations of cell frequencies, the weighted kappa statistic, κ_w, and the exact hypergeometric point probability value under the null hypothesis, $p(n_{ijk}|R_i, C_j, S_k, N)$, are calculated, where

$$p(n_{ijk}|R_i, C_j, S_k, N) = \frac{\left(\prod_{i=1}^{c} R_i!\right)\left(\prod_{j=1}^{c} C_j!\right)\left(\prod_{k=1}^{c} S_k!\right)}{(N!)^2 \prod_{i=1}^{c} \prod_{j=1}^{c} \prod_{k=1}^{c} n_{ijk}!} \tag{6.11}$$

[54].

If κ_o denotes the value of the observed weighted kappa test statistic, the exact probability value of κ_o under the null hypothesis is given by

$$P(\kappa_o|H_0) = \sum_{l=1}^{M} \Psi_l\left(n_{ijk}|R_i, C_j, S_k, N\right) ,$$

where

$$\Psi_l\left(n_{ijk}|R_i, C_j, S_k, N\right) = \begin{cases} p(n_{ijk}|R_i, C_j, S_k, N) & \text{if } \kappa_w \geq \kappa_o , \\ 0 & \text{otherwise} , \end{cases}$$

and M denotes the total number of possible, equally-likely cell frequency arrangements given fixed observed marginal frequency totals. When the reference set of M possible arrangements is very large, as is typical with multi-way contingency tables, exact tests are impractical and Monte Carlo resampling procedures become necessary. Under resampling, a random sample of size L drawn from the M possible arrangements of cell frequencies provides for a comparison of κ_w test statistics calculated on the L random tables with the κ_w test statistic calculated on the observed table.

6.5.5 Algorithm for $r \times c \times s$ Contingency Tables

An efficient resampling algorithm to generate random cell frequency arrangements for multi-way contingency tables with fixed marginal frequency totals was developed by Mielke, Berry, and Johnston in 2007 [59, pp. 19–20]. For a three-way contingency table with r rows, c columns, and s slices, the Monte Carlo resampling algorithm is given in 12 simple steps.

STEP 1. Construct an $r \times c \times s$ contingency table from the observed data.

STEP 2. Obtain the fixed marginal frequency totals $R_1, \ldots, R_r, C_1, \ldots, C_c, S_1, \ldots, S_s$, and frequency total N. Set the resampling counter $JL = 0$, and set L equal to the number of samples desired.

STEP 3. Set the resampling counter $JL = JL + 1$.

STEP 4. Set the marginal frequency counters $JR_i = R_i$ for $i = 1, \ldots, r$; $JC_j = C_j$ for $j = 1, \ldots, c$; $JS_k = S_k$ for $k = 1, \ldots, s$, and $M = N$.

STEP 5. Set $n_{ijk} = 0$ for $i = 1, \ldots, r$, $j = 1, \ldots, c$, and $k = 1, \ldots, s$, and set row, column, and slice counters *IR*, *IC*, and *IS* equal to zero.

STEP 6. Create cumulative probability distributions PR_i, PC_j, and PS_k from the adjusted marginal frequency totals JR_i, JC_j, and JS_k for $i = 1, \ldots, r$, $j = 1, \ldots, c$, and $k = 1, \ldots, s$, where

$$PR_1 = JR_1/M \quad \text{and} \quad PR_i = PR_{i-1} + JR_i/M$$

for $i = 1, \ldots, r$,

$$PC_1 = JC_1/M \quad \text{and} \quad PC_j = PC_{j-1} + JC_j/M$$

for $j = 1, \ldots, c$, and

$$PS_1 = JS_1/M \quad \text{and} \quad PS_k = PS_{k-1} + JS_k/M$$

for $k = 1, \ldots, s$.

STEP 7. Generate three uniform pseudorandom numbers U_r, U_c, and U_s over $[0, 1)$ and set row, column, and slice indices $i = j = k = 1$, respectively.

STEP 8. If $U_r \leq PR_i$, then $IR = i$, $JR_i = JR_i - 1$, and go to STEP 9; otherwise, $i = i + 1$ and repeat STEP 8.

STEP 9. If $U_c \leq PC_j$, then $IC = j$, $JC_j = JC_j - 1$, and go to STEP 10; otherwise, $j = j + 1$ and repeat STEP 9.

STEP 10. If $U_s \leq PS_k$, then $IS = k$, $JS_k = JS_k - 1$, and go to STEP 11; otherwise, $k = k + 1$ and repeat STEP 10.

STEP 11. Set $M = M - 1$ and $n_{IR,IC,IS} = n_{IR,IC,IS} + 1$. If $M > 0$, go to STEP 4; otherwise, obtain the required test statistic and go to STEP 12.

STEP 12. If $JL < L$, go to STEP 3; otherwise, stop.

At the conclusion of the resampling algorithm, κ_w, as given in Eq. (6.10) on p. 342, is obtained for each of the L random three-way contingency tables, given the observed marginal frequency distributions. Under the null hypothesis, the resampling approximate probability value for the observed value of κ_w, κ_o, is given by

$$P(\kappa_o) = \frac{1}{L} \sum_{l=1}^{L} \Psi_l(\kappa_w) \ ,$$

where

$$\Psi_l(\kappa_w) = \begin{cases} 1 & \text{if } \kappa_w \geq \kappa_o \ , \\ 0 & \text{otherwise} \ . \end{cases}$$

Example

The calculation of weighted kappa and the Monte Carlo resampling procedure for obtaining a probability value with multiple raters can be illustrated with a small example data set. Consider $b = 3$ independent journal reviewers for $N = 93$ submitted manuscripts over a five-year period. Each reviewer classified each manuscript into one of $c = 3$ disjoint, ordered categories: reject, revise and resubmit, or accept. Table 6.35 lists the c^3 cross-classified observed frequencies

Table 6.35 Article recommendations by three independent reviewers for $N = 93$ manuscripts: reject, revise, and accept

Reviewer 1	Reviewer 2	Reviewer 3: Reject	Reviewer 3: Revise	Reviewer 3: Accept
Reject	Reject	6 (0) [0]	4 (2) [2]	2 (4) [8]
	Revise	3 (2) [2]	5 (2) [2]	4 (4) [6]
	Accept	2 (4) [8]	3 (4) [6]	4 (4) [8]
Revise	Reject	4 (2) [2]	5 (2) [2]	3 (4) [6]
	Revise	5 (2) [2]	8 (0) [0]	4 (2) [2]
	Accept	3 (4) [6]	2 (2) [2]	3 (2) [2]
Accept	Reject	1 (4) [8]	3 (4) [6]	4 (4) [8]
	Revise	3 (4) [6]	2 (2) [2]	2 (2) [2]
	Accept	1 (4) [8]	2 (2) [2]	5 (0) [0]

Note—Linear cell weights are in parentheses and quadratic cell weights are in brackets

and corresponding linear and quadratic weights, where the linear cell weights are given in parentheses and the quadratic cell weights are given in brackets.

Linear Weighting

For the observed data listed in Table 6.35 with linear cell disagreement weights, the observed value of weighted kappa is $\kappa_w = +0.1000$, indicating 10% agreement above that expected by chance, and the approximate Monte Carlo resampling probability value based on $L = 1{,}000{,}000$ random arrangements of cell frequencies with fixed marginal frequency totals is

$$P(\kappa_w \geq \kappa_o | H_0) = \frac{\text{number of } \kappa_w \text{ values } \geq \kappa_o}{L} = \frac{21{,}949}{1{,}000{,}000} = 0.0219 ,$$

where κ_o denotes the observed value of κ_w with linear weighting.

Quadratic Weighting

For the observed data listed in Table 6.35 with quadratic cell disagreement weights, the observed value of weighted kappa is $\kappa_w = +0.1036$, indicating approximately 10% agreement above that expected by chance, and the approximate Monte Carlo resampling probability value based on $L = 1{,}000{,}000$ random arrangements of cell frequencies with fixed marginal frequency totals is

$$P(\kappa_w \geq \kappa_o | H_0) = \frac{\text{number of } \kappa_w \text{ values } \geq \kappa_o}{L} = \frac{48{,}926}{1{,}000{,}000} = 0.0489 ,$$

where κ_o denotes the observed value of κ_w with quadratic weighting.

6.5.6 Advantages of Linear Weighting

In practice, linear and quadratic weighting schemes are the most widely used, to the point of near exclusivity [89, p. 162]. For two judges, linear *disagreement* weights and quadratic *disagreement* weights are given by

$$w_{ij} = |i - j| \quad \text{and} \quad w_{ij} = (i - j)^2 ,$$

respectively, for $i, j = 1, \ldots, c$. On the other hand, Cicchetti and Allison [11] proposed using linear *agreement* weights and Fleiss and Cohen [29] proposed using quadratic *agreement* weights given by

$$w_{ij} = 1 - \frac{|i - j|}{c - 1} \quad \text{and} \quad w_{ij} = 1 - \frac{(i - j)^2}{c - 1} ,$$

respectively, for $i, j = 1, \ldots, c$.

Cohen showed that if the marginal distributions of the two judges are the same and quadratic weights are used, weighted kappa is equivalent to Pearson's product-moment correlation coefficient [14]. Moreover, Fleiss and Cohen showed that, using quadratic weights, weighted kappa has the same interpretation as the intraclass correlation coefficient [29]. Fleiss and Cohen noted that the use of quadratic weights was "admittedly arbitrary," but argued that the scaling of errors by the means of their squares was so common that the convention required little justification [29, p. 617]. On the other hand, a number of researchers have argued that linear weighting is simpler and more intuitive than quadratic weighting [48].

Writing in *Statistical Methodology* in 2008, Vanbelle and Albert provided support for linear weighting, showing that using linear agreement weights for c ordered categories is equivalent to deriving unweighted kappa coefficients from $c-1$ embedded 2×2 contingency tables [89]. Given a $c \times c$ agreement table where p_{ij} denotes a cell proportion, $i, j = 1, \ldots, c$, $p_{i.}$ denotes a row marginal proportion, $i = 1, \ldots, c$, and $p_{.j}$ denotes a column marginal proportion, $j = 1, \ldots, c$, a weighted kappa coefficient can be defined in terms of linear agreement weights by

$$\kappa_w = \frac{p_o - p_e}{1 - p_e} ,$$

where

$$p_o = \sum_{i=1}^{c} \sum_{j=1}^{c} w_{ij} p_{ij} \quad \text{and} \quad p_e = \sum_{i=1}^{c} \sum_{j=1}^{c} w_{ij} p_{i.} p_{.j} ,$$

with $0 \le w_{ij} \le 1$, $w_{ii} = 1$ for $i = 1, \ldots, c$, and linear agreement weights given by

$$w_{ij} = 1 - \frac{|i - j|}{c - 1}$$

for $i, j = 1, \ldots, c$.

6.5.7 Embedded 2×2 Tables

Consider the notation of Vanbelle and Albert given in Table 6.36. Denote by a dot $(\cdot)$ the partial sum of all rows or all columns, depending on the position of the $(\cdot)$ in the subscript list. If the $(\cdot)$ is in the first subscript position, the sum is over all rows, and if the $(\cdot)$ is in the second subscript position, the sum is over all columns. Thus, $n_{i.}$ denotes the marginal frequency total of the ith row, $i = 1, \ldots, c$, summed over all columns, and $n_{.j}$ denotes the marginal frequency total of the jth column, $j = 1, \ldots, c$, summed over all rows. For any "cut-off" value k, $k = 1, \ldots, c-1$, the $c \times c$ classification table in Table. 6.36 can be reduced to a 2×2 contingency table by summing up all observations below and above the first k rows and the first k columns, as shown in Table 6.37, where

$$n_{11}(k) = \sum_{i=1}^{k} \sum_{j=1}^{k} n_{ij} \,, \quad n_{12}(k) = \sum_{i=1}^{k} \sum_{j=k+1}^{c} n_{ij} \,,$$

$$n_{21}(k) = \sum_{i=k+1}^{c} \sum_{j=1}^{k} n_{ij} \,, \quad n_{22}(k) = \sum_{i=k+1}^{c} \sum_{j=k+1}^{c} n_{ij} \,.$$

Example

To illustrate the Vanbelle and Albert procedure, consider the frequency data given in Table 6.38 where $N = 500$ objects have been placed into one of $c = 5$ disjoint, ordered categories by $b = 2$ independent judges; linear agreement cell weights are

Table 6.36 Notation for a two-way classification table resulting from the classification of N items by two judges on an ordinal scale with c categories

	Judge 2					
Judge 1	1	$\cdots$	j	$\cdots$	c	Total
1	n_{11}	$\cdots$	n_{1j}	$\cdots$	n_{1c}	$n_{1.}$
$\vdots$	$\vdots$	$\ddots$	$\vdots$	$\ddots$	$\vdots$	$\vdots$
i	n_{i1}	$\cdots$	n_{ij}	$\cdots$	n_{ic}	$n_{i.}$
$\vdots$	$\vdots$	$\ddots$	$\vdots$	$\ddots$	$\vdots$	$\vdots$
c	n_{c1}	$\cdots$	n_{cj}	$\cdots$	n_{cc}	$n_{c.}$
Total	$n_{.1}$	$\cdots$	$n_{.j}$	$\cdots$	$n_{.c}$	N

Table 6.37 Notation for the cross-classification of two categorical variables with $c = 2$ disjoint categories

	Judge 2		
Judge 1	$\leq k$	$> k$	Total
$\leq k$	$n_{11}(k)$	$n_{12}(k)$	$n_{1.}(k)$
$> k$	$n_{21}(k)$	$n_{22}(k)$	$n_{2.}(k)$
Total	$n_{.1}(k)$	$n_{.2}(k)$	N

given in parentheses. Using linear agreement weights, $p_o = 0.6350$, $p_e = 0.5858$, and weighted kappa for the frequency data given in Table 6.38 is

$$\kappa_w = \frac{p_o - p_e}{1 - p_r} = \frac{0.6350 - 0.5858}{1 - 0.5858} = +0.1188 ,$$

indicating approximately 12% agreement above that expected by chance.

Since $c = 5$, $c - 1 = 4$ embedded 2×2 tables can be constructed. The four embedded tables are given in Table 6.39. For the first 2×2 embedded table ($\leq 1, > 1$), $p_o(1) = 0.6400$, $p_e(1) = 0.5896$, and unweighted $\kappa(1)$ is

$$\kappa(1) = \frac{p_o(1) - p_e(1)}{1 - p_e(1)} = \frac{0.6400 - 0.5896}{1 - 0.5896} = +0.1228 ;$$

for the second 2×2 embedded table ($\leq 2, > 2$), $p_o(2) = 0.5080$, $p_e(2) = 0.5096$, and unweighted $\kappa(2)$ is

$$\kappa(2) = \frac{p_o(2) - p_e(2)}{1 - p_e(2)} = \frac{0.5080 - 0.5096}{1 - 0.5096} = -0.0033 ;$$

Table 6.38 Example two-way contingency table with two independent judges and $c = 5$ disjoint, ordered categories

	Judge 2					
Judge 1	1	2	3	4	5	Total
1	45 (1.00)	2 (0.75)	23 (0.50)	8 (0.25)	12 (0.00)	90
2	22 (0.75)	23 (1.00)	28 (0.75)	31 (0.50)	16 (0.25)	120
3	32 (0.50)	5 (0.75)	14 (1.00)	7 (0.75)	2 (0.50)	60
4	45 (0.25)	6 (0.50)	41 (0.75)	42 (1.00)	16 (0.75)	150
5	36 (0.00)	4 (0.25)	4 (0.50)	2 (0.75)	34 (1.00)	80
Total	180	40	110	90	80	500

Note—Linear agreement cell weights are in given parentheses

Table 6.39 All possible embedded 2×2 tables derived from the original 5×5 classification table given in Table 6.38

	Judge 2				Judge 2		
Judge 1	≤ 1	> 1	Total	Judge 1	≤ 2	> 2	Total
≤ 1	45	45	90	≤ 2	92	118	210
> 1	135	275	410	> 2	128	162	290
Total	180	320	500	Total	220	280	500
	Judge 2				Judge 2		
Judge 1	≤ 3	> 3	Total	Judge 1	≤ 4	> 4	Total
≤ 3	194	76	270	≤ 4	374	46	420
> 3	136	94	230	> 4	46	34	80
Total	330	170	500	Total	420	80	500

for the third 2×2 embedded table ($\leq 3, > 3$), $p_{\text{o}}(3) = 0.5760$, $p_{\text{e}}(3) = 0.5128$, and unweighted $\kappa(3)$ is

$$\kappa(3) = \frac{p_{\text{o}}(3) - p_{\text{e}}(3)}{1 - p_{\text{e}}(3)} = \frac{0.5760 - 0.5128}{1 - 0.5128} = +0.1297 ;$$

and for the fourth 2×2 embedded table ($\leq 4, > 4$), $p_{\text{o}}(4) = 0.8160$, $p_{\text{e}}(4) = 0.7312$, and unweighted $\kappa(4)$ is

$$\kappa(4) = \frac{p_{\text{o}}(4) - p_{\text{e}}(4)}{1 - p_{\text{e}}(4)} = \frac{0.8160 - 0.7312}{1 - 0.7312} = +0.3155 .$$

Then, averaging the observed and expected proportions yields,

$$p'_{\text{o}} = \frac{1}{c-1} \sum_{k=1}^{c-1} p_{\text{o}}(k) = \frac{0.64 + 0.5080 + 0.5760 + 0.8160}{5-1} = 0.6350$$

and

$$p'_{\text{e}} = \frac{1}{c-1} \sum_{k=1}^{c-1} p_{\text{e}}(k) = \frac{0.5896 + 0.5096 + 0.5128 + 0.7312}{5-1} = 0.5858 .$$

As expected, the p'_{o} and p'_{e} average values obtained from the $c - 1$ embedded 2×2 tables are equal to the p_{o} and p_{e} values obtained from the full 5×5 classification table given in Table 6.38.[10]

It should be noted that the average unweighted kappa coefficient derived from the 2×2 tables, namely

$$\bar{\kappa} = \frac{1}{c-1} \sum_{k=1}^{c-1} \kappa(k) = \frac{+0.1228 - 0.0033 + 0.1297 + 3155}{5-1} = +0.5647 ,$$

is not equal to $\kappa_w = +0.1188$ calculated on the full 5×5 classification table.

In this manner, Vanbelle and Albert showed that the observed and expected weighted agreements are merely the mean values of the corresponding proportions of all possible 2×2 embedded tables obtained by collapsing the first c categories and last $c - 1$ categories ($k = 1, \ldots, c - 1$) of the original $c \times c$ classification table. Thus, the linearly weighted kappa coefficient for a $c \times c$ ordinal table can simply be derived from non-weighted observed and expected agreements (or disagreements) computed from $c - 1$ embedded 2×2 tables.

[10]When using linear disagreement weights, instead of linear agreement weights, the weighted observed and expected disagreements are obtained by the sum rather than the average of the corresponding elements of the 2×2 contingency tables.

6.5.8 Embedded 2×2×2 Tables

Utilizing the linear agreement weights suggested by Cicchetti and Allison [11], Vanbelle and Albert [89] demonstrated that weighted kappa for $b = 2$ independent judges and $c \geq 3$ ordered categories is equivalent to deriving the weighted kappa coefficient from unweighted kappa coefficients computed on $c - 1$ embedded 2×2 classification tables. In 2009 Mielke and Berry generalized the results of Vanbelle and Albert to $b \geq 2$ independent judges [56]. While the generalized procedure is appropriate for any number of judges, in this section the description of the procedure and the example are confined to $b = 3$ independent judges to simplify presentation.

Consider N items classified into c disjoint, ordered categories by $b = 3$ independent judges. Judge 1 assigns the N items to the c ordered categories and Judges 2 and 3 independently assign the same N items to the same c ordered categories. Arrange the assignments of the $b = 3$ judges in a 3-way classification table dimensioned as c rows, c columns, and c slices, and index the assignments of Judges 1, 2, and 3 by $i, j, k = 1, \ldots, c$, respectively. The layout of a 3-way classification table with $c = 2$ rows, $c = 2$ columns, and $c = 2$ slices is portrayed in Table 6.40, where a dot $(\cdot)$ indicates a partial sum over either all rows, all columns, or all slices depending on the position of the $(\cdot)$ in the subscript list. If the $(\cdot)$ is in the first subscript position, the sum is over all rows, if the $(\cdot)$ is in the second subscript position, the sum is over all columns, and if the $(\cdot)$ is in the third subscript position, the sum is over all slices. Thus, $n_{i..}$ denotes the marginal frequency total of the ith row, $i = 1, \ldots, c$, summed over all columns and all slices, $n_{.j.}$ denotes the marginal frequency total of the jth column, $j = 1, \ldots, c$, summed over all rows and all slices, and $n_{..k}$ denotes the marginal frequency total of the kth slice, $k = 1, \ldots, c$, summed over all rows and all columns.

For any "cut-off" value ℓ for $\ell = 1, \ldots, c - 1$ a $c{\times}c{\times}c$ classification table can be reduced to a distinct 2×2×2 table by summing the observations below and above the first ℓ rows, the first ℓ columns, and the first ℓ slices, where the 2×2×2 table contains eight cells indexed by

$$n_{111}(\ell) = \sum_{i=1}^{\ell} \sum_{j=1}^{\ell} \sum_{k=1}^{\ell} n_{ijk}\,, \qquad n_{112}(\ell) = \sum_{i=1}^{\ell} \sum_{j=1}^{\ell} \sum_{k=1}^{\ell} n_{ijk}\,,$$

$$n_{121}(\ell) = \sum_{i=1}^{\ell} \sum_{j=1}^{\ell} \sum_{k=1}^{\ell} n_{ijk}\,, \qquad n_{211}(\ell) = \sum_{i=1}^{\ell} \sum_{j=1}^{\ell} \sum_{k=1}^{\ell} n_{ijk}\,,$$

Table 6.40 Example layout of a 3-way classification table with $c = 2$ rows, $c = 2$ columns, and $c = 2$ slices

	Slice 1			Slice 2		
	Col 1	Col 2	Total	Col 1	Col 2	Total
Row 1	n_{111}	n_{121}	$n_{1.1}$	n_{112}	n_{122}	$n_{1.2}$
Row 2	n_{211}	n_{221}	$n_{2.1}$	n_{212}	n_{222}	$n_{2.2}$
Total	$n_{.11}$	$n_{.21}$	$n_{..1}$	$n_{.12}$	$N_{.22}$	$n_{..2}$

$$n_{221}(\ell) = \sum_{i=1}^{\ell}\sum_{j=1}^{\ell}\sum_{k=1}^{\ell} n_{ijk} , \qquad n_{212}(\ell) = \sum_{i=1}^{\ell}\sum_{j=1}^{\ell}\sum_{k=1}^{\ell} n_{ijk} ,$$

$$n_{122}(\ell) = \sum_{i=1}^{\ell}\sum_{j=1}^{\ell}\sum_{k=1}^{\ell} n_{ijk} , \qquad n_{222}(\ell) = \sum_{i=1}^{\ell}\sum_{j=1}^{\ell}\sum_{k=1}^{\ell} n_{ijk} .$$

Let

$$f_{ijk(\ell)} = \frac{1}{N} n_{ijk}(\ell) ,$$

$$f_{i..(\ell)} = \frac{1}{N} n_{i..}(\ell) ,$$

$$f_{.j.(\ell)} = \frac{1}{N} n_{.j.}(\ell) ,$$

and

$$f_{..k(\ell)} = \frac{1}{N} n_{..k}(\ell) ,$$

represent the corresponding joint and marginal frequency totals for $i, j, k = 1, \ldots, c$ and $\ell = 1, \ldots, c-1$. Finally, denote by

$$p_{\text{o}}(\ell) = f_{111}(\ell) + f_{222}(\ell)$$

and

$$p_{\text{e}}(\ell) = f_{1..}(\ell) f_{.1.}(\ell) f_{..1}(\ell) + f_{2..}(\ell) f_{.2.}(\ell) f_{..2}(\ell)$$

the observed and expected proportions of agreement, respectively, corresponding to Table 6.41.

Table 6.41 Reduction of a $c \times c \times c$ classification table into a $2 \times 2 \times 2$ classification table utilizing cut-off level ℓ for $\ell = 1, \ldots, c-1$

	Judge 2			
	$\leq \ell$		$> \ell$	
	Judge 3		Judge 3	
Judge 1	$\leq \ell$	$> \ell$	$\leq \ell$	$> \ell$
$\leq \ell$	$n_{111}(\ell)$	$n_{112}(\ell)$	$n_{121}(\ell)$	$n_{122}(\ell)$
$> \ell$	$n_{211}(\ell)$	$n_{212}(\ell)$	$n_{221}(\ell)$	$n_{222}(\ell)$

Table 6.42 Three-way classification table with $b = 3$ judges, $c = 4$ disjoint, ordered categories, and $N = 56$ observations, with linear agreement weights in parentheses

		Judge 3			
Judge 1	Judge 2	1	2	3	4
1	1	3 (1.000)	0 (0.667)	0 (0.333)	1 (0.000)
	2	0 (0.667)	0 (0.667)	1 (0.333)	1 (0.000)
	3	0 (0.333)	1 (0.333)	1 (0.333)	0 (0.000)
	4	0 (0.000)	1 (0.000)	2 (0.000)	3 (0.000)
2	1	0 (0.667)	1 (0.667)	1 (0.333)	0 (0.000)
	2	1 (0.667)	3 (1.000)	1 (0.667)	0 (0.333)
	3	0 (0.333)	1 (0.667)	4 (0.667)	1 (0.333)
	4	0 (0.000)	0 (0.333)	1 (0.333)	2 (0.333)
3	1	0 (0.333)	0 (0.333)	1 (0.333)	1 (0.000)
	2	0 (0.333)	1 (0.667)	1 (0.667)	0 (0.333)
	3	1 (0.333)	0 (0.667)	1 (1.000)	0 (0.667)
	4	1 (0.000)	0 (0.333)	1 (0.667)	4 (0.667)
4	1	1 (0.000)	0 (0.000)	1 (0.000)	0 (0.000)
	2	1 (0.000)	2 (0.333)	1 (0.333)	0 (0.333)
	3	0 (0.000)	1 (0.333)	1 (0.667)	1 (0.667)
	4	0 (0.000)	1 (0.333)	1 (0.667)	3 (1.000)

Note—Linear cell agreement weights are in parentheses

Example

Consider $N = 56$ items classified by $b = 3$ independent judges into $c = 4$ disjoint, ordered categories and arranged in a 4×4×4 classification table. Table 6.42 lists the raw frequency data and the corresponding linear agreement weights in parentheses.

For the frequency data given in Table 6.42, $p_{\text{o}} = 0.9815$, and $p_{\text{e}} = 0.9780$, yielding

$$\kappa_w = \frac{p_{\text{o}} - p_{\text{e}}}{1 - p_{\text{e}}} = \frac{0.9815 - 0.9780}{1 - 0.9780} = +0.1594 ,$$

indicating approximating 16% agreement above that expected by chance. Since $c = 4$, $c - 1 = 3$ embedded 2×2×2 classification tables can be constructed from the full 4×4×4 classification table given in Table 6.42. Tables 6.43, 6.44, and 6.45 contain the three embedded 2×2×2 classification tables constructed from the frequency data given in Table 6.42.

For the first 2×2×2 embedded table, given in Table 6.43, $p_{\text{o}}(1) = 0.9866$, $p_{\text{e}}(1) = 0.9834$, and unweighted $\kappa(1)$ is

$$\kappa(1) = \frac{p_{\text{o}}(1) - p_{\text{e}}(1)}{1 - p_{\text{e}}(1)} = \frac{0.9866 - 0.9834}{1 - 0.9834} = +0.1945 ;$$

Table 6.43 First embedded 2×2×2 classification table

	Judge 2			
	≤ 1		> 1	
	Judge 3		Judge 3	
Judge 1	≤ 1	> 1	≤ 1	> 1
≤ 1	3	1	1	5
> 1	0	10	4	32

Table 6.44 Second embedded 2×2×2 classification table

	Judge 2			
	≤ 2		> 2	
	Judge 3		Judge 3	
Judge 1	≤ 2	> 2	≤ 2	> 2
≤ 2	8	5	5	5
> 2	3	14	4	12

Table 6.45 Third embedded 2×2×2 classification table

	Judge 2			
	≤ 3		> 3	
	Judge 3		Judge 3	
Judge 1	≤ 3	> 3	≤ 3	> 3
≤ 3	23	4	8	1
> 3	6	9	2	3

for the second 2×2×2 embedded table, given in Table 6.44, $P_o(2) = 0.9770$, $P_e(2) = 0.9809$, and unweighted $\kappa(2)$ is

$$\kappa(2) = \frac{p_o(2) - p_e(2)}{1 - p_e(2)} = \frac{0.9770 - 0.9809}{1 - 0.9809} = +0.1377\ ;$$

and for the third 2×2×2 embedded table, given in Table 6.45, $P_o(3) = 0.9809$, $P_e(3) = 0.9772$, and unweighted $\kappa(3)$ is

$$\kappa(3) = \frac{p_o(3) - p_e(3)}{1 - p_e(3)} = \frac{0.9809 - 0.9772}{1 - 0.9772} = +0.1592\ .$$

For the three 2×2×2 embedded tables in Tables 6.43, 6.44, and 6.45, define

$$p_o' = \frac{1}{c-1}\sum_{\ell=1}^{c-1} p_o(\ell) = \frac{0.9866 + 0.9770 + 0.9809}{4-1} = 0.9815$$

and

$$p_e' = \frac{1}{c-1}\sum_{\ell=1}^{c-1} p_e(\ell) = \frac{0.9834 + 0.9734 + 0.9772}{4-1} = 0.9870\ .$$

As expected, the p_o' and p_e' averaged values obtained from the $c - 1$ embedded $2 \times 2 \times 2$ tables are equal to the p_o and p_e values obtained from the full $4 \times 4 \times 4$ classification table given in Table 6.42. Finally, the average unweighted kappa coefficient derived from the embedded $2 \times 2 \times 2$ classification tables,

$$\bar{\kappa} = \frac{1}{c-1} \sum_{\ell=1}^{c-1} \kappa(\ell) = \frac{0.1945 + 0.1377 + 0.1592}{4-1} = +0.1638 \,,$$

is not equal to $\kappa_w = +0.1594$.

6.6 Alternative Approaches for Multiple Judges

In this section, five methods for determining probability values for kappa with multiple independent judges are compared and contrasted. Although the five methods are appropriate for any number of independent judges, the descriptions of the methods and the examples are confined to three judges to simplify presentation. Extension to more than three judges is straightforward for all five methods.

Consider b independent judges/raters, each of which classifies N objects into c disjoint categories. The five methods for calculating weighted kappa with $b \geq 2$ independent judges and $c \geq 2$ disjoint, ordered categories are (1) an exact variance method, (2) a resampling contingency table method, (3) an intraclass correlation method, (4) a randomized-block method, and (5) a resampling-block method [3]. A sixth method based on agreement values among all possible pairs of b judges is sometimes advanced; see articles by Fleiss [27], Light [51], Landis and Koch [50], Conger [15], Schouten [74, 75, 76], Kramer and Feinstein [47], Epstein, Dalinka, Kaplan, Aronchick, Marinelli, and Kundel [23], Herman, Khan, Kallman, Rojas, Carmody, and Bodenheimer [36], Taplin, Rutter, Elmore, Seger, White, and Brenner [86], Kundel and Polansky [49], and Schorer and Weiss [73]. However, the paired-judges agreement method is not considered here as the pairwise probability values are not orthogonal and cannot be combined into a single probability value [61].

6.6.1 *Exact Variance Method*

In 1968 Brian Everitt [24] derived the exact variance of weighted kappa for $b = 2$ independent judges under the null hypothesis that was suitable for any weighting scheme, but the calculations were deemed too complicated to be practical for routine use [28]. In 2005 Mielke, Berry, and Johnston reformulated the exact variance presented by Everitt for $b = 2$ independent judges into a form conducive to computation and provided a programming algorithm for $b = 2$ judges [57]. In 2007

Mielke, Berry, and Johnston extended the exact variance result developed by Everitt to include the classification of N objects by $b \geq 2$ independent judges with fixed marginal frequency totals [55]. Because any weighting scheme is allowed, asymmetric weighting schemes are permitted. For detailed discussions regarding choices of weighting schemes, see articles by Maclure and Willett [52], Graham and Jackson [33], Banerjee, Capozzoli, McSweeney, and Sinha [2], Kundel and Polansky [49], and Schuster and Smith [78].

Since

$$z = \frac{\kappa_w - \mathrm{E}[\kappa_w]}{\left[\mathrm{Var}(\kappa_w)\right]^{1/2}} ,$$

approaches the $N(0, 1)$ distribution as $N \to \infty$ with fixed positive marginal proportions, the approximate probability value (P) under the null hypothesis is given by $P(z \geq z_o)$, where

$$z_o = \frac{\kappa_o - \mathrm{E}[\kappa_w]}{\left[\mathrm{Var}(\kappa_w)\right]^{1/2}} ,$$

κ_o denotes the observed value of κ_w, and $\mathrm{E}[\kappa_w] = 0$.

6.6.2 Resampling Contingency Table Method

In the context of a multi-way contingency table with N objects cross-classified by $b \geq 2$ independent judges, a Monte Carlo resampling procedure generates L random samples, drawn with replacement, from all M possible, equally-likely arrangements of cell frequencies, given fixed marginal frequency totals, where L is usually set to a large number, e.g., $L = 1{,}000{,}000$ [39]. Mielke, Berry, and Johnston [58] developed Monte Carlo resampling algorithms to generate random contingency table cell frequency arrangements with fixed marginal frequency totals that permit any $b \geq 2$ independent judges, and Mielke, Berry, and Johnston [60] developed a resampling algorithm for weighted kappa that accommodates $b \geq 2$ independent judges (see Sect. 6.5.4). The resampling probability value (P) is simply the proportion of κ_w values among the L sampled κ_w values equal to or greater than κ_o, i.e.,

$$P = \frac{\text{number of } \kappa_w \text{ values } \geq \kappa_o}{L} .$$

If the exact probability value is not too small and L is large, Monte Carlo resampling methods provide highly accurate probability values. The Monte Carlo resampling contingency table method also allows for any weighting scheme as well as symmetric and asymmetric weights.

6.6.3 *Intraclass Correlation Method*

Provided that weighted kappa is confined to symmetric quadratic weights, Fleiss and Cohen [29] showed that a specific form of the intraclass correlation coefficient is identical to weighted kappa for $B = 2$ independent judges.[11] Extension of the Fleiss and Cohen intraclass correlation coefficient to B independent judges is straightforward [67, 68, 69]. Specifically, for a randomized-block design with $B \geq 2$ judges and N subjects, the intraclass correlation coefficient given by

$$ICC = \frac{MS_{\text{BS}} - MS_{\text{B}\times\text{S}}}{MS_{\text{BS}} + (B-1)MS_{\text{B}\times\text{S}} + B(MS_{\text{B}})/(N-1)} \tag{6.12}$$

is equivalent to weighted kappa with symmetric quadratic weighting, where MS_{BS}, MS_{B}, and $MS_{\text{B}\times\text{S}}$ refer to the subject, judge, and error mean squares, respectively. The approximate probability value is based on

$$F = \frac{MS_{\text{BS}}}{MS_{\text{B}\times\text{S}}} ,$$

which follows Snedecor's F distribution with $N-1$ and $(B-1)(N-1)$ degrees of freedom [67]. While there are many variations of the intraclass correlation coefficient described in the literature [53, 79], only the intraclass correlation coefficient defined in Eq. (6.12) yields the symmetric quadratic weighting version of weighted kappa.

6.6.4 *Randomized-Block Method*

In 1982 Mielke and Iyer [62] presented a permutation method to analyze randomized-block designs. The test statistic developed by Mielke and Iyer represents the observed proportion of disagreements and, for $b \geq 2$ and $c \geq 2$ disjoint, ordered categories, is given by

$$\delta = \left[N\binom{b}{2}\right]^{-1} \sum_{i=1}^{N} \sum_{j<k} \left[\sum_{l=1}^{c} \left(x_{ijl} - x_{ikl}\right)^2\right]^{v/2} , \tag{6.13}$$

where b is the number of independent judges, N is the number of subjects, x_{ijl} denotes the lth score of the jth judge for the ith of N subjects, x_{ikl} denotes the lth of c scores of the kth of b judges for the ith subject, $\sum_{j<k}$ is the sum over all

[11] In this section, the number of independent judges is denoted by an upper case B to be consistent with conventional randomized-block analysis of variance notation.

j and k such that $1 \leq j < k \leq b$, and $v > 0$ yields a symmetric weighting function. Under the null hypothesis, there are $M = (N!)^b$ equally-likely allocations of the N subjects to the b judges. Symmetric linear and quadratic weightings follow by setting $v = 1$ for linear weighting and $v = 2$ for quadratic weighting in Eq. (6.13). It is easily shown that statistics κ_w and δ are simple linear transformations of each other, i.e.,

$$\kappa_w = 1 - \frac{\delta}{\mu_\delta} \quad \text{and} \quad \delta = \mu_\delta(1 - \kappa_w) ,$$

where μ_δ is the average δ value under the null hypothesis. The exact probability value (P) is the proportion of κ_w values equal to or greater than the observed value of κ_w. Thus,

$$P = \frac{\text{number of } \kappa_w \text{ values } \geq \kappa_o}{M} ,$$

where κ_o denotes the observed value of κ_w.

6.6.5 Resampling-Block Method

The resampling-block method for multiple independent judges is identical to the randomized-block method, except for the calculation of the probability value. Thus, the same class of symmetric weighting functions is allowed. A Monte Carlo resampling procedure for $b \geq 2$ independent judges generates L random samples, drawn with replacement from all $M = (N!)^b$ possible, equally-likely arrangements of the classification values under the null hypothesis. The resampling probability value (P) is the proportion of κ_w values among the L sampled values of κ_w equal to or greater than the observed value of κ_w. Thus,

$$P = \frac{\text{number of } \kappa_w \text{ values } \geq \kappa_o}{L} ,$$

where κ_o denotes the observed value of κ_w.

6.6.6 Example with Three Judges

In this section the five methods to obtain probability values for Cohen's kappa with $b = 3$ independent judges are illustrated and compared, utilizing a small example data set. Symmetric unweighted, linear weighted, and quadratic weighted values are used to illustrate the five methods. Consider a data set with $b = 3$ independent judges, $N = 9$ subjects, and $c = 3$ disjoint, categories. The raw data are listed in Table 6.46 and the results of the five analyses are given in Table 6.47.

Exact permutation probability values to four places are listed in the last row of Table 6.47 for comparison purposes. It should be noted that calculation of exact probability values is not possible for the $b = 3$ data listed in Table 6.46 due to the large number of possible arrangements of subjects, i.e., $M = 131{,}681{,}894{,}400$. Thus, the "exact permutation" probability values listed in Table 6.47 are based on $L = 10{,}000{,}000{,}000$ randomizations of the $b = 3$ data listed in Table 6.46. Under a worst-case scenario with $P = 0.5$, the 95% confidence bounds are

$$\pm 2\left[\frac{P(1-P)}{L}\right]^{1/2} = \pm 2\left[\frac{(0.5)(0.5)}{10{,}000{,}000{,}000}\right]^{1/2} = \pm 1.00\times 10^{-5}\ ,$$

implying that the exact probability values reported in Table 6.47 are very likely accurate to four decimal places, since $P < 0.02$ for each weighting scheme [39].

Table 6.46 Example data set for kappa with multiple judges with $b = 3$ independent judges, $N = 9$ subjects, and $c = 3$ categories

	Judge		
Subject	*A*	*B*	*C*
1	1	1	1
2	1	1	2
3	1	2	1
4	2	2	2
5	2	3	2
6	3	2	3
7	3	3	3
8	3	3	3
9	3	3	1

Table 6.47 Cohen's kappa probability values (P) calculated with exact variance, resampling three-way contingency, intraclass correlation, randomized-block, resampling-block, and exact permutation procedures for $b = 3$ independent judges for symmetric unweighted, linear, and quadratic weightings

	Weighting					
	Unweighted		Linear		Quadratic	
Method	κ	P	κ_w	P	κ_w	P
Exact variance	0.3721	0.0012	0.5091	0.0008	0.5740	0.0021
Contingency table	0.3721	0.0159	0.5091	0.0043	0.5740	0.0062
Intraclass correlation					0.5740	0.0025
Randomized-block			0.5091	0.0035	0.5740	0.0061
Resampling-block			0.5091	0.0045	0.5740	0.0065
Exact permutation	0.3721	0.0161	0.5091	0.0043	0.5740	0.0063

6.6.7 Strengths and Limitations of the Five Methods

The five methods differ greatly in strengths and limitations. No single method is sufficiently flexible to address all important aspects of unweighted and weighted kappa for multiple judges. However, for a specific application, a researcher may well find one of the methods to be very satisfactory, despite its general limitations. The five summaries provided below are numbered for comparison purposes, where (1) considers weighting schemes, (2) considers the number of disjoint categories, (3) considers symmetric/asymmetric weights, (4) considers suitability for unweighted kappa, (5) considers suitability for weighted kappa, (6) considers the number of possible judges, (7) considers the nature of the probability value, (8) considers assumptions about the probability distribution, and (9) considers assumptions about the data distribution.

Exact Variance Method

1. Permits any weighting scheme.
2. Allows for $c \geq 2$ disjoint, ordered categories.
3. Accommodates both symmetric and asymmetric weights.
4. Is appropriate for unweighted kappa.
5. Is appropriate for weighted kappa.
6. Is highly cumbersome for $b \geq 5$ judges.
7. Provides an approximate asymptotic probability value.
8. Approaches the $N(0, 1)$ probability distribution of the standardized test statistic with fixed positive marginal proportions as $N \to \infty$.
9. Requires no distributional assumptions for the data.

Resampling Contingency Table Method

1. Permits any weighting scheme.
2. Allows for $c \geq 2$ disjoint, ordered categories.
3. Accommodates both symmetric and asymmetric weights.
4. Is appropriate for unweighted kappa.
5. Is appropriate for weighted kappa.
6. Is computationally intensive for $b \geq 7$ judges.
7. Provides a highly accurate Monte Carlo resampling probability value when the exact probability value is not too small.
8. Makes no assumptions about the probability distribution of the statistic.
9. Requires no distributional assumptions for the data.

Intraclass Correlation Method

1. Is restricted to quadratic weighting.
2. Allows for $c \geq 2$ disjoint categories.
3. Is limited to symmetric quadratic weights and is not appropriate for linear weighting.
4. Is not suitable for unweighted kappa.
5. Is appropriate for a specified weighted kappa.
6. Easily accommodates large numbers of judges.
7. Provides an approximate probability value if assumptions are not excessively violated.
8. Assumes the probability distribution of the statistic is Snedecor's F.
9. Assumes that the data were independently drawn from a normal distribution.

Randomized-Block Method

1. Permits any symmetric weighting scheme based on $v > 0$.
2. Allows for $c \geq 2$ disjoint categories.
3. Is limited to symmetric weights that include linear and quadratic weights when $v = 1$ and $v = 2$, respectively.
4. Is specifically suited for unweighted kappa when $b = 2$.
5. Is appropriate for a particular class of weighted kappa with $b \geq 2$.
6. Easily accommodates any number of judges for weighted kappa.
7. Provides an approximate probability value.
8. Makes no assumptions about the probability distribution of the statistic.
9. Requires no distributional assumptions for the data.

Resampling-Block Method

1. Permits any symmetric weighting scheme based on $v > 0$.
2. Allows for $c \geq 2$ disjoint categories.
3. Is limited to symmetric weights that include linear and quadratic weights when $v = 1$ and $v = 2$, respectively.
4. Is specifically suited for unweighted kappa when $b = 2$.
5. Is appropriate for a particular class of weighted kappa with $b \geq 2$.
6. Easily accommodates any number of judges for weighted kappa.
7. Provides a highly accurate Monte Carlo resampling probability value when the exact probability value is not too small.
8. Makes no assumptions about the probability distribution of the statistic.
9. Requires no distributional assumptions for the data.

6.6.8 Discussion

Fisher in 1935 [26] was the first to propose a permutation test that employed a reference set of test statistic values based on the actual observations, rather than their ranks [46]. Further work by Eden and Yates in 1933 [22], Hotelling and Pabst in 1936 [38], Pitman in 1937 and 1938 [64, 65, 66], Wald and Wolfowitz in 1944 [90], Hoeffding in 1952 [37], Box and Anderson in 1955 [8], Kempthorne in 1955 [40], Feinstein in 1973 [25], and others extended permutation tests to a wide variety of analytic problems. The initial motivation for permutation statistical methods was to validate asymptotic tests. Consequently, permutation methods have become the gold standard against which conventional parametric tests are tested and evaluated [1, 70]. Thus, the Monte Carlo resampling permutation contingency table method is the most versatile and accurate of the five methods for univariate data, provided that the number of judges is not too large. As summarized, *vide supra*, the resampling contingency table method permits any weighting scheme, accommodates both symmetric and asymmetric weights, is suitable for both unweighted and weighted kappa, makes no assumptions about the data distribution, and makes no assumptions about the probability distribution.

Finally, there are some concerns about the intraclass correlation method, in general, and quadratic symmetric weighting, in particular. Cicchetti and Fleiss [12, p. 200] noted that the intraclass correlation method, based as it is on the analysis of variance, assumes that the data are continuous. In addition, Graham and Jackson [33] observed that the use of symmetric quadratic weights for weighted kappa results in a measure of association, not agreement.

6.7 Ridit Analysis

In 1958 I.D.J. Bross introduced ridit scoring for the analysis of ordered categorical data where "ridit" is an acronym for *R*elative to an *I*dentified *D*istribution and the "it" represents a type of transformation similar to logit and probit [10]. Two applications of ridit analysis are common. The first compares treatment and control groups where the observed control group serves as a reference group and ridits are calculated for the c disjoint, ordered categories of the control group and applied to the c disjoint, ordered categories of the treatment group.

In the first application, the control group and corresponding ridits are treated as an infinite population and population parameters, respectively. The second application compares two independent treatment groups where neither treatment group is considered to be a reference group and ridits are calculated for the c disjoint, ordered category frequencies of each treatment group and applied to the c disjoint, ordered categories of the other treatment group. In this application, the $k = 2$ treatment groups are considered as independent finite samples, with neither identified as a reference group. The assumption of the second application that both groups are finite is more realistic. In 2009 Mielke, Long, Berry, and Johnston generalized ridit analysis for $k \geq 2$ independent treatment groups [63].

Consider a $c \times k$ cross-classification contingency table with c disjoint, ordered response categories and k unordered treatment groups. Following the notation of Bross, let m_{ij} denote the observed cell frequency of the ith row and jth column for $i = 1, \ldots, c$ and $j = 1, \ldots, k$, let

$$M_j = \sum_{i=1}^{c} m_{ij}$$

denote the unordered treatment frequency totals for $j = 1, \ldots, k$, and let

$$N = \sum_{i=1}^{c} \sum_{j=1}^{k} m_{ij}$$

denote the table frequency total for all ck cells. The ridit scores for the jth observed treatment, $j = 1, \ldots, k$, are given by

$$R_{1j} = \frac{m_{ij}}{2M_j}, \quad R_{2j} = \frac{m_{1j} + \dfrac{m_{2j}}{2}}{M_j}, \quad \ldots, \quad R_{cj} = \frac{m_{1j} + \cdots + m_{c-1,j} + \dfrac{m_{cj}}{2}}{M_j} .$$

Thus, the ridit score R_{ij} for the ith of c categories in the jth of k treatments is the proportion of observations in the categories below the ith category in the jth treatment, plus half the proportion of observations in the ith category of the jth treatment.

6.7.1 Example Calculations

For an example illustrating the calculation of ridit scores, consider the data given in Table 6.48. The graded categories in Table 6.48 refer to a scale of injuries suffered in automobile accidents. Column 1 of Table 6.48 is the frequency distribution in an identified treatment group. Column 2 is one-half of the corresponding entry in Column 1, e.g., for category None, $17/2 = 8.5$. Column 3 is the cumulative frequency of Column 1, displaced by one category downward, e.g., the frequency of 17 for category None in Column 1 is added to the frequency of 54 for category Minor in Column 1 and the frequency of 71 for Moderate in Column 3 is the sum of 17 and 54. Column 4 is the sum of Columns 2 and 3, e.g., for category Minor, $27.0 + 17 = 44.0$. Column 5 contains the ridit scores that are the entries in Column 4 divided by N, e.g., for category None, $8.5/179 = 0.0475$.

Table 6.48 Example calculation of ridit scores

	Column				
Category	1	2	3	4	5
None	17	8.5	0	8.5	0.0475
Minor	54	27.0	17	44.0	0.2458
Moderate	60	30.0	71	101.0	0.5642
Severe	19	9.5	131	140.5	0.7849
Serious	9	4.5	150	154.5	0.8631
Critical	6	3.0	159	162.0	0.9050
Fatal	14	7.0	165	172.0	0.9609
Total	179		179		

Define test statistic T as

$$T = \sum_{i=1}^{k-1} \sum_{j=i+1}^{k} \left| x_{ij} - x_{ji} \right| ,$$

where

$$x_{ij} = \sum_{k=1}^{c} \frac{R_{ki} m_{kj}}{M_j}$$

for $i, j = 1, \ldots, k$.

In the context of a k-treatment ridit analysis, exact permutation procedures examine all possible, equally-likely assignments of the N subjects to the c disjoint, ordered categories. Alternatively, Monte Carlo resampling permutation procedures examine a random subset selected from all possible assignments of the N subjects to the c disjoint, ordered categories. The null hypothesis of a permutation test specifies that all possible outcomes of the ridit analysis are equally likely.

Exact Permutation Procedures

The M_j subjects of the jth treatment group, $j = 1, \ldots, k$, are classified into c disjoint, ordered categories. Among the c^N equally-likely distinguishable assignment configurations under the null hypothesis, there are

$$W = \prod_{j=1}^{k} \binom{M_j + c - 1}{c - 1}$$

distinguishable partitions of the c^N assignment configurations of the k treatment groups. In a typical application, W and c^N are usually very large, e.g., with $c = k = 4$ and $M_1 = M_2 = M_3 = M_4 = 20$,

$$W = 9{,}837{,}262{,}146{,}481 \quad \text{and} \quad c^N = 1.4615 \times 10^{48} \ .$$

Therefore, an exact permutation analysis is generally not practical for ridit analyses with $k > 2$ treatments and Monte Carlo permutation procedures are recommended.

Resampling Permutation Procedures

A Monte Carlo resampling permutation procedure generates L sets of N random assignments selected with replacement from the c^N equally-likely assignment configurations of the k treatment groups. In general, $L = 1{,}000{,}000$ is sufficient to ensure three decimal places of accuracy [39]. For each of the L sets, counters for the c disjoint, ordered categories indexed by $i = 1, \ldots, c$ are set to zero and an independent uniform random variable U_j over $[0, 1)$ is generated for $j = 1, \ldots, N$. If U_j belongs to

$$\left[\frac{i-1}{c}, \frac{i}{c}\right) ,$$

the ith of c counters is increased by 1. The ridit test statistic T is then calculated for each of the L sets of N random assignments of the ordered category frequencies. Let T_o denote the observed value of T. Then given the resampling ridit statistics, $T_1, \ldots, T_L$, the resampling upper-tail probability value of T_o under the null hypothesis is given by

$$P = \frac{1}{L} \sum_{i=1}^{L} \Psi(T_i) \ ,$$

where

$$\Psi(T_i) = \begin{cases} 1 & \text{if } T_i \geq T_o \ , \\ 0 & \text{otherwise} \ . \end{cases}$$

6.7.2 *Example Ridit Analysis*

Consider an example ridit analysis with $c = 5$ disjoint, ordered categories and $k = 4$ treatment groups. Suppose that a medical researcher evaluates four post-surgery medications on $N = 149$ patients in a large hospital over a period of one year. Each patient received a robotic-assisted laparoscopic radical prostatectomy and was randomly assigned to one of $k = 4$ post-surgery groups. Patients in each treatment group were administered standard doses of one of four opioids: Fentanyl, Codeine, Oxycodone, or Morphine. Four hours after recovery, patients rated the effectiveness of the pain medication on a $c = 5$ point scale from Excellent to Poor. Table 6.49 lists the rating frequencies and associated ridit scores for each opioid, i.e., m_{ij} and R_{ij} for $i = 1, \ldots, c = 5$ and $j = 1, \ldots, k = 4$. At the completion of the research trial, for Fentanyl $M_1 = 36$, for Codeine $M_2 = 38$, for Oxycodone $M_3 = 38$, for Morphine $M_4 = 37$, and $N = 149$. For the ridit data listed in Table 6.49, based on $L = 1{,}000{,}000$ random arrangements of the observed data, the observed value of T is $T_o = 0.8420$ with an upper-tail probability value of $P = 0.0359$.

Once the k-treatment analysis is completed, researchers often look to compare all possible pairs of treatments. In this example, there are

$$\binom{k}{2} = \frac{k(k-1)}{2} = \frac{4(4-1)}{2} = 6$$

possible treatment pairs. Table 6.50 summarizes the results of the pairwise comparisons, where the probability values (in parentheses) for each comparison are based on $L = 1{,}000{,}000$ random arrangements of the observed data given in Table 6.49.

Table 6.49 Observed frequencies and associated ridit scores (in parentheses) for four post-surgery opioids

	Opioid			
Rating	Fentanyl	Codeine	Oxycodone	Morphine
Excellent	5 (0.0694)	4 (0.0526)	2 (0.0263)	3 (0.0405)
Good	9 (0.2639)	8 (0.2105)	16 (0.2632)	17 (0.3108)
Adequate	2 (0.4167)	3 (0.3553)	7 (0.5658)	4 (0.5946)
Weak	3 (0.4861)	15 (0.5921)	5 (0.7237)	5 (0.7162)
Poor	17 (0.7639)	8 (0.8947)	8 (0.8947)	8 (0.8919)
Sum	36	38	38	37

Table 6.50 Test statistic T and associated P values (in parentheses) for six pairwise treatment comparisons

Opioid	Codeine	Oxycodone	Morphine
Fentanyl	0.1031 (0.1160)	0.1674 (0.1301)	0.1944 (0.0925)
Codeine	–	0.1537 (0.1275)	0.1743 (0.1110)
Oxycodone	–	–	0.0491 (0.5037)

6.8 Coda

While Chap. 5 applied permutation statistical methods to measures of association designed for two ordinal-level variables based on pairwise comparisons between rank scores, Chap. 6 applied exact and Monte Carlo resampling permutation statistical methods to measures of association designed for two ordinal-level variables that are based on criteria other than pairwise comparisons between rank scores. Included in Chap. 6 were Spearman's rank-order correlation coefficient, Spearman's footrule measure of inter-rater agreement, Kendall's coefficient of concordance, Kendall's u measure of chance-corrected agreement, Cohen's weighted kappa measure of inter-rater agreement with linear and quadratic weightings, Vanbelle and Albert's analysis of embedded 2×2 contingency tables, and Bross's ridit analysis.

Chapter 7 examines exact and Monte Carlo resampling statistical permutation methods applied to measures of association for two variables at the interval level of measurement. Included in Chap. 7 are discussions of ordinary least squares (OLS regression), least absolute deviation (LAD) regression, point-biserial correlation, biserial correlation, intraclass correlation, and Fisher's z transform for skewed distributions.

References

1. Bakeman, R., Robinson, B.F., Quera, V.: Testing sequential association: Estimating exact p values using sampled permutations. Psychol. Methods **1**, 4–15 (1996)
2. Banerjee, M., Capozzoli, M., McSweeney, L., Sinha, D.: Beyond kappa: A review of interrater agreement measures. Can. J. Stat. **27**, 3–23 (1999)
3. Berry, K.J., Johnston, J.E., Mielke, P.W.: Weighted kappa for multiple raters. Percept. Motor Skill **107**, 837–848 (2008)
4. Berry, K.J., Mielke, P.W.: A generalization of Cohen's kappa agreement measure to interval measurement and multiple raters. Educ. Psychol. Meas. **48**, 921–933 (1988)
5. Berry, K.J., Mielke, P.W.: Extension of Spearman's footrule to multiple rankings. Psychol. Rep. **82**, 376–378 (1998)
6. Berry, K.J., Mielke, P.W.: Probabilities of the sum of N ranks assigned to one of K objects by N independent judges. Percept. Motor Skill **93**, 154–156 (2001)
7. Biggs, N.L.: The roots of combinatorics. Hist. Math. **6**, 109–136 (1979)
8. Box, G.E.P., Andersen, S.L.: Permutation theory in the derivation of robust criteria and the study of departures from assumption (with discussion). J. R. Stat. Soc. B Meth. **17**, 1–34 (1955)
9. Brenner, H., Kliebsch, U.: Dependence of weighted kappa coefficients on the number of categories. Epidemiology **7**, 199–202 (1996)
10. Bross, I.D.J.: How to use ridit analysis. Biometrics **14**, 18–38 (1958)
11. Cicchetti, D.V., Allison, A.: A new procedure for assessing reliability of scoring EEG sleep recordings. Am. J. EEG Technol. **11**, 101–109 (1971)
12. Cicchetti, D.V., Fleiss, J.L.: Comparison of the null distribution of weighted kappa and the C ordinal statistic. Appl. Psychol. Meas. **1**, 195–201 (1977)
13. Cohen, J.: A coefficient of agreement for nominal scales. Educ. Psychol. Meas. **20**, 37–46 (1960)

14. Cohen, J.: Weighted kappa: Nominal scale agreement with provision for scaled disagreement or partial credit. Psychol. Bull. **70**, 213–220 (1968)
15. Conger, A.J.: Integration and generalization of kappas for multiple raters. Psychol. Bull. **88**, 322–328 (1980)
16. Cowles, M.: Statistics in Psychology: An Historical Perspective, 2nd edn. Lawrence Erlbaum, Mahwah, NJ (2001)
17. David, F.N.: Studies in the history of probability and statistics: I. Dicing and gaming. Biometrika **42**, 1–15 (1955)
18. David, F.N.: Games, Gods, and Gambling: The Origin and History of Probability and Statistical Ideas from the Earliest Times to the Newtonian Era. Hafner, New York (1962)
19. de Moivre, A.: De mensura sortis, seu, de probabilitate eventuum in ludis a casu fortuito pendentibus. Phil. Trans. Roy. Soc. Lond. **27**(329), 213–264 (1711)
20. de Moivre, A.: Miscellanea Analytica de Seriebus et Quadraturis. Tonson & Watts, London (1730)
21. de Moivre, A.: The Doctrine of Chances or, A Method of Calculating the Probabilities of Events in Play, 2nd edn. Woodfall, London (1738)
22. Eden, T., Yates, F.: On the validity of Fisher's z test when applied to an actual example of non-normal data. J. Agric. Sci. **23**, 6–17 (1933)
23. Epstein, D.M., Dalinka, M.K., Kaplan, F.S., Aronchick, J.M., Marinelli, D.L., Kundel, H.L.: Observer variation in the detection of osteopenia. Skeletal. Radiol. **15**, 347–349 (1986)
24. Everitt, B.S.: Moments of the statistics kappa and weighted kappa. Brit. J. Math. Stat. Psy. **21**, 97–103 (1968)
25. Feinstein, A.R.: Clinical Biostatistics XXIII: The role of randomization in sampling, testing, allocation, and credulous idolatry (Part 2). Clin. Pharmacol. Ther. **14**, 898–915 (1973)
26. Fisher, R.A.: The Design of Experiments. Oliver and Boyd, Edinburgh (1935)
27. Fleiss, J.L.: Measuring nominal scale agreement among many raters. Psych. Bull. **76**, 378–382 (1971)
28. Fleiss, J.L., Cohen, J., Everitt, B.S.: Large sample standard errors of kappa and weighted kappa. Psychol. Bull. **72**, 323–327 (1969)
29. Fleiss, J.L., J, C.: The equivalence of weighted kappa and the intraclass coefficient as measures of reliability. Educ. Psychol. Meas. **33**, 613–619 (1973)
30. Fleiss, J.L., Levin, B., Paik, M.C.: Statistical Methods for Rates and Proportions, 5th edn. Wiley, New York (2003)
31. Franklin, L.A.: Exact tables of Spearman's footrule for $n = 11(1)18$ with estimate of convergence and errors for the normal approximation. Stat. Probab. Lett. **6**, 399–406 (1988)
32. Friedman, M.: The use of ranks to avoid the assumption of normality implicit in the analysis of variance. J. Am. Stat. Assoc. **32**, 675–701 (1937)
33. Graham, P., Jackson, R.: The analysis of ordinal agreement data: Beyond weighted kappa. J. Clin. Epidemiol. **46**, 1055–1062 (1993)
34. Hacking, I.: The Emergence of Probability: A Philosophical Study of Early Ideas About Probability, Induction and Statistical Inference. Cambridge University Press, Cambridge, UK (1975)
35. Hald, A.: A de Moivre: 'De mensura sortis' or 'On the measurement of chance'. Int. Stat. Rev. **52**, 229–262 (1984)
36. Herman, P.G., Khan, A., Kallman, C.E., Rojas, K.A., Carmody, D.P., Bodenheimer, M.M.: Limited correlation of left ventricular end-diastolic pressure with radiographic assessment of pulmonary hemodynamics. Radiology **174**, 721–724 (1990)
37. Hoeffding, W.: The large-sample power of tests based on permutations of observations. Ann. Math. Stat. **23**, 169–192 (1952)
38. Hotelling, H., Pabst, M.R.: Rank correlation and tests of significance involving no assumption of normality. Ann. Math. Stat. **7**, 29–43 (1936)
39. Johnston, J.E., Berry, K.J., Mielke, P.W.: Permutation tests: Precision in estimating probability values. Percept. Motor Skill **105**, 915–920 (2007)

40. Kempthorne, O.: The randomization theory of experimental inference. J. Am. Stat. Assoc. **50**, 946–967 (1955)
41. Kendall, M.G.: Studies in the history of probability and statistics: II. The beginnings of a probability calculus. Biometrika **43**, 1–14 (1956)
42. Kendall, M.G.: Rank Correlation Methods, 3rd edn. Griffin, London (1962)
43. Kendall, M.G., Babington Smith, B.: The problem of m rankings. Ann. Math. Stat. **10**, 275–287 (1939)
44. Kendall, M.G., Babington Smith, B.: On the method of paired comparisons. Biometrika **31**, 324–345 (1940)
45. Kendall, M.G., Kendall, S.F.H., Babington Smith, B.: The distribution of Spearman's coefficient of rank correlation in a universe in which all rankings occur an equal number of times. Biometrika **30**, 251–273 (1939)
46. Kennedy, P.E.: Randomization tests in econometrics. J. Bus. Econ. Stat. **13**, 85–94 (1995)
47. Kramer, M.S., Feinstein, A.R.: Clinical biostatistics: LIV. The biostatistics of concordance. Clin. Pharm. Therap. **29**, 111–123 (1981)
48. Krippendorff, K.: Bivariate agreement coefficients for reliability of data. In: Borgatta, E.F. (ed.) Sociological Methodology, pp. 139–150. Jossey–Bass, San Francisco (1970)
49. Kundel, H.L., Polansky, M.: Measurement of observer agreement. Radiology **228**, 303–308 (2003)
50. Landis, J.R., Koch, G.G.: The measurement of observer agreement for ordinal data. Biometrics **33**, 159–174 (1977)
51. Light, R.J.: Measures of response agreement for qualitative data: Some generalizations and alternatives. Psychol. Bull. **76**, 365–377 (1971)
52. Maclure, M., Willett, W.C.: Misinterpretation and misuse of the kappa statistic. Am. J. Epidemiol. **126**, 161–169 (1987)
53. McGraw, K.O., Wong, S.P.: Forming inferences about some intraclass correlation coefficients. Psychol. Meth. **1**, 30–46 (1996)
54. Mielke, P.W., Berry, K.J.: Cumulant methods for analyzing independence of r-way contingency tables and goodness-of-fit frequency data. Biometrika **75**, 790–793 (1988)
55. Mielke, P.W., Berry, K.J.: Permutation Methods: A Distance Function Approach, 2nd edn. Springer–Verlag, New York (2007)
56. Mielke, P.W., Berry, K.J.: A note on Cohen's weighted kappa coefficient of agreement with linear weights. Stat. Methodol. **6**, 439–446 (2009)
57. Mielke, P.W., Berry, K.J., Johnston, J.E.: A FORTRAN program for computing the exact variance of weighted kappa. Percept. Motor Skill **101**, 468–472 (2005)
58. Mielke, P.W., Berry, K.J., Johnston, J.E.: The exact variance of weighted kappa with multiple raters. Psychol. Rep. **101**, 655–660 (2007)
59. Mielke, P.W., Berry, K.J., Johnston, J.E.: Resampling programs for multiway contingency tables with fixed marginal frequency totals. Psychol. Rep. **101**, 18–24 (2007)
60. Mielke, P.W., Berry, K.J., Johnston, J.E.: Resampling probability values for weighted kappa with multiple raters. Psychol. Rep. **102**, 606–613 (2008)
61. Mielke, P.W., Berry, K.J., Johnston, J.E.: Unweighted and weighted kappa as measures of agreement for multiple judges. Int. J. Manag. **26**, 213–223 (2009)
62. Mielke, P.W., Iyer, H.K.: Permutation techniques for analyzing multi-response data from randomized block experiments. Commun. Stat. Theor. M **11**, 1427–1437 (1982)
63. Mielke, P.W., Long, M.A., Berry, K.J., Johnston, J.E.: g-treatment ridit analysis: Resampling permutation methods. Stat. Methodol. **6**, 223–229 (2009)
64. Pitman, E.J.G.: Significance tests which may be applied to samples from any populations. Suppl. J. R. Stat. Soc. **4**, 119–130 (1937)
65. Pitman, E.J.G.: Significance tests which may be applied to samples from any populations: II. The correlation coefficient test. Suppl. J. R. Stat. Soc. **4**, 225–232 (1937)
66. Pitman, E.J.G.: Significance tests which may be applied to samples from any populations: III. The analysis of variance test. Biometrika **29**, 322–335 (1938)

67. Rae, G.: On measuring agreement among several judges on the presence or absence of a trait. Educ. Psychol. Meas. **44**, 247–253 (1984)
68. Rae, G.: The equivalence of multiple rater kappa statistics and intraclass correlation coefficients. Educ. Psychol. Meas. **48**, 367–374 (1988)
69. Rajaratnam, N.: Reliability formulas for independent decision data when reliability data are matched. Psychometrika **25**, 261–271 (1960)
70. Read, T.R.C., Cressie, N.A.C.: Goodness-of-Fit for Discrete Multivariate Data. Springer–Verlag, New York (1988)
71. Salama, I.A., Quade, D.: A note on Spearman's footrule. Commun. Stat. Simul. C **19**, 591–601 (1990)
72. Savage, I.R.: Nonparametric statistics. J. Am. Stat. Assoc. **52**, 331–344 (1957)
73. Schorer, J., Weiss, C.: A weighted kappa coefficient for three observers as a measure for reliability of expert ratings on characteristics in handball throwing patterns. Meas. Physic. Educ. Exer. Sci. **11**, 177–187 (2007)
74. Schouten, H.J.A.: Measuring pairwise agreement among many observers. Biometrical J. **22**, 497–504 (1980)
75. Schouten, H.J.A.: Measuring pairwise agreement among many observers: II. Some improvements and additions. Biometrical J. **24**, 431–435 (1982)
76. Schouten, H.J.A.: Measuring pairwise interobserver agreement when all subjects are judged by the same observers. Stat. Neerl. **36**, 45–61 (1982)
77. Schuster, C.: A note on the interpretation of weighted kappa and its relations to other rater agreement statistics for metric scales. Educ. Psychol. Meas. **64**, 243–253 (2004)
78. Schuster, C., Smith, D.A.: Dispersion-weighted kappa: An integrative framework for metric and nominal scale agreement coefficients. Psychometrika **70**, 135–146 (2005)
79. Shrout, P.E., Fleiss, J.L.: Intraclass correlations: Uses in assessing rater reliability. Psychol. Bull. **86**, 420–428 (1979)
80. Siegel, S., Castellan, N.J.: Nonparametric Statistics for the Behavioral Sciences, 2nd edn. McGraw–Hill, New York (1988)
81. Spearman, C.E.: General intelligence, objectively determined and measured. Am. J. Psychol. **15**, 201–293 (1904)
82. Spearman, C.E.: The proof and measurement of association between two things. Am. J. Psychol. **15**, 72–101 (1904)
83. Spearman, C.E.: 'Footrule' for measuring correlation. Brit. J. Psychol. **2**, 89–108 (1906)
84. Strode, T.: An Arithmetical Treatise of the Combinations, Permutations, Elections, and Composition of Quantities: Illustrated by Several Examples, with a New Speculation of the Differences of the Powers of Numbers. Taylor, London (1693)
85. Stuart, A.: Spearman-like computation of Kendall's tau. Brit. J. Math. Stat. Psy. **30**, 104–112 (1977)
86. Taplin, S.H., Rutter, C.M., Elmore, J.G., Seger, D., White, D., Brenner, R.J.: Accuracy of screening mammography using single versus independent double interpretation. Am. J. Roentgenol. **174**, 1257–1262 (2000)
87. Todhunter, I.: A History of the Mathematical Theory of Probability: From the Time of Pascal to That of Laplace. Chelsea, Bronx, NY (1965/1865). [A 1965 textually-unaltered reprint of the 1865 original]
88. Ury, H.K., Kleinecke, D.C.: Tables of the distribution of Spearman's footrule. J. R. Stat. Soc. C Appl. **28**, 271–275 (1979)
89. Vanbelle, S., Albert, A.: A note on the linearly weighted kappa coefficient for ordinal scales. Stat. Methodol. **6**, 157–163 (2008)
90. Wald, A., Wolfowitz, J.: Statistical tests based on permutations of the observations. Ann. Math. Stat. **15**, 358–372 (1944)
91. Wallis, W.A.: The correlation ratio for ranked data. J. Am. Stat. Assoc. **34**, 533–538 (1939)

Chapter 7
Interval-Level Variables

Chapter 7 of *The Measurement of Association* applies exact and Monte Carlo permutation statistical methods to measures of association designed for two or more interval-level variables. While permutation statistical methods are commonly associated with non-parametric statistics and, therefore, thought by many to be limited to nominal- and ordinal-level measurements, such is certainly not the case, as noted by Feinstein in 1973 [12]. In fact, a great strength of exact and Monte Carlo permutation statistical methods is in the analysis of interval-level measurements [6]. Chapter 7 begins with a discussion and comparison of simple and multiple ordinary least squares (OLS) regression and simple and multiple least absolute deviation (LAD) regression using permutation statistical methods. Multiple regression with multiple independent variables and multivariate dependent variables is described and illustrated. Point-biserial and biserial correlation coefficients are described and analyzed with exact and Monte Carlo permutation methods. Fisher's z transform is examined and evaluated as to its utility in transforming skewed distributions for both hypothesis testing and confidence intervals. Chapter 7 concludes with a discussion of permutation statistical methods applied to Pearson's intraclass correlation coefficient.

7.1 Ordinary Least Squares (OLS) Linear Regression

Ordinary least squares (OLS) regression with a single predictor is a popular statistical measure of the degree of association (correlation) between two interval-level variables, usually denoted as x and y. The assumption of normality comes into play when the null hypothesis is tested by conventional means. Permutation statistical methods do not assume normality and, therefore, are often more useful than conventional statistical methods, especially when the sample size is small. Let r_{xy} denote the Pearson product-moment correlation coefficient for variables x and y

K. J. Berry et al., *The Measurement of Association*,
https://doi.org/10.1007/978-3-319-98926-6_7

given by

$$r_{xy} = \frac{\sum_{i=1}^{N}(x_i - \bar{x})(y_i - \bar{y})}{\sqrt{\left[\sum_{i=1}^{N}(x_i - \bar{x})^2\right]\left[\sum_{i=1}^{N}(y_i - \bar{y})^2\right]}} ,$$

where $\bar{x}$ and $\bar{y}$ denote the arithmetic means of variables x and y, respectively, and N is the number of bivariate measurements. The conventional test of significance is given by

$$t = \frac{r_{xy}\sqrt{N-2}}{\sqrt{1 - r_{xy}^2}} ,$$

which is distributed as Student's t with $N - 2$ degrees of freedom, under the assumption of normality.

More useful than simple OLS regression and correlation is multiple OLS regression with p predictors, $x_1, x_2, \ldots, x_p$. Let $R_{y.x_1,x_2,\ldots,x_p}$ indicate the multiple correlation coefficient for variables y and $x_1, x_2, \ldots, x_p$ given by

$$R^2_{x_1,x_2,\ldots,x_p} = \boldsymbol{\beta}'\mathbf{r}_y ,$$

where $\boldsymbol{\beta}'$ is the transposed vector of standardized regression weights and $\mathbf{r}_y$ is the vector of zero-order correlation coefficients of y with $x_1, x_2, \ldots, x_p$. The conventional test of significance is given by

$$F = \frac{(N - p - 1)R^2_{y.x_1,x_2,\ldots,x_p}}{p(1 - R^2_{y.x_1,x_2,\ldots,x_p})} ,$$

which is distributed as Snedecor's F with p and $N - p - 1$ degrees of freedom, under the assumption of normality.

7.1.1 Univariate Example of OLS Regression

Consider the example set of bivariate data listed in Table 7.1 for $N = 11$ subjects. For the bivariate data listed in Table 7.1, the Pearson product-moment correlation coefficient is $r_{xy} = +0.8509$. An exact permutation analysis requires random shuffles of either the x or the y values with the other set of values held constant.

Table 7.1 Example bivariate OLS correlation data on $N = 11$ subjects

Subject	x	y
1	11	4
2	18	11
3	12	1
4	27	16
5	15	5
6	21	9
7	25	10
8	15	2
9	18	8
10	23	7
11	12	3

For this small example there are

$$M = N! = 11! = 39{,}916{,}800$$

possible, equally-likely arrangements in the reference set of all permutations of the observed bivariate data, making an exact permutation analysis feasible. Monte Carlo resampling methods are generally preferred for permutation correlation analyses since $N!$ is usually a very large number, e.g., with $N = 13$ there are $13! = 6{,}227{,}020{,}800$ possible arrangements. Let r_o indicate the observed value of r_{xy}. Then, based on $L = 1{,}000{,}000$ random arrangements of the observed data under the null hypothesis, there are 861 $|r_{xy}|$ values equal to or greater than $|r_o| = 0.8509$, yielding a Monte Carlo resampling two-sided probability value of $P = 861/1{,}000{,}000 = 0.8610{\times}10^{-3}$.

While $M = 39{,}916{,}800$ possible arrangements of the observed data makes an exact permutation analysis impractical, it is not impossible. Based on the $M = 39{,}916{,}800$ arrangements of the observed data under the null hypothesis, there are 35,216 $|r_{xy}|$ values equal to or greater than $|r_o| = 0.8509$, yielding an exact two-sided probability value of $P = 35{,}216/39{,}916{,}800 = 0.8822{\times}10^{-3}$. For comparison, for the data listed in Table 7.1 $t = 4.8591$ and the two-sided probability value of $|r_o| = 0.8509$ based on Student's t distribution with $N - 2 = 11 - 2 = 9$ degrees of freedom is $P = 0.8969{\times}10^{-3}$.

7.1.2 Multivariate Example of OLS Regression

For a multivariate example of OLS linear regression, consider the small example data set with $p = 2$ predictors listed in Table 7.2 where variable y is Weight in pounds, variable x_1 is Height in inches, and variable x_2 is Age in years for $N = 12$ school children. For the multivariate data listed in Table 7.2, the unstandardized

Table 7.2 Example multivariate OLS correlation data on $N = 12$ children

Child	x_1	x_2	y
1	57	8	64
2	59	10	71
3	49	6	53
4	62	11	67
5	51	8	55
6	50	7	58
7	55	10	77
8	48	9	57
9	52	6	56
10	42	12	51
11	61	9	76
12	57	9	68

OLS regression coefficients are

$$\hat{\beta}_1 = +1.1973 \quad \text{and} \quad \hat{\beta}_2 = +1.1709\,,$$

and the squared OLS multiple correlation coefficient is $R^2_{y.x_1,x_2} = 0.7301$ (henceforth, simply R^2). An exact permutation analysis of multiple correlation requires random shuffles of either the x or the y values. It is important to note that the predictor variables must be shuffled as a unit, i.e., $x_1, \ldots, x_p$. Otherwise, a researcher may end up with a combination of predictor variables that make no sense, e.g., 4-year-old child, married, with two children. Thus, it is advisable to simply shuffle the y values. Even with this very small example there are

$$M = N! = 12! = 479{,}001{,}600$$

possible, equally-likely arrangements of the observed data, making an exact permutation analysis impractical. Based on $L = 1{,}000{,}000$ random arrangements of the observed data, the Monte Carlo resampling probability of $R^2 = 0.7301$ is

$$P(R^2 \geq R^2_{\text{o}} | H_0) = \frac{\text{number of } R^2 \text{ values } \geq R^2_{\text{o}}}{L} = \frac{2{,}370}{1{,}000{,}000} = 0.2370 \times 10^{-2}\,,$$

where R^2_{o} denotes the observed value of R^2.

While $M = 479{,}001{,}600$ possible arrangements makes an exact permutation analysis impractical, it is not impossible. If the reference set of all possible permutations of the observed scores in Table 7.2 occur with equal chance, the exact probability of $R^2 = 0.7301$ under the null hypothesis is

$$P(R^2 \geq R_o^2 | H_0) = \frac{\text{number of } R^2 \text{ values } \geq R_o^2}{M} = \frac{1{,}147{,}714}{479{,}001{,}600} = 0.2396 \times 10^{-2} ,$$

where R_o^2 denotes the observed value of R^2. For comparison, for the data listed in Fig. 7.2, $F = 12.1728$ and the probability value of $R^2 = 0.7301$ based on Snedecor's F distribution with $p, N - p - 1 = 2, 12 - 2 - 1 = 2, 9$ degrees of freedom is approximately $P = 0.2757 \times 10^{-2}$, under the null hypothesis.

7.2 Least Absolute Deviation (LAD) Regression

Ordinary least squares (OLS) linear regression has long been recognized as a useful tool in many areas of research. The optimal properties of OLS linear regression are well known when the errors are normally distributed. In practice, however, the assumption of normality is rarely justified. Least absolute deviation (LAD) linear regression is often superior to OLS linear regression when the errors are not normally distributed [8, 9, 29, 44, 55]. Estimators of OLS regression parameters can be severely affected by unusual values in either the criterion variable or in one or more of the predictor variables, which is largely due to the weight given to each data point when minimizing the sum of squared errors. In contrast, LAD regression is less sensitive to the effects of unusual values because the errors are not squared. The comparison between OLS and LAD linear regression is analogous to the effect of extreme values on the mean and median as measures of location [8]. In this section, the robust nature of least absolute linear regression is illustrated with a simple example and the effects of distance, leverage, and influence are examined. For clarity and efficiency, the illustration and ensuing discussion are limited to simple linear regression with one predictor variable (x) and one criterion variable (y), with no loss of generality.

Consider N paired x_i and y_i observed values for $i = 1, \ldots, N$. For the OLS regression equation given by

$$\hat{y}_i = \hat{\alpha}_{yx} + \hat{\beta}_{yx} x_i ,$$

where $\hat{y}_i$ is the ith of N predicted criterion values and x_i is the ith of N predictor values, $\hat{\alpha}_{yx}$ and $\hat{\beta}_{yx}$ are the OLS parameter estimates of the intercept (α_{yx}) and slope

(β_{yx}), respectively, and are given by

$$\hat{\beta}_{yx} = \frac{\sum_{i=1}^{N} (y_i - \bar{y})(x_i - \bar{x})}{\sum_{i=1}^{N} (x_i - \bar{x})^2} \tag{7.1}$$

and

$$\hat{\alpha}_{yx} = \bar{y} - \hat{\beta}_{yx}\bar{x} \ , \tag{7.2}$$

where $\bar{x}$ and $\bar{y}$ are the sample means of variables x and y, respectively. Estimates of OLS regression parameters minimize the sum of the squared differences between the observed and predicted criterion values, i.e.,

$$\sum_{i=1}^{N} (y_i - \hat{y}_i)^2 \ .$$

For the LAD regression equation given by

$$\tilde{y}_i = \tilde{\alpha}_{yx} + \tilde{\beta}_{yx} x_i \ ,$$

where $\tilde{y}_i$ is the ith of N predicted criterion values and x_i is the ith of N predictor values, $\tilde{\alpha}_{yx}$ and $\tilde{\beta}_{yx}$ are the LAD parameter estimates of the intercept (α_{yx}) and slope (β_{yx}), respectively.[1] Unlike OLS regression, no simple expressions can be given for $\tilde{\alpha}_{yx}$ and $\tilde{\beta}_{yx}$, as for OLS regression in Eqs. (7.1) and (7.2). However, values for $\tilde{\alpha}_{yx}$ and $\tilde{\beta}_{yx}$ may be found through an efficient linear programming algorithm, such as provided by Barrodale and Roberts [1, 2]. In contrast to estimates of OLS regression parameters, estimates of LAD regression parameters minimize the sum of the absolute differences between the observed and predicted criterion values, i.e.,

$$\sum_{i=1}^{N} |y_i - \tilde{y}_i| \ .$$

[1]In this chapter, a caret (∧) over a symbol such as $\hat{\alpha}$ or $\hat{\beta}$ indicates an OLS regression model predicted value of a corresponding population parameter, while a tilde (~) over a symbol such as $\tilde{\alpha}$ or $\tilde{\beta}$ indicates a LAD regression model predicted value of a corresponding population parameter.

It is convenient to have a measure of agreement, not correlation, between the observed and predicted y values. Let

$$\delta = \frac{1}{N} \sum_{i=1}^{N} \left| y_i - \tilde{y}_i \right| .$$

Then, the expected value of δ is given by

$$\mu_\delta = \frac{1}{N^2} \sum_{i=1}^{N} \sum_{j=1}^{N} \left| y_i - \tilde{y}_j \right| ,$$

and a measure of agreement between the observed y values and the predicted $\tilde{y}$ values is given by

$$\Re = 1 - \frac{\delta}{\mu_\delta} .$$

$\Re$ is a chance-corrected measure of agreement and/or effect size, reflecting the amount of agreement in excess of what would be expected by chance. $\Re$ attains a maximum value of unity when the agreement between the observed y values and the predicted $\tilde{y}$ values is perfect, i.e., y_i and $\tilde{y}_i$ values are identical for $i = 1, \ldots, N$. $\Re$ is zero when the agreement between the observed y values and predicted $\tilde{y}$ values is equal to what is expected by chance, i.e., $\mathrm{E}[\Re | H_0] = 0$. Like all chance-corrected measures, $\Re$ will occasionally be slightly negative when agreement is less than what is expected by chance.

7.2.1 Illustration of Effects of Extreme Values

Three useful diagnostics for assessing the potential effects of extreme values on regression estimators are distance, leverage, and influence. In general terms, *distance* refers to the possible presence of unusual values in the criterion variable and is typically measured as the deviation of a value from the measured center of the criterion variable (y). *Leverage* refers to the possible presence of unusual values in a predictor variable. In the case of a single predictor, leverage is typically measured as the deviation of a value from the measured center of the predictor variable (x). *Influence* incorporates both distance and leverage and refers to the possible presence of unusual values in some combination of the criterion and predictor variables.

For OLS regression, the measure of distance for any data point is simply an error term or residual, i.e., $e_i = y_i - \hat{y}_i$ and is sometimes standardized and sometimes Studentized. Leverage is a measure of the importance of the ith observation in determining the model fit and is usually designated as h_i. More specifically, h_i is the ith diagonal element of the $N \times N$ matrix

$$\mathbf{H} = \mathbf{X}\left(\mathbf{X}'\mathbf{X}\right)^{-1}\mathbf{X}'$$

called the "hat matrix," since $\hat{\mathbf{y}} = \mathbf{H}\mathbf{y}$ in which $\hat{\mathbf{y}}$ is the transposed column vector

$$\hat{\mathbf{y}} = \left(\hat{y}_1, \hat{y}_2, \ldots, \hat{y}_N\right)' \quad \text{and} \quad \mathbf{y} = (y_1, y_2, \ldots, y_N)' .$$

In the case of only one predictor, leverage is simply a function of the deviation of an x score on that predictor from the prediction mean and is given by

$$h_i = \frac{1}{N} + \frac{(x_i - \bar{x})^2}{(N-1)s_x^2} \qquad \text{for } i = 1, \ldots, N ,$$

where s_x^2 is the estimated population variance for variable x given by

$$s_x^2 = \frac{1}{N-1}\sum_{i=1}^{N}\left(x_i - \bar{x}\right)^2 .$$

Influence combines both leverage and distance, measured as a Studentized residual, to identify unusually influential observations. Residuals are sometimes standardized and sometimes Studentized. Standardized residuals are given by

$$z_i = \frac{e_i}{s_{y.x}} \qquad \text{for } i = 1, \ldots, N ,$$

where $e_i = y_i - \hat{y}_i$ for $i = 1, \ldots, N$ is the unstandardized residual and

$$s_{y.x} = \left(\frac{1}{N-p-1}\sum_{i=1}^{N} e_i^2\right)^{1/2}$$

is the standard error of estimate. Standardized residuals have a mean of zero and a variance of one. Studentized residuals are given by

$$r_i = \frac{e_i}{s_{y.x}\sqrt{1-h_i}} = \frac{z_i}{\sqrt{1-h_i}} \qquad \text{for } i = 1, \ldots, N .$$

Studentized residuals follow Student's t distribution with mean near zero and variance slightly greater than one.

The most common measure of influence is Cook's distance given by

$$d_i = \left(\frac{1}{p+1}\right) r_i^2 \left(\frac{h_i}{1-h_i}\right) ,$$

where r_i^2 denotes the squared Studentized residual and p is the number of predictor variables.

To illustrate the effects of extreme values on the estimates of OLS and LAD regression parameters, consider an example of linear regression with one predictor and a single extreme data point. This simplified example permits the isolation and assessment of distance, leverage, and influence and allows comparison of the effects of an atypical value on estimates of OLS and LAD regression parameters. The data for a linear regression with one predictor variable are listed in Table 7.3. The bivariate data listed in Table 7.3 consist of nine data points with $x_i = i$ and $y_i = 10 - i$ for $i = 1, \ldots, 9$ and describe a perfect negative linear relationship. Figure 7.1 displays the example bivariate data listed in Table 7.3 and indicates the directions of unusual values implicit in distance (D), leverage (L), and influence (I).

Table 7.3 Example bivariate data on $N = 9$ objects for a perfect negative linear regression with one predictor variable

	Object								
Variable	1	2	3	4	5	6	7	8	9
x	3	6	1	8	5	9	2	4	7
y	7	4	9	2	5	1	8	6	3

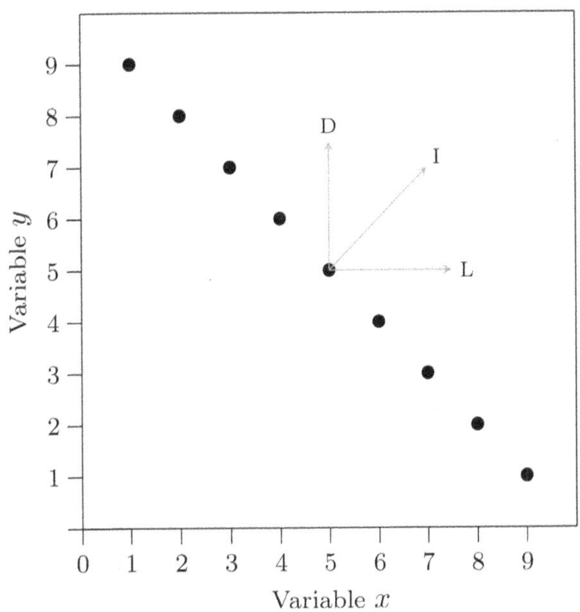

Fig. 7.1 Scatterplot of the data given in Table 7.3 with the directions of extreme values indicated by D, I, and L for distance, influence, and leverage, respectively

Distance

If a tenth bivariate value is added to the nine bivariate values given in Table 7.3 where $(x_{10}, y_{10}) = (5, 5)$, the new data point is located at the common mean and median of both variable x and variable y and, therefore, does not affect the perfect linear relationship between the variables. If x_{10} is held constant at $x_{10} = 5$, but y_{10} takes on the added values of 6, 7, …, 30, 40, 60, 80, and 100, then the effects of distance on the two regression models can be observed. The vertical movement of y_{10} with variable x held constant at $x_{10} = 5$ is depicted by the directional arrow labeled "D" in Fig. 7.1 and by the four white circles in Fig. 7.2, illustrating an additional data point moving vertically away from location $(x_5, y_5) = (5, 5)$ by increments of one y unit, i.e., (5, 6), (5, 7), (5, 8), and so on.

Table 7.4 lists the values for x_{10} and y_{10} in the first two columns, the $\hat{\alpha}_{yx}$ and $\hat{\beta}_{yx}$ estimates of the OLS regression parameters in the next two columns, and the $\tilde{\alpha}_{yx}$ and $\tilde{\beta}_{yx}$ estimates of the LAD regression parameters in the last two columns. The $\tilde{\alpha}_{yx}$ and $\tilde{\beta}_{yx}$ parameter estimates in the last two columns of Table 7.4 were obtained using the linear program of Barrodale and Roberts [2]. The estimates of the OLS regression parameters listed in Table 7.4 demonstrate that $\hat{\alpha}_{yx}$ systematically changes with increases in distance, but $\hat{\beta}_{yx}$ remains constant at −1.00. In contrast, estimates of the LAD regression parameters are unaffected by changes in distance, remaining constant at $\tilde{\alpha}_{yx} = 10.00$ and $\tilde{\beta}_{yx} = -1.00$ for $x_{10} = 5$ and any value of y_{10}. Given the nine bivariate data points listed in Table 7.3 and an additional

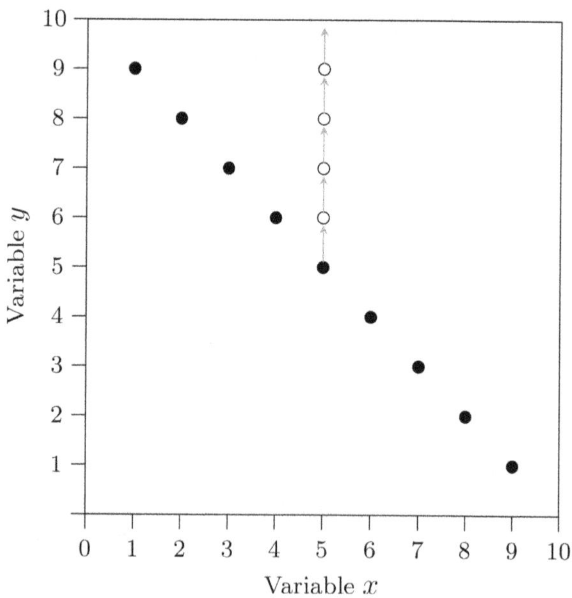

Fig. 7.2 Scatterplot of the data given in Table 7.3 with the locations of an added tenth value indicated by four white circles

Table 7.4 Effects of distance on intercepts and slopes of OLS and LAD linear regression models

		OLS model		LAD model	
x_{10}	y_{10}	$\hat{\alpha}_{yx}$	$\hat{\beta}_{yx}$	$\tilde{\alpha}_{yx}$	$\tilde{\beta}_{yx}$
5	5	+10.0000	−1.0000	+10.0000	−1.0000
5	6	+10.1000	−1.0000	+10.0000	−1.0000
5	7	+10.2000	−1.0000	+10.0000	−1.0000
5	8	+10.3000	−1.0000	+10.0000	−1.0000
5	9	+10.4000	−1.0000	+10.0000	−1.0000
5	10	+10.5000	−1.0000	+10.0000	−1.0000
5	11	+10.6000	−1.0000	+10.0000	−1.0000
5	12	+10.7000	−1.0000	+10.0000	−1.0000
5	13	+10.8000	−1.0000	+10.0000	−1.0000
5	14	+10.9000	−1.0000	+10.0000	−1.0000
5	15	+11.0000	−1.0000	+10.0000	−1.0000
5	16	+11.1000	−1.0000	+10.0000	−1.0000
5	17	+11.2000	−1.0000	+10.0000	−1.0000
5	18	+11.3000	−1.0000	+10.0000	−1.0000
5	19	+11.4000	−1.0000	+10.0000	−1.0000
5	20	+11.5000	−1.0000	+10.0000	−1.0000
5	21	+11.6000	−1.0000	+10.0000	−1.0000
5	22	+11.7000	−1.0000	+10.0000	−1.0000
5	23	+11.8000	−1.0000	+10.0000	−1.0000
5	24	+11.9000	−1.0000	+10.0000	−1.0000
5	25	+12.0000	−1.0000	+10.0000	−1.0000
5	26	+12.1000	−1.0000	+10.0000	−1.0000
5	27	+12.2000	−1.0000	+10.0000	−1.0000
5	28	+12.3000	−1.0000	+10.0000	−1.0000
5	29	+12.4000	−1.0000	+10.0000	−1.0000
5	30	+12.5000	−1.0000	+10.0000	−1.0000
5	40	+13.5000	−1.0000	+10.0000	−1.0000
5	60	+15.5000	−1.0000	+10.0000	−1.0000
5	80	+17.5000	−1.0000	+10.0000	−1.0000
5	100	+19.5000	−1.0000	+10.0000	−1.0000

bivariate data point with $x_{10} = 5$, it follows that

$$\sum_{i=1}^{10} |y_i - \tilde{y}_i| = |y_{10} - 5| \;.$$

Leverage

If a tenth bivariate value is added to the nine bivariate values given in Table 7.3 where $y_{10} = 5$ and x_{10} takes on the added values of 6, 7, …, 30, 40, 60, 80, and 100, then the effects of leverage on the two regression models can be observed.

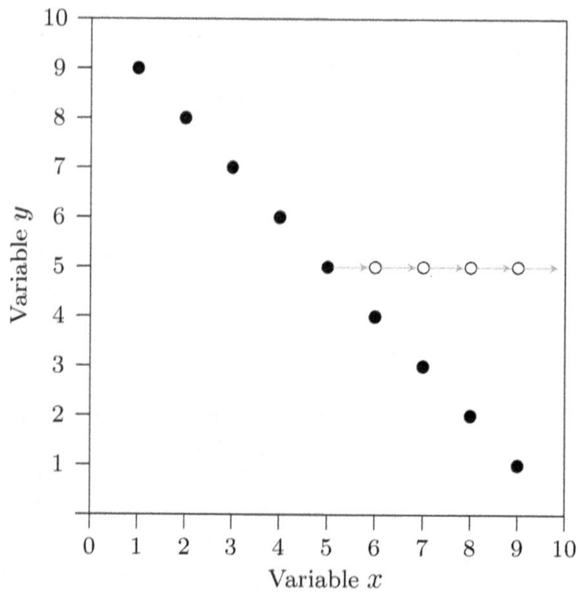

Fig. 7.3 Scatterplot of the data given in Table 7.3 with the locations of an added tenth value indicated by four white circles

The horizontal movement of x_{10} with y_{10} held constant at $y_{10} = 5$ is depicted by the directional arrow labeled "L" in Fig. 7.1 and by the four white circles in Fig. 7.3, illustrating an additional data point moving horizontally away from $(x_5, y_5) = (5, 5)$ by increments of one x unit, i.e., $(6, 5)$, $(7, 5)$, $(8, 5)$, and so on.

Table 7.5 lists the values of x_{10} and y_{10} in the first two columns, the $\hat{\alpha}_{yx}$ and $\hat{\beta}_{yx}$ estimates of the OLS regression parameters in the next two columns, and the $\tilde{\alpha}_{yx}$ and $\tilde{\beta}_{yx}$ estimates of the LAD regression parameters in the last two columns. The $\tilde{\alpha}_{yx}$ and $\tilde{\beta}_{yx}$ estimates were again obtained using the linear program of Barrodale and Roberts [2]. The estimates of the OLS regression parameters listed in Table 7.5 demonstrate that both $\hat{\alpha}_{yx}$ and $\hat{\beta}_{yx}$ exhibit complex changes with increases in leverage. Note the dramatic changes in the intercept from $\hat{\alpha}_{yx} = +10.00$ to $\hat{\alpha}_{yx} = +5.1063$, approaching the mean of y (+5.00), and the slope from $\hat{\beta}_{yx} = -1.00$ to $\hat{\beta}_{yx} = -0.0073$, approaching a slope of zero. In contrast, $\tilde{\alpha}_{yx}$ and $\tilde{\beta}_{yx}$ are unaffected for $y_{10} = 5$ and $5 \leq x_{10} \leq 24$. For $y_{10} = 5$ and $x_{10} \geq 26$, the LAD estimated regression parameters change from $\tilde{\alpha}_{yx} = +10.00$ and $\tilde{\beta}_{yx} = -1.00$ to $\tilde{\alpha}_{yx} = +5.00$ and $\tilde{\beta}_{yx} = 0.00$.

Given the bivariate data listed in Table 7.3 on p. 379 and an additional bivariate data point with variable y held constant at $y_{10} = 5$, it follows that

$$\sum_{i=1}^{10} \left| y_i - \tilde{y}_i \right| \leq 20.00$$

Table 7.5 Effects of leverage on intercepts and slopes of OLS and LAD linear regression models

		OLS model		LAD model	
x_{10}	y_{10}	$\hat{\alpha}_{yx}$	$\hat{\beta}_{yx}$	$\tilde{\alpha}_{yx}$	$\tilde{\beta}_{yx}$
5	5	+10.0000	−1.0000	+10.0000	−1.0000
6	5	+10.0246	−0.9852	+10.0000	−1.0000
7	5	+9.9057	−0.9434	+10.0000	−1.0000
8	5	+9.6696	−0.8811	+10.0000	−1.0000
9	5	+9.3548	−0.8065	+10.0000	−1.0000
10	5	+9.0000	−0.7273	+10.0000	−1.0000
11	5	+8.6364	−0.6494	+10.0000	−1.0000
12	5	+8.2853	−0.5764	+10.0000	−1.0000
13	5	+7.9592	−0.5102	+10.0000	−1.0000
14	5	+7.6637	−0.4515	+10.0000	−1.0000
15	5	+7.4000	−0.4000	+10.0000	−1.0000
16	5	+7.1670	−0.3552	+10.0000	−1.0000
17	5	+6.9620	−0.3165	+10.0000	−1.0000
18	5	+6.7822	−0.2829	+10.0000	−1.0000
19	5	+6.6244	−0.2538	+10.0000	−1.0000
20	5	+6.4857	−0.2286	+10.0000	−1.0000
21	5	+6.3636	−0.2066	+10.0000	−1.0000
22	5	+6.2559	−0.1874	+10.0000	−1.0000
23	5	+6.1604	−0.1706	+10.0000	−1.0000
24	5	+6.0756	−0.1559	+10.0000	−1.0000
25	5	+6.0000	−0.1429	+10.0000	−1.0000
26	5	+5.9324	−0.1313	+5.0000	0.0000
27	5	+5.8717	−0.1211	+5.0000	0.0000
28	5	+5.8170	−0.1119	+5.0000	0.0000
29	5	+5.7676	−0.1037	+5.0000	0.0000
30	5	+5.7229	−0.0964	+5.0000	0.0000
40	5	+5.4387	−0.0516	+5.0000	0.0000
60	5	+5.2264	−0.0216	+5.0000	0.0000
80	5	+5.1464	−0.0117	+5.0000	0.0000
100	5	+5.1063	−0.0073	+5.0000	0.0000

for $x_{10} \leq 25$ and

$$\sum_{i=1}^{10} \left| y_i - \tilde{y}_i \right| = 20.00$$

for $x_{10} \geq 25$. When $x_{10} \leq 25$, the LAD regression line defined by $\tilde{\alpha}_{yx} = +10.00$ and $\tilde{\beta}_{yx} = -1.00$ yields the minimum sum of absolute differences. However, when $x_{10} \geq 25$ the LAD regression line defined by $\tilde{\alpha}_{yx} = +5.00$ and $\tilde{\beta}_{yx} = 0.00$ that passes through the data point located at (x_{10}, y_{10}) yields the minimum sum of absolute differences. For $x_{10} = 25$, the LAD regression line is not unique. While

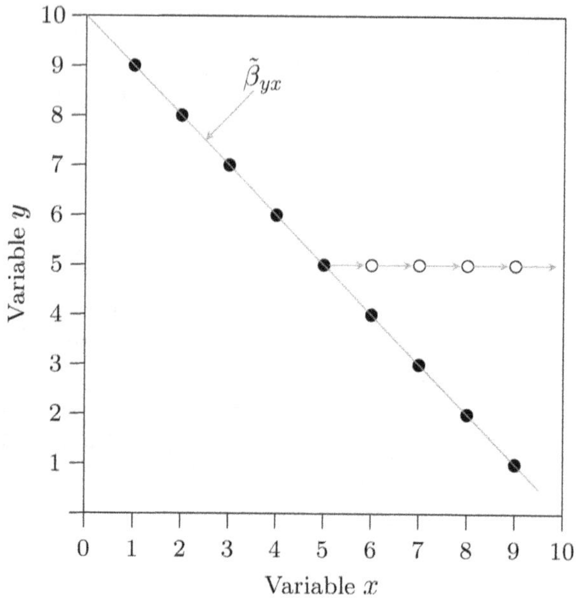

Fig. 7.4 Scatterplot of the data given in Table 7.3 with the regression line $\tilde{\beta}_{yx}$ depicted and the locations of an added tenth value indicated by four white circles

this is an interesting property of LAD regression and can easily be demonstrated with one predictor and a small number of data points, in practice any extreme value would have to be so far removed from the measured center of the distribution of variable x to be considered a "grossly aberrant" value [47, p. 871].

The fact that when $y_{10} = 5$ and $x_{10} = 25$, the solution is not unique and either of the two LAD regression lines is appropriate, deserves some additional explanation. Consider the data points in Fig. 7.4 where the additional tenth point is indicated at locations

$$(x_6, y_5), (x_7, y_5), \ldots, (x_9, y_5)$$

and the LAD regression line for the original nine data points with $\tilde{\alpha} = +10.00$ and $\tilde{\beta} = -1.00$ is depicted. If only the original nine data points are considered, the sum of absolute deviations is zero, i.e.,

$$\sum_{i=1}^{9} |y_i - \tilde{y}_i| = |9-9| + |8-8| + |7-7| + |6-6| + |5-5| + |4-4|$$

$$+ |3-3| + |2-2| + |1-1| = 0.00\,.$$

The addition of a tenth data point at location (x_6, y_5), the first white circle to the right of the regression line in Fig. 7.4, increases the sum of absolute deviations by one, i.e., $|y_i - \hat{y}_i| = |6-5| = 1$. Moving the new data point horizontally to location (x_7, y_5), the second white circle to the right of the regression line in

Fig. 7.4, increases the sum of absolute deviations by two, i.e., $|y_i - \tilde{y}_i| = |7 - 5| = 2$. Continuing to move the new data point horizontally increments the sum of absolute deviations by increasing amounts. Consider locations (x_{24}, y_5), (x_{25}, y_5), and (x_{26}, y_5), where

$$\left|y_i - \tilde{y}_i\right| = \left|24 - 5\right| = 19 \,, \quad \left|y_i - \tilde{y}_i\right| = \left|25 - 5\right| = 20 \,,$$

and

$$\left|y_i - \tilde{y}_i\right| = \left|26 - 5\right| = 21 \,,$$

respectively.

Thus, for an additional value up to location (x_{25}, y_5) the sum of absolute deviations will be equal to or less than 20, and for an additional value beyond location (x_{25}, y_5) the sum of absolute deviations will be equal to or greater than 20. However, when a data point is added at location (x_{25}, y_5) something interesting happens, which is readily apparent in Table 7.5. At this point a dramatic shift in the LAD regression line occurs, from $\tilde{\alpha}_{yx} = +10.00$ and $\tilde{\beta}_{yx} = -1.00$ to $\tilde{\alpha}_{yx} = +5.00$ and $\tilde{\beta}_{yx} = 0.00$. The regression line is leveraged and forced through the new data point location at (x_{25}, y_5). The new regression line is depicted in Fig. 7.5 with the absolute errors indicated by dashed lines. The sum of the absolute errors around the

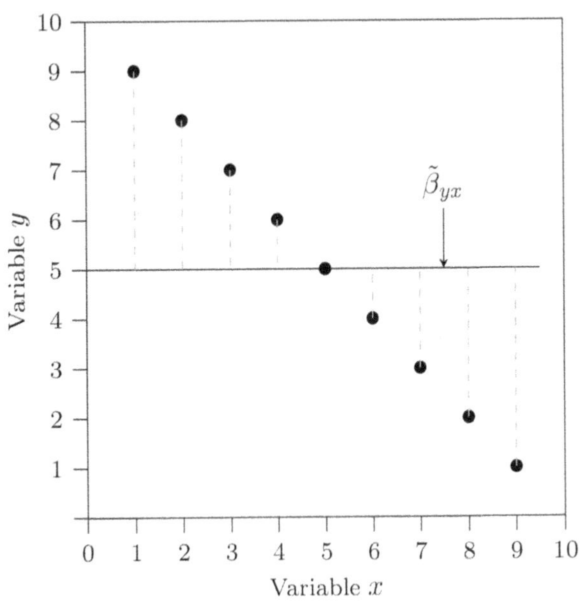

Fig. 7.5 Scatterplot of the data given in Table 7.3 with absolute errors indicated by dashed lines

new regression line is

$$\sum_{i=1}^{10} |y_i - \tilde{y}_i| = |9-5| + |8-5| + |7-5| + |6-5| + |5-5| + |4-5|$$

$$+ |3-5| + |2-5| + |1-5| + |5-5| = 20.00\,.$$

Thus both regression lines given by $\tilde{\alpha}_{yx} = +10.00$ and $\tilde{\beta}_{yx} = -1.00$ and $\tilde{\alpha}_{yx} = +5.00$ and $\tilde{\beta}_{yx} = 0.00$ minimize the sum of absolute deviations when an additional data point is located at (x_{25}, y_5). Note, however, that the additional data point is far to the right and is a very extreme value, unlikely to be encountered in everyday research. Specifically, for this minimalist example, a tenth value at location (x_{25}, y_5) is almost three times the range and over seven standard deviations above the mean—too extreme to be of concern in practice. Thus, LAD regression is highly stable under all but the most extreme cases.

Influence

If a tenth bivariate value is added to the nine bivariate values given in Table 7.3 on p. 379 where $x_{10} = y_{10}$ takes on the added values of 6, 7, ..., 30, 40, 60, 80, and 100, then the effects of influence on the two regression models can be observed. The diagonal movement of (x_{10}, y_{10}) is depicted by the directional arrow labeled "I" in Fig. 7.3 and by the four white circles in Fig. 7.6, illustrating an additional data point

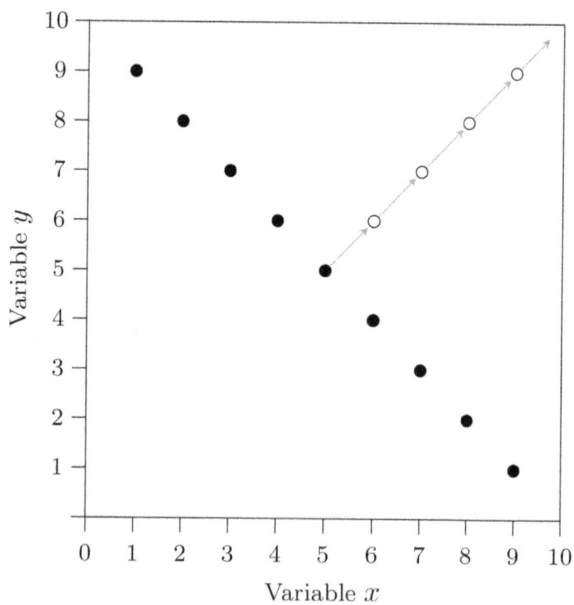

Fig. 7.6 Scatterplot of the data given in Table 7.3 with the locations of an added tenth value indicated by four white circles

moving diagonally away from $(x_5, y_5) = (5, 5)$ by increments of one x and one y unit, i.e., $(6, 6)$, $(7, 7)$, $(8, 8)$, and so on.

Table 7.6 lists the values of x_{10} and y_{10} in the first two columns, the $\hat{\alpha}_{yx}$ and $\hat{\beta}_{yx}$ estimates of the OLS regression parameters in the next two columns, and the $\tilde{\alpha}_{yx}$ and $\tilde{\beta}_{yx}$ estimates of the LAD regression parameters in the last two columns. The estimates of the OLS regression parameters listed in Table 7.4 demonstrate that both $\hat{\alpha}_{yx}$ and $\hat{\beta}_{yx}$ exhibit complex changes with increases in influence, quickly becoming unstable with changes in the intercept from $\hat{\alpha}_{yx} = +10.00$ to $\hat{\alpha}_{yx} = +0.2126$ and changes in the slope from $\hat{\beta}_{yx} = -1.00$ to $\hat{\beta}_{yx} = +0.9853$. Note that $\hat{\beta}_{yx}$ is negative from $x_{10} = 5$ up to $x_{10} = 13$, then changes to positive for $x_{10} = 14$ up to $x_{10} = 100$.

Table 7.6 Effects of influence on intercepts and slopes of OLS and LAD linear regression models

		OLS modell		LAD modell	
x_{10}	y_{10}	$\hat{\alpha}_{yx}$	$\hat{\beta}_{yx}$	$\tilde{\alpha}_{yx}$	$\tilde{\beta}_{yx}$
5	5	+10.0000	−1.0000	+10.0000	−1.0000
6	6	+10.0493	−0.9704	+10.0000	−1.0000
7	7	+9.8113	−0.8868	+10.0000	−1.0000
8	8	+9.3392	−0.7621	+10.0000	−1.0000
9	9	+8.7097	−0.6129	+10.0000	−1.0000
10	10	+8.0000	−0.4545	+10.0000	−1.0000
11	11	+7.2727	−0.2987	+10.0000	−1.0000
12	12	+6.5706	−0.1527	+10.0000	−1.0000
13	13	+5.9184	−0.0204	+10.0000	−1.0000
14	14	+5.3273	+0.0971	+10.0000	−1.0000
15	15	+4.8000	+0.2000	+10.0000	−1.0000
16	16	+4.3339	+0.2895	+10.0000	−1.0000
17	17	+3.9241	+0.3671	+10.0000	−1.0000
18	18	+3.5644	+0.4342	+10.0000	−1.0000
19	19	+3.2487	+0.4924	+10.0000	−1.0000
20	20	+2.9714	+0.5429	+10.0000	−1.0000
21	21	+2.7273	+0.5868	+10.0000	−1.0000
22	22	+2.5117	+0.6251	+10.0000	−1.0000
23	23	+2.3208	+0.6587	+10.0000	−1.0000
24	24	+2.1512	+0.6882	+10.0000	−1.0000
25	25	+2.0000	+0.7143	0.0000	+1.0000
26	26	+1.8647	+0.7374	0.0000	+1.0000
27	27	+1.7433	+0.7579	0.0000	+1.0000
28	28	+1.6340	+0.7762	0.0000	+1.0000
29	29	+1.5353	+0.7925	0.0000	+1.0000
30	30	+1.4458	+0.8072	0.0000	+1.0000
40	40	+0.8774	+0.8968	0.0000	+1.0000
60	60	+0.4528	+0.9569	0.0000	+1.0000
80	80	+0.2928	+0.9766	0.0000	+1.0000
100	100	+0.2126	+0.9853	0.0000	+1.0000

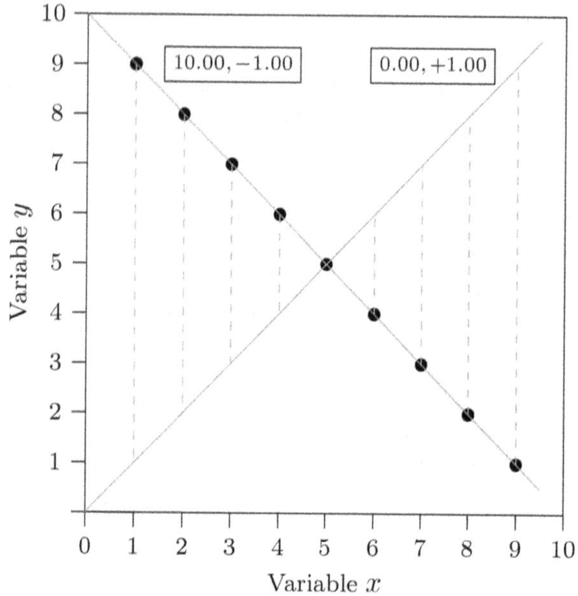

Fig. 7.7 Scatterplot of the data given in Table 7.3 with the regression lines minimizing the sum of absolute errors

Note also that the range of changes in $\hat{\beta}_{yx}$ is from $\hat{\beta}_{yx} = -1.00$ for $x_{10} = 5$ approaching $\hat{\beta}_{yx} = +1.00$ for $x_{10} = 100$; actually, $\hat{\beta}_{yx} = +0.9853$ for $x_{10} = 100$. In contrast, $\tilde{\alpha}_{yx}$ and $\tilde{\beta}_{yx}$ do not change for $5 \leq x_{10} = y_{10} \leq 24$. For $x_{10} = y_{10} \geq 26$, the estimates of the LAD regression parameters change from $\tilde{\alpha}_{yx} = +10.00$ and $\tilde{\beta}_{yx} = -1.00$ to $\tilde{\alpha}_{yx} = 0.00$ and $\tilde{\beta}_{yx} = +1.00$. When $x_{10} = y_{10} = 25$, either of the two LAD regression lines holds since the solution is not unique. Thus, two LAD regression lines minimize the sum of absolute errors: one with $\tilde{\alpha}_{yx} = +10.00$ and $\tilde{\beta}_{yx} = -1.00$ and the other with $\tilde{\alpha}_{yx} = 0.00$ and $\tilde{\beta}_{yx} = +1.00$.

Figure 7.7 depicts the two LAD regression lines, labeled with the values for $\tilde{\alpha}_{yx}$ and $\tilde{\beta}_{yx}$, and dashed lines indicating the errors around the regression line with $\tilde{\alpha}_{yx} = 0.00$ and $\tilde{\beta}_{yx} = +1.00$. As shown in Fig. 7.7, the sum of absolute errors is

$$\sum_{i=1}^{10} |y_i - \tilde{y}_i| = |9-1| + |8-2| + |7-3| + |6-4| + |5-5| + |4-6|$$
$$+ |3-7| + |2-8| + |1-9| + |25-25| = 40.00\,.$$

Given the bivariate data listed in Table 7.3 on p. 379 and an additional bivariate data point $x_{10} = y_{10}$, it follows that

$$\sum_{i=1}^{10} |y_i - \tilde{y}_i| \leq 40.00$$

for $5 \leq x_{10} = y_{10} \leq 25$ and

$$\sum_{i=1}^{10} |y_i - \tilde{y}_i| = 40.00$$

for $x_{10} = y_{10} \geq 25$. When $x_{10} = y_{10} \leq 25$, the LAD regression line defined by $\tilde{\alpha}_{yx} = +10.00$ and $\tilde{\beta}_{yx} = -1.00$ yields the minimum sum of absolute differences between y_i and $\tilde{y}_i$ for $i = 1, \ldots, N$. However, when $x_{10} = y_{10} \geq 25$, the LAD regression line defined by $\tilde{\alpha}_{yx} = 0.00$ and $\tilde{\beta}_{yx} = +1.00$ that passes through the data point located at (x_{10}, y_{10}) yields the minimum sum of absolute differences between y_i and $\tilde{y}_i$ for $i = 1, \ldots, N$. For $x_{10} = y_{10} = 25$, the LAD regression line is not unique. It should be noted that the shift in the LAD regression line is a consequence of only the leverage component of influence. For these data, the LAD regression line is defined by $\tilde{\alpha}_{yx} = +10.00$ and $\tilde{\beta}_{yx} = -1.00$ if $|x_{10} - 5| \leq 20.00$ and the regression line is unique if $|x_{10} - 5| < 20.0$ or $y_{10} = 10 - x_{10}$.

LAD linear regression is a robust alternative to OLS linear regression, especially when errors are generated by fat-tailed distributions [10, 52]. Fat-tailed distributions mean an abundance of extreme values and OLS linear regression gives disproportionate weight to extreme values. In practice, LAD linear regression is virtually unaffected by the presence of a few extreme values. While the effects of distance, leverage, and influence are illustrated with only a simplified example of perfect linear regression with one predictor, the results extend to more general regression models. If a less-than-perfect regression model with p predictors is considered, then the estimators of the LAD regression parameters are unaffected by unusual y_i values, when the leverage effect is absent. In addition, only exceedingly extreme values of the predictors $x_1, \ldots, x_p$ have any effect on the estimation of the LAD regression parameters.

7.2.2 *Univariate Example of LAD Regression*

Consider the small example set of bivariate data listed in Table 7.7 for $N = 10$ subjects. For the bivariate data listed in Table 7.7, the LAD regression coefficient is $\tilde{\beta} = +2.1111$, $\delta = 5.9889$, $\mu_\delta = 9.2267$, and the LAD chance-corrected measure of agreement between the observed y values and the predicted $\tilde{y}$ values is

$$\Re = 1 - \frac{\delta}{\mu_\delta} = 1 - \frac{5.9889}{9.2267} = +0.3509 \ .$$

Since there are $M = N! = 10! = 3{,}628{,}800$ possible arrangements of the observed data, an exact permutation analysis may not be practical. Based on $L = 1{,}000{,}000$ random arrangements of the observed data, the Monte Carlo resampling probability

Table 7.7 Example bivariate LAD correlation data on $N = 10$ subjects

Subject	x	y
1	14	25
2	8	23
3	5	21
4	2	10
5	1	12
6	3	11
7	9	19
8	2	13
9	3	13
10	9	16

value of $\Re = +0.3509$ is

$$P(\Re \geq \Re_o | H_0) = \frac{\text{number of } \Re \text{ values } \geq \Re_o}{L} = \frac{6{,}679}{1{,}000{,}000} = 0.6679 \times 10^{-2} ,$$

where $\Re_o$ denotes the observed value of $\Re$.

While $M = 3{,}628{,}800$ possible arrangements makes an exact permutation analysis impractical, it is not impossible. If the reference set of all possible permutations of the observed scores in Table 7.7 occur with equal chance, the exact probability of $\Re = +0.3509$ under the null hypothesis is

$$P(\Re \geq \Re_o | H_0) = \frac{\text{number of } \Re \text{ values } \geq \Re_o}{M} = \frac{26{,}966}{3{,}628{,}800} = 0.7431 \times 10^{-2} ,$$

where $\Re_o$ denotes the observed value of $\Re$.

7.2.3 Multivariate Example of LAD Regression

To illustrate a multivariate LAD linear regression analysis, an application of the LAD regression model to forecasting African rainfall in the western Sahel is utilized [38]. For the multivariate data listed in Table 7.8, the first column lists $N = 15$ calendar years from 1950 to 1964 and the second through fourth columns (U_{50}, U_{30}, and $|U_{50} - U_{30}|$) contain values based on the quasibiennial oscillation of equatorial east/west winds. U_{50} is the zonal wind measured in meters per second at 50 millibars (approximately 20 km in altitude) and U_{30} is the zonal wind measured

Table 7.8 Regional rainfall precipitation by years with predictors U_{50}, U_{30}, $|U_{50} - U_{30}|$, R_s, and R_g

	Predictor					
Year	U_{50}	U_{30}	$\|U_{50} - U_{30}\|$	R_s	R_g	Rainfall
1950	−3	−3	0	−0.14	+1.07	+1.05
1951	−4	−13	9	+1.68	−0.66	+0.74
1952	−23	−26	3	+0.49	+0.65	+1.45
1953	0	−18	18	+0.93	+0.41	+0.99
1954	−23	−32	9	+0.20	−0.16	+1.12
1955	0	−4	4	+0.60	+0.64	+1.07
1956	−19	−33	14	+1.00	+0.41	+0.36
1957	−2	−3	1	+0.47	−0.36	+0.87
1958	−12	−28	16	+0.58	+1.03	+0.86
1959	−9	−5	4	+1.45	−0.74	+0.30
1960	−6	−21	15	+0.25	+0.12	+0.24
1961	−3	−3	0	+0.23	+1.05	+0.20
1962	−12	−32	20	+0.48	−0.74	+0.41
1963	−17	−3	14	+0.28	+0.73	+0.22
1964	−4	−18	14	−0.12	+1.18	+0.76

in meters per second at 30 millibars (approximately 23 km is altitude).[2] The R_s values in the fifth column are standard deviations from the mean rainfall for the western Sahel region. The values for R_g in the sixth column are standard deviations from the mean rainfall for the Gulf of Guinea. The dependent variable in the seventh column is the April to October rainfall in the western Sahel region based on recordings from 20 stations in the region.

For the multivariate data listed in Table 7.8, the LAD regression coefficients are

$$\tilde{\beta}_1 = -0.0021\,, \quad \tilde{\beta}_2 = -0.0364\,, \quad \tilde{\beta}_3 = -0.0325\,,$$

$$\tilde{\beta}_4 = +0.5328\,, \quad \text{and} \quad \tilde{\beta}_5 = +0.5215\,,$$

$\delta = 0.3439$, $\mu_\delta = 0.4756$, and the LAD chance-corrected measure of agreement between the observed y values and the predicted $\tilde{y}$ values is

$$\Re = 1 - \frac{\delta}{\mu_\delta} = 1 - \frac{0.3439}{0.4756} = +0.2768.$$

Even with a small sample of observations such as this, there are

$$M = N! = 15! = 1{,}307{,}674{,}368{,}000$$

[2]For comparison, the top of Mount Everest is approximately 8.85 km with a pressure of about 300 millibars.

possible, equally-likely arrangements of the observed to be considered, far too many for an exact permutation analysis. Based on $L = 1{,}000{,}000$ random arrangements of the observed data, the Monte Carlo resampling probability value of $\mathfrak{R} = +0.2768$ is

$$P(\mathfrak{R} \geq \mathfrak{R}_{\text{o}}|H_0) = \frac{\text{number of } \mathfrak{R} \text{ values } \geq \mathfrak{R}_{\text{o}}}{L} = \frac{42{,}279}{1{,}000{,}000} = 0.0423 ,$$

where $\mathfrak{R}_{\text{o}}$ denotes the observed value of $\mathfrak{R}$.

7.3 LAD Multivariate Multiple Regression

An extension of LAD multiple linear regression to include multiple response variables, coupled with multiple predictor variables, is developed in this section [36, 37]. The extension was prompted by a multivariate Least Sum of Euclidean Distances (LSED) algorithm developed by Kaufman, Taylor, Mielke, and Berry in 2002 [24].

Consider the multivariate multiple linear regression model given by

$$y_{ik} = \sum_{j=1}^{m} x_{ij}\beta_{jk} + e_{ik}$$

for $i = 1, \ldots, N$ and $k = 1, \ldots, r$, where y_{ik} represents the ith of N measurements for the kth of r response variables, possibly affected by a treatment; x_{ij} is the jth of m covariates associated with the ith response, where $x_{i1} = 1$ if the model includes an intercept; β_{jk} denotes the jth of m regression parameters for the kth of r response variables; and e_{ik} designates the error associated with the ith of N measurements for the k of r response variables.

If estimates of β_{jk} that minimize

$$\sum_{i=1}^{N} \left(\sum_{k=1}^{r} e_{ik}^2 \right)^{1/2}$$

are denoted by $\tilde{\beta}_{jk}$ for $j = 1, \ldots, m$ and $k = 1, \ldots, r$, then the N r-dimensional residuals of the LSED multivariate multiple linear regression model are given by

$$e_{ik} = y_{ik} - \sum_{j=1}^{m} x_{ij}\tilde{\beta}_{jk}$$

for $i = 1, \ldots, N$ and $k = 1, \ldots, r$.

Let the N r-dimensional residuals, $e_{i1}, \ldots, e_{ir}$ for $i = 1, \ldots, N$, obtained from a LSED multivariate multiple linear regression model, be partitioned into g

treatment groups of sizes $n_1, \ldots, n_g$, where $n_i \geq 2$ for $i = 1, \ldots, g$ and

$$N = \sum_{i=1}^{g} n_i \; .$$

The analysis of the multivariate multiple regression residuals depends on test statistic

$$\delta = \sum_{i=1}^{g} C_i \xi_i \; , \tag{7.3}$$

where $C_i = n_i / N$ is a positive weight for the ith of g treatment groups and ξ_i is the average pairwise Euclidean distance among the n_i r-dimensional residuals in the ith of g treatment groups defined by

$$\xi_i = \binom{n_i}{2}^{-1} \sum_{k=1}^{N-1} \sum_{l=k+1}^{N} \left[\sum_{j=1}^{r} \left(e_{kj} - e_{lj} \right)^2 \right]^{1/2} \Psi_{ki} \Psi_{li} \; , \tag{7.4}$$

where

$$\Psi_{ki} = \begin{cases} 1 & \text{if } (e_{k1}, \ldots, e_{kr}) \text{ is in the } i\text{th treatment group} \; , \\ 0 & \text{otherwise} \; . \end{cases}$$

The null hypothesis specifies that each of the

$$M = \frac{N!}{\displaystyle\prod_{i=1}^{g} n_i!}$$

possible allocations of the N r-dimensional residuals to the g treatment groups is equally-likely. Under the null hypothesis, an exact probability value associated with the observed value of δ, δ_o, is given by

$$P(\delta \leq \delta_o | H_0) = \frac{\text{number of } \delta \text{ values } \leq \delta_o}{M} \; .$$

As with LAD univariate multiple regression models, the criterion for fitting LSED multivariate multiple regression models based on δ is the chance-corrected measure of effect size between the observed and predicted response measurement values given by

$$\Re = 1 - \frac{\delta}{\mu_\delta} \; , \tag{7.5}$$

where μ_δ is the expected value of δ over the $N!$ possible pairings under the null hypothesis, given by

$$\mu_\delta = \frac{1}{M} \sum_{i=1}^{M} \delta_i \ . \tag{7.6}$$

Note that $\Re = 1$ implies perfect agreement between the observed and model-predicted response vectors and the expected value of $\Re$ is 0 under the null hypothesis, i.e., chance-corrected.

7.3.1 Example of Multivariate Multiple Regression

To illustrate a multivariate LSED multiple regression analysis, consider an unbalanced two-way randomized-block experimental design in which $N = 16$ subjects are tested over $a = 3$ levels of Factor A, the experiment is repeated $b = 2$ times for Factor B, and there are $r = 2$ response measurement scores for each subject. The data are listed in Table 7.9. The design is intentionally kept small to illustrate the multivariate multiple regression procedure.

Analysis of Factor *A*

A design matrix of dummy codes (0, 1) for a regression analysis of Factor A is given in Table 7.10, where the first column of 1 values provides for an intercept, the next column contains the dummy codes for Factor B, and the third and fourth columns contain the bivariate response measurement scores listed according to the original random assignment of the $N = 16$ subjects to the $a = 3$ levels of Factor A, with the first $n_{A_1} = 5$ scores, the next $n_{A_2} = 7$ scores, and the last $n_{A_3} = 4$ scores associated with the $a = 3$ levels of Factor A, respectively. The analysis of

Table 7.9 Example data for a two-way randomized-block design with $a = 3$ blocks, $b = 2$ treatments, and $N = 16$ subjects

	Factor A		
Factor B	A_1	A_2	A_3
B_1	(49, 102)	(63, 84)	(45, 107)
		(60, 89)	(50, 100)
			(42, 111)
			(46, 104)
B_2	(48, 103)	(27, 114)	
	(58, 94)	(66, 83)	
	(51, 100)	(74, 79)	
	(55, 97)	(69, 88)	
		(71, 82)	

Table 7.10 Example design matrix and bivariate response measurement scores for a multivariate LSED multiple regression analysis of Factor A with $N = 16$ subjects

Matrix		Scores	
1	1	49	102
1	0	48	103
1	0	58	94
1	0	51	100
1	0	55	97
1	1	63	84
1	1	60	89
1	0	27	114
1	0	66	83
1	0	74	79
1	0	69	88
1	0	71	82
1	1	45	107
1	1	50	100
1	1	42	111
1	1	46	104

the data listed in Table 7.10 examines the $N = 16$ regression residuals for possible differences among the $a = 3$ treatment levels of Factor A; consequently, no dummy codes are provided for Factor A as this information is implicit in the ordering of the $a = 3$ levels of Factor A in the last two columns of Table 7.10.

Because there are only

$$M = \frac{N!}{\prod_{i=1}^{a} n_{A_i}!} = \frac{16!}{5!\ 7!\ 4!} = 1{,}441{,}440$$

possible, equally-likely arrangements of the $N = 16$ bivariate response measurement scores listed in Table 7.10, an exact permutation analysis is feasible. The analysis of the $N = 16$ LAD regression residuals calculated on the bivariate response measurement scores for Factor A in Table 7.10 yields estimated LAD regression coefficients of

$$\tilde{\beta}_{1,1} = +58.00\ , \quad \tilde{\beta}_{2,1} = -9.00\ , \quad \tilde{\beta}_{1,2} = +94.00\ , \quad \text{and} \quad \tilde{\beta}_{2,2} = +8.00$$

for Factor A. Table 7.11 lists the observed y_{ik} values, LAD-predicted $\tilde{y}_{ik}$ values, and residual e_{ik} values for $i = 1, \ldots, 16$ subjects and $k = 1, 2$ response variables.

Following Eq. (7.4) on p. 393 and employing ordinary Euclidean distance between residuals, the $N = 16$ LAD regression residuals listed in Table 7.11 yield $a = 3$ average distance-function values of

$$\xi_{A_1} = 7.2294\ , \quad \xi_{A_2} = 20.0289\ , \quad \text{and} \quad \xi_{A_3} = 7.3475\ .$$

Table 7.11 Observed, predicted, and residual values for a multivariate LSED multiple regression analysis of Factor A with $N = 16$ subjects

y_{i1}	y_{i2}	$\tilde{y}_{i1}$	$\tilde{y}_{i2}$	e_{i1}	e_{i2}
49	102	49.00	102.00	0.00	0.00
48	103	58.00	94.00	−10.00	+9.00
58	94	58.00	94.00	0.00	0.00
51	100	58.00	94.00	−7.00	+6.00
55	97	58.00	94.00	−3.00	+3.00
63	84	49.00	102.00	+14.00	−18.00
60	89	49.00	102.00	+11.00	−13.00
27	114	58.00	94.00	−31.00	+20.00
66	83	58.00	94.00	+8.00	−11.00
74	79	58.00	94.00	+16.00	−15.00
69	88	58.00	94.00	+11.00	−6.00
71	82	58.00	94.00	+13.00	−12.00
45	107	49.00	102.00	−4.00	+5.00
50	100	49.00	102.00	+1.00	−2.00
42	111	49.00	102.00	−7.00	+9.00
46	104	49.00	102.00	−3.00	+2.00

Following Eq. (7.3) on p. 393, the observed value of test statistic δ calculated on the $N = 16$ LAD regression residuals listed in Table 7.11 with treatment group weights

$$C_j = \frac{n_{A_j}}{N} \qquad \text{for } j = 1, 2, 3$$

is

$$\delta_A = \sum_{j=1}^{a} C_j \xi_j = \frac{1}{16}\big[(5)(7.2294) + (7)(20.0289) + (4)(7.3475)\big] = 12.8587\,.$$

If all M arrangements of the $N = 16$ observed LAD regression residuals listed in Table 7.11 occur with equal chance, the exact probability value of $\delta_A = 12.8587$ computed on the $M = 1{,}441{,}440$ possible arrangements of the observed LAD regression residuals with $n_{A_1} = 5$, $n_{A_2} = 7$, and $n_{A_3} = 4$ preserved for each arrangement is

$$P(\delta \leq \delta_A | H_0) = \frac{\text{number of } \delta \text{ values } \leq \delta_A}{M} = \frac{6{,}676}{1{,}441{,}440} = 0.0046\,.$$

Following Eq. (7.6) on p. 394, the exact expected value of the $M = 1{,}441{,}440$ δ values is

$$\mu_\delta = \frac{1}{M}\sum_{i=1}^{M} \delta_i = \frac{26{,}092{,}946.8800}{1{,}441{,}440} = 18.1020$$

and, following Eq. (7.5) on p. 393, the observed chance-corrected measure of effect size for the y_i and $\tilde{y}_i$ values, $i = 1, \ldots, N$, is

$$\Re_A = 1 - \frac{\delta_A}{\mu_\delta} = 1 - \frac{12.8587}{18.1020} = +0.2897\,,$$

indicating approximately 29% agreement between the observed and predicted values above that expected by chance.

Analysis of Factor *B*

A design matrix of dummy codes (0, 1) for a regression analysis of Factor B is given in Table 7.12, where the first column of 1 values provides for an intercept, the next two columns contain the dummy codes for Factor A, and the fourth and fifth columns contain the bivariate response measurement scores listed according to the original random assignment of the $N = 16$ subjects to the $b = 2$ levels of Factor B, with the first $n_{B_1} = 7$ scores and the last $n_{B_2} = 9$ scores associated with the $b = 2$ levels of Factor B, respectively. The analysis of the data listed in Table 7.12 examines the $N = 16$ regression residuals for possible differences between the $b = 2$ treatment levels of Factor B; consequently, no dummy codes are provided for Factor B as this information is implicit in the ordering of the $b = 2$ levels of Factor B in the last two columns of Table 7.12.

Table 7.12 Example design matrix and bivariate response measurement scores for a multivariate LSED multiple regression analysis of Factor B with $N = 16$ subjects

Matrix			Scores	
1	1	0	49	102
1	0	1	63	84
1	0	1	60	89
1	0	0	45	107
1	0	0	50	100
1	1	0	42	111
1	1	0	46	104
1	0	0	48	103
1	0	0	58	94
1	0	0	51	100
1	0	0	55	97
1	0	1	27	114
1	1	1	66	83
1	1	1	74	79
1	1	1	69	88
1	1	1	71	82

Because there are only

$$M = \frac{N!}{\prod_{i=1}^{b} n_{B_i}!} = \frac{16!}{7!\,9!} = 11{,}440$$

possible, equally-likely arrangements of the $N = 16$ response measurement scores listed in Table 7.12, an exact permutation analysis is feasible. The analysis of the $N = 16$ LAD regression residuals calculated on the bivariate response measurement scores for Factor B in Table 7.12 yields estimated LAD regression coefficients of

$$\tilde{\beta}_{1,1} = +46.00\,, \quad \tilde{\beta}_{2,1} = +5.00\,, \quad \tilde{\beta}_{3,1} = +20.00\,, \quad \tilde{\beta}_{1,2} = +104.00\,,$$
$$\tilde{\beta}_{2,2} = -4.00\,, \quad \text{and} \quad \tilde{\beta}_{3,2} = -20.00$$

for Factor B. Table 7.13 lists the observed y_{ik} values, LAD-predicted $\tilde{y}_{ik}$ values, and residual e_{ik} values for $i = 1, \ldots, 16$ subjects and $k = 1, 2$ response variables.

Following Eq. (7.4) on p. 393 and employing ordinary Euclidean distance between residuals, the $N = 16$ LAD regression residuals listed in Table 7.13 yield $b = 2$ average distance-function values of

$$\xi_{B_1} = 6.0229 \quad \text{and} \quad \xi_{B_2} = 16.7440\,.$$

Table 7.13 Observed, predicted, and residual values for a multivariate LSED multiple regression analysis of Factor A with $N = 16$ subjects

y_{i1}	y_{i2}	$\tilde{y}_{i1}$	$\tilde{y}_{i2}$	e_{i1}	e_{i2}
49	102	51.00	100.00	−2.00	+2.00
63	84	66.00	84.00	−3.00	0.00
60	89	66.00	84.00	−6.00	+5.00
45	107	46.00	104.00	−1.00	+3.00
50	100	46.00	104.00	+4.00	−4.00
42	111	46.00	104.00	−4.00	+7.00
46	104	46.00	104.00	0.00	0.00
48	103	51.00	100.00	−3.00	+3.00
58	94	51.00	100.00	+7.00	−6.00
51	100	51.00	100.00	0.00	0.00
55	97	51.00	100.00	+4.00	−3.00
27	114	66.00	84.00	−39.00	+30.00
66	83	66.00	84.00	0.00	−1.00
74	79	66.00	84.00	−8.00	−5.00
69	88	66.00	84.00	+3.00	+4.00
71	82	66.00	84.00	+5.00	−2.00

Following Eq. (7.3) on p. 393, the observed value of test statistic δ calculated on the $N = 16$ LAD regression residuals listed in Table 7.13 with treatment group weights

$$C_i = \frac{n_{B_i}}{N} \qquad \text{for } i = 1, 2 ,$$

is

$$\delta_B = \sum_{i=1}^{b} C_i \xi_i = \frac{1}{16}\big[(7)(6.0229) + (9)(16.7440)\big] = 12.0535 .$$

If all M arrangements of the $N = 16$ observed LAD regression residuals listed in Table 7.13 occur with equal chance, the exact probability value of $\delta_B = 12.0535$ computed on the $M = 11{,}440$ possible arrangements of the observed LAD regression residuals with $n_{B_1} = 7$ and $n_{B_2} = 9$ preserved for each arrangement is

$$P(\delta \leq \delta_B | H_0) = \frac{\text{number of } \delta \text{ values } \leq \delta_B}{M} = \frac{2{,}090}{11{,}440} = 0.1827 .$$

Following Eq. (7.6) on p. 394, the exact expected value of the $M = 11{,}440$ δ values is

$$\mu_\delta = \frac{1}{M} \sum_{i=1}^{M} \delta_i = \frac{140{,}623.9120}{11{,}440} = 12.2923$$

and, following Eq. (7.5) on p. 393, the observed chance-corrected measure of effect size for the y_i and $\tilde{y}_i$ values, $i = 1, \ldots, N$, is

$$\Re_B = 1 - \frac{\delta_B}{\mu_\delta} = 1 - \frac{12.0535}{12.2923} = +0.0194 ,$$

indicating approximately 2% agreement between the observed and predicted values above that expected by chance.

For another example of LAD multiple multivariate example, see an informative and widely cited article by Endler and Mielke on "Comparing entire colour patterns as birds see them" in *Biological Journal of the Linnean Society* [11].

7.4 Comparison of OLS and LAD Linear Regression

In this section, OLS and LAD linear regression analyses are illustrated and compared on two example data sets—one with $p = 2$ predictors and no extreme

Table 7.14 Example multivariate correlation data on $N = 12$ families with $p = 2$ predictors

Family	x_1	x_2	y
A	1	12	1
B	1	14	2
C	1	16	3
D	1	16	5
E	2	18	3
F	2	16	1
G	3	12	5
H	3	12	0
I	4	10	6
J	4	12	3
K	5	10	7
L	5	16	4

values and one with $p = 2$ predictors and a single extreme value.[3] Consider first the small example data set with $p = 2$ predictors listed in Table 7.14 where variable y is Hours of Housework done by husbands per week, variable x_1 is Number of Children, and variable x_2 is husband's Years of Education for $N = 12$ families.

7.4.1 Ordinary Least Squares (OLS) Analysis

For the multivariate data listed in Table 7.14, the unstandardized OLS regression coefficients are

$$\hat{\beta}_1 = +0.6356 \quad \text{and} \quad \hat{\beta}_2 = -0.0649 ,$$

and the observed squared OLS multiple correlation coefficient is $R_o^2 = 0.2539$. Based on $L = 1{,}000{,}000$ random arrangements of the observed data, the Monte Carlo resampling probability value of $R_o^2 = 0.2539$ is

$$P\left(R^2 \geq R_o^2 | H_0\right) = \frac{\text{number of } R^2 \text{ values } \geq R_o^2}{L} = \frac{268{,}026}{1{,}000{,}000} = 0.2680 ,$$

where R_o^2 denotes the observed value of R^2. For comparison, the exact probability value of $R_o^2 = 0.2539$ based on $M = N! = 12! = 479{,}001{,}600$ possible arrangements of the data listed in Table 7.14 is $P = 0.2681$.

[3]For real-life applications and comparisons of OLS and LAD regression applied to meteorological forecasting, see two articles in *Weather and Forecasting* by Mielke, Berry, Landsea, and Gray [39, 40].

7.4.2 Least Absolute Deviation (LAD) Analysis

For the multivariate data listed in Table 7.14, the LAD regression coefficients are

$$\tilde{\beta}_1 = +0.4138 \quad \text{and} \quad \tilde{\beta}_2 = +0.1207 \;,$$

$\delta = 1.5000$, $\mu_\delta = 1.8084$, and the LAD chance-corrected measure of agreement between the observed y values and the predicted $\tilde{y}$ values is

$$\mathfrak{R}_{\text{o}} = 1 - \frac{\delta}{\mu_\delta} = 1 - \frac{1.5000}{1.8084} = +0.1706 \;.$$

Based on $L = 1{,}000{,}000$ random arrangements of the observed data, the Monte Carlo resampling probability value of $\mathfrak{R} = +0.1706$ is

$$P(\mathfrak{R} \geq \mathfrak{R}_{\text{o}}|H_0) = \frac{\text{number of } \mathfrak{R} \text{ values } \geq \mathfrak{R}_{\text{o}}}{L} = \frac{19{,}176}{1{,}000{,}000} = 0.0192 \;,$$

where $\mathfrak{R}_{\text{o}}$ denotes the observed value of $\mathfrak{R}$. For comparison, the exact probability value of $\mathfrak{R}_{\text{o}} = +0.1706$ based on $M = N! = 12! = 479{,}001{,}600$ possible arrangements of the data listed in Table 7.14 is $P = 0.0221$.

Now, suppose that the husband in family "L" was a stay-at-home house-husband and instead of contributing just four hours of housework per week, he actually contributed 40 hours, as in Table 7.15.

Table 7.15 Example multivariate correlation data on $N = 12$ families with $p = 2$ predictors, where the husband in Family L contributed 40 hours of housework per week

Family	x_1	x_2	y
A	1	12	1
B	1	14	2
C	1	16	3
D	1	16	5
E	2	18	3
F	2	16	1
G	3	12	5
H	3	12	0
I	4	10	6
J	4	12	3
K	5	10	7
L	5	16	40

7.4.3 Ordinary Least Squares (OLS) Analysis

For the multivariate data listed in Table 7.15, the unstandardized OLS regression coefficients are

$$\hat{\beta}_1 = +5.7492 \quad \text{and} \quad \hat{\beta}_2 = +2.3896 ,$$

and the observed squared OLS multiple correlation coefficient is $R_o^2 = 0.5786$. Based on $L = 1{,}000{,}000$ random arrangements of the observed data, the Monte Carlo resampling probability value of $R_o^2 = 0.5786$ is

$$P(R^2 \geq R_o^2 | H_0) = \frac{\text{number of } R^2 \text{ values } \geq R_o^2}{L} = \frac{15{,}215}{1{,}000{,}000} = 0.0152 ,$$

where R_o^2 denotes the observed value of R^2. For comparison, the exact probability value of $R_o^2 = 0.5786$ based on $M = N! = 12! = 479{,}001{,}600$ possible arrangements of the data listed in Table 7.15 is $P = 0.0153$.

7.4.4 Least Absolute Deviation (LAD) Analysis

For the multivariate data listed in Table 7.15, the LAD regression coefficients are

$$\tilde{\beta}_1 = +1.3000 \quad \text{and} \quad \tilde{\beta}_2 = +0.0500 ,$$

$\delta_o = 4.0333$, $\mu_\delta = 5.2194$, and the LAD chance-corrected measure of agreement between the observed y values and the predicted $\tilde{y}$ values is

$$\Re_o = 1 - \frac{\delta_o}{\mu_\delta} = 1 - \frac{4.0333}{5.2194} = +0.2272 .$$

Based on $L = 1{,}000{,}000$ random arrangements of the observed data, the Monte Carlo resampling probability value of $\Re_o = +0.2272$ is

$$P(\Re \geq \Re_o | H_0) = \frac{\text{number of } \Re \text{ values } \geq \Re_o}{L} = \frac{4{,}517}{1{,}000{,}000} = 0.4571 \times 10^{-2} ,$$

where $\Re_o$ denotes the observed value of $\Re$. For comparison, the exact probability value of $\Re_o = +0.2272$ based on $M = N! = 12! = 479{,}001{,}600$ possible arrangements of the data listed in Table 7.14 is $P = 0.5630 \times 10^{-2}$.

The results of the comparison of OLS and LAD analyses with 4 and 40 hours of housework by the husband in family "L" are summarized in Table 7.16. The value

Table 7.16 Comparison of OLS and LAD analyses for the data given in Table 7.14 with 4 hours of housework for the husband in family L and the data given in Table 7.15 with 40 hours of housework for the husband in family L

	OLS analysis		LAD analysis	
Hours	R^2	Probability	$\Re$	Probability
4	0.2539	0.2680	0.1706	0.0192
40	0.5786	0.0152	0.2272	0.0046
$\|\Delta\|$	0.3247	0.2528	0.0566	0.0146

of 40 hours of housework by the husband in family "L" is, by any definition, an extreme value. It is six times the mean of $\bar{y} = 6.3333$ and three standard deviations above the mean. It is readily apparent that the extreme value of 40 hours had a profound impact on the results of the OLS analysis. The OLS multiple correlation coefficient more than doubled from $R_o^2 = 0.2539$ to $R_o^2 = 0.5786$, a difference of $R^2 = 0.3247$, and the corresponding probability value decreased from $P = 0.2680$ to $P = 0.0152$, a difference of $P = 0.2528$. The impact of 40 hours of housework on the LAD analysis is more modest with the LAD chance-corrected measure of agreement increasing only slightly from $\Re_o = 0.1706$ to $\Re_o = 0.2272$, a difference of $\Re = 0.0566$, and the probability value decreasing from $P = 0.0192$ to $P = 0.0046$, a difference of only $P = 0.0146$.

7.5 Fisher's r_{xy} to z Transformation

In order to attach a probability statement to inferences about the Pearson product-moment correlation coefficient, it is necessary to know the sampling distribution of a statistic that relates the sample correlation coefficient, r_{xy}, to the population parameter, ρ_{xy}. Because $-1.0 \leq r_{xy} \leq +1.0$, the sampling distribution of statistic r_{xy} is asymmetric whenever $\rho_{xy} \neq 0.0$.[4] Given two random variables that follow the bivariate normal distribution with population parameter ρ_{xy}, the sampling distribution of statistic r_{xy} approaches normality as the sample size increases; however, it converges very slowly for $|\rho_{xy}| \geq 0.6$, even with samples as large as $N = 400$ [7, p. xxxiii]. Fisher [13, 14] obtained the basic distribution of r_{xy} and showed that, when bivariate normality is assumed, a logarithmic transformation of r_{xy} (henceforth referred to as the Fisher z transform),

$$z = \frac{1}{2} \ln \left(\frac{1 + r_{xy}}{1 - r_{xy}} \right) = \tanh^{-1}(r_{xy}) \ ,$$

[4] It is probably safe to assume that in any actual research situation, the population correlation coefficient is always not equal to zero.

becomes normally distributed with a mean of approximately

$$\frac{1}{2}\ln\left(\frac{1+\rho_{xy}}{1-\rho_{xy}}\right) = \tanh^{-1}(\rho_{xy})$$

and the standard error approaches

$$\frac{1}{\sqrt{N-3}}$$

as $N \to \infty$.

The Fisher r_{xy} to z transform is presented in most textbooks and is available in a wide array of statistical software packages. In this section, the precision and accuracy of the Fisher z transform are examined for a variety of bivariate distributions, sample sizes, and values of ρ_{xy} [5]. If $\rho_{xy} \neq 0.0$ and the distribution is not bivariate normal, then the desired properties of the Fisher z transform generally fail.

There are two general applications of the Fisher z transform. The first application comprises the computation of the confidence limits for ρ_{xy} and the second involves the testing of hypotheses about specified values of $\rho_{xy} \neq 0.0$. The second application is more tractable than the first application as a hypothesized value of ρ_{xy} is available. The next part of this section describes the bivariate distributions to be examined, followed by an exploration of confidence intervals and an examination of hypothesis testing. The last part of the section provides some general conclusions about the propriety of uncritically using the Fisher z transform in actual research.

7.5.1 Distributions

Seven bivariate distributions are utilized to test the Fisher z transform. In addition, two related methods by Gayen [17] and Jeyaratnam [22] are also examined. The Gayen and Jeyaratnam techniques are characterized by simplicity, accuracy, and ease of use. For other interesting approaches, see David [7]; Hotelling [21]; Kraemer [25]; Liu, Woodward, and Bonett [28]; Mudholkar and Chaubey [41]; Pillai [45]; Ruben [48]; and Samiuddin [49].

Normal Distribution

The density function of the standardized normal, $N(0, 1)$, distribution is given by

$$f(x) = (2\pi)^{-1/2}\exp(-x^2/2) .$$

Generalized Logistic Distribution

The density function of the generalized logistic (GL) distribution is given by

$$f(x) = \left[\exp(\theta x)/\theta\right]^{1/\theta}\left[1 + \exp(\theta x)/\theta\right]^{-(\theta+1)/\theta}$$

for $\theta > 0$ [34]. The generalized logistic distribution is positively skewed for $\theta < 1$ and negatively skewed for $\theta > 1$. When $\theta = 1.0$, $GL(\theta)$ is a logistic distribution that closely resembles the normal distribution, with somewhat lighter tails. When $\theta = 0.10$, $GL(\theta)$ is a generalized logistic distribution with positive skewness. When $\theta = 0.01$, $GL(\theta)$ is a generalized logistic distribution with even greater positive skewness.

Symmetric Kappa Distribution

The density function of the symmetric kappa (SK) distribution is given by

$$f(x) = 0.5\lambda^{-1/\lambda}\left(1 + |x|^{\lambda}/\lambda\right)^{-(\lambda+1)/\lambda}$$

for $\lambda > 0$ [34, 35]. The shape of the symmetric kappa distribution ranges from an exceedingly heavy-tailed distribution as λ approaches zero to a uniform distribution as λ goes to infinity. When $\lambda = 2$, $SK(\lambda)$ is a peaked, heavy-tailed distribution, identical to Student's t distribution with 2 degrees of freedom. Thus, the variance of $SK(2)$ does not exist. When $\lambda = 3$, $SK(\lambda)$ is also a heavy-tailed distribution, but the variance does exist. When $\lambda = 25$, $SK(\lambda)$ is a loaf-shaped distribution resembling a uniform distribution with the addition of very light tails. These distributions provide a variety of populations from which to sample and evaluate the Fisher z transformation and the Gayen [17] and Jeyaratnam [22] modifications.

Seven bivariate correlated distributions were constructed in the following manner. Let x and y be independent identically distributed univariate random variables from each of seven univariate distributions, i.e., $N(0, 1)$, $GL(1.0)$, $GL(0.1)$, $GL(0.01)$, $SK(2)$, $SK(3)$, and $SK(25)$, and define the correlated random variables U_1 and U_2 of each bivariate distribution by

$$U_1 = x(1 - \rho_{xy}^2)^{1/2} + \rho_{xy}y$$

and $U_2 = y$, where ρ_{xy} is the desired Pearson product-moment correlation coefficient of random variables U_1 and U_2. Then a Monte Carlo procedure obtains random samples, corresponding to x and y, from the normal, generalized logistic, and symmetric kappa distributions.

7.5.2 Confidence Intervals

In this section, Monte Carlo confidence intervals are based on the seven distributions: $N(0, 1)$, $GL(1.0)$, $GL(0.1)$, $GL(0.01)$, $SK(2)$, $SK(3)$, and $SK(25)$. Each simulation is based on $L = 1{,}000{,}000$ bivariate random samples, U_1 and U_2, of size $N = 10$, 20, 40, and 80 for $\rho_{xy} = 0.00, +0.40, +0.60$, and $+0.80$ with $1 - \alpha = 0.90$, 0.95, and 0.99. Confidence intervals obtained from two methods are considered. The first confidence interval is based on the Fisher z transform and is defined by

$$\tanh\left[\tanh^{-1}(r_{xy}) - \frac{z_{\alpha/2}}{\sqrt{N-3}}\right] \leq \rho_{xy} \leq \tanh\left[\tanh^{-1}(r_{xy}) + \frac{z_{\alpha/2}}{\sqrt{N-3}}\right] ,$$

where $z_{\alpha/2}$ is the upper 0.50α probability point of the $N(0, 1)$ distribution. The second confidence interval is based on a method proposed by Jeyaratnam [22] and is defined by

$$\frac{r_{xy} - w}{1 - r_{xy}w} \leq \rho_{xy} \leq \frac{r_{xy} + w}{1 + r_{xy}w} ,$$

where

$$w = \frac{\left(t_{\alpha/2,N-2}\right)/\sqrt{N-2}}{\left[1 + \left(t_{\alpha/2,N-2}\right)^2/\sqrt{N-2}\right]^{1/2}}$$

and $t_{\alpha/2,N-2}$ is the upper 0.50α probability point of Student's t distribution with $N - 2$ degrees of freedom.

The results of the Monte Carlo analyses are summarized in Tables 7.17, 7.18, 7.19, 7.20, 7.21, 7.22, 7.23, which contain simulated containment probability values for the seven bivariate distributions with specified nominal values of $1 - \alpha$ (0.90, 0.95, 0.99), ρ_{xy} (0.00, +0.40, +0.60, +0.80), and N (10, 20, 40, 80) for the Fisher (F) and Jeyaratnam (J) confidence intervals. Table 7.17 analyzes data obtained from the $N(0, 1)$ distribution; Tables 7.18, 7.19, and 7.20 analyze data obtained from the generalized logistic distribution with $\theta = 1.0$, 0.1, and 0.01, respectively; and Tables 7.21, 7.22, and 7.23 analyze data obtained from the symmetric kappa distribution with $\lambda = 2$, 3, and 25, respectively.

In each of the seven tables, the Monte Carlo containment probability values for a $1 - \alpha$ confidence interval based on the Fisher z transform and a $1 - \alpha$ confidence interval based on the Jeyaratnam technique were obtained from the same $L = 1{,}000{,}000$ bivariate random samples of size N drawn with replacement from the designated bivariate distribution characterized by the specified population correlation ρ_{xy}. If the Fisher and Jeyaratnam transforms are appropriate for the

Table 7.17 Containment probability values for a bivariate $N(0, 1)$ distribution with Fisher (F) and Jeyaratnam (J) $1 - \alpha$ correlation confidence intervals

		$\rho_{xy} = 0.00$		$\rho_{xy} = +0.40$		$\rho_{xy} = +0.60$		$\rho_{xy} = +0.80$	
$1 - \alpha$	N	F	J	F	J	F	J	F	J
0.90	10	0.9014	0.8992	0.9026	0.9004	0.9037	0.9015	0.9048	0.9025
	20	0.9012	0.9005	0.9015	0.9008	0.9009	0.9002	0.9020	0.9014
	40	0.9004	0.9001	0.9012	0.9009	0.9009	0.9006	0.9011	0.9009
	80	0.9002	0.9001	0.9000	0.9000	0.9006	0.9005	0.9008	0.9007
0.95	10	0.9491	0.9501	0.9490	0.9501	0.9497	0.9508	0.9516	0.9516
	20	0.9495	0.9502	0.9493	0.9501	0.9500	0.9507	0.9500	0.9507
	40	0.9495	0.9499	0.9497	0.9501	0.9493	0.9497	0.9502	0.9506
	80	0.9595	0.9498	0.9497	0.9499	0.9501	0.9503	0.9498	0.9500
0.99	10	0.9875	0.9900	0.9877	0.9900	0.9877	0.9901	0.9880	0.9904
	20	0.9889	0.9900	0.9888	0.9900	0.9890	0.9901	0.9891	0.9902
	40	0.9893	0.9899	0.9896	0.9901	0.9894	0.9900	0.9895	0.9901
	80	0.9896	0.9899	0.9897	0.9900	0.9897	0.9900	0.9897	0.9900

Table 7.18 Containment probability values for a bivariate $GL(1.0)$ distribution with Fisher (F) and Jeyaratnam (J) $1 - \alpha$ correlation confidence intervals

		$\rho_{xy} = 0.00$		$\rho_{xy} = +0.40$		$\rho_{xy} = +0.60$		$\rho_{xy} = +0.80$	
$1 - \alpha$	N	F	J	F	J	F	J	F	J
0.90	10	0.9011	0.8990	0.8930	0.8907	0.8833	0.8809	0.8710	0.8684
	20	0.9009	0.9002	0.8894	0.8886	0.8742	0.8734	0.8565	0.8557
	40	0.9007	0.9004	0.8873	0.8871	0.8701	0.8698	0.8484	0.8481
	80	0.9005	0.9004	0.8851	0.8850	0.8677	0.8676	0.8438	0.8437
0.95	10	0.9485	0.9496	0.9425	0.9437	0.9359	0.9372	0.9273	0.9287
	20	0.9491	0.9498	0.9407	0.9415	0.9313	0.9322	0.9170	0.9181
	40	0.9491	0.9496	0.9402	0.9406	0.9274	0.9279	0.9116	0.9121
	80	0.9497	0.9499	0.9394	0.9396	0.9266	0.9269	0.9082	0.9085
0.99	10	0.9873	0.9897	0.9852	0.9880	0.9827	0.9858	0.9794	0.9832
	20	0.9886	0.9897	0.9855	0.9870	0.9821	0.9838	0.9764	0.9785
	40	0.9891	0.9897	0.9861	0.9867	0.9815	0.9823	0.9744	0.9755
	80	0.9895	0.9898	0.9860	0.9864	0.9808	0.9812	0.9729	0.9735

simulated data, the containment probability values should agree with the nominal $1 - \alpha$ values.

Some general observations can be made about the Monte Carlo results contained in Tables 7.17 through 7.23. First, in each of the tables there is little difference between the Fisher and Jeyaratnam Monte Carlo containment probability values and both techniques provide values close to the nominal $1 - \alpha$ values for the $N(0, 1)$ distribution analyzed in Table 7.17 with any value of ρ_{xy} and for any of the other distributions analyzed in Tables 7.18 through 7.23 when $\rho_{xy} = 0.00$. Second, for the skewed and heavy-tailed distributions, i.e., $GL(0.1)$, $GL(0.01)$, $SK(2)$, and

Table 7.19 Containment probability values for a bivariate $GL(0.1)$ distribution with Fisher (F) and Jeyaratnam (J) $1-\alpha$ correlation confidence intervals

		$\rho_{xy}=0.00$		$\rho_{xy}=+0.40$		$\rho_{xy}=+0.60$		$\rho_{xy}=+0.80$	
$1-\alpha$	N	F	J	F	J	F	J	F	J
0.90	10	0.9016	0.8995	0.8878	0.8854	0.8729	0.8704	0.8544	0.8516
	20	0.9013	0.9006	0.8821	0.8813	0.8593	0.8584	0.8321	0.8313
	40	0.9010	0.9007	0.8780	0.8777	0.8510	0.8507	0.8174	0.8170
	80	0.9006	0.9004	0.8760	0.8759	0.8459	0.8457	0.8081	0.8079
0.95	10	0.9486	0.9497	0.9389	0.9401	0.9281	0.9295	0.9150	0.9165
	20	0.9495	0.9502	0.9354	0.9362	0.9197	0.9206	0.8982	0.8993
	40	0.9495	0.9499	0.9335	0.9340	0.9136	0.9141	0.8871	0.8877
	80	0.9498	0.9500	0.9320	0.9323	0.9100	0.9102	0.8797	0.8800
0.99	10	0.9871	0.9895	0.9835	0.9865	0.9793	0.9830	0.9744	0.9787
	20	0.9882	0.9895	0.9833	0.9850	0.9770	0.9790	0.9674	0.9700
	40	0.9890	0.9895	0.9833	0.9841	0.9752	0.9763	0.9623	0.9637
	80	0.9895	0.9898	0.9828	0.9832	0.9737	0.9743	0.9585	0.9592

Table 7.20 Containment probability values for a bivariate $GL(0.01)$ distribution with Fisher (F) and Jeyaratnam (J) $1-\alpha$ correlation confidence intervals

		$\rho_{xy}=0.00$		$\rho_{xy}=+0.40$		$\rho_{xy}=+0.60$		$\rho_{xy}=+0.80$	
$1-\alpha$	N	F	J	F	J	F	J	F	J
0.90	10	0.9019	0.8996	0.8860	0.8837	0.8693	0.8667	0.8485	0.8457
	20	0.9015	0.9008	0.8798	0.8790	0.8545	0.8537	0.8243	0.8234
	40	0.9012	0.9009	0.8754	0.8752	0.8454	0.8450	0.8084	0.8080
	80	0.9002	0.9001	0.8726	0.8724	0.8394	0.8393	0.7984	0.7982
0.95	10	0.9485	0.9496	0.9375	0.9388	0.9255	0.9269	0.9106	0.9121
	20	0.9496	0.9503	0.9337	0.9346	0.9160	0.9170	0.8921	0.8932
	40	0.9495	0.9499	0.9317	0.9321	0.9092	0.9097	0.8797	0.8803
	80	0.9500	0.9502	0.9296	0.9298	0.9055	0.9057	0.8713	0.8716
0.99	10	0.9869	0.9893	0.9829	0.9860	0.9782	0.9820	0.9725	0.9771
	20	0.9881	0.9893	0.9825	0.9842	0.9752	0.9774	0.9644	0.9671
	40	0.9889	0.9895	0.9825	0.9833	0.9732	0.9743	0.9584	0.9600
	80	0.9897	0.9897	0.9821	0.9825	0.9712	0.9718	0.9540	0.9548

$SK(3)$, with N held constant, the differences between the Monte Carlo containment probability values and the nominal $1-\alpha$ values become greater as $|\rho_{xy}|$ increases. Third, the differences between the Monte Carlo containment probability values and the nominal $1-\alpha$ values increase with increasing N and $|\rho_{xy}| > 0.00$ for all the distributions except $N(0, 1)$ and $SK(25)$. This is especially evident with the skewed and heavy-tailed distributions $GL(0.1)$, $GL(0.01)$, $SK(2)$, and $SK(3)$.

Table 7.21 Containment probability values for a bivariate $SK(2)$ distribution with Fisher (F) and Jeyaratnam (J) $1-\alpha$ correlation confidence intervals

		$\rho_{xy} = 0.00$		$\rho_{xy} = +0.40$		$\rho_{xy} = +0.60$		$\rho_{xy} = +0.80$	
$1-\alpha$	N	F	J	F	J	F	J	F	J
0.90	10	0.8961	0.8942	0.8054	0.8029	0.7487	0.7457	0.6806	0.6774
	20	0.9002	0.8996	0.7582	0.7573	0.6650	0.6641	0.5733	0.5723
	40	0.9050	0.9048	0.6968	0.6965	0.5755	0.5752	0.4784	0.4781
	80	0.9097	0.9096	0.6192	0.6191	0.4884	0.4883	0.3942	0.3941
0.95	10	0.9403	0.9413	0.8670	0.8687	0.8198	0.8217	0.7612	0.7634
	20	0.9415	0.9421	0.8257	0.8269	0.7442	0.7457	0.6522	0.6538
	40	0.9436	0.9439	0.7726	0.7732	0.6543	0.6551	0.5521	0.5528
	80	0.9461	0.9463	0.6982	0.6986	0.5630	0.5634	0.4599	0.4602
0.99	10	0.9797	0.9828	0.9357	0.9420	0.9068	0.9152	0.8697	0.8810
	20	0.9789	0.9803	0.9065	0.9102	0.8523	0.8577	0.7761	0.7829
	40	0.9788	0.9794	0.8694	0.8715	0.7748	0.7780	0.6733	0.6768
	80	0.9794	0.9797	0.8107	0.8121	0.6819	0.6835	0.5721	0.5738

Table 7.22 Containment probability values for a bivariate $SK(3)$ distribution with Fisher (F) and Jeyaratnam (J) $1-\alpha$ correlation confidence intervals

		$\rho_{xy} = 0.00$		$\rho_{xy} = +0.40$		$\rho_{xy} = +0.60$		$\rho_{xy} = +0.80$	
$1-\alpha$	N	F	J	F	J	F	J	F	J
0.90	10	0.9007	0.8985	0.8707	0.8707	0.8451	0.8424	0.8145	0.8117
	20	0.9009	0.9002	0.8508	0.8499	0.8068	0.8060	0.7575	0.7566
	40	0.9015	0.9012	0.8284	0.8280	0.7670	0.7667	0.7027	0.7023
	80	0.9016	0.9015	0.8022	0.8021	0.7246	0.7245	0.6490	0.6488
0.95	10	0.9474	0.9485	0.9248	0.9262	0.9052	0.9067	0.8810	0.8827
	20	0.9479	0.9486	0.9095	0.9105	0.8751	0.8762	0.8306	0.8318
	40	0.9482	0.9485	0.8920	0.8925	0.8382	0.8388	0.7803	0.7810
	80	0.9490	0.9491	0.8697	0.8700	0.8010	0.8013	0.7275	0.7279
0.99	10	0.9863	0.9888	0.9758	0.9796	0.9660	0.9708	0.9536	0.9596
	20	0.9869	0.9881	0.9682	0.9705	0.9488	0.9518	0.9217	0.9257
	40	0.9873	0.9879	0.9588	0.9601	0.9256	0.9275	0.8825	0.8849
	80	0.9878	0.9880	0.9455	0.9462	0.8968	0.8980	0.8387	0.8401

7.5.3 Hypothesis Testing

In this section, Monte Carlo tests of hypotheses are based on the same seven distributions: $N(0, 1)$, $GL(1.0)$, $GL(0.1)$, $GL(0.01)$, $SK(2)$, $SK(3)$, and $SK(25)$. Each simulation is based on L = 1,000,000 bivariate random samples of size $N = 20$ and $N = 80$ for $\rho_{xy} = 0.00$ and $\rho_{xy} = +0.60$ and compared to seven nominal upper-tail probability values of $P = 0.99, 0.90, 0.75, 0.50, 0.25, 0.10$, and 0.01. Two tests of $\rho_{xy} \neq 0.00$ are considered. The first test is based on the Fisher z

Table 7.23 Containment probability values for a bivariate *SK*(25) distribution with Fisher (*F*) and Jeyaratnam (*J*) $1-\alpha$ correlation confidence intervals

		$\rho_{xy} = 0.00$		$\rho_{xy} = +0.40$		$\rho_{xy} = +0.60$		$\rho_{xy} = +0.80$	
$1-\alpha$	*N*	*F*	*J*	*F*	*J*	*F*	*J*	*F*	*J*
0.90	10	0.9009	0.8988	0.9134	0.9114	0.9288	0.9270	0.9485	0.9471
	20	0.9010	0.9003	0.9151	0.9145	0.9322	0.9317	0.9556	0.9552
	40	0.9006	0.9004	0.9159	0.9157	0.9340	0.9338	0.9590	0.9589
	80	0.9005	0.9004	0.9157	0.9156	0.9347	0.9346	0.9605	0.9604
0.95	10	0.9476	0.9487	0.9551	0.9561	0.9648	0.9657	0.9759	0.9765
	20	0.9489	0.9496	0.9577	0.9583	0.9691	0.9696	0.9817	0.9821
	40	0.9496	0.9496	0.9592	0.9595	0.9704	0.9707	0.9844	0.9845
	80	0.9494	0.9496	0.9599	0.9600	0.9716	0.9717	0.9853	0.9854
0.99	10	0.9862	0.9888	0.9889	0.9910	0.9919	0.9935	0.9950	0.9960
	20	0.9881	0.9892	0.9911	0.9921	0.9943	0.9950	0.9973	0.9976
	40	0.9891	0.9897	0.9923	0.9927	0.9951	0.9954	0.9981	0.9982
	80	0.9896	0.9898	0.9925	0.9928	0.9959	0.9960	0.9985	0.9986

transform and uses the standardized test statistic given by

$$T = \frac{z - \mu_z}{\sigma_z} ,$$

where

$$z = \tanh^{-1}(r_{xy}) , \quad \mu_z = \tanh^{-1}(\rho_{xy}) , \quad \text{and} \quad \sigma_z = \frac{1}{\sqrt{N-3}} .$$

The second test is based on corrected values proposed by Gayen [17], where

$$z = \tanh^{-1}(r_{xy}) ,$$

$$\mu_z = \tanh^{-1}(\rho_{xy}) + \frac{\rho_{xy}}{2(N-1)} \left[1 + \frac{5 - \rho_{xy}^2}{4(N-1)} \right] ,$$

and

$$\sigma_z = \left\{ \frac{1}{N-1} \left[1 + \frac{4 - \rho_{xy}^2}{2(N-1)} + \frac{22 - 6\rho_{xy}^2 - 3\rho_{xy}^4}{6(N-1)^2} \right] \right\}^{1/2} .$$

The results of the Monte Carlo analyses are summarized in Tables 7.24, 7.25, 7.26, 7.27, 7.28, 7.29, 7.30, which contain simulated upper-tail probability values for the seven distributions with specified nominal probability values of *P* (0.99, 0.95, 0.75, 0.50, 0.25, 0.10, 0.01), ρ_{xy} (0.00, +0.60), and *N* (20, 80) for the Fisher

Table 7.24 Upper-tail probability values compared with nominal values (P) for a bivariate $N(0, 1)$ distribution with Fisher (F) and Gayen (G) tests of hypotheses on $\rho_{xy} = 0.00$ and $\rho_{xy} = 0.60$

	$N = 20$				$N = 80$			
	$\rho_{xy} = 0.00$		$\rho_{xy} = 0.60$		$\rho_{xy} = 0.00$		$\rho_{xy} = +0.60$	
P	F	G	F	G	F	G	F	G
0.99	0.9894	0.9893	0.9915	0.9895	0.9898	0.9898	0.9908	0.9899
0.90	0.9016	0.9014	0.9147	0.9022	0.9009	0.9009	0.9065	0.9005
0.75	0.7531	0.7529	0.7754	0.7525	0.7514	0.7514	0.7622	0.7512
0.50	0.5001	0.5001	0.5281	0.4997	0.5008	0.5008	0.5141	0.5006
0.25	0.2464	0.2466	0.2685	0.2471	0.2495	0.2496	0.2601	0.2494
0.10	0.0983	0.0985	0.1098	0.0986	0.0999	0.1000	0.1054	0.0995
0.01	0.0108	0.0108	0.0126	0.0110	0.0102	0.0102	0.0110	0.0101

Table 7.25 Upper-tail probability values compared with nominal values (P) for a bivariate $GL(1.0)$ distribution with Fisher (F) and Gayen (G) tests of hypotheses on $\rho_{xy} = 0.00$ and $\rho_{xy} = +0.60$

	$N = 20$				$N = 80$			
	$\rho_{xy} = 0.00$		$\rho_{xy} = 0.60$		$\rho_{xy} = 0.00$		$\rho_{xy} = 0.60$	
P	F	G	F	G	F	G	F	G
0.99	0.9892	0.9891	0.9878	0.9853	0.9897	0.9897	0.9851	0.9838
0.90	0.9019	0.9016	0.9020	0.8888	0.9011	0.9011	0.8880	0.8817
0.75	0.7539	0.7537	0.7638	0.7419	0.7518	0.7518	0.7451	0.7348
0.50	0.4999	0.4999	0.5324	0.5060	0.5004	0.5004	0.5158	0.5037
0.25	0.2457	0.2460	0.2895	0.2688	0.2495	0.2495	0.2815	0.2715
0.10	0.0981	0.0983	0.1314	0.1197	0.1000	0.1000	0.1290	0.1228
0.01	0.0109	0.0109	0.0195	0.0173	0.0102	0.0102	0.0190	0.0177

Table 7.26 Upper-tail probability values compared with nominal values (P) for a bivariate $GL(0.1)$ distribution with Fisher (F) and Gayen (G) tests of hypotheses on $\rho_{xy} = 0.00$ and $\rho_{xy} = +0.60$

	$N = 20$				$N = 80$			
	$\rho_{xy} = 0.00$		$\rho_{xy} = 0.60$		$\rho_{xy} = 0.00$		$\rho_{xy} = 0.60$	
P	F	G	F	G	F	G	F	G
0.99	0.9918	0.9918	0.9869	0.9841	0.9916	0.9916	0.9819	0.9804
0.90	0.9059	0.9056	0.8954	0.8818	0.9026	0.9026	0.8774	0.8710
0.75	0.7502	0.7499	0.7560	0.7342	0.7484	0.7484	0.7347	0.7247
0.50	0.2436	0.4908	0.5297	0.5045	0.4937	0.4937	0.5144	0.5027
0.25	0.1016	0.2438	0.2982	0.2784	0.2470	0.2470	0.2921	0.2824
0.10	0.0137	0.1018	0.1441	0.1323	0.1016	0.1016	0.1435	0.1373
0.01	0.0000	0.0138	0.0257	0.0231	0.0122	0.0122	0.0265	0.0250

Table 7.27 Upper-tail probability values compared with nominal values (P) for a bivariate $GL(0.01)$ distribution with Fisher (F) and Gayen (G) tests of hypotheses on $\rho_{xy} = 0.00$ and $\rho_{xy} = +0.60$

	$N = 20$				$N = 80$			
	$\rho_{xy} = 0.00$		$\rho_{xy} = 0.60$		$\rho_{xy} = 0.00$		$\rho_{xy} = 0.60$	
P	F	G	F	G	F	G	F	G
0.99	0.9924	0.9923	0.9865	0.9837	0.9920	0.9920	0.9890	0.9792
0.90	0.9060	0.9058	0.8940	0.8803	0.9030	0.9030	0.8740	0.8675
0.75	0.7491	0.7488	0.7544	0.7329	0.7481	0.7481	0.7311	0.7210
0.50	0.4893	0.4893	0.5301	0.5054	0.4921	0.4921	0.5135	0.5018
0.25	0.2429	0.2431	0.3010	0.2810	0.2469	0.2469	0.2947	0.2850
0.10	0.1019	0.1021	0.1476	0.1357	0.1019	0.1019	0.1476	0.1416
0.01	0.0141	0.0142	0.0279	0.0250	0.0128	0.0128	0.0285	0.0268

Table 7.28 Upper-tail probability values compared with nominal values (P) for a bivariate $SK(2)$ distribution with Fisher (F) and Gayen (G) tests of hypotheses on $\rho_{xy} = 0.00$ and $\rho_{xy} = +0.60$

	$N = 20$				$N = 80$			
	$\rho_{xy} = 0.00$		$\rho_{xy} = 0.60$		$\rho_{xy} = 0.00$		$\rho_{xy} = 0.60$	
P	F	G	F	G	F	G	F	G
0.99	0.9842	0.9841	0.9487	0.9423	0.9852	0.9852	0.8480	0.8442
0.90	0.9096	0.9094	0.8159	0.8016	0.9167	0.9167	0.7162	0.7111
0.75	0.7739	0.7737	0.6918	0.6750	0.7838	0.7837	0.6221	0.6165
0.50	0.5001	0.5001	0.5327	0.5163	0.5002	0.5002	0.5121	0.5064
0.25	0.2263	0.2265	0.3797	0.3662	0.2172	0.2172	0.4060	0.4011
0.10	0.0905	0.0907	0.2650	0.2548	0.0834	0.0834	0.3224	0.3182
0.01	0.0159	0.0160	0.1333	0.1284	0.0151	0.0151	0.2099	0.2071

Table 7.29 Upper-tail probability values compared with nominal values (P) for a bivariate $SK(3)$ distribution with Fisher (F) and Gayen (G) tests of hypotheses on $\rho_{xy} = 0.00$ and $\rho_{xy} = +0.60$

	$N = 20$				$N = 80$			
	$\rho_{xy} = 0.00$		$\rho_{xy} = 0.60$		$\rho_{xy} = 0.00$		$\rho_{xy} = 0.60$	
P	F	G	F	G	F	G	F	G
0.99	0.9883	0.9883	0.9766	0.9726	0.9887	0.9887	0.9463	0.9437
0.90	0.9034	0.9032	0.8731	0.8595	0.9031	0.9031	0.8215	0.8152
0.75	0.7559	0.7557	0.7394	0.7192	0.7553	0.7553	0.6941	0.6854
0.50	0.4998	0.4998	0.5348	0.5119	0.4998	0.4998	0.5169	0.5076
0.25	0.2440	0.2442	0.3249	0.3067	0.2450	0.2451	0.3394	0.3315
0.10	0.0967	0.0970	0.1790	0.1672	0.0973	0.0973	0.2107	0.2051
0.01	0.0118	0.0119	0.0506	0.0471	0.0112	0.0112	0.0807	0.0783

Table 7.30 Upper-tail probability values compared with nominal values (P) for a bivariate $SK(25)$ distribution with Fisher (F) and Gayen (G) tests of hypotheses on $\rho_{xy} = 0.00$ and $\rho_{xy} = +0.60$

	$N = 20$				$N = 80$			
	$\rho_{xy} = 0.00$		$\rho_{xy} = 0.60$		$\rho_{xy} = 0.00$		$\rho_{xy} = 0.60$	
P	F	G	F	G	F	G	F	G
0.99	0.9890	0.9889	0.9955	0.9943	0.9899	0.9899	0.9958	0.9953
0.90	0.9014	0.9017	0.9337	0.9217	0.9006	0.9006	0.9292	0.9237
0.75	0.7538	0.7536	0.7928	0.7679	0.7512	0.7512	0.7831	0.7714
0.50	0.5005	0.5005	0.5179	0.4861	0.5004	0.5004	0.5076	0.4924
0.25	0.2463	0.2465	0.2354	0.2133	0.2493	0.2493	0.2295	0.2184
0.10	0.0975	0.0978	0.0830	0.0734	0.0999	0.0999	0.0785	0.0734
0.01	0.0111	0.0112	0.0072	0.0062	0.0103	0.0103	0.0054	0.0049

(F) and Gayen (G) test statistics. Table 7.24 analyzes data obtained from the $N(0, 1)$ distribution; Tables 7.25, 7.26, and 7.27 analyze data obtained from the generalized logistic distribution with $\theta = 1.0, 0.1$, and 0.01, respectively; and Tables 7.28, 7.29, and 7.30 analyze data obtained from the symmetric kappa distribution with $\lambda = 2$, 3, and 25, respectively.

In each table, the Monte Carlo upper-tail probability values for tests of hypotheses based on the Fisher and Gayen approaches were obtained from the same $L = 1{,}000{,}000$ bivariate random samples of size N drawn with replacement from the designated bivariate distribution characterized by the specified population correlation ρ_{xy}. If the Fisher [14] and Gayen [17] techniques are appropriate for the simulated data, the upper-tail probability values should agree with the nominal upper-tail values, P.

Considered as a set, some general statements can be made about the Monte Carlo results contained in Tables 7.24 through 7.30. First, both the Fisher z transform and the Gayen correction provide very satisfactory results for the $N(0, 1)$ distribution analyzed in Table 7.24 with any value of ρ_{xy} and for any of the other distributions analyzed in Tables 7.25 through 7.30 when $\rho_{xy} = 0.00$. Second, in general the Monte Carlo upper-tail probability values obtained with the Gayen correction are better than those obtained with the uncorrected Fisher z transform, especially near $P = 0.50$. Where differences exist, the Fisher z transform is somewhat better than the Gayen correction with $P > 0.75$ and the Gayen correction performs better when $P < 0.75$. Third, discrepancies between the Monte Carlo upper-tail probability values and the nominal probability values are noticeably larger for $N = 80$ than for $N = 20$ and for $\rho_{xy} = 0.60$ than for $\rho_{xy} = 0.00$, especially for the skewed and heavy-tailed distributions, i.e., $GL(0.1)$, $GL(0.01)$, $SK(2)$, and $SK(3)$. Fourth, the Monte Carlo upper-tail probability values in Tables 7.24 through 7.30 are consistently closer to the nominal values for $\rho_{xy} = 0.00$ than for $\rho_{xy} = +0.60$.

To illustrate the difference in results among the seven distributions, consider the first and last values in the last column in each table, i.e., the two Gayen values corresponding to $P = 0.99$ and $P = 0.01$ for $N = 80$ and $\rho_{xy} = +0.60$ in

Tables 7.25 to 7.30, inclusive. If an investigator was to test the null hypothesis $H_0\colon \rho_{xy} = +0.60$ with a two-tailed test at $\alpha = 0.02$, then given the $N(0, 1)$ distribution analyzed in Table 7.24, the investigator would reject the null hypothesis at a rate of 0.0202 or about 2.02% of the time, i.e., $1.0000 - 0.9899 + 0.0101 = 0.0202$, which is very close to $\alpha = 0.02$. For the light-tailed $GL(1.0)$ or generalized logistic distribution analyzed in Table 7.25, the investigator would reject $H_0\colon \rho_{xy} = 0.60$ at a rate of 0.0339 or about 3.39% of the time, i.e., $1.0000-0.9838+0.0177 = 0.0339$, compared with the specified $\alpha = 0.02$. For the skewed $GL(0.1)$ distribution analyzed in Table 7.26, the investigator would reject $H_0\colon \rho_{xy} = +0.60$ at a rate of 0.0446 or about 4.46% of the time, and for the $GL(0.01)$ distribution analyzed in Table 7.27, which has a more pronounced skewness than $GL(0.1)$, the rejection rate is 0.0476 or about 4.76%, compared to $\alpha = 0.02$. The heavy-tailed distributions, $SK(2)$ and $SK(3)$, analyzed in Tables 7.28 and 7.29, respectively, yield rejection rates of 0.3629 and 0.1346, respectively, which are not the least bit close to $\alpha = 0.02$. Finally, the very light-tailed distribution, $SK(25)$, analyzed in Table 7.30 yields a reversal with a very conservative rejection rate of 0.0096, compared to $\alpha = 0.02$.

7.5.4 Discussion

The Fisher z transform of the sample correlation coefficient, r_{xy}, is widely used in a variety of disciplines for both estimating population ρ_{xy} values and for testing hypothesized values of $\rho_{xy} \neq 0.00$. The transform is presented in most textbooks and is a standard feature of many statistical software packages. The assumptions underlying the use of the Fisher z transform are (1) a simple random sample drawn with replacement from (2) a bivariate normal distribution. It is commonly believed that the Fisher z transform is robust to non-normality. For example, in 1929 Karl Pearson observed:

> [T]he normal bivariate surface can be mutilated and distorted to a remarkable degree without affecting the frequency distribution of r in samples as small as 20 [43, p. 357].

Given correlated non-normal bivariate distributions, these Monte Carlo analyses demonstrate that the Fisher z transform is not at all robust.

In general, while the Fisher z transform and the alternative techniques proposed by Gayen [17] and Jeyaratnam [22] provide accurate results for a bivariate normal distribution with any value of ρ_{xy} and for non-normal bivariate distributions when $\rho_{xy} = 0.0$, serious problems surface with non-normal bivariate distributions when $|\rho_{xy}| > 0.0$. The results for the light-tailed $SK(25)$ distribution are, in general, slightly conservative when $|\rho_{xy}| > 0.0$; cf. Liu, Woodward, and Bonett [28, p. 508]. This is usually not seen as a serious problem in practice as conservative results imply possible failure to reject the null hypothesis and a potential increase in type II error. In comparison, the results for the heavy-tailed distributions, $SK(2)$ and $SK(3)$, and the skewed distributions, $GL(0.1)$ and $GL(0.01)$ are quite liberal when $|\rho_{xy}| > 0.0$.

Also, $GL(1.0)$ is a light-tailed distribution that yields slightly liberal results. Liberal results are much more serious than conservative results, as they imply possible rejection of the null hypothesis and a potential increase in type I error.

Most surprisingly, from a statistical perspective, for the heavy-tailed and skewed distributions, small samples provide better estimates than large samples. Table 7.31 extends the analyses of Tables 7.21, 7.22, 7.23, and 7.24 to larger sample sizes. In Table 7.31 the investigation is limited to Monte Carlo containment probability values obtained from the Fisher z transform for the skewed bivariate distributions based on $GL(0.1)$ and $GL(0.01)$ and for the heavy-tailed bivariate distributions based on $SK(2)$ and $SK(3)$, with $\rho_{xy} = 0.00$ and $\rho_{xy} = 0.60$, and for $N = 10$, 20, 40, 80, 160, 320, and 640. Inspection of Table 7.31 confirms that the trend observed in Tables 7.19 through 7.22 continues with larger sample sizes, producing increasingly smaller containment probability values with increasing N for $|\rho_{xy}| > 0.00$, where $\rho_{xy} = +0.60$ is considered representative of larger ρ_{xy} values.

The impact of large sample sizes is most pronounced in the heavy-tailed bivariate distribution based on $SK(2)$ and the skewed bivariate distribution based on $GL(0.01)$ where, with $\rho_{xy} = +0.60$, the divergence between the containment probability values and the nominal $1 - \alpha$ values for $N = 10$ and $N = 640$ is quite extreme. For example, $SK(2)$ with $1 - \alpha = 0.90$, $\rho_{xy} = +0.60$, and $N = 10$ yields a containment probability value of $P = 0.7487$, whereas $N = 640$ for this case yields a containment probability value of $P = 0.2677$, compared with $1 - \alpha = 0.90$. Obviously, large samples have a greater chance of selecting rare extreme values than small samples. Consequently, the Monte Carlo containment probability values become worse with increasing sample size when heavy-tailed distributions are encountered.

It is clear that the Fisher z transform provides very good results for the bivariate normal distribution and any of the other distributions when $\rho_{xy} = 0.00$. However, if a distribution is not bivariate normal and $\rho_{xy} > 0.00$, then the Fisher z random variable does not follow a normal distribution. Geary [18, p. 241] admonished: "Normality is a myth; there never was, and never will be, a normal distribution." In the absence of bivariate normality and in the presence of correlated heavy-tailed bivariate distributions, such as those contaminated by extreme values, or correlated skewed bivariate distributions, the Fisher z transform and related techniques can yield highly inaccurate results.

Given that normally distributed populations are rarely encountered in actual research situations [18, 33] and that both heavy-tailed symmetrical distributions and heavy-tailed skewed distributions are prevalent in much research, considerable caution should be exercised when using the Fisher z transform or related techniques such as those proposed by Gayen [17] and Jeyaratnam [22], as these methods clearly are not robust to deviations from normality when $|\rho_{xy}| \neq 0.0$. In general, there is no easy answer to this problem. However, a researcher cannot simply ignore a problem just because it is annoying. Unfortunately, given a non-normal population with $\rho_{xy} \neq 0.0$, there appear to be no published alternative tests of significance nor viable options for the construction of confidence intervals.

Table 7.31 Containment probability values for the bivariate $GL(0.1)$, $GL(0.01)$, $SK(2)$, and $SK(3)$ distributions with Fisher (F) $1-\alpha$ correlation confidence intervals

		Distribution							
		$GL(0.1)$		$GL(0.01)$		$SK(2)$		$SK(3)$	
$1-\alpha$	N	$\rho_{xy}=0.00$	$\rho_{xy}=0.60$	$\rho_{xy}=0.00$	$\rho_{xy}=0.60$	$\rho_{xy}=0.00$	$\rho_{xy}=+0.60$	$\rho_{xy}=0.00$	$\rho_{xy}=+0.60$
0.90	10	0.9016	0.8729	0.9019	0.8693	0.8961	0.7487	0.9007	0.8451
	20	0.9013	0.8593	0.9015	0.8545	0.9002	0.6650	0.9009	0.8068
	40	0.9010	0.8510	0.9012	0.8454	0.9050	0.5755	0.9015	0.7670
	80	0.9006	0.8459	0.9002	0.8394	0.9097	0.4884	0.9016	0.7246
	160	0.9004	0.8431	0.9004	0.8366	0.9138	0.4060	0.9021	0.6822
	320	0.9003	0.8405	0.9003	0.8338	0.9173	0.3314	0.9025	0.6369
	640	0.9002	0.8400	0.9001	0.8332	0.9204	0.2677	0.9016	0.5934
0.95	10	0.9486	0.9281	0.9485	0.9255	0.9403	0.8217	0.9474	0.9052
	20	0.9495	0.9197	0.9496	0.9160	0.9415	0.7457	0.9479	0.8751
	40	0.9495	0.9136	0.9495	0.9092	0.9436	0.6551	0.9482	0.8382
	80	0.9498	0.9100	0.9500	0.9055	0.9461	0.5634	0.9490	0.8010
	160	0.9504	0.9075	0.9503	0.9025	0.9490	0.4714	0.9495	0.7590
	320	0.9500	0.9063	0.9500	0.9011	0.9514	0.3889	0.9497	0.7164
	640	0.9498	0.9053	0.9499	0.9001	0.9535	0.3147	0.9500	0.6714
0.99	10	0.9871	0.9793	0.9869	0.9782	0.9797	0.9152	0.9863	0.9660
	20	0.9882	0.9770	0.9881	0.9752	0.9789	0.8577	0.9869	0.9488
	40	0.9890	0.9752	0.9889	0.9732	0.9788	0.7780	0.9873	0.9256
	80	0.9895	0.9737	0.9897	0.9712	0.9794	0.6835	0.9878	0.8968
	160	0.9896	0.9726	0.9896	0.9702	0.9802	0.5854	0.9877	0.8639
	320	0.9899	0.9721	0.9899	0.9697	0.9811	0.4901	0.9883	0.8272
	640	0.9900	0.9721	0.9899	0.9696	0.9817	0.4020	0.9885	0.7877

Finally, to paraphrase a line from Thompson regarding the use of tiltmeters in volcanology [53, p. 258],

1. Do not use the Fisher z transformation.
2. If you do use it, don't believe it.
3. If you do believe it, don't publish it.
4. If you do publish it, don't be the first author.

7.6 Point-Biserial Linear Correlation

The point-biserial correlation coefficient measures the association between a dichotomous variable and an interval-level variable. Applications of the point-biserial correlation abound in fields such as education and educational psychology. The point-biserial correlation may be thought of simply as the Pearson product-moment correlation between an interval-level variable and a variable with two disjoint, unordered categories.

7.6.1 Example

To illustrate the point-biserial correlation coefficient, consider the dichotomous data listed in Table 7.32 for $N = 13$ subjects where variable x is a dichotomous variable coded (0, 1) and variable y is an interval-level variable. The point-biserial correlation is usually computed as

$$r_{pb} = \frac{\bar{y}_1 - \bar{y}_0}{s_y} \sqrt{\frac{n_0 n_1}{N(N-1)}} ,$$

Table 7.32 Example bivariate data for point-biserial correlation on $N = 13$ subjects

Subject	x	y
1	0	19
2	1	17
3	0	18
4	0	18
5	1	26
6	1	28
7	0	20
8	1	19
9	0	22
10	1	23
11	1	26
12	0	25
13	1	30

where n_0 and n_1 denote the number of y values coded 0 and 1, respectively, $N = n_0 + n_1$, $\bar{y}_0$ and $\bar{y}_1$ denote the means of the y values coded 0 and 1, respectively, and s_y is the sample standard deviation of the y values given by

$$s_y = \sqrt{\frac{1}{N-1}\sum_{i=1}^{N}\left(y_i - \bar{y}\right)^2} \; .$$

For the data listed in Table 7.32, $n_0 = 6$, $n_1 = 7$, $\bar{y}_0 = 20.3333$, $\bar{y}_1 = 24.1429$, $s_y = 4.2728$, and the point-biserial correlation is

$$r_{pb} = \frac{\bar{y}_1 - \bar{y}_0}{s_y}\sqrt{\frac{n_0 n_1}{N(N-1)}} = \frac{24.1429 - 20.3333}{4.2728}\sqrt{\frac{(6)(7)}{13(13-1)}} = +0.4626 \; .$$

However, r_{pb} can also be calculated simply as the Pearson product-moment correlation (r_{xy}) between dichotomous variable x and interval variable y. For the data listed in Table 7.32, $N = 13$,

$$\sum_{i=1}^{N} x_i = \sum_{i=1}^{N} x_i^2 = 7 \, , \quad \sum_{i=1}^{N} y_i = 291 \, , \quad \sum_{i=1}^{N} y_i^2 = 6{,}733 \, , \quad \sum_{i=1}^{N} x_i y_i = 169 \, ,$$

and

$$r_{xy} = \frac{N\sum_{i=1}^{N} x_i y_i - \sum_{i=1}^{N} x_i \sum_{i=1}^{N} y_i}{\sqrt{\left[N\sum_{i=1}^{N} x_i^2 - \left(\sum_{i=1}^{N} x_i\right)^2\right]\left[N\sum_{i=1}^{N} y_i^2 - \left(\sum_{i=1}^{N} y_i\right)^2\right]}}$$

$$= \frac{(13)(169) - (7)(291)}{\sqrt{\left[(13)(7) - 7^2\right]\left[(13)(6{,}733) - 291^2\right]}} = +0.4626 \; .$$

Approaching the calculation of the probability value from a product-moment perspective, there are

$$M = N! = 13! = 6{,}227{,}020{,}800$$

possible, equally-likely arrangements in the reference set of all permutations of the observed bivariate data, making an exact permutation analysis impractical. Let r_o denote the observed value of r_{pb}. Then, based on $L = 1{,}000{,}000$ random arrangements of the observed data under the null hypothesis, there are 121,667 $|r_{pb}|$

values equal to or greater than $|r_o| = 0.4626$, yielding a Monte Carlo resampling two-sided probability value of $P = 121{,}667/1{,}000{,}000 = 0.121667$.

In general, $L = 1{,}000{,}000$ ensures three decimal places of accuracy. However, it requires an increase of two orders of magnitude, i.e., $L = 100{,}000{,}000$, to ensure four decimal places of accuracy [23]. Based on $L = 100{,}000{,}000$ random arrangements of the observed bivariate data, the two-sided Monte Carlo resampling probability value of $r_{pb} = +0.4626$ to six decimal places is $P = 12{,}121{,}600/100{,}000{,}000 = 0.121216$.

However, because variable x is composed of only two categories, an alternative procedure exists for establishing the probability value of r_{pb}. The relationships between r_{pb} and Student's two-sample t test are

$$r_{pb} = \sqrt{\frac{t^2}{t^2 + N - 2}} \quad \text{and} \quad t = \frac{r_{pb}\sqrt{N-2}}{\sqrt{1 - r_{pb}^2}} \; .$$

Thus, the probability value for a specified point-biserial correlation coefficient can be calculated much more efficiently as the probability value of a two-sample t test with $N - 2$ degrees of freedom. Consider the data in Table 7.32 rearranged into two groups coded 0 and 1 as in Table 7.33.

For the observed data listed in Table 7.33, Student's t test statistic is

$$t = \frac{r_{pb}\sqrt{N-2}}{\sqrt{1 - r_{pb}^2}} = \frac{+0.4626\sqrt{13-2}}{\sqrt{1 - (+0.4626)^2}} = +1.7307 \; .$$

For the data listed in Table 7.33, there are only

$$M = \frac{N!}{n_0!\, n_1!} = \frac{13!}{6!\; 7!} = 1{,}716$$

possible, equally-likely arrangements in the reference set of all permutations of the observed scores, compared with

$$M = N! = 13! = 6{,}227{,}020{,}800$$

Table 7.33 Example data on $N = 13$ subjects for Student's t test

0	1
19	17
18	26
18	28
20	19
22	23
25	26
	30

in the initial set, making an exact permutation analysis possible. If all arrangements of the $N = 13$ observed scores occur with equal chance, the exact two-sided probability value of $t = +1.7307$ to six places computed on the $M = 1{,}716$ possible arrangements of the observed data with $n_0 = 6$ and $n_1 = 7$ preserved for each arrangement is $208/1{,}716 = 0.121212$.

The Monte Carlo resampling probability value of $P = 0.121667$ based on $L = 1{,}000{,}000$ and the Monte Carlo resampling probability value of $P = 0.121216$ based on $L = 100{,}000{,}000$ both compare favorably with the exact probability value of $P = 0.121212$. For comparison, the two-sided probability value of $t = +1.7303$ based on Student's t distribution with $N - 2 = 13 - 2 = 11$ degrees of freedom is $P = 0.111421$.

7.6.2 Problems with the Point-Biserial Coefficient

Whenever a dichotomous variable is correlated with an interval-level variable, as in point-biserial correlation, there are potential problems with proper norming between ± 1. In brief, it is not possible to obtain a perfect correlation, positive or negative, between a dichotomous variable and a continuous variable [42, p. 145]. The reason is simply that it is not possible for a dichotomous variable and a continuous variable to have the same shape, as illustrated in Fig. 7.8 where a dichotomous variable (x) is correlated with a continuous variable (y) that is comprised of a uniform distribution, i.e, $y = 1, 2, \ldots, 10$. In order to achieve a perfect correlation of $r_{pb} = +1.00$, it

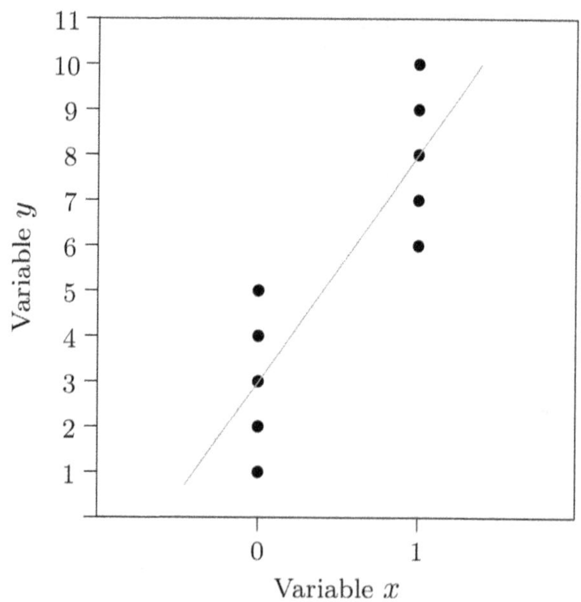

Fig. 7.8 Scatterplot of a uniform distribution of y values with the regression line overlaid

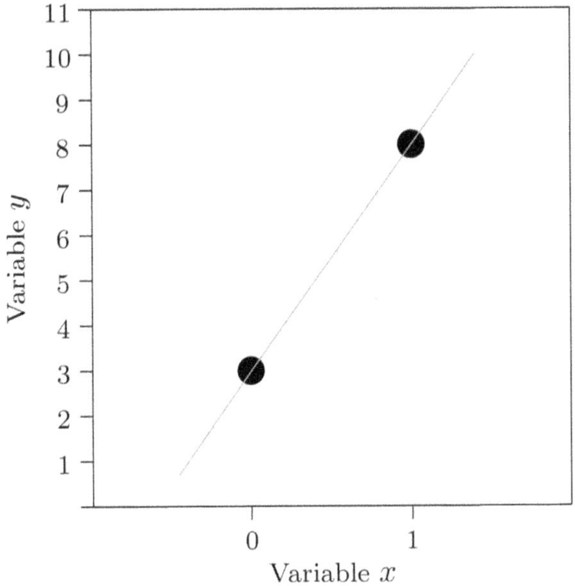

Fig. 7.9 Scatterplot of clusters of y values located at $x = 0$ and $x = 1$ with the regression line overlaid

would be necessary for all the scores at the two points of variable x ($x = 0$ and $x = 1$) to fall exactly on two points on variable y, as depicted in Fig. 7.9 where the larger black circles represent a cluster of points at $x = 0$ and $x = 1$. Since variable y is assumed to be continuous, this is not possible. Consequently, values of variable y at either of the two points on variable x (the dichotomous variable) must correspond to a range of points on variable y (the continuous variable).

As Jum Nunnally showed in 1978, the maximum value of r_{pb} between a dichotomous variable and a normally distributed variable is approximately $r_{pb} = \pm 0.80$, which occurs only when $p = n_0/N = 0.50$ [42]. As p deviates from 0.50 in either direction, the maximum value of r_{pb} is further reduced. Consequently, when $p = 0.25$ or $p = 0.75$, the maximum value of r_{pb} is approximately $r_{pb} = \pm 0.75$, and when $p = 0.90$ or $p = 0.10$, the maximum value of r_{pb} is only approximately $r_{pb} = \pm 0.58$.[5]

The problem can be illustrated with a small empirical example. Table 7.34 contains 10 scores $(1, 2, \ldots, 10)$ with frequencies corresponding to an expanded binomial distribution, which approximates a normal distribution with $N = 512$. For

[5]The problem is not confined to r_{pb}. In general, the problem is called the base-rate problem or the marginal-dependent problem. See two excellent discussions of the problem by Goodman [19] and McGrath and Meyer [31].

Table 7.34 Example binomial distribution on $N = 512$ subjects with $p = 0.50$

x	y	f	fy	y^2	fy^2
0	1	1	1	1	1
0	2	9	18	4	36
0	3	36	108	9	324
0	4	84	336	16	1,344
0	5	126	630	25	3,150
1	6	126	756	36	4,536
1	7	84	588	49	4,116
1	8	36	288	64	2,304
1	9	9	81	81	729
1	10	1	10	100	100
Sum		512	2,816		16,640

the binomial data listed in Table 7.34 with $p = 0.50$,

$$\bar{y}_0 = \left(\sum_{i=1}^{n_0} f_i \right)^{-1} \sum_{i=1}^{n_0} f_i y_i = \frac{1 + 18 + 108 + 336 + 630}{1 + 9 + 36 + 84 + 126} = 4.2695 \; ,$$

$$\bar{y}_1 = \left(\sum_{i=1}^{n_1} f_i \right)^{-1} \sum_{i=1}^{n_1} f_i y_i = \frac{756 + 588 + 288 + 81 + 10}{126 + 84 + 36 + 9 + 1} = 6.7305 \; ,$$

$$s_y = \sqrt{\frac{\displaystyle\sum_{i=1}^{N} fy^2 - \frac{\left(\displaystyle\sum_{i=1}^{N} fy \right)^2}{N}}{N - 1}} = \sqrt{\frac{16{,}640 - \dfrac{(2{,}816)^2}{512}}{512 - 1}} = 1.5015 \; ,$$

and

$$r_{pb} = \frac{\bar{y}_1 - \bar{y}_0}{s_y} \sqrt{\frac{n_0 n_1}{N(N-1)}} = \frac{6.7305 - 4.2695}{1.5015} \sqrt{\frac{(256)(256)}{512(512-1)}}$$

$$= +0.8203 \; ,$$

which approximates Nunnally's estimate of $r_{pb} = +0.80$.

Table 7.35 illustrates a binomial distribution with $N = 512$ and $p \simeq 0.25$, i.e.,

$$p = \frac{1}{N} \sum_{i=1}^{n_0} f_i = \frac{1 + 9 + 36 + 84}{512} = 0.2539 \; .$$

Table 7.35 Example binomial distribution on $N = 512$ subjects with $p \simeq 0.25$

x	y	f	fy	y^2	fy^2
0	1	1	1	1	1
0	2	9	18	4	36
0	3	36	108	9	324
0	4	84	336	16	1,344
1	5	126	630	25	3,150
1	6	126	756	36	4,536
1	7	84	588	49	4,116
1	8	36	288	64	2,304
1	9	9	81	81	729
1	10	1	10	100	100
Sum		512	2,816		16,640

For the binomial data in Table 7.35 with $p \simeq 0.25$,

$$\bar{y}_0 = \left(\sum_{i=1}^{n_0} f_i \right)^{-1} \sum_{i=1}^{n_0} f_i y_i = \frac{1 + 18 + 108 + 336}{1 + 9 + 36 + 84} = 3.5615 \; ,$$

$$\bar{y}_1 = \left(\sum_{i=1}^{n_1} f_i \right)^{-1} \sum_{i=1}^{n_1} f_i y_i = \frac{630 + 756 + 588 + 288 + 81 + 10}{126 + 126 + 84 + 36 + 9 + 1} = 6.1597 \; ,$$

the standard deviation of the y values is unchanged at $s_y = 1.5015$ and

$$r_{pb} = \frac{\bar{y}_1 - \bar{y}_0}{s_y} \sqrt{\frac{n_0 n_1}{N(N-1)}} = \frac{6.1597 - 3.5615}{1.5015} \sqrt{\frac{(130)(382)}{512(512-1)}}$$

$$= +0.7539 \; ,$$

which approximates Nunnally's estimate of $r_{pb} = +0.75$.

While it is not convenient to take exactly 10% of $N = 512$ cases, as arranged in Table 7.34, it is possible to take 9% of $N = 512$ cases. Thus,

$$p = \frac{1}{N} \sum_{i=1}^{n_0} = \frac{1 + 9 + 36}{512} = \frac{46}{512} = 0.0898 .$$

Table 7.36 Example binomial distribution on $N = 512$ subjects with $p = 0.09$

x	y	f	fy	y^2	fy^2
0	1	1	1	1	1
0	2	9	18	4	36
0	3	36	108	9	324
1	4	84	336	16	1,344
1	5	126	630	25	3,150
1	6	126	756	36	4,536
1	7	84	588	49	4,116
1	8	36	288	64	2,304
1	9	9	81	81	729
1	10	1	10	100	100
Sum		512	2,816		16,640

Table 7.36 illustrates a binomial distribution with $N = 512$ and $p = 0.09$. For the binomial data listed in Table 7.36 with $p \simeq 0.10$,

$$\bar{y}_0 = \left(\sum_{1=1}^{n_0} f_i \right)^{-1} \sum_{i=1}^{n_0} f_i y_i = \frac{1 + 18 + 108}{1 + 9 + 36} = 2.7609 ,$$

$$\bar{y}_1 = \left(\sum_{i=1}^{n_1} f_i \right)^{-1} \sum_{i=1}^{n_1} f_i y_i = \frac{336 + 630 + 756 + 588 + 288 + 81 + 10}{84 + 126 + 126 + 84 + 36 + 9 + 1}$$
$$= 5.7704 ,$$

the standard deviation of the y values is unchanged at $s_y = 1.5015$ and

$$r_{pb} = \frac{\bar{y}_1 - \bar{y}_0}{s_y} \sqrt{\frac{n_0 n_1}{N(N-1)}} = \frac{5.7704 - 2.7609}{1.5015} \sqrt{\frac{(46)(466)}{512(512-1)}}$$
$$= +0.5737 ,$$

which approximates Nunnally's estimate of $r_{pb} = +0.58$.

7.7 Biserial Linear Correlation

Point-biserial correlation measures the degree of association between an interval-level variable and a dichotomous variable that is a true dichotomy, such as right and wrong, true and false, or left and right. On the other hand, biserial correlation measures the degree of association between an interval-level variable and a dichotomous variable that has been created from a variable that is assumed to be continuous and normally distributed, such as grades that have been dichotomized into "pass" and "fail" or weight that has been classified into "normal" and "obese."[6] Biserial correlation has long been difficult to compute, requiring the ordinate of a unit-normal distribution. Some approximating methods have been suggested to simplify computation [16], but these are unnecessary with permutation methods.

Let x represent the dichotomous variable and y represent the continuous interval-level variable, then the biserial correlation coefficient is given by

$$r_b = \frac{(\bar{y}_1 - \bar{y}_0)pq}{uS_y} ,$$

where p and $q = 1 - p$ denote the proportions of all y values coded 0 and 1, respectively, $\bar{y}_0$ and $\bar{y}_1$ denote the arithmetic means of the y values coded 0 and 1, respectively, S_y is the standard deviation of the y values given by[7]

$$S_y = \sqrt{\frac{1}{N}\sum_{i=1}^{N}(y_i - \bar{y})^2} ,$$

and u is the ordinate of the unit normal curve at the point of division between the p and q proportions under the curve given by

$$u = \frac{\exp(-z^2/2)}{\sqrt{2\pi}} .$$

Written in raw terms without the p and q proportions,

$$r_b = \frac{(\bar{y}_0 - \bar{y}_1)n_0n_1}{N^2uS_y} ,$$

where n_0 and n_1 denote the number of y values coded 0 and 1, respectively, and $N = n_0 + n_1$. The biserial correlation may also be written in terms of the point-biserial correlation coefficient,

$$r_b = \frac{r_{pb}\sqrt{pq}}{u} = \frac{r_{pb}\sqrt{n_0n_1}}{Nu} ,$$

[6]For many years height has been considered as normally distributed, but recent research indicates that this is not necessarily the case [30, pp. 205–207].

[7]Note that the sum of squared deviation is divided by N, not $N-1$ and the symbol for the standard deviation is S_y with an uppercase letter S to distinguish it from the usual sample standard deviation denoted by s_y.

where the point-biserial correlation coefficient is given by

$$r_{pb} = \frac{(\bar{y}_1 - \bar{y}_0)\sqrt{pq}}{S_y} \; .$$

7.7.1 Example

To illustrate the calculation of the biserial correlation coefficient, consider the set of data given in Table 7.37 where $N = 15$ subjects are scored on interval-level variable y and are classified into types on dichotomous variable x. For the data listed in Table 7.37, $n_0 = 6$, $n_1 = 9$, $p = 6/15 = 0.40$, $q = 9/15 = 0.60$,

$$\bar{y}_0 = \frac{1}{n_0}\sum_{i=1}^{n_0} y_i = \frac{12+15+11+18+13+11}{6} = 13.3333 \; ,$$

$$\bar{y}_1 = \frac{1}{n_1}\sum_{i=1}^{n_1} y_i = \frac{10+33+19+21+29+12+19+23+16}{9} = 20.2222 \; ,$$

$$S_y = \sqrt{\frac{1}{N}\sum_{i=1}^{N}(y_i - \bar{y})^2} = \sqrt{\frac{649.7333}{15}} = 6.5815 \; ,$$

the standard score that defines the lower $p = 0.40$ of the unit-normal distribution is $z = -0.2533$,

$$u = \frac{\exp(-z^2/2)}{\sqrt{2\pi}} = \frac{\exp[-(-0.2533)^2/2]}{\sqrt{(2)(3.1416)}} = 0.3863 \; ,$$

and

$$r_b = \frac{(\bar{y}_1 - \bar{y}_0)pq}{uS_y} = \frac{(20.2222 - 13.3333)(0.40)(0.60)}{(0.3863)(6.5815)} = +0.6503 \; .$$

For the data listed in Table 7.37, the point-biserial correlation coefficient is

$$r_{pb} = \frac{(\bar{y}_1 - \bar{y}_0)\sqrt{pq}}{S_y} = \frac{(20.2222 - 13.3333)\sqrt{(0.40)(0.60)}}{6.5815} = +0.5128 \; ,$$

and in terms of the point-biserial correlation coefficient, the biserial correlation coefficient is

$$r_b = \frac{r_{pb}\sqrt{pq}}{u} = \frac{+0.5128\sqrt{(0.40)(0.60)}}{0.3863} = +0.6503 \; .$$

Table 7.37 Example biserial correlation data on $N = 15$ subjects

Subject	x	y
1	0	12
2	0	15
3	0	11
4	0	18
5	0	13
6	0	11
7	1	10
8	1	33
9	1	19
10	1	21
11	1	29
12	1	12
13	1	19
14	1	23
15	1	16

For the $N = 15$ scores listed in Table 7.37, there are only

$$M = \frac{N!}{n_0!\, n_1!} = \frac{15!}{6!\, 9!} = 5{,}005$$

possible, equally-likely arrangements in the reference set of all permutations of the observed scores, making an exact permutation analysis easily accomplished. Note that in the formula for the biserial correlation coefficient,

$$r_b = \frac{\bar{y}_1 - \bar{y}_0 pq}{u S_y}$$

p, q, u, and S_y are invariant under permutation. Therefore, the permutation distribution can efficiently be based entirely on $\bar{y}_1 - \bar{y}_0$. If all $M = 5{,}005$ arrangements of the $N = 15$ observed values occur with equal chance, the exact two-sided probability value of $|r_b| = +0.6503$ computed on the $M = 5{,}005$ possible arrangements of the observed data with $n_0 = 6$ and $n_1 = 9$ preserved for each arrangement is $P = 263/5{,}005 = 0.0525$.

7.8 Intraclass Correlation

There exists an extensive, and controversial, literature on the intraclass correlation coefficient and its uses. The standard reference is by E.A. Haggard, *Intraclass Correlation and the Analysis of Variance* [20], although it has been heavily criticized for both its exposition and its statistical accuracy [51]. See also discussions by

Bartko [3, 2, 4], Kraemer [27], Kraemer and Thiemann [26, pp. 32–34, 54–56], Shrout and Fleiss [50], von Eye and Mun [54, pp. 116-122], and Winer [56, pp. 289–296].

The intraclass correlation coefficient is most often used for measuring the level of agreement among judges. The coefficient represents concordance, where $+1$ indicates perfect agreement and 0 indicates no agreement. While the maximum value of the intraclass correlation coefficient is $+1$, the minimum is given by $-1/(k-1)$, where k is the number of judges. Thus, for $k = 2$ judges the lower limit is -1, but for $k = 3$ judges the lower limit is $-1/2$, for $k = 4$ judges the lower limit is $-1/3$, for $k = 5$ judges the lower limit is $-1/4$, and so on, approaching zero as the number of judges increases. A number of authors recommend that when the intraclass correlation coefficient is negative, it should be interpreted as zero [4, 20, p. 71], but this seems intuitively wrong.

In many ways the intraclass correlation coefficient is a special form of the Pearson product-moment (interclass) correlation coefficient. Consider the small set of data given in Table 7.38 with $N = 5$ subjects and measurements on Height (x) and Weight (y). For the bivariate data given in Table 7.38 with $N = 5$ subjects,

$$\sum_{i=1}^{N} x_i = 15\,,\quad \sum_{i=1}^{N} x_i^2 = 55\,,\quad \sum_{i=1}^{N} y_i = 25\,,\quad \sum_{i=1}^{N} y_i^2 = 135\,,\quad \sum_{i=1}^{N} x_i y_i = 83\,,$$

and the Pearson product-moment correlation coefficient is $r_{xy} = +0.80$.

Now consider $N = 5$ sets of twins and let the variable under consideration be Weight, as in Table 7.39. The question is, which of the two variables labeled Weight is to be considered variable x and which is to be considered variable y? The problem can be solved by the intraclass correlation coefficient using double entries. The intraclass correlation between N pairs of observations on two variables, x and y, is by definition the ordinary Pearson product-moment (interclass) correlation between $2N$ pairs of observations, the first N of which are the original observations, and the

Table 7.38 Example bivariate correlation data on $N = 5$ subjects

Subject	Height (x)	Weight (y)
A	1	4
B	2	3
C	3	5
D	4	7
E	5	6

Table 7.39 Example bivariate correlation data on $N = 5$ twins

Twins	Weight	Weight
A	1	4
B	2	3
C	3	5
D	4	7
E	5	6

second N the original observations with variable x replacing variable y and vice versa [15, Sect. 38]. Table 7.40 illustrates the arrangement. For the bivariate data given in Table 7.40 with $2N = 10$ subjects,

$$\sum_{i=1}^{N} x_i = \sum_{i=1}^{N} y_i = 40 \,, \quad \sum_{i=1}^{N} x_i^2 = \sum_{i=1}^{N} y_i^2 = 190 \,, \quad \sum_{i=1}^{N} x_i y_i = 166 \,,$$

and the intraclass correlation coefficient is $r_I = +0.20$. Note that certain computational simplifications follow from the reversal of the variables, mainly because the reversals make the marginal distributions for the new variables the same and, therefore, the means and variances of the new variables are also the same [46, p. 20].

For cases with $k > 2$, the construction of a table suitable for calculating the intraclass correlation coefficient is more laborious. For example, given $k = 3$ judges, designate the three values for each subject as x_1, x_2, and x_3. The three values are entered into the table as six observations, each being one of the six permutations of two values that can be made from the original three values. That is, the values of the three values x_1, x_2, and x_3 for each subject are entered into a bivariate correlation table with coordinates (x_1, x_2), (x_1, x_3), (x_2, x_3), (x_2, x_1), (x_3, x_1), and (x_3, x_2), and the Pearson product-moment correlation coefficient is computed for the resulting table, yielding the intraclass correlation coefficient.

To illustrate, consider the small data set given in Table 7.41 with $N = 3$ subjects and $k = 3$ judges. The permutations of the observations in Table 7.41 are listed in the correlation matrix given in Table 7.42. For the bivariate data listed in Table 7.42

Table 7.40 Example bivariate correlation data on $2N = 10$ twins

Twins	Weight (x)	Weight (y)
A	1	4
B	2	3
C	3	5
D	4	7
E	5	6
A′	4	1
B′	3	2
C′	5	3
D′	7	4
E′	6	5

Table 7.41 Example correlation data with $k = 3$ judges and $N = 3$ subjects

Subject	x_1	x_2	x_3
A	1	2	3
B	6	4	5
C	8	9	7

Table 7.42 Bivariate permutation matrix for $k = 3$ judges and $N = 3$ subjects

Ss	1	2	3	4	5	6	7	8	9	10	11	12	13	14	15	16	17	18
x	1	1	2	6	6	4	8	8	9	3	3	2	5	5	4	7	7	9
y	2	3	3	4	5	5	9	7	7	1	2	1	4	6	6	9	8	8

Table 7.43 Example data for Case 1, Form 1, with $N = 6$ subjects (S) and $k = 4$ judges (A)

	Judge (A)			
Subject (S)	1	2	3	4
1	9	2	5	8
2	6	1	3	2
3	8	4	6	8
4	7	1	2	6
5	10	5	6	9
6	6	2	4	7

with $N = 18$ subjects,

$$\sum_{i=1}^{N} x_i = \sum_{i=1}^{N} y_i = 90 \,, \quad \sum_{i=1}^{N} x_i^2 = \sum_{i=1}^{N} y_i^2 = 570 \,, \quad \sum_{i=1}^{N} x_i y_i = 552 \,,$$

and the intraclass correlation coefficient obtained via the Pearson product-moment correlation coefficient is $r_{\text{I}} = r_{xy} = +0.85$.

Because of the complexity of double entries with $k > 2$, the intraclass correlation coefficient is usually formulated as an analysis of variance with variable A a random variable. There are actually three different intraclass correlation coefficients, and two forms of each [32, 50, 57]. The three types and two forms are designated as:

$$\text{ICC}(1,1) \text{ and } \text{ICC}(1,k),$$
$$\text{ICC}(2,1) \text{ and } \text{ICC}(2,k),$$
$$\text{ICC}(3,1) \text{ and } \text{ICC}(3,k).$$

Case 1, Form 1: ICC(1, 1) For Case 1, Form 1, there exists a pool of judges. For each subject, a researcher randomly samples k judges from the pool to evaluate each subject. The k judges who rate Subject 1 are not necessarily the same judges who rate Subject 2. To illustrate Case 1, Form 1, Table 7.43 lists example data for $k = 4$ judges (A) and $N = 6$ subjects (S).

Now consider the data given in Table 7.43 as a one-way randomized-block analysis of variance, given in Table 7.44. For the summary data given in Table 7.44, let a indicate the number of levels of Factor A, then the sum-of-squares Total is

$$SS_{\text{Total}} = \sum_{i=1}^{N} x_i^2 - \frac{\left(\displaystyle\sum_{i=1}^{N} x_i\right)^2}{Na} = 841 - \frac{(127)^2}{(6)(4)} = 168.9583 \,,$$

Table 7.44 Example data for Case 1, Form 1, prepared for an analysis of variance with $N = 6$ subjects (S) and $k = 4$ judges (A)

	Judge (A)				
Subject (S)	1	2	3	4	T_S
1	9	2	5	8	24
2	6	1	3	2	12
3	8	4	6	8	26
4	7	1	2	6	16
5	10	5	6	9	30
6	6	2	4	7	19
N	6	6	6	6	24
T_A	46	15	26	40	127
Σx^2	366	51	126	298	841

the sum-of-squares Between Subjects (BS) is

$$SS_{\text{BS}} = \frac{\displaystyle\sum_{i=1}^{N} T_{S_i}^2}{a} - \frac{\left(\displaystyle\sum_{i=1}^{N} x_i\right)^2}{Na} = \frac{(24)^2 + (12)^2 + \cdots + (19)^2}{4} - \frac{(127)^2}{(6)(4)} = 56.2083 \,,$$

the sum-of-squares for Factor A is

$$SS_{\text{A}} = \frac{\displaystyle\sum_{j=1}^{a} T_{A_j}^2}{N} - \frac{\left(\displaystyle\sum_{i=1}^{N} x_i\right)^2}{Na} = \frac{(46)^2 + (15)^2 + (26)^2 + (40)^2}{6} - \frac{(127)^2}{(6)(4)} = 97.4583 \,,$$

the sum-of-squares Within Subjects (WS) is

$$SS_{\text{WS}} = SS_{\text{Total}} - SS_{\text{BS}} = 168.9583 - 56.2083 = 112.7500 \,,$$

and the sum-of-squares Error is

$$SS_{\text{Error}} = SS_{\text{A}\times\text{S}} = SS_{\text{WS}} - SS_{\text{A}} = 112.7500 - 97.4583 = 15.2917 \,.$$

Table 7.45 Analysis of variance source table for the data given in Table 7.44 with $k = 4$ judges and $N = 6$ subjects

Source	*SS*	*df*	*MS*	*F*
Between *S*	56.2083	5	11.2417	
Within *S*	112.7500	18	6.2639	
Factor *A*	97.4583	3	32.4861	31.87
Error ($A \times S$)	15.2917	15	1.0194	
Total	168.9583	23		

The analysis of variance source table is given in Table 7.45. For Case 1, Form 1, the intraclass correlation coefficient is given by

$$\mathrm{ICC}(1,1) = \frac{MS_{\mathrm{BS}} - MS_{\mathrm{WS}}}{MS_{\mathrm{BS}} + (a-1)MS_{\mathrm{WS}}}$$

$$= \frac{11.2417 - 6.2639}{11.2417 + (4-1)(6.2639)} = +0.1659\ .$$

Case 1, Form *k*: ICC(1,*k*) If each judge is replaced with a group of k judges, such as a team of clinicians, and the score is the average score of the k judges, then for Case 1, Form k, the intraclass correlation coefficient is

$$\mathrm{ICC}(1,k) = \frac{MS_{\mathrm{BS}} - MS_{\mathrm{WS}}}{MS_{\mathrm{BS}}} = \frac{11.2417 - 6.2639}{11.2417} = +0.4428\ .$$

Case 2, Form 1: ICC(2, 1) If the same set of k judges rate each subject and the k judges are considered a random sample from a population of potential judges, then the intraclass correlation coefficient is designated ICC(2, 1). Because this is the most common case/form, it is usually designated simply as r_{I} in the literature.

$$\mathrm{ICC}(2,1) = \frac{MS_{\mathrm{BS}} - MS_{\mathrm{A\times S}}}{MS_{\mathrm{BS}} + (a-1)MS_{\mathrm{A\times S}} + \dfrac{a(MS_{\mathrm{A}} - MS_{\mathrm{A\times S}})}{N}}$$

$$= \frac{11.2417 - 1.0194}{11.2417 + (4-1)(1.0194) + \dfrac{(4)(32.4861 - 1.0194)}{6}} = +0.2898\ .$$

Case 2, Form *k*: ICC(2, *k*) If each judge is replaced with a team of k judges, and the score is the average score of the k judges, then for Case 2, Form k, the intraclass correlation coefficient is

$$\mathrm{ICC}(2,k) = \frac{MS_{\mathrm{BS}} - MS_{\mathrm{A\times S}}}{MS_{\mathrm{BS}} + \dfrac{MS_{\mathrm{A}} - MS_{\mathrm{A\times S}}}{N}}$$

$$= \frac{11.2417 - 1.0194}{11.2417 + \dfrac{32.4861 - 1.0194}{6}} = +0.6200\ .$$

Case 3, Form 1: ICC(3, 1) Case 3, Form 1 is the same as Case 2, Form 1, except that the raters are considered as fixed, not random. For Case 3, Form 1, the intraclass correlation coefficient is

$$\text{ICC}(3,1) = \frac{MS_{\text{BS}} - MS_{\text{A}\times\text{S}}}{MS_{\text{BS}} + (a-1)MS_{\text{A}\times\text{S}}}$$

$$= \frac{11.2417 - 1.0194}{11.2417 + (4-1)(1.0194)} = +0.7148\,.$$

Case 3, Form k: ICC(3, k) If each judge is replaced with a team of k judges and the teams are considered as fixed, not random, the intraclass correlation coefficient is

$$\text{ICC}(3,k) = \frac{MS_{\text{BS}} - MS_{\text{A}\times\text{S}}}{MS_{\text{BS}}} = \frac{11.2417 - 1.0194}{11.2417} = +0.9093\,.$$

7.8.1 Example

For another example of the intraclass correlation coefficient, consider Case 2, Form 1, the most common in the literature, with k judges randomly selected from a pool of potential judges. Table 7.46 contains data for $k = 3$ judges and $N = 5$ subjects. Table 7.47 contains the analysis of variance source table for the data given in Table 7.46. Given the analysis of variance source table in Table 7.47, the intraclass

Table 7.46 Example data for Case 2, Form 1, with $N = 5$ subjects (S) and $k = 3$ judges (A)

	Judge (A)		
Subject (S)	1	2	3
1	12	10	8
2	15	11	7
3	9	9	6
4	6	5	4
5	8	5	5

Table 7.47 Analysis of variance source table for the data given in Table 7.46 with $k = 3$ judges and $N = 5$ subjects

Source	SS	df	MS	F
Between S	78.00	4	19.50	
Within S	54.00	10	5.40	
Factor A	40.00	2	20.00	11.43
Error ($A\times S$)	14.00	8	1.75	
Total	132.00	14		

correlation coefficient is

$$r_{\mathrm{I}} = \frac{MS_{\mathrm{BS}} - MS_{\mathrm{A\times S}}}{MS_{\mathrm{BS}} + (a-1)MS_{\mathrm{A\times S}} + \dfrac{a(MS_{\mathrm{A}} - MS_{\mathrm{A\times S}})}{N}}$$

$$= \frac{19.50 - 1.75}{19.50 + (3-1)(1.75) + \dfrac{(3)(20.00 - 1.75)}{5}} = 0.5228\ .$$

7.8.2 A Permutation Analysis

Permutation analyses are completely data-dependent and do not depend on random sampling and/or fixed- or random-effects models. For the data given in Table 7.46 for $k = 3$ judges and $N = 5$ subjects there are only

$$M = \left(k!\right)^N = \left(3!\right)^5 = 7{,}776$$

possible, equally-likely arrangements in the reference set of all permutations of the observed data, making an exact permutation analysis possible. If r_{o} denotes the observed value of r_{I}, the exact upper-tail probability value of the observed value of r_{I} is

$$P\left(r_{\mathrm{I}} \geq r_{\mathrm{o}} | H_0\right) = \frac{\text{number of } r_{\mathrm{I}} \text{ values } \geq r_{\mathrm{o}}}{M} = \frac{24}{7{,}776} = 0.0031\ .$$

7.8.3 Interclass and Intraclass Linear Correlation

In the special case of $k = 2$ the relationship between the Pearson product-moment (interclass) correlation coefficient and the Pearson intraclass correlation coefficient can easily be demonstrated. Given $k = 2$ judges, the value of the intraclass correlation depends in part upon the corresponding Pearson product-moment correlation, but it also depends upon the differences between the means and standard deviations of the two variables. Thus,

$$r_{\mathrm{I}} = \frac{\left[\left(\sigma_x^2 + \sigma_y^2\right) - \left(\sigma_x - \sigma_y\right)^2\right] r_{xy} - (\bar{x} - \bar{y})^2/2}{(\sigma_x^2 + \sigma_y^2) + (\bar{x} - \bar{y})^2/2}\ ,$$

Table 7.48 Example bivariate correlation data on $N = 5$ subjects

Subject	Height (x)	Weight (y)
A	1	4
B	2	3
C	3	5
D	4	7
E	5	6

where $\bar{x}$ and $\bar{y}$ denote the means, σ_x^2 and σ_y^2 the variances, and r_{xy} the Pearson product-moment correlation of variables x and y. Thus, for the bivariate data given in Table 7.38 on p. 428, replicated in Table 7.48 for convenience,

$$\bar{x} = 3.00 \,, \quad \bar{y} = 5.00 \,, \quad \sigma_x = \sigma_y = 1.4142 \,, \quad \sigma_x^2 = \sigma_y^2 = 2.00 \,,$$

$r_{xy} = +0.80$, and

$$r_I = \frac{\left[2.00 + 2.00 - (1.4142 - 1.4142)^2\right] 0.80 - (3.00 - 5.00)^2/2}{(2.00 + 2.00) + (3.00 - 5.00)^2/2}$$

$$= \frac{1.20}{6.00} = +0.20 \,,$$

the same value found with $2N$ pairs of observations.

7.9 Coda

Chapter 7 applied permutation statistical methods to measures of association for two variables at the interval level of measurement. Included in Chap. 7 were discussions of ordinary least squares (OLS) regression, least absolute deviation (LAD regression), multivariate multiple regression, point-biserial correlation, biserial correlation, intraclass correlation, and Fisher's z transform for skewed distributions.

Chapter 8 applies exact and Monte Carlo resampling permutation statistical methods to measures of association for two variables at different levels of measurement, e.g., a nominal-level variable and an ordinal-level variable, a nominal-level variable and an interval-level variable, and an ordinal-level variable and an interval-level variable. Included in Chap. 8 are permutation statistical methods applied to Freeman's θ, Agresti's $\hat{\delta}$, Piccarreta's $\hat{\tau}$, Whitfield's S, Cureton's r_{rb}, Pearson's η^2, Kelley's ϵ^2, Hays' $\hat{\omega}^2$, and Jaspen's multiserial correlation coefficient.

References

1. Barrodale, I., Roberts, F.D.K.: A improved algorithm for discrete ℓ_1 linear approximation. J. Num. Anal. **10**, 839–848 (1973)
2. Barrodale, I., Roberts, F.D.K.: Solution of an overdetermined system of equations in the ℓ_1 norm. Commun. ACM **17**, 319–320 (1974)
3. Bartko, J.J.: The intraclass correlation coefficient as a measure of reliability. Psychol. Rep. **19**, 3–11 (1966)
4. Bartko, J.J.: On various intraclass correlation reliability coefficients. Psychol. Bull. **83**, 762–765 (1976)
5. Berry, K.J., Mielke, P.W.: A Monte Carlo investigation of the Fisher Z transformation for normal and nonnormal distributions. Psychol. Rep. **87**, 1101–1114 (2000)
6. Berry, K.J., Mielke, P.W., Johnston, J.E.: Permutation Statistical Methods: An Integrated Approach. Springer–Verlag, Cham, CH (2016)
7. David, F.N.: Tables of the Distribution of the Correlation Coefficient. Cambridge University Press, Cambridge, UK (1938)
8. Dielman, T.E.: A comparison of forecasts from least absolute and least squares regression. J. Forecasting **5**, 189–195 (1986)
9. Dielman, T.E.: Corrections to a comparison of forecasts from least absolute and least squares regression. J. Forecasting **8**, 419–420 (1989)
10. Dielman, T.E., Pfaffenberger, R.: Least absolute value regression: Necessary sample sizes to use normal theory inference procedures. Dec. Sci. **19**, 734–743 (1988)
11. Endler, J.A., Mielke, P.W.: Comparing entire colour patterns as birds see them. Biol. J. Linn. Soc. **86**, 405–431 (2005)
12. Feinstein, A.R.: Clinical Biostatistics XXIII: The role of randomization in sampling, testing, allocation, and credulous idolatry (Part 2). Clin. Pharmacol. Ther. **14**, 898–915 (1973)
13. Fisher, R.A.: Frequency distribution of the values of the correlation coefficient in samples from an indefinitely large population. Biometrika **10**, 507–521 (1915)
14. Fisher, R.A.: Studies in crop variation, I. An examination of the yield of dressed grain from Broadbalk. J. Agric. Sci. **11**, 107–135 (1921)
15. Fisher, R.A.: Statistical Methods for Research Workers, 5th edn. Oliver and Boyd, Edinburgh (1934)
16. Flanagan, J.C.: General considerations in the selection of test items and a short method of estimating the product-moment coefficient from the data at the tails of the distribution. J. Educ. Psych. **30**, 674–680 (1939)
17. Gayen, A.K.: The frequency distribution of the product-moment correlation coefficient in random samples of any size drawn from non-normal universes. Biometrika **38**, 219–247 (1951)
18. Geary, R.C.: Testing for normality. Biometrika **34**, 209–242 (1947)
19. Goodman, L.A.: Measures, models, and graphical displays in the analysis of cross-classified data. J. Am. Stat. Assoc. **86**, 1085–1111 (1991)
20. Haggard, E.A.: Intraclass Correlation and the Analysis of Variance. Dryden, New York (1958)
21. Hotelling, H.: New light on the correlation coefficient and its transforms. J. R. Stat. Soc. Meth **15**, 193–232 (1953)
22. Jeyaratnam, S.: Confidence intervals for the correlation coefficient. Stat. Probab. Lett. **15**, 389–393 (1992)
23. Johnston, J.E., Berry, K.J., Mielke, P.W.: Permutation tests: Precision in estimating probability values. Percept. Motor Skill **105**, 915–920 (2007)
24. Kaufman, E.H., Taylor, G.D., Mielke, P.W., Berry, K.J.: An algorithm and FORTRAN program for multivariate LAD (ℓ_1 of ℓ_2) regression. Computing **68**, 275–287 (2002)
25. Kraemer, H.C.: Improved approximation to the non-null distribution of the correlation coefficient. J. Am. Stat. Assoc. **68**, 1004–1008 (1973)
26. Kraemer, H.C., Thiemann, S.: How Many Subjects? Sage, Newbury Park, CA (1987)
27. Krause, E.F.: Taxicab Geometry. Addison–Wesley, Menlo Park, CA (1975)

28. Liu, W.C., Woodward, J.A., Bonett, D.G.: The generalized likelihood ratio test for the Pearson correlation. Commun. Stat. Simul. C **25**, 507–520 (1996)
29. Mathew, T., Nordström, K.: Least squares and least absolute deviation procedures in approximately linear models. Stat. Probab. Lett. **16**, 153–158 (1993)
30. Matthews, R.: Beautiful, but dangerous. Significance **13**, 30–31 (2016)
31. McGrath, R.E., Meyer, G.J.: When effect sizes disagree: The case of r and d. Psychol. Meth. **11**, 386–401 (2006)
32. McGraw, K.O., Wong, S.P.: Forming inferences about some intraclass correlation coefficients. Psychol. Meth. **1**, 30–46 (1996)
33. Micceri, T.: The unicorn, the normal curve, and other improbable creatures. Psychol. Bull. **105**, 156–166 (1989)
34. Mielke, P.W.: Asymptotic behavior of two-sample tests based on powers of ranks for detecting scale and location alternatives. J. Am. Stat. Assoc. **67**, 850–854 (1972)
35. Mielke, P.W.: Another family of distributions for describing and analyzing precipitation data. J. Appl. Meteor. **12**, 275–280 (1973). [Corrigendum: J. Appl. Meteor. **13**, 516 (1973)]
36. Mielke, P.W., Berry, K.J.: Multivariate multiple regression analyses: A permutation method for linear models. Psychol. Rep. **91**, 3–9 (2002)
37. Mielke, P.W., Berry, K.J.: Multivariate multiple regression prediction models: A Euclidean distance approach. Psychol. Rep. **92**, 763–769 (2003)
38. Mielke, P.W., Berry, K.J.: Permutation Methods: A Distance Function Approach, 2nd edn. Springer–Verlag, New York (2007)
39. Mielke, P.W., Berry, K.J., Landsea, C.W., Gray, W.M.: Artificial skill and validation in meteorological forecasting. Weather Forecast **11**, 153–169 (1996)
40. Mielke, P.W., Berry, K.J., Landsea, C.W., Gray, W.M.: A single-sample estimate of shrinkage in meteorological forecasting. Weather Forecast **12**, 847–858 (1997)
41. Mudholkar, G.S., Chaubey, Y.P.: On the distribution of Fisher's transformation of the correlation coefficient. Commun. Stat. Simul. C **5**, 163–172 (1976)
42. Nunnally, J.C.: Psychometric Theory, 2nd edn. McGraw–Hill, New York (1978)
43. Pearson, E.S.: Some notes on sampling with two variables. Biometrika **21**, 337–360 (1929)
44. Pfaffenberger, R., Dinkel, J.: Absolute deviations curve-fitting: An alternative to least squares. In: David, H.A. (ed.) Contributions to Survey Sampling and Applied Statistics, pp. 279–294. Academic Press, New York (1978)
45. Pillai, K.C.S.: Confidence interval for the correlation coefficient. Sankhyā **7**, 415–422 (1946)
46. Robinson, W.S.: The statistical measurement of agreement. Am. Sociol. Rev. **22**, 17–25 (1957)
47. Rousseeuw, P.J.: Least median of squares regression. J. Am. Stat. Assoc. **79**, 871–880 (1984)
48. Ruben, H.: Some new results on the distribution of the sample correlation coefficient. J. R. Stat. Soc. **28**, 513–525 (1966)
49. Samiuddin, M.: On a test for an assigned value of correlation in a bivariate normal distribution. Biometrika **57**, 461–464 (1970)
50. Shrout, P.E., Fleiss, J.L.: Intraclass correlations: Uses in assessing rater relaibility. Psychol. Bull. **86**, 420–428 (1979)
51. Sitgreaves, R.: Review of "Intraclass Correlation and the Analysis of Variance" by E. A. Haggard. J. Am. Stat. Assoc. **55**, 384–385 (1960)
52. Taylor, L.D.: Estimation by minimizing the sum of absolute errors. In: Zarembka, P. (ed.) Frontiers in Econometrics, pp. 169–190. Academic Press, New York (1974)
53. Thompson, D.: Volcano Cowboys. St. Martin's Press, New York (2000)
54. von Eye, A., Mun, E.Y.: Analyzing Rater Agreement. Lawrence Erlbaum, Mahwah, NJ (2005)
55. Wilson, H.G.: Least squares versus minimum absolute deviations estimation in linear models. Dec. Sci. **9**, 322–325 (1978)
56. Winer, B.J.: Statistical Principles in Experimental Design, 2nd edn. McGraw–Hill, New York (1971)
57. Wong, S.P., McGraw, K.O.: Confidence intervals and F tests for intraclass correlations based on three-way random effects models. Educ. Psychol. Meas. **59**, 270–288 (1999)

Chapter 8
Mixed-Level Variables

Chapters 3 and 4 of *The Measurement of Association* applied permutation statistical methods to measures of association for two nominal-level (categorical) variables, e.g., Pearson's ϕ^2, Tschuprov's T^2, Cramér's V^2, Pearson's C, Goodman and Kruskal's λ_a, λ_b, t_a, and t_b measures, Cohen's unweighted kappa measure of agreement, McNemar's and Cochran's Q tests for change, and Leik and Gove's d_N^c measure of nominal association. Chapters 5 and 6 applied permutation statistical methods to measures of association for two ordinal-level (ranked) variables, e.g., Kendall's τ_a and τ_b measures, Stuart's τ_c measure, Goodman and Kruskal's γ, Somers' d_{yx} and d_{xy}, Spearman's rank-order correlation coefficient, Spearman's footrule measure, Kendall's coefficient of concordance, Cohen's weighted kappa measure of agreement, and Bross's ridit analysis. Chapter 7 applied permutation statistical methods to measures of association for two interval-level variables, e.g., Pearson's product-moment correlation coefficient, the intraclass correlation coefficient, ordinary least squares (OLS) regression, least absolute deviation (LAD) regression, biserial correlation, and point-biserial correlation.

In this, the eighth chapter of *The Measurement of Association*, exact and Monte Carlo permutation statistical methods are applied to measures of association designed for two variables at different levels of measurement, e.g., a nominal-level independent variable and an ordinal- or interval-level dependent variable, and an ordinal-level independent variable and an interval-level dependent variable. For practical use there is little reason to examine those cases in which the dependent variable is at a lower measurement level than the independent variable because the underlying logic of prediction cannot use the added information contained within the independent variable [47, p. 292].

Chapter 8 begins with discussions of permutation statistical methods for three measures of association for a nominal-level independent variable and an ordinal-level dependent variable: Freeman's θ, Agresti's $\hat{\delta}$, and Piccarreta's $\hat{\tau}$. As special cases for the measurement of nominal-ordinal association, permutation implementations of Whitfield's S measure and Cureton's rank-biserial measure for a

K. J. Berry et al., *The Measurement of Association*,
https://doi.org/10.1007/978-3-319-98926-6_8

dichotomous nominal-level variable and an ordinal-level variable are described. Chapter 8 continues with a discussion of measures of association for a nominal-level variable and an interval-level variable: Pearson's η^2, Kelley's ϵ^2, and Hays' $\hat{\omega}^2$. As special cases for the measurement of nominal-ordinal association, permutation implementations of point-biserial correlation and biserial correlation for a dichotomous nominal-level variable and an interval-level variable are described. Next, permutation statistical methods for Jaspen's multiserial correlation coefficient for an ordinal-level variable and an interval-level variable are presented. Chapter 8 concludes with suggestions for a chance-corrected, generalized measure of association for nominal-, ordinal-, or interval-level variables.

8.1 Freeman's Index of Nominal-Ordinal Association

In 1965 Linton Freeman proposed a new measure of association for a nominal-level independent variable and an ordinal-level dependent variable that he called theta (θ) [20, pp. 108–119].[1] Consider an $r \times c$ contingency table where the r rows are a nominal-level independent variable (x) and the c columns are an ordinal-level dependent variable (y). In the fashion of Goodman and Kruskal [24], let $n_{i.}$, $n_{.j}$, and n_{ij} denote the row marginal frequency totals, column marginal frequency totals, and number of objects in the ijth cell, respectively, for $i = 1, \ldots, r$ and $j = 1, \ldots, c$, and let N denote the total number of objects in the $r \times c$ contingency table, i.e.,

$$n_{i.} = \sum_{j=1}^{c} n_{ij} \;, \quad n_{.j} = \sum_{i=1}^{r} n_{ij} \;, \quad \text{and} \quad N = \sum_{i=1}^{r} \sum_{j=1}^{c} n_{ij} \;.$$

If x and y represent the row and column variables, respectively, the number of concordant pairs (C), i.e., pairs of objects that are ranked in the same order on both variable x and variable y, plus the number of discordant pairs (D), i.e., pairs of objects that are ranked in one order on variable x and the reverse order on variable y, plus the number of pairs tied on variable y but not tied on variable x (T_y) can be shown to be given by

$$C + D + T_y = \frac{1}{2} \left(N^2 - \sum_{i=1}^{r} n_{i.}^2 \right) \;.$$

[1] Unconventionally, Freeman's θ was first presented in an introductory textbook on *Elementary Applied Statistics* and not in a journal article.

Alternatively,

$$C + D + T_y = \sum_{i=1}^{r-1} \sum_{j=i+1}^{r} n_{i.}n_{j.} \; .$$

For Freeman's θ, it is necessary to calculate the absolute sum of the number of concordant pairs and number of discordant pairs for all combinations of rows (the nominal-level independent variable) considered two at a time. Thus, assuming that the c ordered variable (y) is underlying continuous and that ties in ranking result simply from crude classification on that variable [20, p. 113], Freeman's nominal-ordinal measure of association is given by

$$\theta = \frac{\sum_{i=1}^{r-1} \sum_{j=i+1}^{r} \left| C_{ij} - D_{ij} \right|}{C + D + T_y} \; .$$

8.1.1 Example 1

Consider a simple example with $r = 2$ disjoint, unordered categories and $c = 4$ disjoint, ordered categories, such as given in Table 8.1 with $N = 14$ subjects. For the frequency data given in Table 8.1, the number of concordant pairs (C) is obtained by proceeding from the upper-left cell with frequency $n_{11} = 1$ downward and to the right, multiplying each cell frequency by the sum of all cell frequencies below and to the right, and summing the products. The number of discordant pairs (D) is obtained by proceeding from the upper-right cell with frequency $n_{14} = 4$ downward and to the left, multiplying each cell frequency by the sum of all cell frequencies below and to the left, and summing the products. The number of pairs tied on variable y (T_y) is obtained by proceeding from the first row in each column, multiplying each cell frequency by the sum of all cell frequencies below, and summing the products. Thus, the number of concordant pairs is

$$C = \sum_{i=1}^{r-1} \sum_{j=1}^{c-1} x_{ij} \left(\sum_{k=i+1}^{r} \sum_{l=j+1}^{c} x_{kl} \right)$$

$$= (1)(0 + 2 + 0) + (2)(2 + 0) + (3)(0) = 6 \; ,$$

Table 8.1 Listing of example data for Freeman's θ with $N = 14$ subjects classified into $r = 2$ unordered categories of the nominal-level independent variable Gender (x) and $c = 4$ ranks on the ordinal-level dependent variable Social Status (y)

	Social Status (y)				
Gender (x)	4	3	2	1	Total
Female	1	2	3	4	10
Male	2	0	2	0	4
Total	3	2	5	4	14

the number of discordant pairs is

$$D = \sum_{i=1}^{r-1} \sum_{j=1}^{c-1} x_{i,c-j+1} \left(\sum_{k=i+1}^{r} \sum_{l=1}^{c-j} x_{kl} \right)$$

$$= (4)(2+0+2) + (3)(0+2) + (2)(2) = 26 ,$$

the number of pairs tied on variable y is

$$T_y = \sum_{j=1}^{c} \sum_{i=1}^{r-1} n_{ij} \left(\sum_{k=i+1}^{r} n_{kj} \right) = (1)(2) + (2)(0) + (3)(2) + (4)(0) = 8 ,$$

and, since there are only $r = 2$ unordered categories,

$$\theta = \frac{|C - D|}{C + D + T_y} = \frac{|6 - 26|}{6 + 26 + 8} = \frac{20}{40} = 0.50 .$$

The standard error of Freeman's θ is unknown, so a permutation analysis is essential. Usually, a Monte Carlo resampling permutation analysis is recommended for analyzing contingency tables as the number of possible arrangements of cell frequencies may often be very large. However, in this example with $N = 14$ subjects and $rc = (2)(4) = 8$ cell frequencies, there are only $M = 30$ possible arrangements in the reference set of all permutations of the cell frequencies consistent with the observed row and column marginal frequency distributions, $\{10, 4\}$ and $\{3, 2, 5, 4\}$, respectively, making an exact permutation analysis feasible.

Since $M = 30$ is a small number, it will be illustrative to list all M arrangements of the observed data, the values of Freeman's θ, and the associated hypergeometric probability values. The $M = 30$ arrangements of the observed data are listed in Table 8.2, organized by the values of Freeman's θ from high to low. Because the data given in Table 8.1 have only three degrees of freedom, it is sufficient to list only three cell frequency values in Table 8.2, n_{11}, n_{12}, and n_{13}, as the remaining five cell frequency values are determined by the marginal frequency totals. The 11 arrangements in Table 8.2 indicated with asterisks, i.e., arrangements 1 through 11, possess values of θ equal to or greater than the observed value of $\theta = 0.50$. For the

Table 8.2 Listing of $M = 30$ possible arrangements of the data given in Table 8.1 with associated θ values and hypergeometric point probability values; values of θ equal to or greater than $\theta = 0.50$ are indicated by asterisks

	Cell frequency				
Number	n_{11}	n_{12}	n_{13}	θ	Probability
1*	3	2	5	1.0000	0.000999
2*	0	1	5	0.9750	0.001998
3*	1	0	5	0.8500	0.002997
4*	0	2	4	0.8000	0.004995
5*	3	2	4	0.6785	0.019980
6*	1	1	4	0.6750	0.029970
7*	1	1	5	0.6571	0.023976
8*	0	2	5	0.5750	0.003996
9*	2	0	4	0.5500	0.014985
10*	2	0	5	0.5143	0.011988
11*	1	2	3	0.5000	0.029970
12	3	2	3	0.4706	0.059940
13	1	2	4	0.4167	0.059940
14	1	2	5	0.4000	0.017982
15	2	1	2	0.3750	0.059940
16	3	1	5	0.3600	0.007992
17	3	2	2	0.2895	0.039960
18	2	1	4	0.2778	0.119880
19	3	0	3	0.2500	0.009990
20	2	1	5	0.2333	0.035964
21	3	1	4	0.2187	0.059940
22	2	2	2	0.2000	0.029970
23	2	2	5	0.1600	0.011988
24	3	0	4	0.1389	0.019980
25	3	2	1	0.1000	0.004995
26	3	1	3	0.0811	0.079920
27	3	1	2	0.0750	0.019980
28	3	0	5	0.0667	0.005994
29	1	0	1	0.0625	0.089910
30	1	0	2	0.0541	0.119880
Sum					1.000000

data given in Table 8.1, the exact probability value is the sum of the hypergeometric point probability values in Table 8.2 associated with the arrangements of cell frequencies with values of θ equal to or greater than the observed value of $\theta = 0.50$. Based on the underlying hypergeometric probability distribution, the exact upper-tail probability value is $P = 0.000999 + 0.001998 + \cdots + 0.029970 = 0.1459$.

As Jacobson [35] noted, when there are only $r = 2$ categories of the nominal-level independent variable, Freeman's θ is equivalent to Somers' d_{yx}; see Chap. 5, Sect. 5.7. However, the signs may differ due to the fact that $0 \leq \theta \leq 1$ and $-1 \leq d_{yx} \leq +1$.

Table 8.3 Listing of example data for Freeman's θ with $N = 40$ subjects classified into $r = 4$ categories of the nominal-level independent variable Marital Status and $c = 5$ ranks on the ordinal-level dependent variable Social Adjustment

	Rank on Social Adjustment (y)					
Marital Status (x)	5	4	3	2	1	Total
Single	1	2	5	2	0	10
Married	10	5	5	0	0	20
Widowed	0	0	2	2	1	5
Divorced	0	0	0	2	3	5
Total	11	7	12	6	4	40

8.1.2 Example 2

For a second, more realistic, example of Freeman's θ, consider the data given in Table 8.3 with $r = 4$ disjoint, unordered categories and $c = 5$ disjoint, ordered categories. When the number of unordered categories is greater than two, the computation of Freeman's θ is more involved. In such cases, the number of concordant pairs (C) and the number of discordant pairs (D) must be calculated for all $r(r-1)/2$ combinations of row categories. For the frequency data given in Table 8.3, the number of concordant pairs is

$$\begin{aligned} C &= \sum_{i=1}^{r-1}\sum_{j=1}^{c-1} x_{ij}\left(\sum_{k=i+1}^{r}\sum_{l=j+1}^{c} x_{kl}\right) \\ &= (1)(5+5+0+0+0+2+2+1+0+0+2+3) \\ &\quad + (2)(5+0+0+2+2+1+0+2+3) \\ &\quad + \cdots + (2)(2+3) + (2)(3) = 304\ , \end{aligned}$$

the number of discordant pairs is

$$\begin{aligned} D &= \sum_{i=1}^{r-1}\sum_{j=1}^{c-1} x_{i,c-j+1}\left(\sum_{k=i+1}^{r}\sum_{l=1}^{c-j} x_{kl}\right) \\ &= (0)(2+0+0+0+2+2+0+0+0+5+5+10) \\ &\quad + (2)(0+0+0+2+0+0+5+5+10) \\ &\quad + \cdots + (2)(0+0) + (0)(0) = 141\ , \end{aligned}$$

the number of pairs tied on variable y is

$$T_y = \sum_{j=1}^{c} \sum_{i=1}^{r-1} n_{ij} \left(\sum_{k=i+1}^{r} n_{kj} \right)$$

$$= (1)(10+0+0) + (10)(0+0) + (0)(0)$$

$$+ \cdots + (0)(0+1+3) + (1)(1+3) + (1)(3) = 80 \; ,$$

the concordant and discordant pairs for the $r = 4$ rows considered two at a time are

$$C_{12} = (1)(5+5+0+0) + (2)(5+0+0) + (5)(0+0) + (2)(0) = 20 \; ,$$

$$D_{12} = (0)(10+5+5+0) + (2)(10+5+5) + (5)(10+5) + (2)(10) = 135 \; ,$$

$$C_{13} = (1)(0+2+2+1) + (2)(2+2+1) + (5)(2+1) + (2)(1) = 32 \; ,$$

$$D_{13} = (0)(0+0+2+2) + (2)(0+0+2) + (5)(0+0) + (2)(0) = 4 \; ,$$

$$C_{14} = (1)(0+0+2+3) + (2)(0+2+3) + (5)(2+3) + (2)(3) = 46 \; ,$$

$$D_{14} = (0)(0+0+0+2) + (2)(0+0+0) + (5)(0+0) + (2)(0) = 0 \; ,$$

$$C_{23} = (10)(0+2+2+1) + (5)(2+2+1) + (5)(2+1) + (0)(1) = 90 \; ,$$

$$D_{23} = (0)(0+0+2+2) + (0)(0+0+2) + (5)(0+0) + (5)(0) = 0 \; ,$$

$$C_{24} = (10)(0+0+2+3) + (5)(0+2+3) + (5)(2+3) + (0)(3) = 100 \; .$$

$$D_{24} = (0)(0+0+0+2) + (0)(0+0+0) + (5)(0+0) + (5)(0) = 0 \; ,$$

$$C_{34} = (0)(0+0+2+3) + (0)(0+2+3) + (2)(2+3) + (2)(3) = 16 \; ,$$

$$D_{34} = (1)(0+0+0+2) + (2)(0+0+0) + (2)(0+0) + (0)(0) = 2 \; ,$$

and Freeman's θ is

$$\theta = \frac{\displaystyle\sum_{i=1}^{r-1} \sum_{j=i+1}^{r} |C_{ij} - D_{ij}|}{C + D + T_y}$$

$$= \frac{|20-135| + |32-4| + |46-0| + |90-0| + |100-0| + |16-2|}{304 + 141 + 80}$$

$$= 0.7486 \; .$$

There are only $M = 6{,}340{,}588$ possible arrangements in the reference set of all permutations of cell frequencies consistent with the observed row and column marginal frequency distributions, $\{10, 20, 5, 5\}$ and $\{11, 7, 12, 6, 4\}$, respectively, making an exact permutation analysis possible. If all M possible arrangements occur with equal chance, the exact probability value of θ under the null hypothesis is the sum of the hypergeometric point probability values associated with the arrangements of cell frequencies with values of θ equal to or greater than the observed value of $\theta = 0.7486$. Based on the underlying hypergeometric probability distribution, the exact upper-tail probability value of $\theta = 0.7486$ is $P = 0.2105{\times}10^{-10}$.

8.2 Agresti's Index of Nominal-Ordinal Association

In 1981 Alan Agresti proposed a new measure of association for a nominal-level independent variable and an ordinal-level dependent variable that he denoted as $\hat{\delta}$ [1]. Agresti noted that $\hat{\delta}$ was equivalent to Somers' [69] d_{yx} measure of ordinal association when the independent variable was dichotomous, and directly related to the ridit measure introduced by Bross in 1954 [10].[2] Consequently, $\hat{\delta}$ is also equivalent to Freeman's θ when there are $r = 2$ categories of the independent variable. Additionally, a similar approach was put forward by Maravelakis, Perakis, Psarakis, and Panaretos [50] and Perakis, Maravelakis, Psarakis, Xekalaki, and Panaretos [61] in 2003 and 2005, respectively. Agresti's $\hat{\delta}$ measure is based on concordant and discordant pairwise structures, is bounded $0 \leq \hat{\delta} \leq 1$, and possesses a maximum-corrected interpretation.

Let X be a nominal-level independent variable with r disjoint, unordered categories, $x_1, \ldots, x_r$, and Y be an ordinal-level dependent variable with c disjoint, ordered categories, $y_1, \ldots, y_c$, ranging from least to greatest in degree. If N objects are classified on both variables X and Y, the frequency for which objects are characterized by $\{x_i, y_j\}$ is denoted by n_{ij} for $i = 1, \ldots, r$ and $j = 1, \ldots, c$. The row and column marginal frequency distributions of X and Y are denoted by $\{n_{1.}, \ldots, n_{r.}\}$ and $\{n_{.1}, \ldots, n_{.c}\}$, respectively. Agresti's measure of nominal-ordinal association is given by

$$\hat{\delta} = \frac{\displaystyle\sum_{i=1}^{r-1} \sum_{h=i+1}^{r} |\Delta_{ih}|}{\displaystyle\sum_{i=1}^{r-1} \sum_{h=i+1}^{r} n_{i.} n_{h.}} , \tag{8.1}$$

[2]For a discussion of Bross's ridit analysis, see Chap. 6, Sect. 6.7.

where

$$\Delta_{ih} = \sum_{j=1}^{c-1} \sum_{k=j+1}^{c} n_{ji} n_{kh} - \sum_{j=2}^{c} \sum_{k=1}^{j-1} n_{jh} n_{ki} \; . \tag{8.2}$$

8.2.1 Example

Consider an example with $N = 33$ subjects, $r = 3$ disjoint, unordered categories, and $c = 4$ disjoint, ordered categories, as given in Table 8.4. For the frequency data given in Table 8.4, the denominator of $\hat{\delta}$ in Eq. (8.1) is the sum of the pairwise products of the row marginal frequency totals, i.e.,

$$\sum_{i=1}^{r-1} \sum_{h=i+1}^{r} n_{i.} n_{h.}$$

$$= (11)(8) + (11)(14) + (8)(14) = 88 + 154 + 112 = 354 \; .$$

The numerator of $\hat{\delta}$ in Eq. (8.1) is the sum of all possible pairs of concordant (C) minus discordant (D) row frequencies calculated from Eq. (8.2), i.e.,

$$\Delta_{12} = (5)(2+3+2) + (3)(3+2) + (2)(2)$$
$$- (1)(3+2+1) + (2)(2+1) + (3)(1) = 39 \; ,$$

$$\Delta_{13} = (5)(1+6+7) + (3)(6+7) + (2)(7)$$
$$(0)(3+2+1) + (1)(2+1) + (6)(1) = 114 \; ,$$

and

$$\Delta_{23} = (1)(1+6+7) + (2)(6+7) + (3)(7)$$
$$(0)(2+3+2) + (1)(3+2) + (6)(2) = 44 \; .$$

Table 8.4 Example data for Agresti's $\hat{\delta}$ with $N = 33$ subjects, $r = 3$ independent unordered row categories, and $c = 4$ dependent ordered column categories

	Y				
X	1	2	3	4	Total
A	5	3	2	1	11
B	1	2	3	2	8
C	0	1	6	7	14
Total	6	6	11	10	33

Then, the numerator of $\hat{\delta}$ in Eq. (8.1) is $|39| + |114| + |44| = 197$ and

$$\hat{\delta} = \frac{\sum_{i=1}^{r-1} \sum_{h=i+1}^{r} |\Delta_{ih}|}{\sum_{i=1}^{r-1} \sum_{h=i+1}^{r} n_{i.} n_{h.}} = \frac{197}{354} = 0.5565 \; .$$

When analyzing contingency tables, an exact permutation analysis generally is not practical as the number of possible arrangements of cell frequencies in the reference set is usually very large. In such cases, Monte Carlo resampling permutation tests generate a random sample of L arrangements of cell frequencies from the M total possible arrangements with the fixed observed marginal frequency totals of the observed cell frequencies. If $\hat{\delta}_{\text{o}}$ denotes the observed value of Agresti's $\hat{\delta}$, the resampling upper-tail probability value of $\hat{\delta}_{\text{o}}$ is given by

$$P(\hat{\delta} \geq \hat{\delta}_{\text{o}} | H_0) = \frac{1}{L} \sum_{i=1}^{L} \Psi_i(\hat{\delta}) \; ,$$

where

$$\Psi_i(\hat{\delta}) = \begin{cases} 1 & \text{if } \hat{\delta} \geq \hat{\delta}_{\text{o}} \; , \\ 0 & \text{otherwise} \; , \end{cases}$$

and L is set to a large number for accuracy. For the frequency data given in Table 8.4, $\hat{\delta}_{\text{o}} = 0.5565$ and with $L = 1{,}000{,}000$ randomly selected $\hat{\delta}$ values, the Monte Carlo resampling probability of a $\hat{\delta}$ value equal to or greater than the observed value of $\hat{\delta}_{\text{o}} = 0.5565$ is

$$P(\hat{\delta} \geq \hat{\delta}_{\text{o}} | H_0) = \frac{\text{number of } \hat{\delta} \text{ values } \geq \hat{\delta}_{\text{o}}}{L} = \frac{15{,}151}{1{,}000{,}000} = 0.0152 \; .$$

Since, for the frequency data given in Table 8.4, there are only $M = 24{,}641$ possible arrangements of cell frequencies, given the observed row and column marginal frequency totals, $\{11, 8, 14\}$ and $\{6, 6, 11, 10\}$, respectively, an exact permutation analysis is possible. The exact probability value is the sum of the hypergeometric point probability values associated with values of $\hat{\delta}$ equal to or greater than the observed value of $\hat{\delta} = 0.5565$. Based on the underlying hypergeometric probability distribution, the exact upper-tail probability value is $P = 0.0221$.

8.3 Piccarreta's Index of Nominal-Ordinal Association

As noted, *vide supra*, a common problem in data analysis is the measurement of the magnitude of association between a nominal independent variable and an ordinal dependent variable. Some representative examples are the measured association between nominal variables such as religious affiliation (Catholic, Jewish, Protestant, None), voting behavior (Democrat, Independent, Republican), gender (Female, Male), and marital status (Single, Married, Widowed, Divorced, Separated), versus ordinal attitudinal questions that are Likert-scaled (Strongly Agree, Agree, Disagree, Strongly Disagree). In 2001 Raffælla Piccarreta [62] presented a new index of nominal-ordinal association that was a generalization of the Goodman and Kruskal [24] well-known τ index of nominal-nominal association. The Piccarreta $\hat{\tau}$ index is based on the Gini mean difference, is bounded between zero and one, and possesses a proportional-reduction-in-error interpretation.

Following the notation of Piccarreta, let X be a nominal-level independent variable with r disjoint, unordered categories, $x_1, \ldots, x_r$, and let Y be an ordinal-level dependent variable with c disjoint, ordered categories, $y_1, \ldots, y_c$, ranging from least to greatest in degree. If N objects in a sample are classified on both X and Y, the frequency with which objects are characterized by $\{x_i, y_j\}$ is denoted by n_{ij} for $i = 1, \ldots, r$ and $j = 1, \ldots, c$. The row and column marginal frequency distributions of variables X and Y are denoted by $\{n_{1.}, \ldots, n_{r.}\}$ and $\{n_{.1}, \ldots, n_{.c}\}$, respectively. The Piccarreta proportional-reduction-in-error index of nominal-ordinal association is then defined as

$$\hat{\tau} = 1 - \frac{V_{YX}}{V_Y} ,$$

where

$$V_Y = \frac{1}{N} \sum_{j=1}^{c-1} \left(y'_{j+1} - y'_j\right) F_j \left(N - F_j\right) , \tag{8.3}$$

$$V_{YX} = \sum_{i=1}^{r} \frac{1}{n_{i.}} \sum_{j=1}^{c-1} \left(y'_{j+1} - y'_j\right) F_{j|i} \left(N - F_{j|i}\right) , \tag{8.4}$$

F_j denotes the cumulative marginal frequency distribution of Y, defined as

$$F_j = \sum_{k=1}^{j} n_{.k} ,$$

$F_{j|i}$ denotes the cumulative frequency distribution of Y in category i of variable X, defined as

$$F_{j|i} = \sum_{k=1}^{j} n_{ik} \;,$$

and y'_j is an auxiliary variable representing the distances between adjacent categories of Y, $j = 1, \ldots, c$. In the most elementary case where the categories of Y are simply ranked, as in any Likert scale, $y'_j = j$ for $j = 1, \ldots, c$, in which case the term $y'_{j+1} - y'_j = 1$ can be omitted from Eqs. (8.3) and (8.4). The minimum value of $\hat{\tau}$ is 0 and occurs if and only if $F_{j|i} = F_j$ for $i = 1, \ldots, r$ and $j = 1, \ldots, c$, i.e., independence. The maximum value of $\hat{\tau}$ is 1 and occurs if and only if $V_{YX(i)} = 0$ for $i = 1, \ldots, r$.

8.3.1 Example

To illustrate Piccarreta's $\hat{\tau}$ measure of nominal-ordinal association, consider the frequency data for $N = 243$ respondents on a 3-point Likert scale arranged in a 3×3 contingency table as given in Table 8.5. For this example analysis, $r = 3$ disjoint, unordered categories (Single, Married, Divorced) and $c = 3$ disjoint, ordered categories (Agree, Neutral, Disagree). To demonstrate the calculation of Piccarreta's $\hat{\tau}$ for the data given in Table 8.5, assume that the $c = 3$ ordered categories of variable Y are simply ranked as 1, 2, 3, and therefore, y'_j for $j = 1, \ldots, c$ and $y'_{j+1} - y'_j = 1$. Then, $F_1 = n_{.1} = 86$, $F_2 = n_{.1} + n_{.2} = 86 + 81 = 167$, and

$$V_Y = \frac{1}{N} \sum_{j=1}^{c-1} (y'_{j+1} - y'_j) F_j (N - F_j)$$

$$= \frac{1}{243} \big[(1)(86)(243 - 86) + (1)(167)(243 - 167) \big] = 107.7942 \, .$$

Table 8.5 Example data for Piccarreta's $\hat{\tau}$ arranged in a 3×3 contingency table with a nominal-level independent variable (X) and an ordinal level dependent variable (Y)

	Variable Y			
Variable X	Agree	Neutral	Disagree	Total
Single	37	31	19	87
Married	25	32	24	81
Divorced	24	18	33	75
Total	86	81	76	243

V_{YX} is calculated over the $r = 3$ disjoint, unordered categories. For row 1, $F_{1|1} = n_{11} = 37$, $F_{2|1} = n_{11} + n_{12} = 37 + 31 = 68$, and

$$V_{YX(1)} = \sum_{i=1}^{r} \frac{1}{n_{1.}} \sum_{j=1}^{c-1} \left(y'_{j+1} - y'_j\right) F_{j|1}\left(N - F_{j|1}\right)$$

$$= \frac{1}{87}\big[(1)(37)(87 - 37) + (1)(68)(87 - 68)\big] = 36.1149 \; .$$

For row 2, $F_{1|2} = n_{21} = 25$, $F_{2|2} = n_{21} + n_{22} = 25 + 32 = 57$, and

$$V_{YX(2)} = \sum_{i=1}^{r} \frac{1}{n_{2.}} \sum_{j=1}^{c-1} \left(y'_{j+1} - y'_j\right) F_{j|2}\left(N - F_{j|2}\right)$$

$$= \frac{1}{81}\big[(1)(25)(81 - 25) + (1)(57)(877)\big] = 34.1728 \; .$$

For row 3, $F_{1|3} = n_{31} = 24$, $F_{2|3} = n_{31} + n_{32} = 24 + 18 = 42$, and

$$V_{YX(3)} = \sum_{i=1}^{r} \frac{1}{n_{3.}} \sum_{j=1}^{c-1} \left(y'_{j+1} - y'_j\right) F_{j|3}\left(N - F_{j|3}\right)$$

$$= \frac{1}{75}\big[(1)(24)(75 - 24) + (1)(42)(75 - 42)\big] = 34.80 \; .$$

Then

$$V_{YX} = \sum_{i=1}^{r} V_{YX(i)} = 36.1149 + 34.1728 + 34.80 = 105.0878$$

and the observed value of Piccarreta's test statistic is

$$\hat{\tau}_{\text{o}} = 1 - \frac{V_{YX}}{V_Y} = 1 - \frac{105.0878}{107.7942} = 0.0251 \; .$$

In analyzing large contingency tables, an exact permutation analysis generally is not practical. If $\hat{\tau}_{\text{o}}$ denotes the observed value of Piccarreta's $\hat{\tau}$, the Monte Carlo resampling upper-tail probability value of $\hat{\tau}_{\text{o}}$ is given by

$$P(\hat{\tau} \geq \hat{\tau}_{\text{o}} | H_0) = \frac{1}{L} \sum_{i=1}^{L} \Psi_i(\hat{\tau}) \; ,$$

where

$$\Psi_i(\hat{\tau}) = \begin{cases} 1 & \text{if } \hat{\tau} \geq \hat{\tau}_o \,, \\ 0 & \text{otherwise} \,, \end{cases}$$

and L is set to a large number for accuracy. For the frequency data given in Table 8.5, $\hat{\tau}_o = 0.0251$ and with $L = 1{,}000{,}000$ randomly selected $\hat{\tau}$ values, the Monte Carlo resampling probability of a $\hat{\tau}$ value equal to or greater than the observed value of $\hat{\tau}_o = 0.0251$ is

$$P(\hat{\tau} \geq \hat{\tau}_o | H_0) = \frac{\text{number of } \hat{\tau} \text{ values } \geq \hat{\tau}_o}{L} = \frac{255{,}978}{1{,}000{,}000} = 0.0256 \,.$$

8.4 Comparisons Between $\hat{\delta}$ and $\hat{\tau}$

Agresti's $\hat{\delta}$ and Piccarreta's $\hat{\tau}$ measures of nominal-ordinal association are based on entirely different principles and often lead to quite different results. In this section, the two measures are compared and evaluated. For convenience, the necessary notation and equations are reproduced here.

Let X be a nominal-level independent variable with r disjoint, unordered categories, $x_1, \ldots, x_r$, and let Y be an ordinal-level dependent variable with c disjoint, ordered categories, $y_1, \ldots, y_c$, ranging from least to greatest in degree. If N objects are classified on both variables X and Y, the frequency that objects are characterized by $\{x_i, y_j\}$ is denoted by n_{ij} for $i = 1, \ldots, r$ and $j = 1, \ldots, c$. The row and column marginal frequency distributions of X and Y are denoted by $\{n_{1.}, \ldots, n_{r.}\}$ and $\{n_{.1}, \ldots, n_{.c}\}$, respectively. Agresti's $\hat{\delta}$ measure of nominal-ordinal association is given by

$$\hat{\delta} = \frac{\displaystyle\sum_{i=1}^{r-1} \sum_{h=i+1}^{r} |\Delta_{ih}|}{\displaystyle\sum_{i=1}^{r-1} \sum_{h=i+1}^{r} n_{i.} n_{h.}} \,, \tag{8.5}$$

where

$$\Delta_{ih} = \sum_{j=1}^{c-1} \sum_{k=j+1}^{c} n_{ji} n_{kh} - \sum_{j=2}^{c} \sum_{k=1}^{j-1} n_{jh} n_{ki} \,.$$

Piccarreta's $\hat{\tau}$ measure of nominal-ordinal association is given by

$$\hat{\tau} = 1 - \frac{V_{YX}}{V_Y} ,$$

where

$$V_Y = \frac{1}{N} \sum_{j=1}^{c-1} (y'_{j+1} - y'_j) F_j (N - F_j) ,$$

$$V_{YX} = \sum_{i=1}^{r} \frac{1}{n_{i.}} \sum_{j=1}^{c-1} (y'_{j+1} - y'_j) F_{j|i} (N - F_{j|i}) ,$$

F_j denotes the cumulative marginal frequency distribution of Y, defined as

$$F_j = \sum_{k=1}^{j} n_{.k} ,$$

$F_{j|i}$ denotes the cumulative frequency distribution of Y in category i of variable X, defined as

$$F_{j|i} = \sum_{k=1}^{j} n_{ik} ,$$

and y'_j is an auxiliary variable representing the distances between adjacent categories of Y, $j = 1, \ldots, c$.

Both measures, Agresti's $\hat{\delta}$ and Piccarreta's $\hat{\tau}$, are bounded by 0 and 1, as is customary with nominal independent variables, but Agresti's $\hat{\delta}$ is a maximum-corrected measure, i.e., the denominator in Eq. (8.5) is the maximum value that the numerator can attain, given the observed row and column marginal frequency distributions, respectively. In contrast, while Piccarreta's $\hat{\tau}$ is a maximum-corrected measure, it is also a proportional-reduction-in-error measure with a familiar interpretation, i.e., the reduction in error provided by the inclusion of the specified independent variable, compared with knowledge of the dependent variable alone.

One weakness of Agresti's $\hat{\delta}$ is that it ignores the characteristics of the distributions of the dependent variable, Y, conditional on the categories of the explanatory variable, X [3]. Thus, $\hat{\delta} = 1$ whenever one of the conditional distributions is entirely above or below another. Consequently, Agresti's $\hat{\delta}$ is equal to 1 under a variety of cell frequency arrangements. In contrast, Piccarreta's $\hat{\tau}$ is equal to 1 if and only if all the conditional variables, $x_1, \ldots, x_r$, fall into only one level of the dependent variable, Y. Table 8.6 illustrates this deficiency of Agresti's $\hat{\delta}$ with seven $2{\times}4$ contingency tables. The results summarized in Table 8.6 indicate that $\hat{\delta} = 1$ for all seven cell configurations, while $\hat{\tau}$ is more sensitive to the various cell configurations.

Table 8.6 Agresti's $\hat{\delta}$ and Piccarreta's $\hat{\tau}$ values for seven 2×4 contingency tables

Table	X	Y 1	2	3	4	$\hat{\delta}$	$\hat{\tau}$
1	A	2	3	4	0	1.0000	0.2444
	B	0	0	0	1		
2	A	1	0	0	0	1.0000	0.3004
	B	0	2	3	4		
3	A	1	2	0	0	1.0000	0.5591
	B	0	0	3	4		
4	A	1	2	3	0	1.0000	0.5679
	B	0	0	0	4		
5	A	3	4	0	0	1.0000	0.5895
	B	0	0	1	2		
6	A	4	0	0	0	1.0000	0.6667
	B	0	1	2	3		
7	A	4	0	0	0	1.0000	1.0000
	B	0	4	0	0		

8.4.1 Example Analysis

Table 8.7 contains frequency data arranged in a 3×6 contingency table to illustrate a comparison between Agresti's $\hat{\delta}$ and Piccarreta's $\hat{\tau}$ measures of nominal-ordinal association. Variable X is a nominal-level independent variable with $r = 3$ disjoint, unordered categories {A, B, C} and variable Y is an ordinal-level dependent variable with $c = 6$ disjoint, ordered categories $\{1, 2, 3, 4, 5, 6\}$. For the frequency data given in Table 8.7, the observed value of Agresti's $\hat{\delta}$ measure is $\hat{\delta}_{\text{o}} = 0.5210$ and the observed value of Piccarreta's $\hat{\tau}$ measure with $y'_j = 1, 2, \ldots, 6$ and $y'_{j+1} - y'_j = 1$, is $\hat{\tau}_{\text{o}} = 0.1828$, highlighting the two different approaches for measuring the magnitude of nominal-ordinal association.

Two different methods can be considered in establishing probability values for the two measures. First, the delta method [30], advocated by both Agresti and Piccarreta, estimates the mean and variance of the sampling distribution of the selected statistic, which is assumed to be distributed $N(0, 1)$. A z-score is computed and an approximate probability value is obtained by numerical integration of the normal distribution over a finite interval.

Table 8.7 Example 3×6 contingency table to compare Agresti's $\hat{\delta}$ and Piccarreta's $\hat{\tau}$ measures of nominal-ordinal association

X	Y 1	2	3	4	5	6	Total
A	1	2	3	4	0	0	10
B	0	2	3	4	5	0	14
C	0	0	3	4	5	6	18
Total	1	4	9	12	10	6	42

Second, Monte Carlo resampling methods generate L random arrangements of cell frequencies, given the fixed observed marginal frequency totals, where L typically is a large number, e.g., $L = 1{,}000{,}000$. For each random arrangement of cell frequencies, the selected statistic is calculated, resulting in a discrete sampling distribution. The probability of obtaining the observed statistic value, or a more extreme value, is simply the proportion of randomly selected test statistics, $\hat{\delta}$ or $\hat{\tau}$, with values equal to or more extreme than the value of the observed statistic.

Consider the frequency data given in Table 8.7 and Agresti's $\hat{\delta}$ measure of nominal-ordinal association. For the data given in Table 8.7, the delta method is based on a mean of $\mu_{\hat{\delta}} = 0.3605$ and a variance of $\sigma^2_{\hat{\delta}} = 0.0082$; skewness ($\gamma_{\hat{\delta}}$) is not considered in the delta method since the distribution is assumed to be $N(0, 1)$. The standard score for the observed value of $\hat{\delta}_o = 0.5210$ is

$$z = \frac{\hat{\delta}_o - \mu_{\hat{\delta}}}{\sigma_{\hat{\delta}}} = \frac{0.5210 - 0.3605}{\sqrt{0.0082}} = +1.7724$$

and the $N(0, 1)$ upper-tail probability value is $P = 0.0384$. For the frequency data given in Table 8.7, based on $L = 1{,}000{,}000$ randomly selected values, the Monte Carlo resampling probability of a $\hat{\delta}$ value equal to or greater than the observed value of $\hat{\delta}_o = 0.5210$ is

$$P(\hat{\delta} \geq \hat{\delta}_o | H_0) = \frac{\text{number of } \hat{\delta} \text{ values } \geq \hat{\delta}_o}{L} = \frac{55{,}100}{1{,}000{,}000} = 0.0551 \ .$$

Analogously, for the data listed in Table 8.7 and Piccarreta's $\hat{\tau}$ measure of nominal-ordinal association, the delta method is based on a mean of $\mu_{\hat{\tau}} = 0.0488$ and a variance of $\sigma^2_{\hat{\tau}} = 0.8565 \times 10^{-3}$. The standard score for the observed value of $\hat{\tau}_o = 0.1828$ is

$$z = \frac{\hat{\tau}_o - \mu_{\hat{\tau}}}{\sigma_{\hat{\tau}}} = \frac{0.1828 - 0.0488}{\sqrt{0.8565 \times 10^{-3}}} = +4.5787$$

and the $N(0, 1)$ upper-tail probability value is $P = 2.3394 \times 10^{-6}$. For the frequency data given in Table 8.7, based on $L = 1{,}000{,}000$ randomly selected values, the Monte Carlo resampling probability of a $\hat{\tau}$ value equal to or greater than the observed value of $\hat{\tau}_o = 0.1828$ is

$$P(\hat{\tau} \geq \hat{\tau}_o | H_0) = \frac{\text{number of } \hat{\tau} \text{ values } \geq \hat{\tau}_o}{L} = \frac{2{,}300}{1{,}000{,}000} = 0.0023 \ ,$$

which is markedly different than $P = 0.0551$ obtained by resampling permutation methods for Agresti's $\hat{\delta}$ measure.

8.4.2 The Delta Method

The delta method advocated by both Agresti and Piccarreta obtains only the expected mean ($\mu_{\hat{\delta}}$ or $\mu_{\hat{\tau}}$) and variance ($\sigma^2_{\hat{\delta}}$ or $\sigma^2_{\hat{\tau}}$) of the differentiable function of a random variable based on the first and second order terms in a truncated Taylor series, with the third and higher order terms ignored. In the cases of both Agresti's $\hat{\delta}$ and Piccarreta's $\hat{\tau}$, the use of the delta method is problematic, since the method does not consider possible skewness. For the data given in Table 8.7, $\gamma_{\hat{\delta}} = +0.5965$ and $\gamma_{\hat{\tau}} = +1.1500$ for $\hat{\delta}$ and $\hat{\tau}$, respectively. Tables 8.8 and 8.9 examine skewness for Agresti's $\hat{\delta}$ and Piccarreta's $\hat{\tau}$ measures of nominal-ordinal association, respectively. The contingency tables are constructed with $n_{ij} = 3$, $n_{ij} = 9$, and $n_{ij} = 18$ for $i = 1, \ldots, r$ and $j = 1, \ldots, c$, $r = 2, \ldots, 5$,

Table 8.8 Skewness values for Agresti's $\hat{\delta}$ for 48 $r \times c$ contingency tables with cell frequencies of $n_{ij} = 3$, $n_{ij} = 9$, and $n_{ij} = 18$ for $i = 2, \ldots, 5$ and $j = 2, \ldots, 5$

		Columns			
Rows	n_{ij}	2	3	4	5
2	3	+0.4897	+0.7189	+0.8331	+0.8858
	9	+0.7312	+0.8946	+0.9402	+0.9606
	18	+0.8458	+0.9406	+0.9701	+0.9778
3	3	+0.7172	+0.4949	+0.5740	+0.5950
	9	+0.8932	+0.6061	+0.6247	+0.6305
	18	+0.9451	+0.6257	+0.6330	+0.6561
4	3	+0.7168	+0.5327	+0.4443	+0.4647
	9	+0.8926	+0.6089	+0.4842	+0.4930
	18	+0.9404	+0.6294	+0.4959	+0.4981
5	3	+0.7141	+0.5384	+0.4473	+0.3817
	9	+0.8932	+0.6105	+0.4873	+0.4132
	18	+0.9430	+0.6348	+0.4954	+0.4213

Table 8.9 Skewness values for Piccarreta's $\hat{\tau}$ for 48 $r \times c$ contingency tables with cell frequencies of $n_{ij} = 3$, $n_{ij} = 9$, and $n_{ij} = 18$ for $i = 2, \ldots, 5$ and $j = 2, \ldots, 5$

		Columns			
Rows	n_{ij}	2	3	4	5
2	3	+2.4972	+2.1322	+2.1839	+2.2646
	9	+2.7022	+2.3811	+2.3786	+2.4164
	18	+2.7586	+2.4343	+2.4436	+2.4543
3	3	+1.6444	+1.5213	+1.5658	+1.6078
	9	+1.8808	+1.6880	+1.6893	+1.7012
	18	+1.9409	+1.7296	+1.7223	+1.7269
4	3	+1.2820	+1.2354	+1.2782	+1.3168
	9	+1.5245	+1.3716	+1.3783	+1.4023
	18	+1.5844	+1.4069	+1.4042	+1.4206
5	3	+1.0988	+1.0719	+1.1069	+1.1249
	9	+1.3175	+1.2017	+1.2020	+1.2150
	18	+1.3701	+1.2245	+1.2111	+1.2335

$c = 2, \ldots, 5$, and $y_j = j = 1, \ldots, c$, i.e., 16 contingency tables ranging in size from 2×2 to 5×5, ensuring identical uniform marginal frequency distributions with $n_{ij} = 3$, $n_{ij} = 9$, and $n_{ij} = 18$. The 96 skewness terms in Tables 8.8 and 8.9 were obtained by simulation based on $L = 1{,}000{,}000$ random arrangements of cell frequencies and a common seed. One obvious result for both Tables 8.8 and 8.9 is that all the skewness values are substantially greater than zero.

Three skewness patterns for Agresti's $\hat{\delta}$ measure are apparent in Table 8.8: (1) skewness increases as n_{ij} increases from $n_{ij} = 3$ to $n_{ij} = 18$, when r and c are held constant, (2) inconsistent skewness decreasing with increasing r is suggested when n_{ij} and c are held constant, and (3) skewness increases with $c \geq 3$ when n_{ij} and $r = 3$ or $r = 4$ are held constant; however, skewness decreases as $c \geq 3$ increases when n_{ij} and $r = 4$ or $r = 5$ are held constant.

In contrast with the skewness results in Table 8.8 for Agresti's $\hat{\delta}$, the skewness patterns for Piccarreta's $\hat{\tau}$ are far more consistent, as is evident in Table 8.9: (1) skewness increases as n_{ij} increases, when r and c are held constant, (2) skewness decreases as r increases, when n_{ij} and c are held constant, and skewness increases as $c \geq 3$ increases, when n_{ij} and r are held constant.

While both Agresti's $\hat{\delta}$ and Piccarreta's $\hat{\tau}$ measures of nominal-ordinal association possess different strengths and weaknesses, overall Piccarreta's $\hat{\tau}$ appears to be the better of the two measures. Although $\hat{\delta} = 0$ if and only if independence holds, perfect association implies $\hat{\delta} = 1$, but $\hat{\delta} = 1$ does not imply perfect association, i.e., $\hat{\delta} = 1$ under a variety of cell frequency configurations, as demonstrated in Table 8.6 on p. 454. On the other hand, while $\hat{\tau} = 0$ if and only if independence holds, and $\hat{\tau} = 1$ if and only if perfect association holds, $\hat{\tau}$ only achieves unity when $r = c$. Piccarreta's $\hat{\tau}$ possesses a proportional-reduction-in-error interpretation, which is familiar to many researchers, while Agresti's $\hat{\delta}$ is very difficult to interpret, especially when $\hat{\delta} = 1$. Piccarreta's $\hat{\tau}$ is more flexible in that different weights can be assigned to the ordered categories, while Agresti's $\hat{\delta}$ is restricted to y_j' for $j = 1, \ldots, c$. The sampling distributions of both $\hat{\delta}$ and $\hat{\tau}$ possess considerable skewness, $\hat{\tau}$ more than $\hat{\delta}$, but permutation statistical methods easily accommodate for any skewness.

8.5 Dichotomous Nominal-Level Variables

As special cases of nominal-ordinal association, consider two examples: Whitfield's symmetrical measure of association, S, and Cureton's rank-biserial correlation, r_{rb}. Both examine the relationship between a dichotomous variable and an ordinal-level variable where, in this case, the dichotomous variable is considered to be a nominal-level variable with only two disjoint, unordered categories.

Table 8.10 Ranking of a dichotomous variable with $n_A = 5$, $n_B = 3$, and $N = 8$

Rank	1	2	3	4	5	6	7	8
Sample	A	B	A	A	B	B	A	A

8.5.1 Whitfield's τ Measure of Association

In 1947 John Whitfield proposed a measure of correlation between two variables in which one variable was composed of N rank scores and the other variable was dichotomous [72]. Consider the $N = 8$ rank scores listed in Table 8.10 where the dichotomous variable categories are two samples indicated by the letters A and B and the rank scores are from 1 to 8. Let n_A denote the number of rank scores in sample A, let n_B denote the number of rank scores in sample B, and let $N = n_A + n_B$.

Whitfield designed a procedure to calculate a statistic that he labeled S, following Kendall's notation in a 1945 *Biometrika* article on "The treatment of ties in ranking problems" [40]. Given the $N = 8$ rank scores listed in Table 8.10, consider the $n_B = 3$ rank scores in the sample identified by the letter B: 2, 5, and 6.[3] Beginning with rank score 2 with the letter B, there is one rank score with the letter A to the left of $B = 2$ (rank 1) and four rank scores with the letter A to the right of $B = 2$ (ranks 3, 4, 7, and 8); so Whitfield calculated $1 - 4 = -3$. For rank score 5 with the letter B, there are three rank scores to the left of $B = 5$ with the letter A (ranks 1, 3, and 4) and two rank scores to the right of $B = 5$ with the letter A (ranks 7 and 8); so $3 - 2 = +1$. Finally, for rank score 6 with the letter B, there are three rank scores to the left of $B = 6$ with the letter A (ranks 1, 3, and 4) and two rank scores to the right of $B = 6$ with the letter A; so $3 - 2 = +1$. The sum of the three differences between variables A and B is $S = -3 + 1 + 1 = -1$. In this manner, Whitfield's approach accommodated unequal sample sizes as well as tied rank scores.

Since the number of possible pairs of N consecutive integers is given by

$$\frac{N(N-1)}{2} ,$$

Whitfield defined and calculated a measure of rank-order association between a dichotomous variable and an ordinal-level variable as

$$\tau = \frac{2S}{N(N-1)} = \frac{2(-1)}{8(8-1)} = -0.0357 .$$

Alternatively, as Whitfield suggested, arrange the two samples into a contingency table with two rows and columns equal to the frequency distribution of the combined samples, as depicted in Table 8.11. The first row of frequencies in Table 8.11

[3] Sample B simply because it is the smaller of the two samples.

Table 8.11 Contingency table of the frequencies of rank scores in Table 8.10

A	1	0	2	0	2
B	0	1	0	2	0

represents the runs in the list of rank scores in Table 8.10 labeled A, i.e., there is one occurrence of A in rank 1, no occurrence of A in rank 2, two occurrences of A in ranks 3 and 4, no occurrences of A in ranks 5 and 6, and two occurrences of A in ranks 5 and 6. The second row of frequencies in Table 8.11 represents the runs in the list of rank scores in Table 8.10 labeled B, i.e., there is no occurrence of B in rank 1, one occurrence of B in rank 2, no occurrences of B in ranks 3 and 4, two occurrences of B in ranks 5 and 6, and no occurrences of B in ranks 5 and 6.

Given the $r \times c$ contingency table in Table 8.11 with $r = 2$ rows and $c = 5$ columns, let x_{ij} indicate a cell frequency for $i = 1, \ldots, r$ and $j = 1, \ldots, c$. Then, as Kendall showed in 1948 [41], the number of concordant pairs is

$$C = \sum_{i=1}^{r-1} \sum_{j=1}^{c-1} x_{ij} \left(\sum_{k=i+1}^{r} \sum_{l=j+1}^{c} x_{kl} \right)$$
$$= (1)(1+0+2+0) + (0)(0+2+0) + (2)(2+0) + (0)(0)$$
$$= 3+0+4+0 = 7 \;,$$

the number of discordant pairs is

$$D = \sum_{i=1}^{r-1} \sum_{j=1}^{c-1} x_{i,c-j+1} \left(\sum_{k=i+1}^{r} \sum_{l=1}^{c-j} x_{kl} \right)$$
$$= (2)(0+1+0+2) + (0)(0+1+0) + (2)(0+1) + (0)(0)$$
$$= 6+0+2+0 = 8 \;,$$

and $S = C - D = 7 - 8 = -1$.

Thus, Whitfield's S statistic is identical to Kendall's S statistic and is also directly related to the two-sample rank-sum U statistic of Mann and Whitney [49] and, hence, to the two-sample rank-sum W statistic of Wilcoxon [73]. The relationships between Whitfield's S statistic and Mann and Whitney's U statistic are given by

$$S = 2U - n_A n_B \quad \text{and} \quad U = \frac{S + n_A n_B}{2}$$

and the relationships between Whitfield's S statistic and Wilcoxon's W statistic are given by

$$S = n_B(N + 1) - 2W \quad \text{and} \quad W = \frac{n_B(N + 1) - S}{2} .$$

Example

To illustrate Whitfield's τ measure of association, consider the $N = 15$ rank scores listed in Table 8.12 consisting of $n_A = 9$ rank scores in Sample A and $n_B = 6$ rank scores in Sample B. To calculate Whitfield's S statistic for the dichotomous data listed in Table 8.12, there are two A rank scores to the left of $B = 3$ (ranks 1 and 2) and seven A rank scores to the right of $B = 3$ (ranks 4, 5, 6, 9, 10 11, and 12), so $2 - 7 = -5$. There are five A rank scores to the left of $B = 7$ and $B = 8$ (ranks 1, 2, 4, 5, and 6) and four A rank scores to the right of $B = 7$ and $B = 8$ (ranks 9, 10, 11, and 12), so $(5 - 4) + (5 - 4) = +2$. There are nine A rank scores to the left of $B = 13$, 14, and 15 (ranks 1, 2, 4, 5, 6, 9, 10, 11, and 12) and zero A rank scores to the right of $B = 13$, 14, and 15, so $(9 - 0) + (9 - 0) + (9 - 0) = +27$. Then, $S = -5 + 2 + 27 = +24$.

Alternatively, arrange the two samples into a contingency table with two rows and columns equal to the frequency distribution of the combined samples, as depicted in Table 8.13. The first row of frequencies in Table 8.13 represents the runs in the list of rank scores in Table 8.12 labeled A, i.e., there are two occurrences of A in ranks 1 and 2; no occurrence of A in rank 3; three occurrences of A in ranks 4, 5, and 6; no occurrence of A in ranks 7 and 8; four occurrences of A in ranks 10, 11, and 12; and no occurrence of A in ranks 13, 14, and 15. The second row of frequencies in Table 8.13 represents the runs in the list of rank scores in Table 8.12 labeled B, i.e., there are no occurrences of B in ranks 1 and 2, one occurrence of B in rank 3, no occurrences of B in ranks 4, 5 and 6, two occurrences of B in ranks 7 and 8, no occurrence of B in ranks 9, 10, 11, and 12, and three occurrences of B in ranks 13, 14, and 15.

Given the $r \times c$ contingency table in Table 8.13 with $r = 2$ rows and $c = 6$ columns, let x_{ij} indicate a cell frequency for $i = 1, \ldots, r$ and $j = 1, \ldots, c$. The

Table 8.12 Listing of example data for Whitfield's S with $n_A = 9$ and $n_B = 6$ rank scores from samples A and B, respectively

Rank	1	2	3	4	5	6	7	8	9	10	11	12	13	14	15
Sample	A	A	B	A	A	A	B	B	A	A	A	A	B	B	B

Table 8.13 Contingency table of the frequencies of rank scores in Table 8.12

A	2	0	3	0	4	0
B	0	1	0	2	0	3

number of concordant pairs is

$$C = \sum_{i=1}^{r-1} \sum_{j=1}^{c-1} x_{ij} \left(\sum_{k=i+1}^{r} \sum_{l=j+1}^{c} x_{kl} \right)$$
$$= (2)(1+0+2+0+3) + (0)(0+2+0+3)$$
$$+ (3)(2+0+3) + (0)(0+3) + (4)(3)$$
$$= 12+0+15+0+12 = 39 \,,$$

the number of discordant pairs is

$$D = \sum_{i=1}^{r-1} \sum_{j=1}^{c-1} x_{i,c-j+1} \left(\sum_{k=i+1}^{r} \sum_{l=1}^{c-j} x_{kl} \right)$$
$$= (0)(0+1+0+2+0) + (4)(0+1+0+2)$$
$$+ (0)(0+1+0) + (3)(0+1) + (0)(0)$$
$$= 0+12+0+3+0 = 15 \,,$$

$S = C - D = 39 - 15 = +24$, and Whitfield's test statistic is

$$\tau = \frac{2S}{N(N-1)} = \frac{2(+24)}{15(15-1)} = +0.2286 \,.$$

Calculating Mann and Whitney's U statistic for the data listed in Table 8.12, the number of A rank scores to the left of (less than) the first B rank score (rank 3) is 2; the number of A rank scores to the left of the second and third B rank scores (ranks 7 and 8) is 5 each; and the number of A rank scores to the left of the last three B rank scores (ranks 13, 14, and 15) is 9 each. Then $U = 2+5+5+9+9+9 = 39$. Calculating Wilcoxon's W statistic for the rank data listed in Table 8.12, the sum of the rank scores in Sample A is $W = 1+2+4+5+6+9+10+11+12 = 60$.[4]

Then the relationships among Whitfield's S, Mann and Whitney's U, and Wilcoxon's W are given by

$$S = 2U - n_A n_B = 2(39) - (9)(6) = +24 \,,$$

$$U = \frac{S + n_A n_B}{2} = \frac{24 + (9)(6)}{2} = 39 \,,$$

$$S = n_A(N+1) - 2W = 9(15+1) - 2(60) = +24 \,,$$

[4]Coincidentally, in this example the sum of the $n_1 = 9$ rank scores in Sample B is also 60.

and

$$W = \frac{n_A(N+1) - S}{2} = \frac{9(15+1) - 24}{2} = 60\,.$$

For the $N = 15$ rank scores listed in Table 8.12, there are only

$$M = \frac{N!}{n_A!\,n_B!} = \frac{15!}{9!\,6!} = 5{,}005$$

possible, equally-likely arrangements in the reference set of all permutations of the observed rank scores, making an exact permutation analysis possible. Since Whitfield's τ is simply a linear function of Kendall's S, the probability of S is the probability of τ. If all arrangements of the $N = 15$ observed rank scores listed in Table 8.12 occur with equal chance, the exact probability value of $S = +24$ computed on the $M = 5{,}005$ possible arrangements of the observed data with $n_A = 9$ A rank scores and $n_B = 6$ B rank scores preserved for each arrangement is

$$P(S \geq S_{\text{o}}|H_0) = \frac{\text{number of } S \text{ values } \geq S_{\text{o}}}{M} = \frac{906}{5{,}005} = 0.1810\,,$$

where S_{o} denotes the observed value of Kendall's S.

8.5.2 Cureton's r_{rb} Measure of Association

In 1956 Edward Cureton proposed a new measure of correlation for a ranked variable and a dichotomous variable that he labeled r_{rb} for rank-biserial correlation [14]. The rank-biserial correlation coefficient was introduced by Cureton as a measure of effect size for the Wilcoxon–Mann–Whitney two-sample rank-sum test. Twelve years later, in 1968, Cureton extended r_{rb} to include tied ranks [15]. In this section, only non-tied ranks are considered, with no loss of generality. Cureton stated that the new correlation coefficient should norm properly between ± 1 and should be strictly non-parametric, defined solely in terms of inversions and agreements between rank-pairs, without the use of means, variances, covariances, or regression [14, p. 287]. Consequently, as Cureton stated, "clearly r_{rb} is a Kendall-type coefficient" [14, p. 289].

Example

Consider an example data set such as listed in Table 8.14 in which $N = 10$ objects are ranked (variable y) and also classified into two samples coded 0 and 1

Table 8.14 Example (0, 1) coded data for Cureton's rank-biserial correlation coefficient

	Variable	
Object	x	y
1	0	1
2	1	2
3	0	3
4	0	4
5	0	5
6	0	6
7	1	7
8	0	8
9	1	9
10	1	10

(variable x). Cureton defined r_{rb} as

$$r_{rb} = \frac{C - D}{S_{\max}} = \frac{S}{S_{\max}} ,$$

where C is the number of concordant pairs, D is the number of discordant pairs, $S = C - D$ is the test statistic of Kendall [39] and Whitfield [72], and $S_{\max} = n_0 n_1$, where n_0 and n_1 denote the number of objects coded 0 and 1, respectively.

Table 8.15 lists the

$$\binom{N}{2} = \frac{N(N-1)}{2} = \frac{10(10-1)}{2} = 45$$

possible paired comparisons of x_i and x_j with y_i and y_j, where $i < j$ and n_0 and n_1 denote the number of objects coded 0 and 1, respectively. Each paired difference is labeled as concordant (C) or discordant (D). Paired differences not labeled as C or D are irrelevant in the present context as they are tied by either $x_i = x_j = 0$ or $x_i = x_j = 1$. In Table 8.15 there are $C = 18$ concordant and $D = 6$ discordant paired differences; thus, for the paired differences listed in Table 8.15, the observed value of S is $S = C - D = 18 - 6 = +12$.

Alternatively, as suggested by Whitfield, the rank scores listed in Table 8.14 can be rearranged into a contingency table to make calculation of C and D much easier [72]. Consider the data listed in Table 8.14 arranged into a 2×6 contingency table, such as given in Table 8.16. The top row of frequencies given in Table 8.16 represents the runs in the list of rank scores given in Table 8.14 coded 0, i.e., there is one occurrence of a 0 in rank 1 , no occurrence of a 0 in rank 2, four occurrences of a 0 in ranks 3, 4, 5, and 6, no occurrence of a 0 in rank 7, one occurrence of a 0 in rank 8, and no occurrences of a 0 in ranks 9 and 10. The bottom row of frequencies given in Table 8.16 represents the runs in the list of rank scores given in Table 8.14 coded 1, i.e., there is no occurrence of a 1 in rank 1, one occurrence of a 1 in rank 2,

Table 8.15 Paired differences and concordant (C) and discordant (D) values for the rank scores listed in Table 8.14

Pair	$x_i - x_j$	$y_i - y_j$	Type	Pair	$x_i - x_j$	$y_i - y_j$	Type
1	1 − 0	1 − 2	C	24	0 − 1	3 − 10	C
2	0 − 0	1 − 3		25	0 − 0	4 − 5	
3	0 − 0	1 − 4		26	0 − 0	4 − 6	
4	0 − 0	1 − 5		27	0 − 1	4 − 7	C
5	0 − 0	1 − 6		28	0 − 0	4 − 8	
6	0 − 1	1 − 7	C	29	0 − 1	4 − 9	C
7	0 − 0	1 − 8		30	0 − 1	4 − 10	C
8	0 − 1	1 − 9	C	31	0 − 0	5 − 6	
9	0 − 1	1 − 10	C	32	0 − 1	5 − 7	C
10	1 − 0	2 − 3	D	33	0 − 0	5 − 8	
11	1 − 0	2 − 4	D	34	0 − 1	5 − 9	C
12	1 − 0	2 − 5	D	35	0 − 1	5 − 10	C
13	1 − 0	2 − 6	D	36	0 − 1	6 − 7	C
14	1 − 1	2 − 7		37	0 − 0	6 − 8	
15	1 − 0	2 − 8	D	38	0 − 1	6 − 9	C
16	1 − 1	2 − 9		39	0 − 1	6 − 10	C
17	1 − 1	2 − 10		40	1 − 0	7 − 8	D
18	0 − 0	3 − 4		41	1 − 1	7 − 9	
19	0 − 0	3 − 5		42	1 − 1	7 − 10	
20	0 − 0	3 − 6		43	0 − 1	8 − 9	C
21	0 − 1	3 − 7	C	44	0 − 1	8 − 10	C
22	0 − 0	3 − 8		45	1 − 1	9 − 10	
23	0 − 1	3 − 9	C				

Table 8.16 Ranking of a dichotomous variable with $n_0 = 6$, $n_1 = 4$, and $N = n_0 + n_1 = 10$

0	1	0	4	0	1	0
1	0	1	0	1	0	2

no occurrences of a 1 in ranks 3, 4, 5, and 6, one occurrence of a 1 in rank 7, no occurrence of a 1 in rank 8, and two occurrences of a 1 in ranks 9 and 10.

Given the $r \times c$ contingency table presented in Table 8.16 with $r = 2$ rows and $c = 6$ columns, let x_{ij} indicate a cell frequency for $i = 1, \ldots, r$ and $j = 1, \ldots, c$. The number of concordant pairs is

$$C = \sum_{i=1}^{r-1} \sum_{j=1}^{c-1} x_{ij} \left(\sum_{k=i+1}^{r} \sum_{l=j+1}^{c} x_{kl} \right)$$

$$= (1)(1 + 0 + 1 + 0 + 2) + (0)(0 + 1 + 0 + 2)$$

$$+ (4)(1 + 0 + 2) + (0)(0 + 2) + (1)(2)$$

$$= 4 + 0 + 12 + 2 = 18 ,$$

the number of discordant pairs is

$$D = \sum_{i=1}^{r-1} \sum_{j=1}^{c-1} x_{i,c-j+1} \left(\sum_{k=i+1}^{r} \sum_{l=1}^{c-j} x_{kl} \right)$$
$$= (0)(0+1+0+1+0) + (1)(0+1+0+1)$$
$$+ (0)(0+1+0) + (4)(0+1) + (0)(0)$$
$$= 0+2+0+4+0 = 6\ ,$$

$S = C - D = 18 - 6 = +12$, and Cureton's rank-biserial coefficient is

$$r_{rb} = \frac{S}{S_{\max}} = \frac{S}{n_0 n_1} = \frac{+12}{(6)(4)} = +0.50\ .$$

For the rank scores listed in Table 8.14, there are only

$$M = \frac{N!}{n_0!\ n_1!} = \frac{10!}{6!\ 4!} = 210$$

possible, equally-likely arrangements in the reference set of all permutations of the observed scores with $n_0 = 6$ and $n_1 = 4$ preserved for each arrangement, making an exact permutation analysis possible. If all arrangements of the $N = 10$ observed rank scores occur with equal chance, the exact probability value of $r_{rb} = +0.50$ computed on the $M = 210$ possible arrangements of the observed data is

$$P(r_{rb} \geq r_{\text{o}} | H_0) = \frac{\text{number of } r_{rb} \text{ values } \geq r_{\text{o}}}{M} = \frac{54}{210} = 0.2571\ ,$$

where r_{o} denotes the observed value of Cureton's r_{rb}.

Because Cureton developed r_{rb} as a measure of effect size for the Wilcoxon–Mann–Whitney two-sample rank-sum test, it is not surprising that Cureton's r_{rb} is related to Wilcoxon's W and to Mann and Whitney's U. In addition, it can be shown that r_{rb} is also related to Kendall's τ_a when there are no tied values. For the $N = 10$ rank scores listed in Table 8.14, Wilcoxon's W is simply the smaller of the sums of the rank scores of the two samples, i.e.,

$$W = \sum_{i=1}^{n_0} = 1+3+4+5+6+8 = 27\ .$$

The relationships between Wilcoxon's W and Cureton's r_{rb} are given by

$$W = \frac{n_0(N+1) - n_0 n_1 r_{rb}}{2} \quad \text{and} \quad r_{rb} = \frac{n_0(N+1) - 2W}{n_0 n_1}\ ,$$

where n_0 is the number of objects in the group with the smaller of the two sums; in this case, 27. Thus, the observed value of Wilcoxon's W is

$$W_o = \frac{6(10+1) - (6)(4)(0.50)}{2} = 27$$

and the observed value of Cureton's r_{rb} is

$$r_{rb} = \frac{6(10+1) - 2(27)}{(6)(4)} = +0.50 \; .$$

For the $N = 10$ rank scores listed in Table 8.14, Mann and Whitney's U is the sum of the number of values in one sample, preceded by the number of values in the other sample. Thus, for the rank scores listed in Table 8.14, the value of 1 in Sample 0 is less than values 2, 7, 9, and 10 in Sample 1, yielding $U = 4$. Then, the value of 3 in Sample 0 is less than values 7, 9, and 10 in Sample 1, yielding $U = 3 + 4 = 7$. Next, the value of 4 in Sample 0 is less than values 7, 9, and 10 in Sample 1, yielding $U = 3 + 3 + 4 = 10$. Next, the value of 5 in Sample 0 is less than values 7, 9, and 10 in Sample 1, yielding $U = 3 + 3 + 3 + 4 = 13$. Next, the value of 6 in Sample 0 is less than values 7, 9, and 10 in Sample 1, yielding $U = 3 + 3 + 3 + 3 + 4 = 16$. Finally, the value of 8 in Sample 0 is less than values 9 and 10 in Sample 1, yielding $U = 3 + 3 + 3 + 3 + 4 + 2 = 18$. Alternatively,

$$U = n_0 n_1 + \frac{n_0(n_0+1)}{2} - W = (6)(4) + \frac{6(6+1)}{2} - 27 = 18 \; .$$

The relationships between Mann and Whitney's U and Cureton's r_{rb} are given by

$$U = \frac{n_0 n_1 (1 + r_{rb})}{2} \quad \text{and} \quad r_{rb} = \frac{2U}{n_0 n_1} - 1 \; .$$

Thus, the observed value of Mann and Whitney's U is

$$U = \frac{(6)(4)(1+0.50)}{2} = 18$$

and the observed value of Cureton's r_{rb} is

$$r_{rb} = \frac{2(18)}{(6)(4)} - 1 = +0.50 \; .$$

For the $N = 10$ rank scores listed in Table 8.14, Kendall's τ_a is

$$\tau_a = \frac{2S}{N(N-1)} = \frac{2(+12)}{10(10-1)} = +0.2667 \; .$$

The relationships between Kendall's τ_a and Cureton's r_{rb} are given by

$$\tau_a = \frac{2n_0n_1r_{rb}}{N(N-1)} \quad \text{and} \quad r_{rb} = \frac{\tau_a N(N-1)}{2n_0n_1} \ .$$

Thus, the observed value of Kendall's τ_a is

$$\tau_a = \frac{2(6)(4)(+0.50)}{10(10-1)} = +0.2667$$

and the observed value of Cureton's r_{rb} is

$$r_{rb} = \frac{(0.2667)(10)(10-1)}{2(6)(4)} = +0.50 \ .$$

Since Cureton's r_{rb} is related to Mann and Whitney's U and Whitfield's τ is related to Mann and Whitney's U, the relationships are transitive and it follows that r_{rb} and τ must be related. The relationships between Cureton's r_{rb} and Whitfield's τ are given by

$$r_{rb} = \frac{\tau N(N-1)}{2n_0n_1} \quad \text{and} \quad \tau = \frac{2r_{rb}n_0n_1}{N(N-1)} \ ,$$

where n_0 and n_1 denote the number of objects in samples 0 and 1, respectively, and $N = n_0 + n_1$.

Consider the (0, 1) coded data in Table 8.14 on p. 463, replicated for convenience in Table 8.17. For the data given in Table 8.17, $n_0 = 6$, $n_1 = 4$, $N = 10$, $r_{rb} = +0.50$, and $\tau = +0.2667$. Then, Cureton's rank-biserial correlation coefficient is

$$r_{rb} = \frac{(+0.2667)(10)(10-1)}{2(6)(4)} = +0.50$$

Table 8.17 Example (0, 1) coded data for Cureton's rank-biserial correlation coefficient and Whitfield's measure of nominal-ordinal relationship

	Variable	
Object	x	y
1	0	1
2	1	2
3	0	3
4	0	4
5	0	5
6	0	6
7	1	7
8	0	8
9	1	9
10	1	10

and Whitfield's measure of association is

$$\tau = \frac{2(+0.50)(6)(4)}{10(10-1)} = +0.2667 \,.$$

8.6 Measures of Nominal-Interval Association

In this section, permutation statistical methods are described for measures of association designed for a nominal-level independent variable and an interval-level dependent variable. In practice, such measures are usually referred to as measures of effect size, i.e., a measurement of the strength of association as an indicator of the practical effect of the factors under consideration that is independent of the sample size(s). Four measures are considered: Pearson's squared product-moment correlation coefficient r^2, Pearson's squared correlation ratio η^2, Kelley's ϵ^2, and Hays' $\hat{\omega}^2$. A fifth permutation-based measure, $\mathfrak{R}$, is introduced that corrects some of the deficiencies of the four conventional measures. For simplification, dichotomous independent variables are first considered in this section to illustrate the various measures, with no loss of generality.

8.6.1 Product-Moment Correlation Coefficient

The first measure of effect size for a dichotomous nominal-level independent variable is the familiar squared Pearson product-moment correlation coefficient—the coefficient of determination. For Student's two-sample t test, the squared correlation coefficient may be expressed as

$$r^2 = \frac{t^2}{t^2 + N - 2} \,, \tag{8.6}$$

where N is the total number of subjects in the two treatments combined. It is not uncommon for r^2 to be labeled as r_{pb}^2, indicating that this measure of effect size is the point-biserial correlation between the response measurement scores and a dummy-coded (0, 1) variable representing the two treatment groups, i.e., the correlation between the response measurement scores and group membership; see, for example, discussions by Friedman [22], Howell [32, pp. 307–309], Kline [44, pp. 114–116], and Nunnally [56, pp. 143–146]. In other applications, especially in the analysis of variance, r^2 is designated as the "correlation ratio" and expressed as η^2.

The coefficient of determination (r^2) has been heavily criticized in the literature as a measure of effect size. D'Andrade and Dart advocated the use of r instead of r^2, arguing that the usual interpretation of r^2 as "variance accounted for" is inappropriate since variance is a squared measure, no longer corresponding to the dimensionality of the original measurements [16, p. 47]. Kvålseth [45] and Ozer [57] demonstrated that for any model other than a linear model with an intercept, r^2 is inappropriate as a measure of effect size; see also articles by Anderson-Sprecher [2], Draper [17], Hahn [26], Healy [29], and Willett and Singer [74]. Finally, while r^2 is touted as varying between 0 and 1 and therefore has a clear interpretation, as is obvious in Eq. (8.6) r^2 approaches 1 only as t^2 approaches infinity and, thus, the only way that r^2 can equal 1 is when there is only a single object in each treatment, i.e., $N - 2 = 0$.

Blalock [8] and Rosenthal and Rubin [65, 66] showed that values of r^2 underestimate the magnitudes of experimental effects, even though r^2 is biased upward. Rosenthal and Rubin proposed a new measure to replace r^2 that they called the binomial effect size display (BESD). Table 8.18 illustrates binomial effect size displays for various values of r^2 and r.

To illustrate how the BESD is calculated, consider the 2×2 contingency table in Table 8.19. For the frequency data given in Table 8.19, Pearson's chi-squared test statistic is $\chi^2 = 20.4800$ and Pearson's r^2 is

$$r^2 = \frac{\chi^2}{N} = \frac{20.4800}{200} = 0.1024 .$$

As Rosenthal and Rubin explained, $r^2 = 0.1024$ is the correlational equivalent of increasing a success rate from 34% to 66% by means of an experimental treatment

Table 8.18 Binomial effect size displays (BESD) corresponding to various values of r^2 and r

		Success rate increased		
r^2	r	From	To	Difference
0.01	0.10	0.45	0.55	0.10
0.04	0.20	0.40	0.60	0.20
0.09	0.30	0.35	0.65	0.30
0.16	0.40	0.30	0.70	0.40
0.25	0.50	0.25	0.75	0.50
0.36	0.60	0.20	0.80	0.60
0.49	0.70	0.15	0.85	0.70
0.64	0.80	0.10	0.90	0.80
0.81	0.90	0.05	0.95	0.90
1.00	1.00	0.00	1.00	1.00

Table 8.19 Example binomial effect size display accounting for only 10% of the variance

	Outcome		
Condition	Alive	Dead	Total
Treatment	66	34	100
Control	34	66	100
Total	100	100	200

procedure [66, p. 166]. Put another way, a death rate under the control condition is 66%, but is only 34% under the experimental condition, with a decrease in the death rate of 32%. Rosenthal and Rubin argued that this difference in death rates is not reflected in a coefficient of determination of only $r^2 = 0.1024$.

8.6.2 The Correlation Ratio

The correlation ratio was first described by Karl Pearson in 1911 and 1923 [58, 59] and later by R.A. Fisher in 1925 [19, Chap. 8]. For many years the correlation ratio, η^2, was the standard measure of effect size for a nominal-level independent variable and an interval-level dependent variable, such as in a conventional two-sample t test or a one-way analysis of variance F test. In terms of a simple one-way completely randomized analysis of variance,

$$\eta^2 = \frac{SS_{\text{Between}}}{SS_{\text{Total}}} ,$$

i.e., the proportion of the total variability attributable to the treatment or intervention. The measure of effect size, r^2 or η^2, has been criticized repeatedly in the literature for its positive bias, especially for small sample sizes; see, for example, articles by Levine and Hullett [48] and Maxwell, Camp, and Arvey [52]. In addition, η^2 is affected by the size of the design as well as the total sample size. Other things being equal, the larger the total sample size, the smaller η^2 tends to be. On the other hand, the greater the number of treatments in the design, the larger η^2 tends to be [60, p. 506]. Also, see two articles by Murray and Dosser [55] and Strube [70]. Finally, it should be noted that η^2 is sometimes employed as a test of linearity in simple regression problems, where it is compared with the Pearson product-moment correlation coefficient and evaluated with the F distribution. Since η^2 is a coefficient of non-linearity and r^2 is a coefficient of linearity, the difference between them may be used as a test of linearity where a difference of zero implies linearity and a difference greater than zero indicates non-linearity. For the test of linearity with k categories,

$$F = \frac{(\eta^2 - r^2)(N - k)}{(1 - \eta^2)(k - 2)} ,$$

which is distributed as Snedecor's F with $k-2$ and $N-k$ degrees of freedom, under the assumption of normality.

8.6.3 Kelley's ϵ^2

The third measure of effect size is Kelley's ϵ^2 [38] and, defined for Student's two-sample t test, is given by

$$\epsilon^2 = \frac{t^2 - 1}{t^2 + N - 2} . \tag{8.7}$$

In some earlier textbooks, ϵ^2 was designated as $\hat{\eta}^2$, i.e., η^2 adjusted for degrees of freedom, and is typically termed the "unbiased correlation ratio." It has been well established and is widely recognized that ϵ^2 is not, in fact, unbiased, but since the title of Truman Kelley's article was "An unbiased correlation ratio measure," the label has survived for over 80 years.

8.6.4 Hays' $\hat{\omega}^2$

The fourth measure of effect size for a nominal independent variable and an interval dependent variable is Hays' $\hat{\omega}^2$ [28, pp. 323–332]. According to Hays, $\hat{\omega}^2$ estimates the proportion of total variance attributable to treatment [28, p. 325]. Thus, $\hat{\omega}^2$ is a ratio of variance estimates given by

$$\hat{\omega}^2 = \frac{\hat{\sigma}_t^2}{\hat{\sigma}_t^2 + \hat{\sigma}_x^2} ,$$

where $\hat{\sigma}_t^2$ is an estimate of the treatment variance and $\hat{\sigma}_x^2$ is an estimate of the population variance. For Student's two-sample t test, Hays' $\hat{\omega}^2$ is given by

$$\hat{\omega}^2 = \frac{t^2 - 1}{t^2 + N - 1} . \tag{8.8}$$

Hays defined $\hat{\omega}^2$ as the proportion of variance in the observations attributable to group membership and, alternatively, as the relative reduction in uncertainty about the observations given by knowledge of group membership [28, p. 325]. Note the high degree of similarity between Kelley's ϵ^2 as given in Eq. (8.7) and Hays' $\hat{\omega}^2$ as given in Eq. (8.8). It has been shown empirically by Carroll and Nordholm that ϵ^2 and $\hat{\omega}^2$ will ordinarily differ very little for a given set of response measurement scores [11]. In fact, as sample sizes increase, Kelley's ϵ^2 and Hays' $\hat{\omega}^2$ converge to the same value [52].

8.6.5 Mielke and Berry's $\Re$

The permutation-based chance-corrected measure of agreement, $\Re$, is described more completely in Chap. 4, Sect. 4.8.1 and is defined as

$$\Re = 1 - \frac{\delta}{\mu_\delta} ,$$

where δ is the weighted mean of the observed response measurement scores and μ_δ is the arithmetic average of the δ values calculated on all possible, equally-likely arrangements of the observed scores. Defined in terms of Student's two-sample t test,

$$\Re = \frac{t^2 - 1}{t^2 + N - 2} .$$

Under certain conditions the four measures of effect size, r^2 (η^2), ϵ^2 ($\hat{\eta}^2$), $\hat{\omega}^2$, and $\Re$ produce similar results and are directly related to each other and to Student's t test for two independent samples [7, p. 69]. However, the measures r^2, ϵ^2, and $\hat{\omega}^2$ all require homogeneity of variance as they are appropriate only for pooled two-sample t tests. On the other hand, $\Re$ does not require homogeneity of variance and is appropriate for both pooled and non-pooled two-sample t tests [37].

It is widely recognized that r^2 is a positively biased estimate of the squared Pearson population correlation coefficient, ρ^2. An adjusted r^2 coefficient that compensates for degrees of freedom was introduced by M.J.B. Ezekiel in 1930 [18]; see also discussions by Larson [46] and Wherry [71] in 1931. An adjusted r^2 value is produced by most statistical computer programs and is given by

$$\hat{r}^2 = 1 - \frac{(1 - r^2)(N - 1)}{N - 2}$$

for two treatment groups.[5] It can easily be shown that $\epsilon^2 = \hat{r}^2$; see, for example, discussions by Cohen and Cohen [12, p. 188] and Maxwell, Camp, and Arvey [52]. It can also be shown that $\Re = \epsilon^2 = \hat{r}^2$. Thus, since $\Re$ is a chance-corrected measure, ϵ^2 and $\hat{r}^2$ are also chance-corrected measures of effect size. To clarify the relationship and emphasize that the adjustment is for the degrees of freedom, ϵ^2, $\hat{r}^2$, and $\Re$ can be redefined in an analysis of variance context as

$$\Re = \epsilon^2 = \hat{r}^2 = 1 - \left(\frac{N - 1}{N - k} \right) \frac{SS_{\text{Within}}}{SS_{\text{Total}}} \tag{8.9}$$

[5]In the literature, $\hat{r}^2$ is variously termed "adjusted" or "shrunken" r^2.

and expressed in terms of the conventional F-ratio as

$$\Re = \epsilon^2 = \hat{r}^2 = \frac{(F-1)(k-1)}{F(k-1)+N-k} , \tag{8.10}$$

where k denotes the number of treatments.

As is evident in Eq. (8.10), when $F < 1$, $\Re$, ϵ^2, and $\hat{r}^2$ are all negative. It is disconcerting, to say the least, to try to interpret squared coefficients with negative values, as a negative value does not constitute a valid estimate of the population variance [68, p. 344]. In 1968 Friedman noted that ϵ^2 could sometimes be negative [21]. In 1981 Maxwell, Camp, and Arvey also observed that $\hat{r}^2$ could be negative and suggested that negative values of $\hat{r}^2$, $\hat{\omega}^2$, and ϵ^2 be treated as zero [52], failing to recognize that negative values simply represent effect sizes less than expected by chance. As can be seen in Eq. (8.9), when $SS_{\text{Within}} = 0$, $\Re = \epsilon^2 = \hat{r}^2 = 1$; when $SS_{\text{Within}} = SS_{\text{Total}}$, then

$$\Re = \epsilon^2 = \hat{r}^2 = 1 - \frac{N-1}{N-k} = -\left(\frac{k-1}{N-k}\right) ,$$

i.e., the negated ratio of the numerator and denominator degrees of freedom, which is the most extreme negative value that can be obtained for these equivalent chance-corrected measures of effect size; and when $\delta = \mu_\delta$, i.e., the observed result is expected only by chance, $\Re = \epsilon^2 = \hat{r}^2 = 0$. Thus, positive reported values of $\Re$, ϵ^2, and $\hat{r}^2$ are to be interpreted as effect sizes greater than expected by chance, and negative values are to be interpreted as effect sizes less than expected by chance, i.e., the treatment group means are closer together than expected under randomization of the N subjects.

Hays' $\hat{\omega}^2$ also produces negative values—again, seemingly not appropriate for a squared coefficient of effect size. The value of $\hat{\omega}^2$ will be negative whenever the value of the computed F-ratio is less than 1. Defining $\hat{\omega}$ in terms of F makes this clear. For a fixed-effects one-way analysis of variance,

$$\hat{\omega}^2 = \frac{(F-1)(k-1)}{(F-1)(k-1)+N} . \tag{8.11}$$

If $F < 1$, the numerator of Eq. (8.11) will be negative and $\hat{\omega}^2$ will ipso facto be negative. For a random-effects analysis of variance,

$$\hat{\omega}^2 = \frac{F-1}{F+n-1} , \tag{8.12}$$

where n denotes the common number of objects in each of k treatments. Again, if $F < 1$, the numerator of Eq. (8.12) will be negative and $\hat{\omega}^2$ will also be negative.

Negative value of $\hat{\omega}^2$ has led many researchers to advocate treating negative values as zero, including Hays [28, pp. 327, 383]; see also Kenny [42, p. 234].

Although $\hat{\omega}^2$ does not norm properly between 0 and 1, i.e., its minimum value is given by

$$-\left(\frac{k-1}{N-k+1}\right),$$

it is in fact a chance-corrected measure of effect size like $\Re$, ϵ^2, and $\hat{r}^2$. The relationships between the chance-corrected measures of effect size, $\Re$ and Hays' $\hat{\omega}^2$, in terms of F, for a fixed effects one-way analysis of variance, are given by

$$\Re = \hat{\omega}^2\left(\frac{F+N-1}{F+N-2}\right) \quad \text{and} \quad \hat{\omega}^2 = \Re\left(\frac{F+N-2}{F+N-1}\right).$$

8.6.6 *Biased Estimators*

In general, statisticians prefer sample estimates of population parameters that are unbiased, e.g., the sample mean, $\bar{x}$, is an unbiased estimator of the population mean, μ_x, and the sample variance, s_x^2, is an unbiased estimator of the population variance, σ_x^2. It is well known that, under the population model of inference whereby repeated random samples are hypothetically drawn from a normal population, measures of effect size such as r^2, $\hat{r}^2$, η^2, ϵ^2, and $\hat{\omega}^2$ are biased estimators of their respective population parameters [43, 64, 68].

The terms "biased" and "unbiased" possess quite different meanings when used with the permutation model of inference, as there is no population parameter to be estimated. Under the permutation model, an unbiased measure simply means that the average value of the measure of effect size obtained from all M possible arrangements of the observed response measurement scores is zero. In the case of $\epsilon^2 = \hat{r}^2 = \Re$, the expected value of each measure is indeed zero and each of the three chance-corrected measures of effect size is unbiased under the permutation model. On the other hand, while $\hat{\omega}^2$ is a chance-corrected measure of effect size, it is not an unbiased estimator under either the permutation or population models of inference. That said, however, the positive bias of $\hat{\omega}^2$ is typically quite small, within the context of a fixed-effect one-way analysis of variance. Under the permutation model, the expected value of $\hat{\omega}^2$ is given by

$$\mathrm{E}[\hat{\omega}^2] = \frac{1}{M}\sum_{i=1}^{M}\left(\frac{N\delta_i}{\mu_\delta(N-1)+\delta_i}\right),$$

where

$$M = \frac{N!}{\prod_{i=1}^{k} n_i!}$$

and n_i denotes the number of objects in the ith of k treatment groups.

8.6.7 *Homogeneity of Variance*

It is important to note that conventional measures of effect size such as $\hat{r}^2$, ϵ^2, and $\hat{\omega}^2$ depend on the assumption of homogeneity of variance [54, p. 96]. Mitchell and Hartmann documented this dependency and a number of additional weaknesses of measures of effect size, leading them to conclude that:

> [T]he *uncritical* use of magnitude of effects statistics as a cure for the problem of conventional hypothesis testing methods of assessing treatment effectiveness may very well represent a remedy as troublesome as the original problem [54, p. 99].[6]

The assumption of homogeneity of variance underlies many statistical tests and measures. When confounded with unequal sample sizes, serious problems can arise. When sample sizes are unequal and the homogeneity assumption does not hold then, for example, the t and F-ratio test statistics tend to be liberal when large sample variances are associated with small sample sizes, leading to a potential increase in type I error. On the other hand, t or F-ratio test statistics tend to be conservative when large sample variances are associated with large sample sizes, leading to a potential increase in type II error and a corresponding loss of power [9, 25, 27, 31, 33]. In addition, it has been well documented that equal sample sizes provide little protection against inflated error rates for the t and F-ratio tests when variances are unequal [23, 27].

8.7 Dichotomous Nominal-Level Variables

As special cases of nominal-interval association, consider two measures: the point-biserial correlation coefficient (r_{pb}) and the biserial correlation coefficient (r_b). Both examine the relationship between a dichotomous variable and an interval-level variable where, in this case, the dichotomous variable is considered to be a nominal-level variable with only two disjoint, unordered categories. Although both the point-biserial and biserial correlation coefficients were presented in Chap. 7,

[6]Emphasis in the original.

Sects. 7.6 and 7.7, respectively, brief discussions are included here as a dichotomous variable may be considered as a nominal-level variable with only two categories.

8.7.1 Point-Biserial Correlation

The point-biserial correlation coefficient, r_{pb}, measures the association between a true dichotomous variable and an interval-level variable and is an important measure in fields such as education and educational psychology where it is typically used to measure the correlation between test questions scored as correct (1) or incorrect (0) and the overall score on the test for N students. A low or negative point-biserial correlation coefficient indicates that the students with the highest scores on the test answered the question incorrectly and the students with the lowest scores on the test answered the question correctly, alerting the instructor to the possibility that the question failed to discriminate properly and might be faulty.

Example

To illustrate the calculation of a point-biserial correlation coefficient, consider the dichotomous data listed in Table 8.20 for $N = 20$ objects where variable x is the dichotomous variable and variable y is an unspecified interval-level variable. The point-biserial correlation is often expressed as

$$r_{pb} = \frac{\bar{y}_1 - \bar{y}_0}{s_y} \sqrt{\frac{n_0 n_1}{N(N-1)}} \,,$$

where n_0 and n_1 denote the number of y values coded 0 and 1, respectively, $N = n_0 + n_1$, $\bar{y}_0$ and $\bar{y}_1$ denote the means of the y values coded 0 and 1, respectively, and s_y is the sample standard deviation of the y values given by

$$s_y = \sqrt{\frac{1}{N-1} \sum_{i=1}^{N} (y_i - \bar{y})^2} \,.$$

For the example data listed in Table 8.20, $n_0 = n_1 = 10$,

$$\bar{y}_0 = \frac{1}{n_0} \sum_{i=1}^{n_0} y_i = \frac{99 + 99 + \cdots + 89}{10} = 88.40 \,,$$

$$\bar{y}_1 = \frac{1}{n_1} \sum_{i=1}^{n_1} y_i = \frac{98 + 98 + \cdots + 60}{10} = 95.60 \,,$$

$$s_y = \sqrt{\frac{1}{N-1} \sum_{i=1}^{N} (y_i - \bar{y})^2} = \sqrt{\frac{1{,}456}{20 - 1}} = 8.7539 \,,$$

and

$$r_{pb} = \frac{\bar{y}_1 - \bar{y}_0}{s_y}\sqrt{\frac{n_0 n_1}{N(N-1)}} = \frac{95.60 - 88.40}{8.7539}\sqrt{\frac{(10)(10)}{20(20-1)}} = +0.4219 \; .$$

It should be noted that r_{pb} can also be calculated simply as the Pearson product-moment correlation (r_{xy}) between dichotomous variable x and interval variable y. However, using this approach there are

$$M = N! = 20! = 2{,}432{,}902{,}008{,}176{,}640{,}000$$

possible arrangements of the observed data to be considered. A much more efficient approach is to consider the data listed in Table 8.20 as two groups of observations, as shown in Table 8.21 and compute the difference between the means of the groups. Note that it is not necessary that $n_0 = n_1$.

For the grouped scores listed in Table 8.21, there are only

$$M = \frac{N!}{n_0!\; n_1!} = \frac{20!}{10!\; 10!} = 184{,}756$$

Table 8.20 Example (0, 1) coded data for the point-biserial correlation coefficient

	Variable			Variable	
Object	x	y	Object	x	y
1	0	99	11	1	86
2	0	99	12	1	90
3	1	98	13	0	97
4	1	98	14	0	95
5	1	97	15	1	92
6	0	89	16	0	98
7	0	95	17	1	86
8	0	94	18	1	85
9	1	92	19	0	94
10	1	60	20	0	96

Table 8.21 Example data with the y values arranged in two groups of $n_0 = n_1 = 10$

0	1
99	98
99	98
98	97
97	92
96	92
95	92
95	90
94	86
94	86
89	60

possible, equally-likely arrangements in the reference set of all permutations of the observed scores, making an exact permutation analysis possible. If all arrangements of the $N = 20$ observed scores occur with equal chance, the exact probability value of $r_{pb} = +0.4219$ computed on the $M = 184{,}756$ possible arrangements of the observed data with $n_0 = n_1 = 10$ preserved for each arrangement is

$$P(r_{pb} \geq r_o | H_0) = \frac{\text{number of } r_{pb} \text{ values } \geq r_o}{M} = \frac{5{,}648}{184{,}756} = 0.0306 ,$$

where r_o denotes the observed value of r_{pb}.

8.7.2 Biserial Correlation

Whereas the point-biserial correlation measures the association between an interval-level variable and a dichotomous variable that is a true dichotomy, such as correct or incorrect, biserial correlation measures the association between an interval-level variable and a variable that is assumed to be continuous and normally distributed, but has been dichotomized, such as IQ dichotomized into "below 100" and "above 100" or height dichotomized into "below 70 inches" and "above 70 inches." The biserial correlation coefficient is a special case of Jaspen's coefficient of multiserial correlation for an ordinal-level variable and an interval-level variable when the ordinal scale has only two ranks. See Sect. 8.8.1 for a discussion of Jaspen's coefficient of multiserial correlation. The biserial correlation coefficient is given by

$$r_b = \frac{(\bar{y}_1 - \bar{y}_0)pq}{uS_y} ,$$

where p and q denote the proportions of all y values coded 0 and 1, respectively, $\bar{y}_0$ and $\bar{y}_1$ denote the means of the y values coded 0 and 1, respectively, S_y is the standard deviation of the y values given by[7]

$$S_y = \sqrt{\frac{1}{N} \sum_{i=1}^{N} (y_i - \bar{y})^2} ,$$

and u is the ordinate of the unit normal distribution at the point of division between the p and q proportions under the distribution given by

$$u = \frac{\exp(-z^2/2)}{\sqrt{2\pi}} .$$

[7]Note that, in this case, the sum of squared deviations is divided by N, not $N - 1$.

Written in raw terms without the p and q proportions,

$$r_b = \frac{(\bar{y}_0 - \bar{y}_1)n_0 n_1}{N^2 u S_y} ,$$

where n_0 and n_1 denote the number of y values coded 0 and 1, respectively, and $N = n_0 + n_1$. The biserial correlation may also be written in terms of the point-biserial correlation coefficient,

$$r_b = \frac{r_{pb}\sqrt{pq}}{u} = \frac{r_{pb}\sqrt{n_0 n_1}}{Nu} ,$$

where, in this application, the point-biserial correlation coefficient is given by

$$r_{pb} = \frac{(\bar{y}_1 - \bar{y}_0)\sqrt{pq}}{S_y} .$$

Example

To illustrate the calculation of the biserial correlation coefficient, consider the small set of data given in Table 8.22 where $N = 7$ subjects are scored on Work Effectiveness (y) and are classified into Type A (0) and Type B (1) personalities (x). For the data listed in Table 8.22, $n_0 = 3$, $n_1 = 4$, $p = n_0/N = 3/7 = 0.4286$, $q = n_1/N = 4/7 = 0.5714$,

$$\bar{y}_0 = \frac{1}{n_0}\sum_{i=1}^{n_0} y_i = \frac{20 + 40 + 60}{3} = 40.00 ,$$

$$\bar{y}_1 = \frac{1}{n_1}\sum_{i=1}^{n_1} y_i = \frac{63 + 77 + 83 + 57}{4} = 70.00 ,$$

$$S_y = \sqrt{\frac{1}{N}\sum_{i=1}^{N} (y_i - \bar{y})^2} = \sqrt{\frac{2{,}778.8571}{7}} = 19.9243 ,$$

Table 8.22 Example (0, 1) coded data for the biserial correlation coefficient

Subject	Type	Effectiveness
1	0	20
2	0	40
3	0	60
4	1	63
5	1	77
6	1	83
7	1	57

the standard score that defines the lower $p = 0.4286$ of the unit-normal distribution is $z = -0.1799$,

$$u = \frac{\exp(-z^2/2)}{\sqrt{2\pi}} = \frac{\exp[-(-0.1799)^2/2]}{\sqrt{2(3.1416)}} = 0.3925 \,,$$

and

$$r_b = \frac{(\bar{y}_1 - \bar{y}_0)pq}{uS_y} = \frac{(70.00 - 40.00)(0.4286)(0.5714)}{(0.3925)(19.9243)} = +0.9395 \,.$$

For the data listed in Table 8.22, the point-biserial correlation coefficient is

$$r_{pb} = \frac{(\bar{y}_1 - \bar{y}_0)\sqrt{pq}}{S_y} = \frac{(70.00 - 40.00)\sqrt{(0.4286)(0.5714)}}{19.9243} = +0.7451 \,,$$

and in terms of the point-biserial correlation coefficient, the biserial correlation coefficient is

$$r_b = \frac{r_{pb}\sqrt{pq}}{u} = \frac{+0.7451\sqrt{(0.4286)(0.5714)}}{0.3925} = +0.9395 \,.$$

For the scores listed in Table 8.22, there are only

$$M = \frac{N!}{n_0!\, n_1!} = \frac{7!}{3!\, 4!} = 35$$

possible, equally-likely arrangements in the reference set of all permutations of the observed scores, making an exact permutation analysis possible. Since $M = 35$ is a small number, it will be illustrative to list all M arrangements of the observed data and the associated values of r_b in Table 8.23. Note that in the formula for the biserial correlation coefficient,

$$r_b = \frac{(\bar{y}_1 - \bar{y}_0)pq}{uS_y} \,,$$

p, q, u, and S_y are invariant under permutation. Therefore, the permutation distribution can be based entirely on $\bar{y}_1 - \bar{y}_0$. The $M = 35$ arrangements of the observed data, along with associated r_b and $\bar{y}_1 - \bar{y}_0$ values are listed in Table 8.23. The two arrangements in Table 8.23 indicated with an asterisk (i.e., arrangements 1 and 5) possess values of $\bar{y}_1 - \bar{y}_0$ and an r_b value equal to or greater than the observed value of $\bar{y}_1 - \bar{y}_0 = +30.0000$ and $r_b = +0.9395$, respectively. The two values of $\bar{y}_1 - \bar{y}_0$ that are equal to or greater than $\bar{y}_1 - \bar{y}_0 = +30.0000$ are the observed value in Arrangement 1 with $\bar{y}_1 - \bar{y}_0 = +30.0000$ and Arrangement 5 with $\bar{y}_1 - \bar{y}_0 = +31.7500$; the two values of r_b equal to or greater than the observed

Table 8.23 Listing of all $M = 35$ arrangements of the observed data in Table 8.22 and associated r_b and $\bar{y}_1 - \bar{y}_0$ values

Arrangement	$x = 0$	$x = 1$	r_b	$\bar{y}_1 - \bar{y}_0$
1*	20, 40, 60	63, 77, 83, 57	+0.9395	+30.0000
2	20, 40, 63	60, 77, 83, 57	+0.8847	+28.2500
3	20, 40, 77	60, 63, 83, 57	+0.6289	+20.0833
4	20, 40, 83	60, 63, 77, 57	+0.5193	+16.5833
5*	20, 40, 57	60, 63, 77, 83	+0.9943	+31.7500
6	20, 60, 63	40, 77, 83, 57	+0.5193	+16.5833
7	20, 60, 77	40, 63, 83, 57	+0.2636	+8.4167
8	20, 60, 83	40, 63, 77, 57	+0.1540	+4.9167
9	20, 60, 57	40, 63, 77, 83	+0.6289	+20.0833
10	20, 63, 77	40, 60, 83, 57	+0.2413	+6.6667
11	20, 60, 83	40, 60, 77, 57	+0.0992	+3.1667
12	20, 60, 57	40, 60, 77, 83	+0.5741	+18.3333
13	20, 77, 83	40, 60, 63, 57	−0.1566	−5.0000
14	20, 77, 57	40, 60, 63, 83	+0.3184	+10.1667
15	20, 83, 57	40, 60, 63, 77	+0.2088	+6.6667
16	40, 60, 63	20, 77, 83, 57	+0.1540	+4.9167
17	40, 60, 77	20, 63, 83, 57	−0.1018	−3.2500
18	40, 60, 83	20, 63, 77, 57	−0.2114	−6.7500
19	40, 60, 57	20, 63, 77, 83	+0.2636	+8.4167
20	40, 63, 77	20, 60, 83, 57	+0.1566	−5.0000
21	40, 63, 83	20, 60, 77, 57	−0.2662	−8.5000
22	40, 63, 57	20, 60, 77, 83	+0.2088	+6.6667
23	40, 77, 83	20, 60, 63, 57	−0.5219	−16.6667
24	40, 77, 57	20, 60, 63, 83	−0.0470	−1.5000
25	40, 83, 57	20, 60, 63, 77	−0.1566	−5.0000
26	60, 63, 77	20, 40, 83, 57	−0.5219	−16.6667
27	60, 63, 83	20, 40, 77, 57	−0.6315	−20.1667
28	60, 63, 57	20, 40, 77, 83	−0.1566	−5.0000
29	60, 77, 83	20, 40, 63, 57	−0.8873	−28.3333
30	60, 77, 57	20, 40, 63, 83	−0.4123	−13.1667
31	60, 83, 57	20, 40, 63, 77	−0.5219	−16.6667
32	63, 77, 83	20, 40, 60, 57	−0.9421	−30.0833
33	63, 77, 57	20, 40, 60, 83	−0.4671	−14.9167
34	63, 83, 57	20, 40, 60, 77	−0.5767	−18.4167
35	77, 83, 57	20, 40, 60, 63	−0.8325	−26.5833

value of $r_b = +0.9395$ are the observed value in Arrangement 1 with $r_b = +0.9395$ and Arrangement 5 with $r_b = +0.9943$.

If all arrangements of the $N = 7$ observed values occur with equal chance, the exact upper-tail probability value of $r_b = +0.9395$ computed on the $M = 35$ possible arrangements of the observed data with $n_0 = 3$ and $n_1 = 4$ preserved for each arrangement is

$$P(r_b \geq r_o|H_0) = \frac{\text{number of } r_b \text{ values } \geq r_o}{M} = \frac{2}{35} = 0.0571\,,$$

where r_o denotes the observed value of r_b. More efficiently, the exact probability could alternatively be based on $\bar{y}_1 - \bar{y}_0$, as is shown in the last column of Table 8.23.

Asymptotic probability values cannot be expected to be very accurate with only $N = 7$ observations, but it is instructive to compare the exact probability value with the probability value obtained with conventional means. The biserial correlation coefficient is asymptotically distributed as $N(0, 1)$ with standard error given by

$$s_{r_b} = \frac{1}{\sqrt{N}}\left(\frac{\sqrt{pq}}{u} - r_b^2\right) .$$

For the data listed in Table 8.22,

$$s_{r_b} = \frac{1}{\sqrt{7}}\left(\frac{\sqrt{(0.4286)(0.5714)}}{0.3925} - 0.9395^2\right) = 0.1429\,.$$

Then, under the null hypothesis that the population parameter, ρ_b, is zero,

$$z = \frac{r_b - \rho_b}{s_{r_b}} = \frac{+0.9395 - 0.00}{0.1429} = 6.5729\,,$$

yielding an approximate probability value of $P = 2.4672 \times 10^{-11}$. This is, of course, an unfair comparison as asymptotic probability values cannot be expected to yield accurate results with a sample size of $N = 7$. However, the comparison illustrates the application of exact permutation statistical methods to very small samples.

Improper Norming

In extreme cases, the biserial correlation coefficient will sometimes be greater than unity, as is easily demonstrated. Consider the small set of data given in Table 8.24 where $N = 8$ objects are scored on variable y and classified into two types (0 and 1) on variable x. For the example data listed in Table 8.24, $n_0 = 3$, $n_1 = 5$, $N = 8$,

Table 8.24 Example extreme data for the biserial correlation coefficient

Object	x	y
A	0	1
B	0	2
C	0	3
D	1	4
E	1	5
F	1	6
G	1	7
H	1	8

$p = n_0/N = 3/8 = 0.3750, q = n_1/N = 5/8 = 0.6250,$

$$\bar{y}_0 = \frac{1}{n_0} \sum_{i=1}^{n_0} y_i = \frac{1+2+3}{3} = 2.00 \,,$$

$$\bar{y}_1 = \frac{1}{n_1} \sum_{i=1}^{n_1} y_i = \frac{4+5+6+7+8}{5} = 6.00 \,,$$

$$\bar{y} = \frac{1}{N} \sum_{i=1}^{N} y_i = \frac{1+2+3+4+5+6=7+8}{8} = 4.50 \,,$$

$$S_y = \sqrt{\frac{1}{N} \sum_{i=1}^{N} (y_i - \bar{y})^2} = \sqrt{\frac{42.00}{8}} = 2.2913 \,,$$

the standard score that defines the lower 0.3750 proportion of the unit-normal distribution is $z = -0.3186$,

$$u = \frac{\exp(-z^2/2)}{\sqrt{2\pi}} = \frac{\exp[-(-0.3186)^2/2]}{\sqrt{2(3.1416)}} = 0.3792 \,,$$

and

$$r_b = \frac{(\bar{y}_1 - \bar{y}_0)pq}{uS_y} = \frac{(6.00 - 2.00)(0.3750)(0.6250)}{(0.3792)(2.2913)} = +1.0790 \,.$$

8.8 Measures of Ordinal-Interval Association

In many research situations it is desired to find the degree of association between two variables, one measured on an ordinal scale and the second measured on an interval scale. Because the Pearson product-moment correlation is inappropriate in such situations, researchers commonly degrade the interval-level variable to an ordinal-level variable and apply one of the non-parametric rank-order measures of association such as Spearman's ρ or Kendall's τ_b. The dangers of "scaling down" a quantitative variable are well documented [51, p. 205]. The multiserial correlation coefficient, introduced by Nathan Jaspen [36] in 1946, is a widely used procedure designed to provide an estimate of the degree of association between an ordinal-level variable and an interval-level variable.

8.8.1 Jaspen's Index of Ordinal-Interval Association

Jaspen's multiserial correlation coefficient is simply the Pearson product-moment correlation coefficient between an interval-level variable, Y, and a transformation of an ordinal-level variable, X [36]. The procedure requires the assumption that the rank categories of the ordinal variable are based on an underlying normally distributed interval-level scale. Thus, the multiserial coefficient is highly sensitive to the assumption of normality. Once the assumption is satisfied, percentile ranks are converted to standard scores through an inverse normal probability function. For the procedure to be valid, it is necessary to also assume that each score in a given rank category of the ordinal variable is at the mean of that category on the corresponding underlying interval scale. Given N values on the interval variable and k disjoint, ordered categories on the ordinal variable, the mean standard score of the underlying scale for a given category is given by

$$\bar{Z}_j = \frac{Y_{L_j} - Y_{U_j}}{p_j} \qquad \text{for } j = 1, \ldots, k ,$$

where Y_{L_j} and Y_{U_j} are the lower and upper ordinates of the segment of the $N(0, 1)$ distribution corresponding to the jth ordered category, and where p_j is the proportion of cases in the jth of k categories. Given the obtained values of $\bar{Z}_j$, $j = 1, \ldots, k$, and the original N values of the interval-level variable, a standard Pearson product-moment correlation between the Y and $\bar{Z}$ values yields the multiserial correlation.

However, the resulting multiserial correlation coefficient is usually biased. It is possible to estimate, by means of an appropriate transformation, the correlation between the interval-level variable Y and the continuum hypothesized to underlie the ordinal-level variable X. The transformation is essentially a correction for grouping. As a result of classifying the underlying interval-level values into k ordinal categories, the multiserial correlation coefficient obtained from the grouped data will be smaller than the corresponding Pearson product-moment correlation coefficient that would have been obtained had the interval-level values been available for both variables. The appropriate transformation to obtain a corrected multiserial correlation coefficient is to divide the obtained multiserial correlation coefficient by the assumed correlation between the underlying interval-level variable and the midpoints of the k ordinal categories. The assumed correlation is simply the standard deviation of the $\bar{Z}$ scores corresponding to the midpoints of the ordinal categories and is given by

$$S_{\bar{Z}} = \left(\frac{1}{N} \sum_{j=1}^{k} n_j \bar{Z}_j^2 \right)^{1/2} .$$

Table 8.25 Example data for Jaspen's multiserial correlation coefficient with $N = 10$ integer-level values in $k = 4$ ranked categories

Rank category			
4	3	2	1
4	5	2	1
	4	3	
	3	2	
	3		
	3		

Example 1

To illustrate the calculation of Jaspen's multiserial correlation coefficient, consider the small set of data given in Table 8.25 where $N = 10$ interval-level values are listed in $k = 4$ disjoint, ordered categories.

Table 8.26 illustrates the calculation of Jaspen's multiserial correlation. The first column (X_j) in Table 8.26 lists the $k = 4$ ordered categories of variable X. The second column (n_j) lists the number of observations in each category for $j = 1, \ldots, k$. The third column (p_j) lists the proportion of observations in each category for $j = 1, \ldots, k$, e.g., for rank categories 4 and 3,

$$p_4 = \frac{n_4}{N} = \frac{1}{10} = 0.10 \quad \text{and} \quad p_3 = \frac{n_3}{N} = \frac{5}{10} = 0.50 \; .$$

The fourth column (P_j) lists the cumulative proportion of observations in each category for $j = 1, \ldots, k$, e.g., for rank category 3, $P_3 = p_4 + p_3 = 0.10 + 0.50 = 0.60$. The fifth column ($z_j$) lists the standard score that defines the cumulative proportion from the fourth column under the unit-normal distribution for $j = 1, \ldots, k$, e.g., for rank category 4, the standard score that defines the lowest (left tail) of the normal distribution is $z = -1.2816$. The sixth column (Y_{L_j}) lists the height of the ordinate at the standard score listed in the fifth column below the segment in question of the unit-normal distribution for $j = 1, \ldots, k$, e.g., for rank category 3,

$$Y_{L_3} = \frac{\exp(-z^2/2)}{\sqrt{2\pi}} = \frac{\exp[-(-0.2533)^2/2]}{\sqrt{2(3.1416)}} = 0.3863 \; .$$

Table 8.26 Calculation of the mean standard scores for the $k = 4$ ordinal categories in Table 8.25

X_j	n_j	p_j	P_j	z_j	Y_{L_j}	Y_{U_j}	$\bar{Z}_j$
4	1	0.10	0.10	−1.2816	0.1755	0.0000	+1.7550
3	5	0.50	0.60	+0.2533	0.3863	0.1755	+0.4216
2	3	0.30	0.90	+1.2816	0.1755	0.3863	−0.7027
1	1	0.10	1.00	+1.0000	0.0000	0.1755	−1.7550
Total	10	1.00					

The seventh column (Y_{U_j}) lists the height of the ordinate at the standard score listed in the fifth column above the segment in question of the unit-normal distribution for $j = 1, \ldots, k$, e.g., for rank category 3,

$$Y_{U_3} = \frac{\exp(-z^2/2)}{\sqrt{2\pi}} = \frac{\exp[-(-1.2816)^2/2]}{\sqrt{2(3.1416)}} = 0.1755 .$$

The last column ($\bar{Z}_j$) in Table 8.26 lists the average standard scores for the k categories for $j = 1, \ldots, k$, e.g., for rank category 4,

$$\bar{Z}_4 = \frac{Y_{L_4} - Y_{U_4}}{p_4} = \frac{0.1755 - 0.0000}{0.10} = +1.7550 .$$

The multiserial correlation is simply the Pearson product-moment correlation between the Y interval-level values given in Table 8.25 and the $\bar{Z}$ values given in Table 8.26. Table 8.27 lists the Y, $\bar{Z}$, Y^2, $\bar{Z}^2$, and $Y\bar{Z}$ values, along with the corresponding sums. For the summations given in Table 8.27, the Pearson product-moment correlation between the Y interval-level values and the transformed $\bar{Z}$ values is

$$r_{Y\bar{Z}} = \frac{N\sum_{i=1}^{N} Y_i \bar{Z}_i - \sum_{i=1}^{N} Y_i \sum_{i=1}^{N} \bar{Z}_i}{\sqrt{\left[N\sum_{i=1}^{N} Y_i^2 - \left(\sum_{i=1}^{N} Y_i\right)^2\right]\left[N\sum_{i=1}^{N} \bar{Z}_i^2 - \left(\sum_{i=1}^{N} \bar{Z}_i\right)^2\right]}}$$

$$= \frac{(10)(7.9349) - (30)(0.00)}{\sqrt{[(10)(102) - 30^2][(10)(8.5301) - 0.00^2]}} = +0.7843 .$$

Table 8.27 Calculation of the sums needed for the product-moment correlation between variables Y and $\bar{Z}$

Rank	Y	$\bar{Z}$	Y^2	$\bar{Z}^2$	$Y\bar{Z}$
4	4	+1.7550	16	3.0800	+7.0200
3	5	+0.4216	25	0.1777	+2.1080
	4	+0.4216	16	0.1777	+1.6864
	3	+0.4216	9	0.1777	+1.2648
	3	+0.4216	9	0.1777	+1.2648
	3	+0.4216	9	0.1777	+1.2648
2	2	−0.7027	4	0.4938	−1.4054
	3	−0.7027	9	0.4938	−2.1081
	2	−0.7027	4	0.4938	−1.4054
1	1	−1.7550	1	3.0800	−1.7550
Sum	30	0.0000	102	8.5301	+7.9349

Then, the correction for grouping is

$$S_{\bar{Z}} = \left(\frac{1}{N} \sum_{j=1}^{k} n_j \bar{Z}_j^2 \right)^{1/2}$$

$$= \left\{ \frac{1}{10} \Big[(1)(+1.7550)^2 + (5)(+0.4216)^2 + (3)(-0.7027)^2 + (1)(-1.7550)^2 \Big] \right\}^{1/2} = 0.9236$$

and the corrected multiserial correlation coefficient is

$$r_c = \frac{r_{Y\bar{Z}}}{S_{\bar{Z}}} = \frac{+0.7843}{0.9236} = +0.8492 \; .$$

Typically, Monte Carlo resampling permutation methods are utilized for correlation analyses since there are $M = N!$ possible arrangements to be considered, making exact permutation methods impractical. The usual method is to randomly shuffle either the Y values or the $\bar{Z}$ values a large number of times. Alternatively, random samples of size N can be drawn without replacement from either the N observed Y values or the N observed $\bar{Z}$ values. Let r_o indicate the observed value of r_c. Then, based on $L = 1{,}000{,}000$ random arrangements of the observed data under the null hypothesis, there are 12,300 $|r_c|$ values equal to or greater than $|r_o| = 0.8492$, yielding a Monte Carlo resampling two-sided probability value of $P = 12{,}300/1{,}000{,}000 = 0.0123$.

In comparison, for the correlation data listed in Table 8.27 there are only $N! = 10! = 3{,}628{,}800$ possible, equally-likely arrangements in the reference set of all permutations of the observed scores, making an exact permutation analysis possible. If all arrangements of the $N = 10$ observed bivariate scores occur with equal chance, the exact two-sided probability value of $|r_c| = 0.8492$ computed on the $M = 3{,}628{,}800$ possible arrangements of the observed data is $49{,}091/3{,}628{,}800 = 0.0135$.

In contrast to the exact and resampling permutation probability values, r_c is distributed as Student's t under the null hypothesis with $N - 2$ degrees of freedom. If the population parameter, ρ_c, is assumed to be zero, then for the observed data given in Table 8.25 on p. 485,

$$t = \frac{r_c - \rho_c}{\sqrt{\dfrac{1 - r_c^2}{N - 2}}} = \frac{+0.8492 - 0.00}{\sqrt{\dfrac{1 - (0.8492)^2}{10 - 2}}} = +4.5484 \; ,$$

and with $N - 2 = 10 - 2 = 8$ degrees of freedom the approximate two-sided probability value of $r_c = +0.8492$ is $P = 0.1878 \times 10^{-2}$.

Some investigators have recommended that the corrected r_c value be converted to a standard score with Fisher's z transform and evaluated with the $N(0, 1)$ distribution. For the observed value of $r_c = +0.8490$, Fisher's z is

$$z = \frac{\tanh^{-1}(r_c)}{\sqrt{\dfrac{1}{N-3}}} = \frac{\tanh^{-1}(+0.8492)}{\sqrt{\dfrac{1}{10-3}}} = \frac{+1.2533}{0.3780} = +3.3159$$

yielding an approximate two-sided probability value of $P = 0.9135 \times 10^{-3}$.

Example 2

For a second, more realistic, illustration of Jaspen's multiserial correlation coefficient, consider the data listed in Table 8.28 where $N = 32$ interval-level values are listed in $k = 4$ ordered categories.

Table 8.29 illustrates the calculation of Jaspen's multiserial correlation. The first column (X_j) in Table 8.29 lists the $k = 4$ ordered categories of variable X. The second column (n_j) lists the number of observations in each category for $j = 1, \ldots, k$. The third column (p_j) lists the proportion of observations in each

Table 8.28 Intelligence test scores for $k = 4$ ranks in hypnotic susceptibility

Susceptibility			
4	3	2	1
136	144	139	128
131	137	134	111
126	134	133	104
116	131	132	103
	129	130	103
	126	129	101
	122	123	101
	117	117	
	111	116	
	109	112	
		106	

Table 8.29 Calculation of the mean standard scores for the $k = 4$ ordinal categories in Table 8.28

X_j	n_j	p_j	P_j	z_j	Y_{L_i}	Y_{U_i}	$\bar{Z}_j$
4	4	0.1250	0.1250	−1.1503	0.2059	0.0000	+1.6472
3	10	0.3125	0.4375	−0.1573	0.3940	0.2059	+0.6022
2	11	0.3438	0.7813	+0.7766	0.2951	0.3940	−0.2880
1	7	0.2188	1.0000	+1.0000	0.0000	0.2951	−1.3487
Total	32	1.0000					

category for $j = 1, \ldots, k$, e.g., for rank categories 4 and 3,

$$p_4 = \frac{n_4}{N} = \frac{4}{32} = 0.1250 \quad \text{and} \quad p_3 = \frac{n_3}{N} = \frac{10}{32} = 0.3125\,.$$

The fourth column (P_j) lists the cumulative proportion of observations in each category for $j = 1, \ldots, k$, e.g., for rank category 3, $P_3 = p_4 + p_3 = 0.1250 + 0.3125 = 0.4375$. The fifth column ($z_j$) lists the standard score that defines the cumulative proportion from the fourth column under the unit-normal distribution for $j = 1, \ldots, k$, e.g., for rank category 4, the standard score that defines the lowest (left tail) of the normal distribution is $z = -1.1503$. The sixth column (Y_{L_j}) lists the height of the ordinate at the standard score listed in the fifth column below the segment in question of the unit-normal distribution for $j = 1, \ldots, k$, e.g., for rank category 3,

$$Y_{L_3} = \frac{\exp(-z^2/2)}{\sqrt{2\pi}} = \frac{\exp[-(-0.1573)^2/2]}{\sqrt{2(3.1416)}} = 0.3940\,.$$

The seventh column (Y_{U_j}) lists the height of the ordinate at the standard score listed in the fifth column above the segment in question of the unit-normal distribution for $j = 1, \ldots, k$, e.g., for rank category 3,

$$Y_{U_3} = \frac{\exp(-z^2/2)}{\sqrt{2\pi}} = \frac{\exp[-(-1.1503)^2/2]}{\sqrt{2(3.1416)}} = 0.2059\,.$$

The last column ($\bar{Z}_j$) in Table 8.29 lists the average standard scores for the k categories for $j = 1, \ldots, k$, e.g., for rank category 4,

$$\bar{Z}_4 = \frac{Y_{L_4} - Y_{U_4}}{p_4} = \frac{0.2059 - 0.0000}{0.1250} = +1.6472\,.$$

The multiserial correlation is the Pearson product-moment correlation between the Y interval-level values given in Table 8.28 and the $\bar{Z}$ values given in Table 8.29. Table 8.30 lists the Y, $\bar{Z}$, Y^2, $\bar{Z}^2$, and $Y\bar{Z}$ values, along with the corresponding sums. For the summations given in Table 8.30, the Pearson product-moment correlation between the Y interval-level values and the transformed $\bar{Z}$ values is

$$r_{Y\bar{Z}} = \frac{N\sum_{i=1}^{N} Y_i\bar{Z}_i - \sum_{i=1}^{N} Y_i \sum_{i=1}^{N} \bar{Z}_i}{\sqrt{\left[N\sum_{i=1}^{N} Y_i^2 - \left(\sum_{i=1}^{N} Y_i\right)^2\right]\left[N\sum_{i=1}^{N} \bar{Z}_i^2 - \left(\sum_{i=1}^{N} \bar{Z}_i\right)^2\right]}}$$

$$= \frac{(32)(189.4757) - (3{,}891)(0.00)}{\sqrt{\left[(32)(478{,}029) - 3{,}891^2\right]\left[(32)(28.1428) - 0.00^2\right]}} = +0.5094\,.$$

Table 8.30 Calculation of the sums needed for the product-moment correlation between variables Y and $\bar{Z}$

Rank	Y	$\bar{Z}$	Y^2	$\bar{Z}^2$	$Y\bar{Z}$
4	136	+1.6472	18,496	2.7133	+224.0192
	131	+1.6472	17,161	2.7133	+215.7832
	126	+1.6472	15,876	2.7133	+207.5472
	116	+1.6472	13,456	2.7133	+191.0752
3	144	+0.6022	20,736	0.3626	+86.7168
	137	+0.6022	18,769	0.3626	+82.5014
	134	+0.6022	17,956	0.3626	+80.6948
	131	+0.6022	17,161	0.3626	+78.8882
	129	+0.6022	16,641	0.3626	+77.6838
	126	+0.6022	15,876	0.3626	+75.8772
	122	+0.6022	14,884	0.3626	+73.4684
	117	+0.6022	13,689	0.3626	+70.4574
	111	+0.6022	12,321	0.3626	+66.8442
	109	+0.6022	11,881	0.3626	+65.6398
2	139	−0.2880	19,321	0.0829	−40.0320
	134	−0.2880	17,956	0.0829	−38.5920
	133	−0.2880	17,689	0.0829	−38.3040
	132	−0.2880	17,424	0.0829	−38.0160
	130	−0.2880	16,900	0.0829	−37.4400
	129	−0.2880	16,641	0.0829	−37.1520
	123	−0.2880	15,129	0.0829	−35.4240
	117	−0.2880	13,689	0.0829	−33.6960
	116	−0.2880	13,456	0.0829	−33.4080
	112	−0.2880	12,544	0.0829	−32.2560
	106	−0.2880	11,236	0.0829	−30.5280
1	128	−1.3487	16,384	1.8190	−172.6336
	111	−1.3487	12,321	1.8190	−149.7057
	104	−1.3487	10,816	1.8190	−140.2648
	103	−1.3487	10,609	1.8190	−138.9161
	103	−1.3487	10,609	1.8190	−138.9161
	101	−1.3487	10,201	1.8190	−136.2187
	101	−1.3487	10,201	1.8190	−136.2187
Sum	3,891	0.0000	478,029	28.1248	+189.4757

Then, the correction for grouping is

$$S_{\bar{Z}} = \left(\frac{1}{N} \sum_{j=1}^{k} n_j \bar{Z}_j^2 \right)^{1/2}$$

$$= \left\{ \frac{1}{32} \Big[(4)(+1.6472)^2 + (10)(+0.6022)^2 + (11)(-0.2880)^2 + (7)(-1.3487)^2 \Big] \right\}^{1/2} = 0.9375$$

and the corrected multiserial correlation coefficient is

$$r_{\mathrm{c}} = \frac{r_{Y\bar{Z}}}{S_{\bar{Z}}} = \frac{+0.5094}{0.9375} = +0.5434 \; .$$

Because there are

$$M = N! = 32! = 263{,}130{,}836{,}933{,}693{,}530{,}167{,}218{,}012{,}160{,}000{,}000 \; ,$$

or in words, 263 million, billion, billion, billion possible arrangements of the observed values, an exact permutation analysis is not possible and a Monte Carlo resampling analysis is mandated. Let r_{o} indicate the observed value of r_c. Then, based on $L = 1{,}000{,}000$ random arrangements of the observed data under the null hypothesis, there are 3,069 $|r_c|$ values equal to or greater than $|r_{\mathrm{o}}| = 0.5434$, yielding a Monte Carlo resampling two-sided probability value of $P = 3{,}069/1{,}000{,}000 = 0.3069 \times 10^{-2}$.

In contrast to the permutation probability value, r_{c} is distributed as Student's t under the null hypothesis with $N - 2$ degrees of freedom. If the population parameter, ρ_{c}, is assumed to be zero, then for the observed data in Table 8.28,

$$t = \frac{r_{\mathrm{c}} - \rho_{\mathrm{c}}}{\sqrt{\dfrac{1 - r_{\mathrm{c}}^2}{N - 2}}} = \frac{+0.5434 - 0.00}{\sqrt{\dfrac{1 - (0.5434)^2}{32 - 2}}} = +3.5455 \; ,$$

and with $N - 2 = 32 - 2 = 30$ degrees of freedom the approximate two-sided probability value of $r_{\mathrm{c}} = +0.5434$ is $P = 0.1308 \times 10^{-2}$.

If r_{c} is converted to a standard score with Fisher's z transform and evaluated with the $N(0, 1)$ distribution, Fisher's z is

$$z = \frac{\tanh^{-1}(r_{\mathrm{c}})}{\sqrt{\dfrac{1}{N - 3}}} = \frac{\tanh^{-1}(+0.5434)}{\sqrt{\dfrac{1}{32 - 3}}} = \frac{+0.6090}{0.1857} = +3.2796$$

yielding an approximate two-sided probability value of $P = 0.1039 \times 10^{-2}$.

8.9 A Generalized Measure of Association

As noted, *vide supra*, and in previous chapters, a common problem in data analysis is the measurement of the degree of association between a nominal independent variable and a dependent variable that may be nominal, ordinal, or interval. Some representative examples are the measured associations between religious affiliation (Catholic, Jewish, Protestant) and voting behavior (Democrat, Republican, Libertarian, Independent), between Sex (Female, Male) and any attitudinal question that is Likert-scaled (Strongly Agree, Agree, Neutral, Disagree, Strongly Disagree), and between marital status (Divorced, Separated, Married, Single, Widowed) and number of work days missed each year $(0, 1, 2, \ldots)$. Additionally, interest may be in the degree of association between a nominal independent variable and a multivariate dependent variable such as a person's position in a three-dimensional matrix defined by occupational prestige, income in dollars, and years of education, where the researcher may not want to suffer the loss of information engendered by compositing the three measurements into a univariate index such as socioeconomic status (SES). In this section a generalized measure of association for nominal independent variables is presented, in which any number and/or combination of nominal, ordinal, or interval dependent variables can be accommodated.

8.9.1 Interval-Level Dependent Variables

Let $\Omega = \{\omega_1, \ldots, \omega_N\}$ indicate a finite collection of N subjects, let $\mathbf{x}'_I = [x_{1I}, \ldots, x_{rI}]$ denote a vector of r commensurate interval-level response measurements for subject ω_I for $I = 1, \ldots, N$, and let $S_1, \ldots, S_g$ represent an exhaustive a priori partitioning of the N subjects comprising Ω into g disjoint, categories, where $n_i \geq 2$ is the number of subjects in category S_i, $i = 1, \ldots, g$. In addition, let

$$\Delta_{I,J} = \left[\sum_{k=1}^{r} \left(x_{kI} - x_{kJ} \right)^2 \right]^{v/2}$$

be a symmetric difference function value of the r response measurements associated with subjects ω_I and ω_J, where $v > 0$. If $v = 1$, then $\Delta_{I,J}$ is the ordinary Euclidean distance between response measurements. Let

$$\xi_i = \binom{n_i}{2}^{-1} \sum_{I<J} \Delta_{I,J} \Psi_i(\omega_I) \Psi_i(\omega_J)$$

represent the average between-subject difference for all subjects within category S_i, $i = 1, \ldots, g$, where $\sum_{I<J}$ is the sum over all I and J such that $1 \leq I < J$

$\leq N$, and

$$\Psi_i(\omega_I) = \begin{cases} 1 & \text{if } \omega_I \in S_i \ , \\ 0 & \text{otherwise} \ . \end{cases}$$

Then the average within-category difference, weighted by the number of subjects n_i in category i for $i = 1, \ldots, g$ can be defined as

$$\delta = \sum_{i=1}^{g} C_i \xi_i \ ,$$

where

$$C_i = \frac{n_i}{N} \qquad \text{for } i = 1, \ldots, g \ ,$$

and $\sum_{i=1}^{g} C_i = 1$. The null hypothesis states that equal probabilities are assigned to each of the

$$M = \frac{N!}{\prod_{i=1}^{g} n_i!}$$

possible allocations of the N subjects to the g disjoint categories.

Whenever there are multiple response measurements for each subject, the response variables may possess different units of measurement and must be made commensurate, i.e., rescaled to attain a standardization among the multivariate measurements. Let $\mathbf{y}_I' = [y_{1I}, \ldots, y_{rI}]$ for $i = 1, \ldots, N$ denote N non-commensurate r-dimensional values, where $r \geq 2$. The corresponding N Euclidean commensurate r-dimensional values, $\mathbf{x}_I' = [x_{1I}, \ldots, x_{rI}]$ for $I = 1, \ldots, N$, are given by $x_{jI} = y_{jI}/\phi_j$, where

$$\phi_j = \sum_{I<J} \left| y_{jI} - y_{jJ} \right| \ .$$

As defined, the Euclidean commensurated data have the desired property that

$$\sum_{I<J} \left| x_{jI} - x_{jJ} \right| = 1$$

for $j = 1, \ldots, r$. Euclidean commensuration ensures that the resulting inferences are independent of the units of the individual response measurements and invariant to linear transformations of the response measurements.

If δ_j denotes the jth value among the M possible values of δ, then the expected value of δ under the null hypothesis H_0 is defined by

$$\mathrm{E}\big[\delta|H_0\big] = \mu_\delta = \frac{1}{M}\sum_{j=1}^{M}\delta_j$$

and, since δ reflects differences within the g categories, the within-category measure of association is given by

$$\Re = 1 - \frac{\delta}{\mu_\delta} .$$

$\Re$ is a chance-corrected measure of association, reflecting the amount of association in excess of what would be expected by chance. $\Re$ attains a maximum value of unity when the association between the nominal independent variable and the interval dependent variable(s) is perfect, i.e., dependent variable scores are identical within each of the g categories of the nominal independent variable. $\Re$ attains a value of zero when the association is equal to chance, i.e., $\mathrm{E}[\Re|H_0] = 0$. Like all chance-corrected measures, $\Re$ occasionally will be slightly negative when the association is less than what is expected by chance.

Because $\Re$ is based on a permutation structure, it requires no simplifying assumptions about the underlying population distribution. Finally, $\Re$ is completely data dependent, i.e., all the information on which $\Re$ is based is contained within the available sample(s).

Univariate Example

Consider an example where it is desired to measure the degree of association between Sex (a nominal-level independent variable) and Years of Education (an interval-level dependent variable). Let $N = 22$ subjects, let $g = 2$ disjoint, unordered categories with $n_1 = 10$ Females and $n_2 = 12$ Males, and let $r = 1$ dimension (Education) measured in years. The example univariate data are listed in Table 8.31. The results of the data analysis given in Table 8.31 with $C_i = n_i/N$ for $i = 1, 2$ and $v = 1$ are

$$\xi_1 = 5.6000 , \quad \xi_2 = 5.0152 ,$$

$\delta = 5.2810$, $\mu_\delta = 5.7706$, and

$$\Re = 1 - \frac{\delta}{\mu_\delta} = 1 - \frac{5.2810}{5.7706} = +0.0848 ,$$

indicating approximately 8% agreement above that expected by chance.

Table 8.31 Listing of example data with $N = 22$ subjects classified into $g = 2$ categories of the nominal-level independent variable Sex with $n_1 = 10$ Females and $n_2 = 12$ Males and $r = 1$ dimension of the interval-level dependent variable Education, measured in years

Subject	Sex	Education	Subject	Sex	Education
1	Female	6	1	Male	12
2	Female	8	2	Male	12
3	Female	10	3	Male	16
4	Female	11	4	Male	16
5	Female	13	5	Male	16
6	Female	16	6	Male	18
7	Female	17	7	Male	18
8	Female	17	8	Male	21
9	Female	18	9	Male	22
10	Female	20	10	Male	22
			11	Male	22
			12	Male	26

As $\Re$ is a simple linear transformation of δ, a test of significance for δ is also a test of significance for $\Re$. Thus, the exact probability value for an observed value of δ (δ_o) is the probability, under the null hypothesis, given by $P(\delta \leq \delta_o|H_0)$. Under the null hypothesis, each of the M possible arrangements of the N subjects over the g categories of the nominal independent variable is equally probable with n_i fixed, $i = 1, \ldots, g$. The exact probability value of the observed value of $\Re$ is the proportion of M possible values of $\Re$ equal to or greater than the observed value of $\Re$ ($\Re_o$), i.e.,

$$P(\Re \geq \Re_o|H_0) = \frac{\text{number of } \Re \text{ values } \geq \Re_o}{M}$$

or, equivalently, the proportion of δ values equal to or less than the observed value of δ (δ_o), i.e.,

$$P(\delta \leq \delta_o|H_0) = \frac{\text{number of } \delta \text{ values } \leq \delta_o}{M} .$$

There are only

$$M = \frac{N!}{\displaystyle\prod_{i=1}^{g} n_i!} = \frac{22!}{10!\ 12!} = 646{,}646$$

possible, equally-likely arrangements in the reference set of all permutations of the observed univariate, interval-level data, making an exact permutation analysis possible. If all M arrangements of the observed data occur with equal chance, the exact probability value of $\Re_o = +0.0840$ computed on the $M = 646{,}646$ possible arrangements of the observed data with $n_1 = 10$ and $n_2 = 12$ preserved for each arrangement is

$$P(\Re \geq \Re_o | H_0) = \frac{\text{number of } \Re \text{ values } \geq \Re_o}{M} = \frac{26{,}024}{646{,}646} = 0.0402 \,.$$

Multivariate Example

Consider a second example where it is desired to measure the degree of association between Sex (a nominal-level independent variable) and scores on three dimensions of the Semantic Differential (interval-level dependent variables). Let $N = 15$ subjects, let $g = 2$ disjoint, unordered categories with $n_1 = 8$ Females and $n_2 = 7$ Males, and let $r = 3$ dimensions of the Semantic Differential: Evaluative, Potency, and Activity. The example multivariate data are listed in Table 8.32. The results of the analysis of the data given in Table 8.32 with $C_i = n_i/N$ for $i = 1, 2$ and $v = 1$ are

$$\xi_1 = 8.9158\times10^{-3} \,, \quad \xi_2 = 5.9435\times10^{-3} \,,$$

$\delta_o = 7.5287\times10^{-3}$, $\mu_\delta = 1.7259\times10^{-2}$, and

$$\Re_o = 1 - \frac{\delta_o}{\mu_\delta} = 1 - \frac{7.5287\times10^{-3}}{1.7259\times10^{-2}} = +0.5638 \,,$$

indicating approximately 56% agreement above that expected by chance.

Table 8.32 Listing of example data with $N = 15$ subjects classified into $g = 2$ categories of the nominal-level independent variable Sex with $n_1 = 8$ Females and $n_2 = 7$ Males and $r = 3$ dimensions of the interval-level dependent variable Semantic Differential: Evaluative, Potency, and Activity

		Semantic Differential		
Subject	Sex	Evaluative	Potency	Activity
1	Female	4.5	5.5	3.9
2	Female	2.4	6.0	2.7
3	Female	2.7	5.8	3.8
4	Female	3.6	6.5	4.5
5	Female	4.3	5.6	4.0
6	Female	2.5	5.9	2.8
7	Female	2.8	5.7	4.0
8	Female	3.5	6.4	4.4
9	Male	6.4	3.5	6.1
10	Male	5.6	4.2	5.5
11	Male	5.2	3.1	5.6
12	Male	6.2	3.6	6.0
13	Male	5.7	4.3	5.7
14	Male	5.2	3.0	5.8
15	Male	6.1	3.6	6.2

There are only

$$M = \frac{N!}{\prod_{i=1}^{g} n_i!} = \frac{15!}{8!\ 7!} = 6{,}435$$

possible, equally-likely arrangements in the reference set of all permutations of the observed multivariate, interval-level data, making an exact permutation analysis possible. If all M arrangements of the observed data occur with equal chance, the exact probability value of $\Re_{\text{o}} = +0.5638$ computed on the $M = 6{,}435$ possible arrangements of the observed data with $n_1 = 8$ and $n_2 = 7$ preserved for each arrangement is

$$P(\Re \geq \Re_{\text{o}}|H_0) = \frac{\text{number of } \Re \text{ values } \geq \Re_{\text{o}}}{M} = \frac{1}{6{,}435} = 0.1554 \times 10^{-3}\ .$$

8.9.2 Ordinal-Level Dependent Variables

Researchers are often faced with the problem of measuring the degree of association between a nominal-level independent variable and one or more ordinal-level dependent variables. Three measures of association have been advanced specifically for a nominal-level independent variable and a single ordinal-level dependent variable: Cureton's rank-biserial (r_{rb}) correlation coefficient [14, 15], Freeman's θ_{ON} [20], and Crittenden and Montgomery's ν [13], which is simply a modification of Freeman's θ_{ON} to ensure a proportional-reduction-in-error interpretation. None of these measures has gained much popularity in the research literature. Cureton's rank-biserial correlation coefficient is defined only for a dichotomous nominal-level variable; consequently, its utility is limited. As the sampling distributions of both θ_{ON} and ν are unknown, the development of corresponding tests of significance has not been possible. In addition, as these three measures are all Kendall-type coefficients, they are based on unweighted agreements and inversions of pairwise differences between scores. Because the scoring system codes any pairwise difference simply as the sign of the difference and ignores the magnitude of the difference, a substantial amount of information is lost in the process of measuring the association [63].

Although the focus of this section is on measuring the association between a nominal-level independent variable and ordinal-level dependent variables, it should be noted that Hubert has defined θ_{NO}, a modification of Freeman's θ_{ON} for an ordinal-level independent variable and a nominal-level dependent variable [34]. Again, the sampling distribution remains unknown. In addition, a symmetric version of Freeman's θ_{ON} has been independently proposed by Agresti [1], Crittenden and Montgomery [13], Hubert [34], and Särndal [67], which they termed $\hat{\delta}$, I

(Iota), θ_{SYM}, and κ, respectively. Agresti also developed the asymptotic sampling distribution of $\hat{\delta}$ [1].

$\Re$ is directly applicable, without modification, to a nominal-level independent variable and any number of ordinal-level dependent variables. Ordinal variables, in this context, include the range of dependent variables from (1) fully ranked data wherein each subject is assigned a unique rank from 1 to N based on the conversion of original interval-level scores to ranks, to (2) having N subjects associated with a limited number of ordinal categories, i.e., $N > g$. The second case differs from the first in that an investigator does not have original interval-level data to convert to ranks, but encounters only a crude ordering of the subjects into categories, such as Low, Medium, and High, in the data collection process. In such a case, a simple assignment of ordered values, such as 1, 2, and 3, to low, medium, and high, respectively, may be used, rather than the assigned values associated with tied ranks.

Univariate Example

Consider an example where it desired to measure the degree of association between three competing Schools (a nominal-level independent variable) and Placement at the finish of a race over 1,500 meters (an ordinal-level dependent variable). Let $N = 18$ runners, let $g = 3$ disjoint, unordered categories with $n_1 = 6$ competitors from Eton, $n_2 = 8$ competitors from Harrow, and $n_3 = 4$ competitors from Winchester, and let $r = 1$ dimension of the ordinal dependent variable, Placement at the finish of the race. The example univariate data are listed in Table 8.33. The results of the analysis of the data given in Table 8.33 with $C_i = n_i/N$ for $i = 1, 2, 3$ and $v = 1$ are

$$\xi_1 = 3.5333\ , \quad \xi_2 = 5.3571\ , \quad \xi_3 = 7.0000\ ,$$

$\delta_{\text{o}} = 5.1143$, $\mu_\delta = 6.5425$, and

$$\Re_{\text{o}} = 1 - \frac{\delta_{\text{o}}}{\mu_\delta} = 1 - \frac{5.1143}{6.5425} = +0.2183\ ,$$

indicating approximately 22% agreement above that expected by chance.

Table 8.33 Listing of example data with $N = 18$ runners from $g = 3$ Schools with $n_1 = 6$, $n_2 = 8$, $n_3 = 4$ and $r = 1$ dependent variable: Placement at the finish of the race

Eton	Harrow	Winchester
10	1	3
13	2	6
15	4	9
16	5	16
17	7	
18	8	
	11	
	14	

There are only

$$M = \frac{N!}{\prod_{i=1}^{g} n_i!} = \frac{18!}{6!\ 8!\ 4!} = 9{,}189{,}180$$

possible, equally-likely arrangements in the reference set of all permutations of the observed univariate, ordinal-level data, making an exact permutation analysis possible. If all M arrangements of the observed data occur with equal chance, the exact probability value of $\mathfrak{R}_o = +0.2183$ computed on the $M = 9{,}189{,}180$ possible arrangements of the observed data with $n_1 = 6$, $n_2 = 8$, and $n_3 = 4$ preserved for each arrangement is

$$P(\mathfrak{R} \geq \mathfrak{R}_o | H_0) = \frac{\text{number of } \mathfrak{R} \text{ values } \geq \mathfrak{R}_o}{M} = \frac{192{,}034}{9{,}189{,}180} = 0.0209\ .$$

Multivariate Example

Consider a second example where it is desired to measure the degree of association between Political Affiliation (a nominal-level independent variable) and scores on two dimensions of Socioeconomic Status (ordinal-level dependent variables). Let $N = 20$ subjects, let $g = 2$ disjoint, unordered categories with $n_1 = 8$ Democrats and $n_2 = 12$ Republicans, and let $r = 2$ dependent variables where one variable is Years of Education and the other variable is Occupational Prestige, both measured in quintiles. The example multivariate data are listed in Table 8.34. The results of the analysis of the data given in Table 8.34 with $C_i = n_i/N$ for $i = 1, 2$ and $v = 1$ are

$$\xi_1 = 7.9204 \times 10^{-3}\ , \quad \xi_2 = 4.7916 \times 10^{-3}\ ,$$

$\delta_o = 6.0431 \times 10^{-3}$, $\mu_\delta = 8.3422 \times 10^{-3}$ and

$$\mathfrak{R}_o = 1 - \frac{\delta_o}{\mu_\delta} = 1 - \frac{6.0431 \times 10^{-3}}{8.3422 \times 10^{-3}} = +0.2756\ ,$$

indicating approximately 28% agreement above that expected by chance.

There are only

$$M = \frac{N!}{\prod_{i=1}^{g} n_i!} = \frac{20!}{8!\ 12!} = 125{,}970$$

Table 8.34 Listing of example data with $N = 20$ subjects classified into $g = 2$ categories of the nominal-level independent variable Political Affiliation with $n_1 = 8$ Democrats and $n_2 = 12$ Republicans and $r = 2$ dimensions of the ordinal-level dependent variable Socioeconomic Status: Education, and Prestige

		Socioeconomic Status	
Subject	Political Affiliation	Education	Prestige
1	Democrat	5	3
2	Democrat	4	5
3	Democrat	5	4
4	Democrat	2	3
5	Democrat	2	5
6	Democrat	3	4
7	Democrat	4	2
8	Democrat	2	4
9	Republican	2	1
10	Republican	2	1
11	Republican	1	2
12	Republican	3	1
13	Republican	1	2
14	Republican	2	1
15	Republican	1	2
16	Republican	1	1
17	Republican	3	1
18	Republican	1	2
19	Republican	2	3
20	Republican	3	2

possible, equally-likely arrangements in the reference set of all permutations of the observed multivariate, ordinal-level data, making an exact permutation analysis possible. If all M arrangements of the observed data occur with equal chance, the exact probability value of $\Re_o = +0.2756$ computed on the $M = 125{,}970$ possible arrangements of the observed data with $n_1 = 8$ and $n_2 = 12$ preserved for each arrangement is

$$P(\Re \geq \Re_o | H_0) = \frac{\text{number of } \Re \text{ values } \geq \Re_o}{M} = \frac{2}{125{,}970} = 0.1588 \times 10^{-4} .$$

8.9.3 Nominal-Level Dependent Variables

While nominal-nominal measures of association would ordinarily be outside the purview of this chapter, $\Re$ is such a versatile measure of association, not only in terms of levels of measurement but also in terms of multiple dependent variables, that a brief example is included illustrating nominal-level dependent variables. $\Re$ is easily adapted to measure the degree of association between a nominal-level independent variable and a nominal-level dependent variable.

If the categories of the dependent variable are considered as r dimensions of that variable, then each subject can be assigned a binary vector of length r with $r - 1$ values of 0 and a single value of 1 corresponding to the category of the dependent variable in which the subject is classified, e.g., for four categories labeled "A," "B," "C," and "D" and a subject who is classified into category "C," $\mathbf{x}' = [\,0\,0\,1\,0\,]$.

An alternative form of nominal-level data is the result of a question where the subject is asked to "Check all categories that apply" [6]. In this case, a vector is constructed in which a value of 1 is assigned to each checked category and a 0 is assigned to each unchecked category, e.g., for four categories labeled "A,' "B," "C," and "D" and a subject who has checked "A" and "C," $\mathbf{x}' = [\,1\,0\,1\,0\,]$ [5, 6].

Univariate Example

Consider an example where it is desired to measure the degree of association between rural/urban Residence (a nominal-level independent variable) and Marital Status (a nominal-level dependent variable). Let $N = 24$ subjects, let $g = 2$ disjoint categories with $n_1 = 10$ Rural residents and $n_2 = 14$ Urban residents, and let $r = 4$ dimensions of Marital Status: Divorced, Married, Single, and Widowed. The example univariate data are listed in Table 8.35. The results of the analysis of the data given in Table 8.35 with $C_i = n_i/N$ for $i = 1, 2$ and $v = 1$ are

$$\xi_1 = 4.9841\times10^{-3}\ , \quad \xi_2 = 1.1814\times10^{-2}\ ,$$

$\delta_o = 8.9683\times10^{-3}$, $\mu_\delta = 1.0445\times10^{-2}$, and

$$\Re_o = 1 - \frac{\delta_o}{\mu_\delta} = 1 - \frac{8.9683\times10^{-3}}{1.0445\times10^{-2}} = +0.1414\ ,$$

indicating approximately 14% agreement above that expected by chance.

There are only

$$M = \frac{N!}{\displaystyle\prod_{i=1}^{g} n_i!} = \frac{24!}{10!\ 14!} = 1{,}961{,}256$$

possible, equally-likely arrangements in the reference set of all permutations of the observed nominal-level data, making an exact permutation analysis possible. If all M arrangements of the observed data occur with equal chance, the exact probability value of $\Re_o = +0.1414$ computed on the M possible arrangements of the observed data with $n_1 = 10$ and $n_2 = 14$ preserved for each arrangement is

$$P(\Re \geq \Re_o|H_0) = \frac{\text{number of } \Re \text{ values } \geq \Re_o}{M} = \frac{7{,}192}{1{,}961{,}256} = 0.3667\times10^{-2}\ .$$

Table 8.35 Listing of example data with $N = 24$ subjects classified into $g = 2$ categories of the nominal-level independent variable Rural/Urban Residence with $n_1 = 10$ Rural residents and $n_2 = 14$ Urban residents and $r = 4$ dimensions of the ordinal-level dependent variable Marital Status: Single, Married, Widowed, and Divorced

		Marital Status			
Subject	Residence	Single	Married	Widowed	Divorced
1	Rural	0	0	0	1
2	Rural	0	1	0	0
3	Rural	0	1	0	0
4	Rural	0	1	0	0
5	Rural	0	1	0	0
6	Rural	0	1	0	0
7	Rural	0	1	0	0
8	Rural	0	1	0	0
9	Rural	0	1	0	0
10	Rural	1	0	0	0
11	Urban	0	0	0	1
12	Urban	0	0	0	1
13	Urban	0	0	0	1
14	Urban	0	1	0	0
15	Urban	0	1	0	0
16	Urban	1	0	0	0
17	Urban	1	0	0	0
18	Urban	1	0	0	0
19	Urban	1	0	0	0
20	Urban	1	0	0	0
21	Urban	0	0	1	0
22	Urban	0	0	1	0
23	Urban	0	0	1	0
24	Urban	0	0	1	0

8.9.4 Mixed Dependent Variables

A distinctive advantage of the permutation approach to measuring association is the ability to analyze sets of dependent variables that are mixed: nominal-, ordinal-, and/or interval-level. Each interval-level or ordinal-level dependent variable contributes one dimension to the analysis and, as explained in Sect. 8.9.3, each nominal-level dependent variable contributes one dimension for each category of the variable.

Multivariate Example

Consider an example where it is desired to measure the degree of association between Religious Affiliation (a nominal-level independent variable) and Birth Experience, measured as a mixture of three dependent variables: one interval-level, one ordinal-level, and one nominal-level. Let $N = 15$ first-time mothers who have recently given birth, let $g = 3$ disjoint, unordered categories with $n_1 = 4$ Protestant mothers, $n_2 = 5$ Catholic mothers, and $n_3 = 6$ Jewish mothers. In addition, let $r = 5$ dimensions of the birth experience with Hours in Labor constituting the interval-level dependent variable, Birth Weight (measured as Above-normal, Normal, and Below-normal) constituting the ordinal-level dependent variable, and type of Anesthesia (Local, General, and None) constituting the nominal-level dependent variable. One of the $r = 5$ dimensions represents the interval-level dependent variable, one dimension represents the ordinal-level dependent variable, and three dimensions (one for each category) represent the nominal-level dependent variable. The example multivariate data are listed in Table 8.36. The results of the analysis of the data given in Table 8.36 with $C_i = n_i/N$ for $i = 1, 2, 3$ and $v = 1$ are

$$\xi_1 = 3.0327\times10^{-2}\;, \quad \xi_2 = 2.0490\times10^{-2}\;, \quad \xi_3 = 1.8444\times10^{-2}\;,$$

$\delta_o = 2.2295\times10^{-2}$, $\mu_\delta = 2.8029\times10^{-2}$, and

$$\Re_o = 1 - \frac{\delta_o}{\mu_\delta} = 1 - \frac{2.2295\times10^{-1}}{2.8029\times10^{-2}} = +0.2046\;,$$

indicating approximately 20% agreement above that expected by chance.

There are only

$$M = \frac{N!}{\prod_{i=1}^{g} n_i!} = \frac{15!}{4!\;5!\;6!} = 630{,}630$$

possible, equally-likely arrangements in the reference set of all permutations of the observed multivariate, mixed-level data, making an exact permutation analysis possible. If all M arrangements of the observed data occur with equal chance, the exact probability value of $\Re_o = +0.2046$ computed on the M possible arrangements of the observed data with $n_1 = 4$, $n_2 = 5$, and $n_3 = 6$ preserved for each arrangement is

$$P(\Re \geq \Re_o|H_0) = \frac{\text{number of } \Re \text{ values } \geq \Re_o}{M} = \frac{1{,}792}{630{,}630} = 0.2842\times10^{-2}\;.$$

Table 8.36 Listing of example data with $N = 15$ subjects classified into $g = 3$ categories of the nominal-level independent variable Religion with $n_1 = 4$ Protestant mothers, $n_2 = 5$ Catholic mothers, and $n_3 = 6$ Jewish mothers and $r = 5$ dimensions of the mixed-level dependent variables Hours in Labor, Birth Weight measured as Above-normal (1), Normal (2), and Below-normal (3), and Anesthesia: Local, General, and None

				Anesthesia		
Subject	Religion	Hours of labor	Birth weight	Local	General	None
1	Protestant	20	Below	0	0	1
2	Protestant	15	Below	0	1	0
3	Protestant	10	Normal	0	0	1
4	Protestant	8	Below	0	1	0
5	Catholic	10	Below	0	1	0
6	Catholic	8	Normal	0	1	0
7	Catholic	8	Normal	0	1	0
8	Catholic	6	Above	0	1	0
9	Catholic	5	Above	0	0	1
10	Jewish	12	Below	1	0	0
11	Jewish	10	Normal	1	0	0
12	Jewish	5	Above	0	1	0
13	Jewish	5	Above	1	0	0
14	Jewish	5	Above	1	0	0
15	Jewish	4	Above	1	0	0

8.10 $\Re$ and Existing Statistics

As is the case with any new statistical method, there exist certain relationships between $\Re$ and existing methods. It should be noted that the choice of

$$C_i = \frac{n_i}{N} \qquad \text{for } i = 1, \ldots, g$$

is simply the number of subjects in the ith category of the nominal-level independent variable divided by the total number of subjects. In the subsequent comparisons with existing methods, the maximum likelihood argument based on the normal distribution dictates that

$$C_i = \frac{n_i - 1}{N - g} \qquad \text{for } i = 1, \ldots, g\ .$$

This alternative representation of C_i represents the number of degrees of freedom associated with the ith category of the nominal-level independent variable divided by the total degrees of freedom over all g disjoint categories. In a permutation analysis, degrees of freedom are not relevant, as they are a consequence of fitting parameters in a maximum likelihood context. In addition, it should be noted that

$v = 1$, which is associated with ordinary Euclidean distances, is now replaced with $v = 2$, which also results from the maximum likelihood argument based on the normal distribution. Since the normal distribution assumption is irrelevant to a permutation analysis, the use of $v = 2$ is unjustified. Finally, it should be noted that $\Re$ is a median-based measure of association when $v = 1$, whereas $\Re$ is a mean-based measure of association when $v = 2$.

For clarification, consider the pairwise sum of univariate ($r = 1$) symmetric distance functions given by

$$\sum_{I<J} \Delta_{I,J} = \sum_{I<J} \left| x_I - x_J \right|^v ,$$

where $x_1, \ldots, x_N$ are univariate response variables and $\sum_{I<J}$ is the sum over all I and J such that $1 \leq I < J \leq N$. Let $x_{1,N} \leq \cdots \leq x_{N,N}$ be the order statistics associated with $x_1, \ldots, x_N$. If $v = 1$, then the inequality given by

$$\sum_{I=1}^{N} |N - 2I + 1| \left| x_{I,N} - \theta \right| \geq \sum_{I<J} \left| x_I - x_J \right|$$

holds for all θ and equality holds if θ is the median of $x_1, \ldots, x_N$. If $v = 2$, then the inequality given by

$$N \sum_{I=1}^{N} (x_I - \theta)^2 \geq \sum_{I<J} (x_I - x_J)^2$$

holds for all θ and equality holds if θ is the mean of $x_1, \ldots, x_N$.

8.10.1 Interval-Level Dependent Variable

The permutation version of one-way analysis of variance (ANOVA) is a special case of the permutation method with a single interval-level dependent variable. Specifically,

$$\Re = \frac{(F - 1)(g - 1)}{F(g - 1) + N - g} ,$$

where $r = 1$, $v = 2$, and

$$C_i = \frac{n_i - 1}{N - g} \qquad \text{for } i = 1, \ldots, g .$$

In addition, the putative unbiased correlation ratio ϵ^2 [38] is identical to $\mathfrak{R}$ when $r = 1$, $v = 2$, and $C_i = (n_i - 1)/(N - g)$. Since ϵ^2, in an analysis of variance context, is identical to the shrunken squared correlation coefficient $\hat{r}^2$ [12, p. 188] in a regression context, then $\hat{r}^2$ is also identical to $\mathfrak{R}$. Finally, the permutation version of one-way multivariate analysis of variance (MANOVA) is a special case of the permutation method when $r \geq 2$, $v = 2$,

$$C_i = \frac{n_i - 1}{N - g} \qquad \text{for } i = 1, \ldots, g ,$$

and

$$\Delta_{I,J} = \left[(\mathbf{x}_I - \mathbf{x}_J)' \, \hat{\Sigma}^{-1} (\mathbf{x}_I - \mathbf{x}_j) \right]^{v/2} ,$$

where $\hat{\Sigma}$ denotes the $r \times r$ variance-covariance matrix [53].

8.10.2 Ordinal-Level Dependent Variable

In the discussion in Sect. 8.10.1 pertaining to an interval-level dependent variable, Kelley's ϵ^2 can be associated with a squared correlation coefficient involving the Kruskal–Wallis test, where the rank-order statistics replace the interval-level observations in the one-way analysis of variance. However, the requirement of a complete ordering of all subjects from 1 to N precludes its use in many applications. Consequently, the more general statistic, $\mathfrak{R}$, which is applicable to either fully ranked or partially ranked observations, is potentially more useful. In addition, since the Kruskal–Wallis test is the rank-order analog of one-way ANOVA, then the rank-order analog of one-way MANOVA is attained by substitution.

8.10.3 Nominal-Level Dependent Variable

If

$$C_i = \frac{n_i - 1}{N - g} \qquad \text{for } i = 1, \ldots, g ,$$

then

$$\mathfrak{R} = \frac{N - 1}{N - g} \left(t_a - \frac{g - 1}{N - 1} \right) ,$$

where t_a is Goodman and Kruskal's test statistic associated with g categories of a nominal-level independent variable (B) and r categories of a nominal-level dependent variable (A) [4].

8.11 Coda

Chapter 8 examined exact and Monte Carlo resampling permutation statistical methods applied to measures of association for two variables at different levels of measurement, e.g., a nominal-level variable and an ordinal-level or interval-level variable, and an ordinal-level variable and an interval-level variable. Included in Chap. 8 were discussions of Freeman's θ, Agresti's $\hat{\delta}$, and Piccarreta's $\hat{\tau}$ measures of association for a nominal-level independent variable and an ordinal-level dependent variable. Two special cases for a dichotomous nominal-level variable and an ordinal-level variable were also considered: Whitfield's S and Cureton's r_{rb} measures. Pearson's η^2, Kelley's ϵ^2, and Hays' $\hat{\omega}^2$ measures of association for a nominal-level variable and an interval-level variable were described. Two special cases for a dichotomous nominal-level variable and an interval-level variable were also considered: point-biserial and biserial correlation.

Also included in Chap. 8 was a discussion of Jaspen's multiserial correlation for an ordinal-level variable and an interval-level variable. Chapter 8 concluded with a discussion of a generalized chance-corrected measure of association suitable for a nominal-level independent variable and a nominal-level dependent variable, a nominal-level independent variable and an ordinal-level dependent variable, a nominal-level independent variable and an interval-level dependent variable, and a nominal-level independent variable and any multivariate combination of nominal-, ordinal-, and interval-level dependent variables.

Chapter 9 describes exact and Monte Carlo permutation statistical methods applied to measures of association either specifically designed for or applied to 2×2 contingency tables. Included in Chap. 9 are discussions of permutation statistical methods for Pearson's ϕ^2, Pearson's tetrachoric correlation, Yule's Q and Yule's Y measures, the odds ratio, Goodman and Kruskal's t_a and t_b asymmetric measures, Somers' d_{yx} and d_{xy} asymmetric measures, simple percentage differences, and Kendall's τ_b measure of association.

References

1. Agresti, A.: Measures of nominal-ordinal association. J. Am. Stat. Assoc. **76**, 524–529 (1981)
2. Anderson-Sprecher, R.: Model comparisons and R^2. Am. Stat. **48**, 113–117 (1994)
3. Berry, K.J., Johnston, J.E., Mielke, P.W.: Nominal-ordinal measures of association: A comparison of two measures. Percept. Motor Skill **109**, 285–294 (2009)
4. Berry, K.J., Mielke, P.W.: An APL function for Radlow and Alf's exact chi-square test. Beh. Res. Meth. Ins. C **17**, 131–132 (1985)

5. Berry, K.J., Mielke, P.W.: Longitudinal analysis of data with multiple binary category choices. Psychol. Rep. **93**, 127–131 (2003)
6. Berry, K.J., Mielke, P.W.: Permutation analysis of data with multiple binary category choices. Psychol. Rep. **92**, 91–98 (2003)
7. Berry, K.J., Mielke, P.W., Johnston, J.E.: Permutation Statistical Methods: An Integrated Approach. Springer–Verlag, Cham, CH (2016)
8. Blaug, M.: The myth of the old Poor Law and the making of the new. J. Econ. Hist. **23**, 151–184 (1963)
9. Box, G.E.P.: Some theorems on quadratic forms applied in the study of analysis of variance problems, I. Effect of inequality of variance in the one-way classification. Ann. Math. Stat. **25**, 290–302 (1954)
10. Bross, I.D.J.: How to use ridit analysis. Biometrics **14**, 18–38 (1958)
11. Carroll, R.M., Nordholm, L.A.: Sampling characteristics of Kelley's ϵ^2 and Hays' $\hat{\omega}^2$. Educ. Psychol. Meas. **35**, 541–554 (1975)
12. Cohen, J., Cohen, P.: Applied Multiple Regression/Correlation Analysis for the Behavioral Sciences. Erlbaum, Hillsdale, NJ (1975)
13. Crittenden, K.S., Montgomery, A.C.: A system of paired asymmetric measures of association for use with ordinal dependent variables. Social Forces **58**, 1178–1194 (1980)
14. Cureton, E.E.: Rank-biserial correlation. Psychometrika **21**, 287–290 (1956)
15. Cureton, E.E.: Rank-biserial correlation when ties are present. Educ. Psychol. Meas. **28**, 77–79 (1968)
16. D'Andrade, R., Dart, J.: The interpretation of r versus r^2 or why percent of variance accounted for is a poor measure of size of effect. J. Quant. Anthro. **2**, 47–59 (1990)
17. Draper, N.R.: The Box–Wetz criterion versus R^2. J. R. Stat. Soc. A Gen. **147**, 100–103 (1984)
18. Ezekiel, M.J.B.: Methods of Correlation Analysis. Wiley, New York (1930)
19. Fisher, R.A.: Statistical Methods for Research Workers. Oliver and Boyd, Edinburgh (1925)
20. Freeman, L.C.: Elementary Applied Statistics. Wiley, New York (1965)
21. Friedman, H.: Magnitude of experimental effect and a table for its rapid estimation. Psychol. Bull. **70**, 245–251 (1968)
22. Friedman, M.: A comparison of alternative tests of significance for the problem of m rankings. Ann. Math. Stat. **11**, 86–92 (1940)
23. Glass, G.V., Peckham, P.D., Sanders, J.R.: Consequences of failure to meet assumptions underlying the fixed effects analysis of variance and covariance. Rev. Educ. Res. **42**, 237–288 (1972)
24. Goodman, L.A., Kruskal, W.H.: Measures of association for cross classifications. J. Am. Stat. Assoc. **49**, 732–764 (1954)
25. Gronow, D.G.C.: Non-normality in two-sample t-tests. Biometrika **40**, 222–225 (1953)
26. Hahn, G.J.: The coefficient of determination exposed! Chem. Tech. **3**, 609–612 (1973)
27. Harwell, M.R., Rubinstein, E.N., Hayes, W.S., Olds, C.C.: Summarizing Monte Carlo results in methodological research: The one- and two-factor fixed effects ANOVA cases. J. Educ. Stat. **17**, 315–339 (1992)
28. Hays, W.L.: Statistics. Holt, Rinehart and Winston, New York (1963)
29. Healy, M.J.R.: The use of R^2 as a measure of goodness of fit. J. R. Stat. Soc. A Gen. **147**, 608–609 (1984)
30. Hildebrand, D.K., Laing, J.D., Rosenthal, H.: Prediction Analysis of Cross Classifications. Wiley, New York (1977)
31. Horsnell, G.: The effect of unequal group variances on the F-test for the homogeneity of group means. Biometrika **40**, 128–136 (1953)
32. Howell, D.C.: Statistical Methods for Psychology, 8th edn. Wadsworth, Belmont, CA (2013)
33. Hsu, P.L.: Contributions to the theory of "Student's" t-test as applied to the problem of two samples. Stat. Res. Mem. **2**, 1–24 (1938)
34. Hubert, L.J.: A note on Freeman's measure of association for relating an ordered to an unordered factor. Psychometrika **39**, 517–520 (1974)

35. Jacobson, P.E.: Applying measures of association to nominal-ordinal data. Pacific. Soc. Rev. **15**, 41–60 (1972)
36. Jaspen, N.: Serial correlation. Psychometrika **11**, 23–30 (1946)
37. Johnston, J.E., Berry, K.J., Mielke, P.W.: A measure of effect size for experimental designs with heterogeneous variances. Percept. Motor Skill **98**, 3–18 (2004)
38. Kelley, T.L.: An unbiased correlation ratio measure. Proc. Natl. Acad. Sci. **21**, 554–559 (1935)
39. Kendall, M.G.: A new measure of rank correlation. Biometrika **30**, 81–93 (1938)
40. Kendall, M.G.: The treatment of ties in ranking problems. Biometrika **33**, 239–251 (1945)
41. Kendall, M.G.: Rank Correlation Methods. Griffin, London (1948)
42. Kenny, D.A.: Statistics for the Social and Behavioral Sciences. Little, Brown, Boston (1987)
43. Kirk, R.E.: Practical significance: A concept whose time has come. Educ. Psychol. Meas. **56**, 746–759 (1996)
44. Kline, R.B.: Beyond Significance Testing: Reforming Data Analysis Methods in Behavioral Research. American Psychological Association, Washington, DC (2004)
45. Kvålseth, T.O.: Cautionary note about R^2. Am. Stat. **39**, 279–285 (1985)
46. Larson, S.C.: The shrinkage of the coefficient of multiple correlation. J. Educ. Psychol. **22**, 45–55 (1931)
47. Leik, R.K., Gove, W.R.: Integrated approach to measuring association. In: Costner, H.L. (ed.) Sociological Methodology, pp. 279–301. Jossey Bass, San Francisco, CA (1971)
48. Levine, T.R., Hullett, C.R.: Eta squared, partial eta squared, and misreporting of effect size in communication research. Hum. Commun. Res. **28**, 612–625 (2002)
49. Mann, H.B., Whitney, D.R.: On a test of whether one of two random variables is stochastically larger than the other. Ann. Math. Stat. **18**, 50–60 (1947)
50. Maravelakis, P.E., Perakis, M., Psarakis, S., Panaretos, J.: The use of indices in surveys. Qual. Quant. **37**, 1–19 (2003)
51. Maxim, P.S.: Quantitative Research Methods in the Social Sciences. Oxford, New York (1999)
52. Maxwell, S.E., Camp, C.J., Arvey, R.D.: Measures of strength of association: A comparative examination. J. Appl. Psychol. **66**, 525–534 (1981)
53. Mielke, P.W.: The application of multivariate permutation methods based on distance functions in the earth sciences. Earth Sci. Rev. **31**, 55–71 (1991)
54. Mitchell, C., Hartmann, D.P.: A cautionary note on the use of omega squared to evaluate the effectiveness of behavioral treatments. Behav. Assess. **3**, 93–100 (1981)
55. Murray, L.W., Dosser, D.A.: How significant is a significant difference? Problems with the measurement of magnitude of effect. J. Counsel. Psych. **34**, 68–72 (1987)
56. Nunnally, J.C.: Psychometric Theory, 2nd edn. McGraw–Hill, New York (1978)
57. Ozer, D.J.: Correlation and the coefficient of determination. Psych. Bull. **97**, 307–315 (1985)
58. Pearson, K.: On a correction needful in the case of the correlation ratio. Biometrika **8**, 254–256 (1911)
59. Pearson, K.: On the correction necessary for the correlation ratio η. Biometrika **14**, 412–417 (1923)
60. Pedhazur, E.J.: Multiple Regression in Behavioral Research: Explanation and Prediction, 3rd edn. Harcourt, Fort Worth, TX (1997)
61. Perakis, M., Maravelakis, P.E., Psarakis, S., Xekalaki, E., Panaretos, J.: On certain indices for ordinal data with unequally weighted classes. Qual. Quant. **39**, 515–536 (2005)
62. Piccarreta, R.: A new measure of nominal-ordinal association. J. Appl. Stat. **28**, 107–120 (2001)
63. Reynolds, H.T.: The Analysis of Cross-Classifications. Free Press, New York (1977)
64. Roberts, J.K., Henson, R.K.: Correcting for bias in estimating effect sizes. Educ. Psychol. Meas. **62**, 241–253 (2002)
65. Rosenthal, R., Rubin, D.B.: A note on percent variance explained as a measure of the importance of effects. J. Appl. Soc. Psych. **9**, 395–396 (1979)
66. Rosenthal, R., Rubin, D.B.: A simple, general purpose display of magnitude of experimental effect. J. Educ. Psych. **74**, 166–169 (1982)

67. Särndal, C.E.: A comparative study of association measures. Psychometrika **39**, 165–187 (1974)
68. Snyder, P., Lawson, S.: Evaluating results using corrected and uncorrected effect size estimates. J. Exp. Educ. **61**, 334–349 (1993)
69. Somers, R.H.: A new asymmetric measure of association for ordinal variables. Am. Sociol. Rev. **27**, 799–811 (1962)
70. Strube, M.J.: Some comments on the use of magnitude-of-effect estimates. J. Counsel. Psych. **35**, 342–345 (1988)
71. Wherry, R.J.: A new formula for predicting the shrinkage of the coefficient of multiple correlation. Ann. Math. Stat. **2**, 440–457 (1931)
72. Whitfield, J.W.: Rank correlation between two variables, one of which is ranked, the other dichotomous. Biometrika **34**, 292–296 (1947)
73. Wilcoxon, F.: Individual comparisons by ranking methods. Biometrics Bull. **1**, 80–83 (1945)
74. Willett, J.B., Singer, J.D.: Another cautionary note about R^2: Its use in weighted least squares regression analysis. Am. Stat. **42**, 236–238 (1988)

Chapter 9
Fourfold Contingency Tables, I

The statistical analysis of fourfold (2×2) contingency tables is so prevalent in the current research literature, in such a wide variety of disciplines, that this chapter is devoted entirely to the application of exact and Monte Carlo permutation statistical methods to 2×2 contingency tables. A subclass of 2×2 contingency tables is comprised of symmetrical 2×2 tables, where each marginal frequency total is equal to $N/2$. The application of permutation statistical methods to symmetrical 2×2 contingency tables is reserved for Chap. 10.

The study of 2×2 contingency tables has a long and controversial history. As far back as 1961, R.G. Francis published an entire book subtitled *A Methodological Discussion of the Two-by-Two Table* [21][1] and as early as 1963 A.W.F. Edwards, writing on measures of association for 2×2 contingency tables, commented that "the literature on the interpretation of the 2×2 contingency table is voluminous" [15, p. 109]. While 2×2 tables appear deceptively simple and uncomplicated at first consideration, the analysis of 2×2 contingency tables is fraught with controversy and has been for over a century. Indeed, so much so that in 2012 Stephen Senn wryly observed in a bit of hyperbole that "statisticians have caused the destruction of whole forests to provide paper to print their disputes regarding the analysis of 2×2 tables" [49, p. 33].

Part of the problem is that there is a plethora of different measures or, as Kraemer et al. put it "there are *just too many* measures of 2×2 association" [36, p. 259].[2] Another part of the problem is the lack of consistency among the various measures. Finally, the various measures are scaled differently when applied to 2×2 contingency tables. Some measures of 2×2 association range between −1 and +1,

[1]The full title of the book by Francis was *The Rhetoric of Science: A Methodological Discussion of the Two-by-Two Table*.

[2]Emphasis added.

K. J. Berry et al., *The Measurement of Association*,
https://doi.org/10.1007/978-3-319-98926-6_9

such as Pearson's ϕ and Goodman and Kruskal's γ.[3] Some measures range between 0 and 1, such as Goodman and Kruskal's t_a and t_b. Some measures range between 0 and infinity, such as the odds ratio. Some measures range from 0 to a value that is indeterminate, but is usually less than 1, such as Tschuprov's T^2 and Cramér's V^2. And some measures are chance-corrected, ranging from a slightly negative value when the association is less than expected by chance to +1, such as Cohen's κ measure of inter-rater agreement.

Several statistical measures of association were specifically developed for the analysis of 2×2 contingency tables, e.g., Yule's Q and Y measures of nominal-level association, while other statistics were designed for larger contingency tables, but often take on new meaning when applied to 2×2 tables, e.g., Somers' d_{yx} and d_{xy} measures of ordinal association. In this chapter both types of statistical measures are considered. However, this approach necessitates some overlap and redundancy with measures of association presented in previous chapters. Included in this chapter are applications of permutation statistical methods to Pearson's ϕ coefficient of contingency, Pearson's tetrachoric correlation coefficient, Yule's Q and Yule's Y measures of nominal association, Leik and Gove's d_N^c measure, the odds ratio, Goodman and Kruskal's t_a and t_b asymmetric measures of nominal association, Somers' d_{yx} and d_{xy} measures of ordinal association, simple percentage differences, and Kendall's τ_b measure of ordinal association.

9.1 Fourfold Point Association

In 1954 Goodman and Kruskal argued that a researcher should choose a measure of association that is conceptually meaningful for a particular analysis [23]. Others including Costner [10], Duggan and Dean [13], Francis [21], Kang [29, 30], Kim [35], and Leik and Gove [37] argued that the selected measure of association should represent the form of the hypothesis as well as the degree of association. Unfortunately, the link between the form of the hypothesis and measure of association has largely been neglected [29].

9.1.1 Logical Models of Association

The basic logical models of a hypothesis structure are most easily demonstrated with simple 2×2 contingency tables.[4] Three logical models are represented in Table 9.1

[3]Depending on how Pearson's ϕ is calculated, it may range between −1 and +1 or between 0 and 1.

[4]Kang [29, 30] demonstrated the logical models of hypotheses structures with 3×3 contingency tables.

Table 9.1 Three 2×2 contingency tables illustrating (1) a necessary and sufficient logical form, (2) a necessary but not sufficient logical form, and (3) a sufficient but not-necessary logical form

Table 1 (N/S)			Table 2 $(N/\bar{S})$			Table 3 $(\bar{N}/S)$		
	A	$\bar{A}$		A	$\bar{A}$		A	$\bar{A}$
B	ab	0	B	ab	0	B	ab	$\bar{a}b$
$\bar{B}$	0	$\bar{a}\bar{b}$	$\bar{B}$	$a\bar{b}$	$\bar{a}\bar{b}$	$\bar{B}$	0	$\bar{a}\bar{b}$

where:

A denotes the presence of independent variable A,
$\bar{A}$ denotes the non-presence of independent variable A,
B denotes the presence of dependent variable B,
$\bar{B}$ denotes the non-presence of dependent variable B,
ab denotes the proportion of cases in the joint category AB,
$\bar{a}b$ denotes the proportion of cases in the joint category $\bar{A}B$,
$a\bar{b}$ denotes the proportion of cases in the joint category $A\bar{B}$, and
$\bar{a}\bar{b}$ denotes the proportion of cases in the joint category $\bar{A}\bar{B}$.

For Table 1 in Table 9.1, A is both a necessary and sufficient condition for B $(A \Longleftrightarrow B)$. Thus, $\bar{a}b = a\bar{b} = 0$, i.e., B if and only if A. For Table 2 in Table 9.1, A is a necessary but not sufficient condition of B $(B \Longrightarrow A)$. Thus, $\bar{a}b = 0$, i.e., A must be present, but B need not always follow from A. For Table 3 in Table 9.1, A is a sufficient but not-necessary condition for B $(A \Longrightarrow B)$. Thus, $a\bar{b} = 0$, i.e., if A, then B; whenever A is present, B must follow, but B may also occur when A is not present [29, p. 358].

9.1.2 *Fourfold Contingency Tables*

Fourfold contingency tables constitute a special case of proper norming. Noting that Pearson's ϕ fails to norm properly unless marginal sets are identical, in 1959 Cureton proposed a modification that possessed always-attainable limits of ± 1 [12]. An alternative solution was developed by Berry, Martin, and Olson in 1974 that not only permitted ϕ to norm properly between ± 1, but also provided intermediate values possessing operational interpretations [2]. Following the notation of Berry et al., Pearson's fourfold point measure of association is usually calculated from a 2×2 contingency table such as presented in Table 9.2. where A and $\bar{A}$ and B and $\bar{B}$ represent the presence and absence of variables A and B, respectively, p and q

Table 9.2 Notation for a 2×2 contingency table

	A	$\bar{A}$	Total
B	α	β	p
$\bar{B}$	γ	δ	q
Total	p'	q'	

represent row proportions, p' and q' represent column proportions, and α denotes the joint-presence proportion for p and p'. Then

$$\phi = \frac{\alpha - pp'}{\sqrt{pqp'q'}} \tag{9.1}$$

is Pearson's mean-square contingency measure of association between variables A and B, [12, 18, p. 421].[5]

The definition of ϕ in Eq. (9.1) has two weaknesses. First, ϕ varies between the limits of ± 1 if and only if $p = q = p' = q'$ [11, p. 283]. When variables A and B possess the same shape, $p = p'$ or $p = q'$, but are asymmetrical, $p \neq p'$ and $p' \neq q'$, one or the other of the limits, -1 or $+1$, may be attained, but not both [18, p. 422].[6] Second, if the marginal sets are unbalanced, i.e., $p \neq p'$ and $p \neq q'$, ϕ necessarily understates the degree of association present. Consequently, its interpretation is problematic; see discussions by Quinn McNemar [40, p. 198] and Joy Guilford [25, p. 342].

As discussed previously in Chap. 3, Sect. 3.1.1, ϕ may be expressed as a function of Pearson's chi-squared test statistic; for a 2×2 contingency table,

$$\phi = \sqrt{\frac{\chi^2}{N}} , \tag{9.2}$$

where N denotes not only the total number of cases, but also the maximum value of chi-squared for a 2×2 contingency table where $p = p'$ or $p = q'$. Therefore, like Tschuprov's T^2 and Cramér's V^2, Pearson's ϕ may be interpreted as a function of the ratio of an empirically determined chi-squared value to its maximum value, computed under conditions required by a logical model [21, p. 98]. In this case, the logical model requires that $p = p'$ or $p = q'$. It is just this restriction on ϕ that limits its utility as a measure of association. Because $\chi^2 = N$ only when $p = p'$ or $p = q'$, the use of ϕ is appropriate only under the same ideal conditions. However, the maximum value of chi-squared need not be determined only under these ideal conditions, except when the logical model demands it. If the form of the logical model changes, the conditions for the maximum value of chi-squared change and, consequently, the conditions for Pearson's ϕ also change.

If the logical form of the research hypothesis, H_1, posits that A is both a necessary and sufficient condition (N/S) for B, $P\{B|A\} = P\{A|B\} = 1$, then by definition $\beta = \gamma = 0$, $p = p'$ or $p = q'$, and $\chi^2_{\max} = N$. The ϕ coefficient of association is then correctly given by Eq. (9.2). If, however, the logical form of H_1 posits that A is a necessary but not sufficient condition $(N/\bar{S})$ for B, then

[5] Because a 2×2 contingency table has only one degree of freedom, it is sufficient to analyze only one cell; in this case, the cell labeled α.

[6] For a discussion of the importance of shape in analyzing contingency tables, see Nunnally [42, p. 145].

$P\{B|\bar{A}\} = \beta = 0$, $p = \alpha$, and $q' = \delta$. The maximum value of chi-squared for a 2×2 contingency table can be shown to be

$$\chi^2_{\max} = \frac{Npq'}{qp'} \ .$$

Then, since

$$\phi = \sqrt{\frac{\chi^2}{\chi^2_{\max}}} \ , \tag{9.3}$$

substitution into Eq. (9.3) yields

$$\phi' = \frac{\alpha - pp'}{pq'} \ . \tag{9.4}$$

If the logical form specifies that A is a sufficient but not-necessary condition ($\bar{N}/S$) for B, then $P\{\bar{B}|A\} = \gamma = 0$ and

$$\phi' = \frac{\alpha - pp'}{qp'} \ .$$

Under each of the three logical models, N/S, $N/\bar{S}$, and $\bar{N}/S$, ϕ' will norm properly between ± 1, attaining $+1$ when the cell proportions agree with those specified by the logical model implicit in H_1; -1 when the cell proportions are in complete disagreement; and 0 when statistical independence, $\alpha = pp'$, is present. Moreover, intermediate values of ϕ' acquire clear and meaningful interpretations.

To illustrate, assume that H_1 posits that the presence of A is a necessary but not sufficient condition for B, i.e., $P\{B|\bar{A}\} = \beta = 0$. Let the Total variation in the table be measured as the difference between (1) the value of $\alpha = pq' + pp'$, and (2) the value of α implied by H_0: $\alpha = pp'$. Thus, the Total variation is given by

$$(pq' + pp') - (pp') = pq' \ ,$$

which is the denominator in Eq. (9.4). The Unexplained variation is the difference between the value of α implied by H_1 and the observed value of α given by

$$(pq' + pp') - \alpha \ .$$

The Explained variation is the Total variation minus the Unexplained variation given by

$$(pq') - (pq' + pp' - \alpha) = \alpha - pp' \ ,$$

which is the numerator in Eq. (9.4). Thus, the ratio of Explained to Total variation is

$$\frac{\alpha - pp'}{pq'} = \phi'$$

and is identical to Eq. (9.4).

This formulation permits ϕ' to be interpreted as the percentage of variation explained or, alternatively, as the proportionate reduction in error in predicting the form of a joint distribution by some logical model, as compared with the distribution implied by statistical independence, a justification espoused by Costner [10, p. 351]. Finally, it should be noted that if the observed value of ϕ' does not fall between the values of α implied by H_0 and H_1, ϕ' will yield a negative value indicating that the observed distribution is contrary in logical form to the one implied by H_1. Thus, valid values of the modified ϕ' test statistic vary only between 0 and 1, in the conventional manner of measures of association for qualitative variables.

9.2 Pearson's Mean-Square Measure of Association

In 1900, in his seventh contribution to the series on "Mathematical contributions to the theory of evolution," Karl Pearson proposed the mean-square contingency coefficient, ϕ [43], although the ϕ coefficient was not made explicit until 1912 when Yule clarified it in his formative article in *Journal of the Royal Statistical Society* titled "On the methods of measuring association between two attributes" [53]. See Chap. 3, Sect. 3.1.1, for a more detailed description of Pearson's ϕ measure of contingency.

The fundamental idea of the ϕ coefficient was to consider a scatterplot of points for two variables, such as for the Pearson product-moment correlation coefficient, then divide the points into quadrants using the means of the two variables, which coincidentally corresponded to the medians of the two variables, as a bivariate normal distribution was assumed. Figure 9.1 illustrates the procedure for variables x and y, resulting in the 2×2 contingency table given in Table 9.3.

Using the notation given in Table 9.4, ϕ is calculated as

$$\phi = \frac{ad - bc}{\sqrt{(a+b)(c+d)(a+c)(b+d)}} \, .$$

The expression $ad - bc$ is used in many measures of association applied to 2×2 contingency tables, where it is sometimes called the "tetra difference." It is, of course, simply a determinant of order two.

For the small set of frequency data given in Table 9.3,

$$\phi = \frac{(2)(2) - (4)(4)}{\sqrt{(6)(6)(6)(6)}} = \frac{-12}{\sqrt{1{,}296}} = -0.3333 \, .$$

Fig. 9.1 Simulated scatterplot of $N = 10$ objects in a two-dimensional space

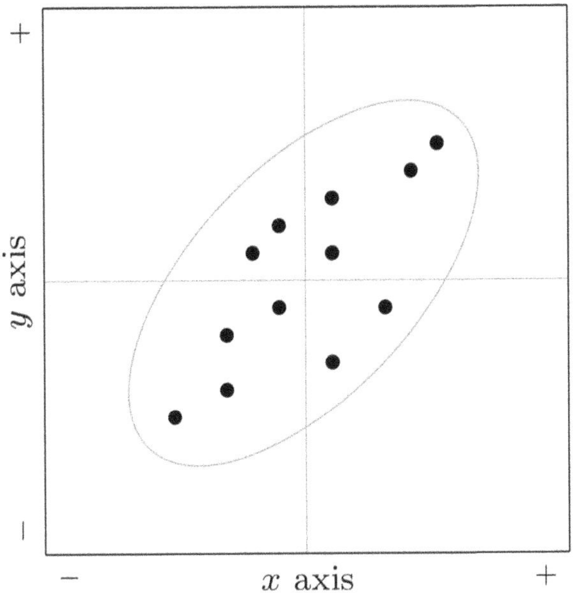

Table 9.3 Example data for variables x and y with categories dummy-coded 0 and 1

	y		
x	0	1	Total
0	2	4	6
1	4	2	6
Total	6	6	12

Table 9.4 Notation for variables x and y with categories dummy-coded 0 and 1

	y		
x	0	1	Total
0	a	b	$a+b$
1	c	d	$c+d$
Total	$a+c$	$b+d$	N

The value for Pearson's ϕ is often squared for ease in interpretation; thus, $\phi^2 = (-0.3333)^2 = 0.1111$.

Pearson's ϕ coefficient is actually a product-moment coefficient of correlation when the two categories of each variable are coded 0 and 1, respectively, as in Table 9.3, and is easily demonstrated. The frequency data given in Table 9.3 are dummy-coded (0, 1) in Table 9.5, where Objects 1 and 2, coded (0, 0), represent the two objects in row 1 and column 1 of Table 9.3; Objects 3 through 6, coded (0, 1), represent the four objects in row 1 and column 2; Objects 7 through 10, coded (1, 0), represent the four objects in row 2 and column 1; and Objects 11 and 12, coded (1, 1), represent the two objects in row 2 and column 2 of Table 9.3. For

Table 9.5 Example dummy-coded (0, 1) values from the 2×2 contingency table given in Table 9.3

	Variable	
Object	x	y
1	0	0
2	0	0
3	0	1
4	0	1
5	0	1
6	0	1
7	1	0
8	1	0
9	1	0
10	1	0
11	1	1
12	1	1

the binary-coded data listed in Table 9.5, $N = 12$,

$$\sum_{i=1}^{N} x_i = \sum_{i=1}^{N} x_i^2 = 6 , \quad \sum_{i=1}^{N} y_i = \sum_{i=1}^{N} y_i^2 = 6 , \quad \sum_{i=1}^{N} x_i y_i = +2 ,$$

and the squared Pearson product-moment correlation coefficient for variables x and y is

$$r_{xy}^2 = \frac{\left(N \sum_{i=1}^{N} x_i y_i - \sum_{i=1}^{N} x_i \sum_{i=1}^{N} y_i \right)^2}{\left[N \sum_{i=1}^{N} x_i^2 - \left(\sum_{i=1}^{N} x_i \right)^2 \right] \left[N \sum_{i=1}^{N} y_i^2 - \left(\sum_{i=1}^{N} y_i \right)^2 \right]}$$

$$= \frac{\left[(12)(+2) - (6)(6) \right]^2}{\left[(12)(6) - 6^2 \right] \left[(12)(6) - 6^2 \right]} = 0.1111 ,$$

which is identical to the value of Pearson's ϕ^2.

It is also widely recognized that ϕ^2 is a simple function of Pearson's chi-squared test of independence, where

$$\phi^2 = \frac{\chi^2}{N} \quad \text{and} \quad \chi^2 = N\phi^2 .$$

For the frequency data given in Table 9.3, the value of χ^2 is given by

$$\chi^2 = \sum_{i=1}^{r} \sum_{j=1}^{c} \frac{\left(O_{ij} - E_{ij} \right)^2}{E_{ij}} ,$$

where O_{ij} denotes the observed cell frequencies, $i = 1, \ldots, r$ and $j = 1, \ldots, c$, and E_{ij} denotes the expected cell values given by

$$E_{ij} = \frac{n_{i.}n_{.j}}{N} \qquad \text{for } i = 1, \ldots, r \text{ and } j = 1, \ldots, c \; ,$$

where $n_{i.}$ denotes a marginal frequency total for the ith row, $i = 1, \ldots, r$, summed over all columns, and $n_{.j}$ denotes a marginal frequency total for the jth column, $j = 1, \ldots, c$, summed over all rows.

For the frequency data given in Table 9.3,

$$E_{11} = E_{12} = E_{21} = E_{22} = \frac{(6)(6)}{12} = 3.00 \; ,$$

$$\chi^2 = \sum_{i=1}^{r} \sum_{j=1}^{c} \frac{\left(O_{ij} - E_{ij}\right)^2}{E_{ij}}$$

$$= \frac{(2-3.00)^2}{3.00} + \frac{(2-3.00)^2}{3.00} + \frac{(4-3.00)^2}{3.00} + \frac{(2-3.00)^2}{3.00} = 1.3333 \; ,$$

and

$$\phi^2 = \frac{\chi^2}{N} = \frac{1.3333}{12} = 0.1111 \; .$$

Because of the manner in which Pearson's ϕ was initially constructed with equivalent marginal frequency totals, *vide supra*, ϕ measures strong monotonicity and can only obtain the limits of -1 and $+1$ indicating perfect negative and positive association, respectively, when the marginal frequency distributions are equivalent, e.g., $\{5, 5\}$ and $\{5, 5\}$ or $\{6, 4\}$ and $\{6, 4\}$ [53, p. 584]. This marginal restriction of Pearson's ϕ greatly limits the interpretation of the test statistic and, consequently, its utility, as noted by Yule in 1912 [53, p. 596].

9.3 Pearson's Tetrachoric Measure of Correlation

In 1900, in the same article on "Mathematical contributions to the theory of evolution" in which he introduced the ϕ measure of mean-square contingency, Karl Pearson proposed the tetrachoric correlation coefficient [43]. The fundamental idea of the tetrachoric correlation coefficient was to consider the $2{\times}2$ contingency table as a double dichotomization of a bivariate standard normal distribution, and then solve for the parameter such that the volumes of the distribution equal the joint probabilities of the contingency table [16]. Pearson considered the tetrachoric correlation coefficient as one of his most important contributions to the theory of statistics, along with his system of continuous curves and the chi-squared test of independence [7].

The tetrachoric correlation coefficient is a product-moment correlation coefficient between two normally distributed variables, each of which is measured on a dichotomous scale [43]. Whereas the tetrachoric correlation coefficient is typically employed to measure the correlation between two independent dichotomous variables, it can also be used to assess the reliability of a single judge when the same two judges independently rate N objects on a dichotomous scale [5, 20]. In addition, the tetrachoric correlation coefficient is often used to measure inter-rater agreement [52] and is preferred by some researchers over Cohen's [9] unweighted kappa measure of inter-rater chance-corrected agreement for this purpose [28].

Because of the extensive calculations necessary to compute the tetrachoric correlation coefficient, it has never been a popular statistic, despite its usefulness. With the advent of high-speed computing, the tetrachoric correlation coefficient has seen a resurrection in fields such as psychology, psychopathology, radiology, and genetics [24]. The tetrachoric correlation coefficient has been especially popular in psychology where quantitative variables measured on a dichotomous scale include test items scored as correct/incorrect, assessment of students having/not-having a learning disability, students passing/not-passing a motor skills or other test, and children classified as having/not-having attention deficit hyperactivity disorder or other emotional or behavioral problems.

An asymptotic approximation to the standard error of the tetrachoric correlation coefficient was given by Pearson in 1913 [44]. However, the accuracy and, therefore, utility of Pearson's standard error has repeatedly been called into question. For example, in 1961 Kendall and Stuart noted that the sampling distribution and the standard error of the tetrachoric correlation coefficient were not known with any precision, and they further observed that it was not known for what sample size the standard error may safely be used [34, p. 306]. Permutation tests have long been used to assess the assumptions of asymptotic tests and the quality of theoretical standard errors [14, 19, 22, 46, 47, 48]. In this section an exact permutation procedure for the tetrachoric correlation coefficient is introduced and the permutation approach is compared with the traditional asymptotic approach [39].

The tetrachoric correlation coefficient is, quite possibly, the single most difficult correlation coefficient to calculate [39, p. 430]. Following Brown [6], denote the four cell frequencies of a 2×2 contingency table as a, b, c, and d as in Table 9.6, where $N = a + b + c + d$. Let z_1 and z_2 denote the standard normal deviates of the

Table 9.6 Notation for variables x and y with categories dummy-coded 0 and 1

	y		
x	0	1	Total
0	a	b	$a+b$
1	c	d	$c+d$
Total	$a+c$	$b+d$	N

marginal probabilities, i.e.,

$$z_1 = \Phi^{-1}\left(\frac{a+c}{N}\right)$$

and

$$z_2 = \Phi^{-1}\left(\frac{a+b}{N}\right) ,$$

where Φ is the cdf of the standard normal distribution. Then Pearson's tetrachoric correlation coefficient, r_{tet}, is the correlation that satisfies

$$\frac{a}{N} = \int_{-\infty}^{z_2} \int_{-\infty}^{z_1} \phi(x_1, x_2, r_{\text{tet}}) dx_1 dx_2 , \tag{9.5}$$

where $\phi(x_1, x_2, r_{\text{tet}})$ is the bivariate normal pdf given by

$$\phi(x_1, x_2, r_{\text{tet}}) = \left[2\pi\left(1 - r_{\text{tet}}^2\right)^{1/2}\right] \exp\left[-\frac{x_1^2 - 2x_1x_2r_{\text{tet}} + x_2^2}{2\left(1 - r_{\text{tet}}^2\right)}\right] ,$$

and where $x_1 = z_1$ and $x_2 = z_2$ define the point that divides the bivariate normal distribution into four quadrants with probabilities corresponding to the probabilities of the four cells in the 2×2 contingency table [8]. When only one cell possesses a zero frequency, the zero is traditionally changed to 0.5 and all other cell frequencies are correspondingly adjusted to maintain the original row and column marginal frequency totals.

When $a = d = 0$, $r_{\text{tet}} = -1$ and when $b = c = 0$, $r_{\text{tet}} = +1$. When $z_1 = z_2 = 0$, then an explicit solution exists where

$$r_{\text{tet}} = -\cos\left(\frac{2\pi a}{N}\right) .$$

In all other cases, r_{tet} must be found by iteration as a root of Eq. (9.5). Pearson [43] and Everitt [17] approximated the bivariate normal integral by the tetrachoric series expansion

$$I = \int_{-\infty}^{z_2} \int_{-\infty}^{z_1} \phi(x_1, x_2, r_{\text{tet}}) dx_1 dx_2$$
$$= \left(\frac{a+b}{N}\right)\left(\frac{a+c}{N}\right) + \sum_{j=1}^{\infty} \frac{r_{\text{tet}}^j}{j!} \phi(z_1, z_2, 0) v_{j-1} w_{j-1} ,$$

where $v_0 = 1$, $v_1 = z_1$, and

$$v_j = z_1 v_{j-1} - (j-1) w_{j-2} \qquad \text{for } j > 1 ,$$

and $w_0 = 1$, $w_1 = z_2$, and

$$w_j = z_2 w_{j-1} - (j-1) w_{j-2} \qquad \text{for } j > 1 \ ,$$

respectively.

The standard error of r_{tet} is given by

$$s_{\text{tet}} = \left[N^{3/2} \phi(z_1, z_2, r_{\text{tet}}) \right]^{-1} \left[\frac{(a+d)(b+c)}{4} + (a+c)(b+d)\Phi_2^2 + (a+b)(c+d)\Phi_1^2 + 2(ad-bc)\Phi_1\Phi_2 - (ab)(cd)\Phi_2 - (ac-bd)\Phi_1 \right]^{1/2} , \tag{9.6}$$

where

$$\Phi_1 = \Phi\left[\frac{z_1 - z_2 r_{\text{tet}}}{\left(1 - r_{\text{tet}}^2\right)^{1/2}} \right] - \frac{1}{2}$$

and

$$\Phi_2 = \Phi\left[\frac{z_2 - z_1 r_{\text{tet}}}{\left(1 - r_{\text{tet}}^2\right)^{1/2}} \right] - \frac{1}{2}$$

[45]. Under the null hypothesis, $\text{E}[r_{\text{tet}}] = 0$, Eq. (9.6) simplifies to

$$s_0 = \left[N^{5/2} \phi(z_1, z_2, 0) \right]^{-1} \left[(a+b)(a+c)(b+c)(b+d) \right]^{1/2} .$$

It is well known that the sampling distributions of correlation coefficients sampled from populations with parameter $\rho \neq 0$ are skewed. Because there is no provision for transforming s_{tet} into a test statistic that is symmetrically distributed, as is true for the Fisher z transformation for the ordinary Pearson product-moment correlation coefficient, the only reasonable approach is the assumption of the null hypothesis $H_0\colon \rho_{\text{tet}} = 0$ [26]. In any case, the Fisher z transformation for the Pearson product-moment correlation coefficient has been shown to perform poorly for skewed and heavy-tailed distributions [1]. Under $H_0\colon \rho_{\text{tet}} = 0$, the test statistic given by

$$T = \frac{r_{\text{tet}}}{s_0}$$

is distributed as Student's t with $N - 2$ degrees of freedom, under the assumption of normality [17].

9.3.1 A Permutation Test for Tetrachoric Correlation

Permutation tests possess certain advantages over conventional statistical tests because permutation tests are completely data-dependent and are free of the usual assumptions associated with traditional asymptotic tests. As noted previously, there are two types of permutation statistical tests: exact permutation tests and Monte Carlo resampling permutation tests. Exact permutation tests consider all possible arrangements of the observed data, whereas Monte Carlo permutation tests consider a random sample of all possible arrangements. Given the observed row and column marginal frequency totals of a 2×2 contingency table, it is necessary to generate only all possible values of a single cell; for example, cell a where the lower and upper limits of cell a are given by

$$L = \max(0, a - d) \quad \text{and} \quad U = \min(a + b, a + c) ,$$

respectively. A tetrachoric correlation coefficient is then calculated for each of the $M = U - L + 1$ possible values of cell a. Let r_o denote the tetrachoric correlation coefficient calculated on the observed data and let r_i denote a tetrachoric correlation coefficient calculated on each possible arrangement of the observed data, $i = L, \ldots, U$. The probability of r_o is given by

$$P = \sum_{i=L}^{U} \Psi(r_i) ,$$

where, if r_o is positive,

$$\Psi(r_i) = \begin{cases} P(a|a+b, a+c, N) & \text{if } r_i \geq r_o , \\ 0 & \text{otherwise} , \end{cases}$$

or, if r_o is negative,

$$\Psi(r_i) = \begin{cases} P(a|a+b, a+c, N) & \text{if } r_i \leq r_o , \\ 0 & \text{otherwise} , \end{cases}$$

and the hypergeometric probability for a 2×2 contingency table is given by

$$P(a|a+b, a+c, N) = \binom{a+c}{a}\binom{b+d}{b}\binom{N}{a+b}^{-1} = \frac{(a+b)!\,(c+d)!\,(a+c)!\,(b+d)!}{N!\,a!\,b!\,c!\,d!} .$$

If $r_o = 0$, $P = 1.00$ as direction is undefined.

9.3.2 Example 1

Consider the example frequency data given in Table 9.7 with $N = 80$ observations, where the observed value of Pearson's tetrachoric correlation coefficient is $r_{\text{tet}} = +0.4027$.

For the frequency data given in Table 9.7,

$$L = \max(0, a - d) = \max(0, 30 - 20) = \max(0, 10) = 10$$

and

$$U = \min(a + b, a + c) = \min(30 + 10, 30 + 20) = \min(40, 50) = 40 \ .$$

Consequently, there are only $M = U - L + 1 = 40 - 10 + 1 = 31$ possible, equally-likely arrangements in the reference set of all permutations of cell frequencies in Table 9.7 given the observed row and column marginal frequency distributions, $\{40, 40\}$ and $\{50, 30\}$, respectively, making an exact permutation analysis feasible. Since $M = 31$ is a reasonable number, it will be illustrative to list the 31 sets of cell frequencies, r_{tet} values, and associated hypergeometric point probability values in Table 9.8, where the rows with hypergeometric point probability values associated with r_{tet} values equal to or greater than the value of the observed test statistic are indicated with asterisks.

If the $M = 31$ possible arrangements in the reference set of all permutations of the frequency data given in Table 9.7 occur with equal chance, the exact probability value of r_{tet} under the null hypothesis is the sum of the hypergeometric point probability values associated with $r_{\text{tet}} = +0.4027$ or greater. Based on the hypergeometric probability distribution, the exact upper-tail probability value is

$$\begin{aligned} P = {} & 0.1317{\times}10^{-1} + 0.4046{\times}10^{-2} + 0.9829{\times}10^{-3} + 0.1865{\times}10^{-3} \\ & + 0.2719{\times}10^{-4} + 0.2984{\times}10^{-5} + 0.2391{\times}10^{-6} + 0.1340{\times}10^{-7} \\ & + 0.4912{\times}10^{-9} + 0.1042{\times}10^{-10} + 0.9555{\times}10^{-13} = 0.0184 \ . \end{aligned}$$

Table 9.7 Example data for variables x and y with categories dummy-coded as 0 and 1

	y		
x	0	1	Total
0	30	10	40
1	20	20	40
Total	50	30	80

Table 9.8 Cell frequencies, r_{tet} values, and exact hypergeometric point probability values for $M = 31$ possible arrangements of the observed data in Table 9.7

Table	Cell frequency				r_{tet}	Probability
	n_{11}	n_{12}	n_{21}	n_{22}		
1*	40	0	10	30	+0.9636	0.9555×10^{-13}
2*	39	1	11	29	+0.9428	0.1042×10^{-10}
3*	38	2	12	28	+0.8999	0.4912×10^{-9}
4*	37	3	13	27	+0.8529	0.1340×10^{-7}
5*	36	4	14	26	+0.8012	0.2391×10^{-6}
6*	35	5	15	25	+0.7447	0.2984×10^{-5}
7*	34	6	16	24	+0.6838	0.2719×10^{-4}
8*	33	7	17	23	+0.6187	0.1865×10^{-3}
9*	32	8	18	22	+0.5499	0.9829×10^{-3}
10*	31	9	19	21	+0.4777	0.4046×10^{-2}
11*	30	10	20	20	+0.4027	0.1317×10^{-1}
12	29	11	21	19	+0.3251	0.3421×10^{-1}
13	28	12	22	18	+0.2456	0.9500×10^{-1}
14	27	13	23	17	+0.1646	0.1204
15	26	14	24	16	+0.8255	0.1644
16	25	15	25	15	0.0000	0.1824
17	24	16	26	14	−0.8255	0.1644
18	23	17	27	13	−0.1646	0.1204
19	22	18	28	12	−0.2456	0.9500×10^{-1}
20	21	19	29	11	−0.3251	0.3421×10^{-1}
21	20	20	30	10	−0.4027	0.1317×10^{-1}
22	19	21	31	9	−0.4777	0.4046×10^{-2}
23	18	22	32	8	−0.5499	0.9829×10^{-3}
24	17	23	33	7	−0.6187	0.1865×10^{-3}
25	16	24	34	6	−0.6838	0.2719×10^{-4}
26	15	25	35	5	−0.7447	0.2984×10^{-5}
27	14	26	36	4	−0.8012	0.2391×10^{-6}
28	13	27	37	3	−0.8529	0.1340×10^{-7}
29	12	28	38	2	−0.8999	0.4912×10^{-9}
30	11	29	39	1	−0.9428	0.1042×10^{-10}
31	10	30	40	0	−0.9636	0.9555×10^{-13}
Sum						1.0000

For comparison, define test statistic $T = r_{tet}/s_0$. The standard error of r_{tet} under the null hypothesis H_0: $\rho_{tet} = 0$ is $s_0 = 0.1789$ and the observed test statistic is

$$T = \frac{r_{tet}}{s_0} = \frac{+0.4027}{0.1789} = +2.2510 \, .$$

Based on Student's t distribution with $N - 2 = 80 - 2 = 78$ degrees of freedom, the asymptotic upper-tail probability value of $T = +2.2510$ is $P = 0.0136$.

9.3.3 Example 2

While the marginal frequency distributions in Example 1 do not differ greatly, given similar row and column marginal frequency distributions, {40, 40} and {50, 30}, respectively, consider a second example where both the row and column marginal frequency distributions are highly skewed, as in Table 9.9 with $N = 80$ observations and row and column marginal frequency distributions, {70, 10} and {70, 10}, respectively. For the frequency data given in Table 9.9, the observed value of Pearson's tetrachoric correlation coefficient is $r_{\text{tet}} = +0.8125$.

There are only

$$M = \min(a+b, a+c) - \max(0, a-d) + 1$$
$$= \min(70, 70) - \max(0, 66-6) + 1 = 70 - 60 + 1 = 11$$

possible, equally-likely arrangements in the reference set of all permutations of cell frequencies in Table 9.9 given the observed row and column marginal frequency distributions, {70, 10} and {70, 10}, respectively, making an exact permutation analysis feasible. Since $M = 11$ is a very small number of arrangements, it will be illustrative to list the 11 sets of cell frequencies, r_{tet} values, and associated hypergeometric point probability values in Table 9.10, where the rows with hypergeometric probability

Table 9.9 Example data for variables x and y with categories dummy-coded as 0 and 1

	y		
x	0	1	Total
0	66	4	70
1	4	6	10
Total	70	10	80

Table 9.10 Cell frequencies, r_{tet} values, and exact hypergeometric point probability values for $M = 11$ possible arrangements of the observed data in Table 9.9

	Cell frequency					
Table	n_{11}	n_{12}	n_{21}	n_{22}	r_{tet}	Probability
1*	70	0	0	10	+1.0000	0.6074×10^{-12}
2*	69	1	1	9	+0.9884	0.4251×10^{-9}
3*	68	2	2	8	+0.9535	0.6600×10^{-7}
4*	67	3	3	7	+0.8951	0.3990×10^{-5}
5*	66	4	4	6	+0.8125	0.1169×10^{-3}
6	65	5	5	5	+0.7046	0.1852×10^{-2}
7	64	6	6	4	+0.5693	0.1672×10^{-1}
8	63	7	7	3	+0.4026	0.8737×10^{-1}
9	62	8	8	2	+0.1956	0.2580
10	61	9	9	1	−0.0777	0.3950
11	60	10	10	0	−0.2697	0.2409
Sum						1.0000

values associated with r_{tet} values equal to or greater than the value of the observed test statistic are indicated with asterisks.

If the $M = 11$ possible arrangements in the reference set of all permutations of the frequency data given in Table 9.9 occur with equal chance, the exact probability value of r_{tet} under the null hypothesis is the sum of the hypergeometric point probability values associated with $r_{\text{tet}} = +0.8125$ or greater. Based on the hypergeometric probability distribution, the exact upper-tail probability value is

$$P = 0.1169\times10^{-3} + 0.3990\times10^{-5} + 0.6600\times10^{-7} + 0.4251\times10^{-9} + 0.6074\times10^{-12} = 0.1210\times10^{-3} .$$

For comparison, the standard error of r_{tet} under the null hypothesis $H_0\colon \rho_{\text{tet}} = 0$ is $s_0 = 0.2886$ and the observed test statistic is

$$T = \frac{r_{\text{tet}}}{s_0} = \frac{+0.8125}{0.2886} = +2.8153 .$$

Based on Student's t distribution with $N - 2 = 80 - 2 = 78$ degrees of freedom, the asymptotic upper-tail probability value of $T = +2.8153$ is $P = 0.3084\times10^{-2}$.

9.4 Exact and Asymptotic Probability Values

It is obvious from the results in Examples 1 and 2 that the marginal distributions can affect the asymptotic probability values of r_{tet} with sample size held constant. In Example 2 with skewed row and column marginal frequency distributions, {70, 10} and {70, 10}, respectively, the ratio of the asymptotic and exact probability values is $0.3084\times10^{-2}/0.1210\times10^{-3} = 25.62$, while in Example 1 with row and column marginal frequency distributions, {40, 40} and {50, 30}, respectively, the ratio of the asymptotic and exact probability values is only $0.0136/0.0184 = 0.74$. Long, Berry, and Mielke investigated the effects of sample sizes and marginal frequency distributions on the exact and asymptotic probability values for r_{tet} [39].

The conventional approach for establishing a probability value for r_{tet} under $H_0\colon \rho_{\text{tet}} = 0$ employs Student's t distribution with $N - 2$ degrees of freedom. The permutation approach provides an alternative to the t distribution that is distribution free. Tables 9.11 and 9.12 present comparisons between exact probability values (P_e) and probability values based on Student's t distribution (P_t) for a variety of marginal proportions and two sample sizes, $N = 10$ and $N = 50$ [39]. The marginal proportions in Tables 9.11 and 9.12 range from 0.5/0.5 to 0.9/0.1 and are identical for both rows and columns. For example, given $N = 10$ and marginal proportions of 0.6/0.4 in Table 9.11, the row and marginal frequency distributions are {6, 4} and {6, 4}, respectively.

Table 9.11 Tetrachoric correlation coefficients (r_{tet}) with marginal proportions, cell frequencies for cell a, exact probability values (P_e), probability values based on Student's t distribution (P_t), and absolute differences between the probability values ($|P_e - P_t|$), with $N = 10$

Marginal proportions	Cell a	r_{tet}	P_e	P_t	$\|P_e - P_t\|$
0.5/0.5	0	−1.0000	0.0040	0.0394	0.1355
	1	−0.8090	0.1032	0.0710	0.0322
	2	−0.3090	0.5000	0.2756	0.2244
	3	+0.3090	0.5000	0.2756	0.2244
	4	+0.8090	0.1032	0.0710	0.0322
	5	+1.0000	0.0040	0.0394	0.0355
0.6/0.4	2	−0.6990	0.0714	0.1032	0.0318
	3	−0.3979	0.4524	0.2282	0.2242
	4	+0.2629	0.5476	0.3095	0.2381
	5	+0.7963	0.1190	0.0780	0.0411
	6	+1.0000	0.0048	0.0424	0.0376
0.7/0.3	4	−0.3449	0.2917	0.2738	0.0179
	5	+0.0817	0.7083	0.4427	0.2656
	6	+0.7482	0.1833	0.1052	0.0782
	7	+1.0000	0.0083	0.0531	0.0448
0.8/0.2	6	+0.1222	1.0000	0.4273	0.5727
	7	+0.6060	0.3778	0.1877	0.1901
	8	+1.0000	0.0222	0.0800	0.0578
0.9/0.1	8	+0.7366	1.0000	0.2242	0.7758
	9	+1.0000	0.1000	0.1554	0.0554

Approximating a skewed discrete probability distribution with a symmetrical continuous distribution is fraught with danger. To illustrate the problems with the use of P_t in assessing tetrachoric correlation, consider the difference between P_e and P_t for $N = 10$ and 0.8/0.2 marginal proportions in Table 9.11. Given the observed row and column marginal frequency totals, $\{8, 2\}$ and $\{8, 2\}$, respectively, there are only three possible arrangements of cell frequencies, i.e., $a = 6, 7$, and 8, with r_{tet} values of +0.1222, +0.6060, and +1.000, respectively. It is obvious that the upper-tail probability of $r_{\text{tet}} = +0.1222$ must be $P = 1.00$ since all three coefficients are positive and $r_{\text{tet}} = +0.1222$ is the smallest of the three coefficients. Specifically, the hypergeometric point probability value for cell $a = 6$ is $p = 0.6222$, for cell $a = 7$ the hypergeometric point probability is $p = 0.3556$, and for cell $a = 8$ the hypergeometric point probability is $p = 0.0222$. Thus, the cumulative probability of an observed r_{tet} value as large or larger than $r_{\text{tet}} = +0.1222$ is

$$P = 0.6222 + 0.3556 + 0.0222 = 1.00 .$$

Table 9.12 Tetrachoric correlation coefficients (r_{tet}) with marginal proportions, cell frequencies for cell a, exact probability values (P_e), probability values based on Student's t distribution (P_t), and absolute differences between the probability values ($|P_e - P_t|$), with $N = 50$

Marginal proportions	Cell a	r_{tet}	P_e	P_t	$\|P_e - P_t\|$
0.5/0.5	0	−1.0000	0.0000	0.0000	0.0000
	5	−0.8090	0.0000	0.0003	0.0003
	10	−0.3090	0.1289	0.0853	0.0436
	15	+0.3090	0.1289	0.0853	0.0436
	20	+0.8090	0.0000	0.0003	0.0003
	25	+1.0000	0.0000	0.0000	0.0000
0.6/0.4	10	−0.9087	0.0000	0.0001	0.0001
	15	−0.3979	0.0692	0.0433	0.0260
	20	+0.2629	0.1883	0.1267	0.0617
	25	+0.7963	0.0000	0.0005	0.0005
	30	+1.0000	0.0000	0.0000	0.0000
0.7/0.3	20	−0.7378	0.0014	0.0021	0.0007
	25	+0.0817	0.4925	0.3704	0.1221
	30	+0.7482	0.0005	0.0019	0.0014
	35	+1.0000	0.0000	0.0001	0.0001
0.8/0.2	30	+0.4662	0.0825	0.0565	0.0261
	35	+0.6060	0.0181	0.0205	0.0024
	40	+1.0000	0.0000	0.0006	0.0006
0.9/0.1	40	0.0000	1.0000	0.5000	0.5000
	45	+1.0000	0.0000	0.0097	0.0097

However,

$$T = \frac{r_{\text{tet}}}{s_0} = \frac{0.1222}{0.6455} = 0.1893$$

and the one-sided probability of $r_{\text{tet}} = +0.1222$, based on Student's t distribution with $N - 2 = 10 - 2 = 8$ degrees of freedom is $P_t = 0.4273$, indicating that only approximately 43% of possible r_{tet} values are as large or larger than $r_{\text{tet}} = +0.1222$, yielding a difference of $|P_e - P_t| = |1.00 - 0.4273| = 0.5727$.

It is abundantly evident from even a cursory inspection of Tables 9.11 and 9.12 that two factors are contributing to the poor performance of Student's t distribution: sample size and disproportionate marginal frequency totals. Tables 9.13 and 9.14 examine these two factors, respectively.

Table 9.13 lists $|P_e - P_t|$ values for five marginal proportions—0.5/0.5, 0.6/0.4, 0.7/0.3, 0.8/0.2, and 0.9/0.1—with common r_{tet} values for $N = 10$, 20, 50, 100, 500, and 1,000. As in Tables 9.11 and 9.12, the marginal proportions in Table 9.13 are identical for both rows and columns. The r_{tet} values for each marginal proportion were chosen simply for convenience and provide illustrations of the

Table 9.13 $|P_e - P_t|$ values for five marginal proportions with common r_{tet} values for $N = 10$, 20, 50, 100, 500, and 1,000

	Marginal proportions (r_{tet})				
N	0.5/0.5 (+0.3090)	0.6/0.4 (+0.2629)	0.7/0.3 (+0.0817)	0.8/0.2 (+0.6060)	0.9/0.1 (+0.2649)
10	0.2244	0.2381	0.2656	0.1901	–
20	0.1329	0.1513	0.1948	0.0616	–
50	0.0436	0.0617	0.1221	0.0024	0.1611
100	0.0097	0.0200	0.0819	0.0012	0.0781
500	0.0000	0.0000	0.0222	0.0000	0.0032
1,000	0.0000	0.0000	0.0083	0.0000	0.0010

Table 9.14 Marginal proportions, cell frequencies for cell d, exact skewness values (γ_{tet}), exact probability values (P_e), probability values based on Student's t distribution (P_t), and absolute differences between the probability values ($|P_e - P_t|$), with $N = 50$

Marginal proportions	Cell d	r_{tet}	γ_{tet}	P_e	P_t	$\lvert P_e - P_t\rvert$
0.50/0.50	0	−1.00	0.0000	0.0011	0.0260	0.0249
0.60/0.40	3	−0.79	0.0296	0.0168	0.0399	0.0231
0.70/0.30	8	−0.58	0.2040	0.0775	0.0771	0.0004
0.80/0.20	18	−0.34	0.5730	0.2267	0.1845	0.0422
0.90/0.10	48	−0.06	1.1653	0.5159	0.4405	0.0754
0.94/0.06	88	+0.09	1.5907	1.0000	0.4118	0.5882
0.95/0.05	108	+0.13	1.7570	1.0000	0.3733	0.6267
0.96/0.04	138	+0.18	1.9766	1.0000	0.3355	0.6645
0.97/0.03	188	+0.23	2.2952	1.0000	0.2993	0.7007
0.98/0.02	288	+0.30	2.8267	1.0000	0.2671	0.7329
0.99/0.01	588	+0.39	4.0270	1.0000	0.2461	0.7539

effect in increasing sample sizes on $|P_e - P_t|$ differences. Inspection of the column values in Table 9.13 reveals that $|P_e - P_t|$ is large with small sample sizes up to $N = 50$ and in some cases even for $N = 100$. The blank values in Table 9.13 under the marginal proportions 0.9/0.1 are missing because there are too few choices with $N = 10$ or 20 and marginal proportions of 0.9/0.1.

Table 9.14 lists $|P_e - P_t|$ values for 11 marginal proportions—0.50/0.50, 0.60/0.40, 0.70/0.30, 0.80/0.20, 0.90/0.10, 0.94/0.06, 0.95/0.05, 0.96/0.04, 0.97/0.03, 0.98/0.02, and 0.99/0.01—and demonstrates the effect of increasingly unequal marginal proportions on $P_e - P_t$. As in Tables 9.11, 9.12, and 9.13, the marginal proportions in Table 9.14 are identical for both rows and columns. For the results given in Table 9.14, a series of 2×2 contingency tables was constructed with cell $a = 0$, cell $b = 6$, cell $c = 6$, and cell d as listed in the second column. The results in Table 9.14 demonstrate that as the marginal proportions become more unequal, $|P_e - P_t|$ increases, indicating that P_t becomes more inaccurate with increasingly unequal marginal proportions, despite increasing sample sizes as indicated in the second column of Table 9.14.

The relationship between marginal proportions and $|P_e - P_t|$ is associated with the level of skewness (γ_{tet}) of r_{tet}. The values of γ_{tet} in the fourth column of Table 9.14 were obtained from the permutation distribution generated from all possible arrangements of cell frequencies with fixed marginal frequency totals. A comparison of the first and fourth columns in Table 9.14 demonstrates the relationship between skewness and marginal proportions; viz., as the marginal proportions become increasingly unequal, γ_{tet} increases. The relationship can be summarized as follows. Given a 2×2 contingency table where either $b = c$ or $a = d$ and N is much larger than $a + b = M$, then the approximate skewness of r_{tet} is either $N^{1/2}/M$ or $-N^{1/2}/M$, respectively. Thus, the skewness of the tetrachoric correlation distribution may be arbitrarily large in either the positive or negative direction. Therefore, as γ_{tet} increases, $|P_e - P_t|$ increases.

Under H_0: $\rho_{\text{tet}} = 0$, the test statistic $T = r_{\text{tet}}/s_0$ is distributed as Student's t distribution with $N-2$ degrees of freedom, under the assumption of normality. The use of the standard error, s_0, and the t distribution was called into question by Kendall and Stuart [32]. In particular, the appropriateness of the t distribution is problematic for small samples and/or widely disproportionate marginal frequency totals. In such cases, an exact permutation test provides a data-dependent distribution-free alternative that is accurate for both small sample sizes and disproportionate marginal frequency distributions.

9.5 Yule's Q Measure of Association

Developed specifically for the measurement of nominal-level association in 2×2 contingency tables, Yule's Q measure entered the statistical literature under a cloud of controversy. In 1912 G. Udny Yule published a paper titled "On the methods of measuring association between two attributes" in *Journal of the Royal Statistical Society* [53].[7] In this formative paper Yule introduced a new statistic for 2×2 contingency tables that he called Q,[8] although Yule had earlier mentioned Q in a paper published in *Philosophical Transactions of the Royal Society of London* in 1900 [53]. Contained within this lengthy paper of 74 pages was strong criticism of the work of Karl Pearson and biometrician David Heron on the analysis of contingency tables. Pearson, in particular, was greatly offended and a vitriolic

[7]Earlier in 1912, on 23 April, Yule had presented a paper on the same topic to the Royal Statistical Society, where the discussants were Francis Ysidro Edgeworth, Charles Percy Sanger, Reginald Hawthorn Hooker, Major Greenwood, and Ernest Charles Snow.

[8]The symbol Q was taken from the initial letter of the surname of Lambert Adolphe Jacques Quetelet, the 19th century Belgium astronomer, mathematician, statistician, and sociologist [53, p. 436].

N/S

	A	$\bar{A}$
B	X	0
$\bar{B}$	0	X

$N/\bar{S}$

	A	$\bar{A}$
B	X	0
$\bar{B}$	X	X

$\bar{N}/S$

	A	$\bar{A}$
B	X	X
$\bar{B}$	0	X

Fig. 9.2 Graphics for necessary and sufficient (N/S), necessary but not sufficient ($N/\bar{S}$), and sufficient but not-necessary ($\bar{N}/S$) conditions

response soon followed from Pearson and Heron in *Biometrika*. The ascerbic rejoinder consisted of a remarkable 157 folio pages [45].

The nature of the controversy involved whether attributes that were dichotomous were truly discrete, such as true and false, or were obtained from some underlying continuous distribution, such as arbitrarily dividing age into young and old. George Udny Yule, a former student of Karl Pearson, favored the approach of an inherently discrete underlying distribution [16]. In his 1912 article Yule criticized Pearson's tetrachoric correlation coefficient and its assumption of underlying continuous variables.[9] The debate was especially caustic with Pearson and Heron responding, in part:

> The recent paper by Mr Yule entitled "On the Methods of Measuring Association between Two Attributes" calls for an early reply on two grounds,—first because of its singularly acrimonious tone is to us wholly inexplicable, not to say unusual, and secondly because we believe that, if Mr. Yule's views are accepted, irreparable damage will be done to the growth of modern statistical theory. Mr Yule has invented a series of statistical methods which are in no case based on a reasoned theory, but which possess the dangerous fascination of very easy and ready application, and therefore are at once seized upon as applicable to all sorts of problems by those who are without adequate training in statistical theory, or without the mathematical knowledge requisite to weigh cautiously their logical basis [45, pp. 159–160].

There was more to the controversy between Yule and Pearson than just the disagreement over discrete and continuous distributions. Yule strongly advocated coefficients of association that could attain ± 1 under all of three conditions, such as illustrated in Fig. 9.2, where a 0 indicates a zero cell frequency and an **X** indicates a non-zero cell frequency. For the first 2×2 table, on the left in Fig. 9.2, A is both a necessary and sufficient condition for B. Thus, $\bar{A}B = A\bar{B} = 0$, i.e., B if and only if A. For the second 2×2 table, in the middle in Fig. 9.2, A is a necessary but not sufficient condition of B. Thus, $\bar{A}B = 0$, i.e., A must be present, but B need not always follow from A. For the third 2×2 table, on the right in Fig. 9.2, A is a sufficient, but not-necessary condition for B. Thus, $A\bar{B} = 0$, i.e., whenever A is present, B must follow, but B may also occur when A is not present.

[9] It should be noted that Pearson's tetrachoric correlation coefficient in question was notoriously difficult to calculate at the time.

Table 9.15 Notation for variables x and y with categories dummy-coded 0 and 1

	y		
x	0	1	Total
0	a	b	$a+b$
1	c	d	$c+d$
Total	$a+c$	$b+d$	N

Yule contended that his statistic, Q, achieved ± 1 under all three conditions, but Pearson's statistic, r_{tet}, could only achieve ± 1 under the conditions in the first table (N/S) in Fig. 9.2, i.e., A is a necessary and sufficient condition of B, arguing that the greatest possible negative value was not in general the same as the greatest possible positive value unless the marginal frequency distributions were identical [53, p. 585]. In addition, Yule was especially proud of the fact that Q was unaltered by multiplying or dividing "either or both of the columns of the table by any arbitrary factor" [53, p. 587] and argued that "this is a most important property" of measures of association [53, p. 587].

It is important to point out that however rancorous the exchange between Yule and Pearson, Yule wrote Pearson's obituary for the Royal Society [54] and, according to Kendall [31], Yule was deeply affected by Pearson's passing on 27 April 1936 [16].[10] The only reference to their controversy in Yule's obituary is a brief mention of their disagreement:

> As concerns the further developments of methods applicable to unmeasured characters, I have been too much engaged in the controversy to give an objective opinion. Through nearly all that work run two assumptions: (1) that the quantitative classification represents a grouping of a scalar variable; (2) that the table of double entry represents a grouping of normally distributed frequency. Both seem to me often false, and consequently dangerous. But that is a personal and may be an uncharitable judgment. Time will settle the question in due course [55, p. 84].

Originally developed for categorical data, Yule's Q is often also used for ordinal-level data [53]. For a 2×2 contingency table, such as given in Table 9.15, Yule's Q is given by

$$Q = \frac{ad - bc}{ad + bc} \ .$$

To illustrate the calculation of Yule's Q measure of association, consider the example frequency data given in Table 9.16 with $N = 100$ observations, where

[10] Karl Pearson was elected Fellow of the Royal Society in 1896. A longer, very detailed, affectionate obituary of 39 pages was written by Yule and Filon in 1936 and is well worth reading to gain insight into the life and accomplishments of Karl Pearson and his relationship to G. Udny Yule [55].

Table 9.16 Example data for variables x and y with categories dummy-coded 0 and 1

	y		
x	0	1	Total
0	30	10	40
1	30	30	60
Total	60	40	100

Yule's Q is

$$Q = \frac{ad - bc}{ad + bd} = \frac{(30)(30) - (10)(30)}{(30)(30 + (10)(30)} = +0.50 \, .$$

For 2×2 contingency tables, Yule's Q is a simple function of Kendall's S test statistic and is identical to Goodman and Kruskal's γ statistic [23]. Thus, Yule's Q is also given by

$$Q = \frac{S}{C + D} \, ,$$

where C and D denote the number of concordant and discordant pairs, respectively, and $S = C - D$. Thus, for the frequency data given in Table 9.16 where

$$C = ad = (30)(30) = 900 \quad \text{and} \quad D = bc = (10)(30) = 300 \, ,$$

the observed value of Yule's Q is

$$Q = \frac{C - D}{C + D} = \frac{S}{C + D} = \frac{900 - 300}{900 + 300} = \frac{600}{1200} = +0.50 \, .$$

For the frequency data given in Table 9.16, there are only

$$M = \min(a + b, a + c) - \max(0, a - d) + 1$$
$$= \min(40, 60) - \max(0, 30 - 30) + 1 = 40 - 0 + 1 = 41$$

possible, equally-likely arrangements in the reference set of all permutations of cell frequencies given the observed row and column marginal frequency distributions, {40, 60} and {60, 40}, respectively, making an exact permutation analysis feasible. Since $M = 41$ is a reasonable number of arrangements, it will be illustrative to list the 41 sets of cell frequencies, Yule's Q coefficients, and the associated hypergeometric point probability values in Table 9.17, where the rows with hypergeometric point probability values associated with Q values equal to or greater than the observed Q value are indicated with asterisks.

If the $M = 41$ possible arrangements given in Table 9.17 occur with equal chance, the exact probability value of Q under the null hypothesis is the sum of the hypergeometric point probability values associated with $Q = +0.50$ or

Table 9.17 Cell frequencies, Q values, and exact hypergeometric point probability values for $M = 41$ possible arrangements of the observed data in Table 9.16

	Cell frequency					
Table	n_{11}	n_{12}	n_{21}	n_{22}	Yule's Q	Probability
1*	40	0	20	40	+1.0000	0.3049×10^{-12}
2*	39	1	21	39	+0.9728	0.2323×10^{-12}
3*	38	2	22	38	+0.9409	0.8032×10^{-9}
4*	37	3	23	37	+0.9040	0.1681×10^{-7}
5*	36	4	24	36	+0.8621	0.2397×10^{-6}
6*	35	5	25	35	+0.8148	0.2485×10^{-5}
7*	34	6	26	34	+0.7622	0.1409×10^{-4}
8*	33	7	27	33	+0.7042	0.1194×10^{-3}
9*	32	8	28	32	+0.6410	0.5803×10^{-3}
10*	31	9	29	31	+0.5728	0.2277×10^{-2}
11*	30	10	30	30	+0.5000	0.7293×10^{-2}
12	29	11	31	29	+0.4230	0.1925×10^{-1}
13	28	12	32	28	+0.3425	0.4215×10^{-1}
14	27	13	33	27	+0.2591	0.7704×10^{-1}
15	26	14	34	26	+0.1736	0.1180
16	25	15	35	25	+0.0870	0.1519
17	24	16	36	24	0.0000	0.1648
18	23	17	37	23	−0.0864	0.1510
19	22	18	38	22	−0.1712	0.1167
20	21	19	39	21	−0.2538	0.7626×10^{-1}
21	20	20	40	20	−0.3333	0.4204×10^{-1}
22	19	21	41	19	−0.4092	0.1953×10^{-1}
23	18	22	42	18	−0.4808	0.7630×10^{-2}
24	17	23	43	17	−0.5477	0.2500×10^{-2}
25	16	24	44	16	−0.6098	0.6841×10^{-3}
26	15	25	45	15	−0.6667	0.1557×10^{-3}
27	14	26	46	14	−0.7184	0.2928×10^{-4}
28	13	27	47	13	−0.7650	0.4523×10^{-5}
29	12	28	48	12	−0.8065	0.5687×10^{-6}
30	11	29	49	11	−0.8431	0.5763×10^{-7}
31	10	30	50	10	−0.8750	0.4649×10^{-8}
32	9	31	51	9	−0.9025	0.2941×10^{-9}
33	8	32	52	8	−0.9259	0.1431×10^{-10}
34	7	33	53	7	−0.9455	0.5238×10^{-12}
35	6	34	54	6	−0.9615	0.1398×10^{-13}
36	5	35	55	5	−0.9744	0.2614×10^{-15}
37	4	36	56	4	−0.9843	0.3242×10^{-17}
38	3	37	57	3	−0.9915	0.2460×10^{-19}
39	2	38	58	2	−0.9964	0.1327×10^{-20}
40	1	39	59	1	−0.9991	0.1746×10^{-24}
41	0	40	60	0	−1.0000	0.7275×10^{-28}
Sum						1.0000

greater. Based on the hypergeometric probability distribution, the exact upper-tail probability value is

$$P = 0.3049\times10^{-12} + 0.2323\times10^{-12} + 0.8032\times10^{-09} + 0.1681\times10$$
$$+ 0.2397\times10^{-06} + 0.2485\times10^{-05} + 0.1409\times10^{-04} + 0.1194\times10^{-03}$$
$$+ 0.5803\times10^{-03} + 0.2277\times10^{-02} + 0.7293\times10^{-02} = 0.0103\ .$$

9.6 Yule's *Y* Measure of Association

In the same 1912 paper, "On the methods of measuring association between two attributes," in which Q was first presented, Yule introduced a second measure of association for 2×2 contingency tables [53, p. 591]. Yule termed the new measure the "coefficient of colligation" and identified it by the lowercase Greek letter omega, ω, although it is customarily labeled as Yule's Y in the current literature.[11] The same acrimonious exchange between Yule, on the one hand, and Pearson and Heron, on the other, continued with the introduction of Y, based largely on the proper approach to analyzing variables versus attributes.

Given the notation for a 2×2 contingency table in Table 9.18, Yule's coefficient of colligation is given by

$$Y = \frac{\sqrt{ad} - \sqrt{bc}}{\sqrt{ad} + \sqrt{bc}}\ .$$

An advantage, noted by Yule, was that, unlike Q, Y could be directly compared with Pearson's product-moment correlation coefficient [53, p. 631].[12]

To illustrate the calculation of Yule's Y measure of association, consider the frequency data given in Table 9.19 with $N = 15$ observations where the observed

Table 9.18 Notation for variables x and y with categories dummy-coded 0 and 1

	y		
x	0	1	Total
0	a	b	$a+b$
1	c	d	$c+d$
Total	$a+c$	$b+d$	N

[11]It should be noted that R.H. Hooker, in his discussion of Yule's paper, took exception to the term "colligation," suggesting that Yule simply call his new coefficient the "coefficient of association" [27].

[12]If N is even and each marginal frequency total is equal to $N/2$, then Yule's Y and Pearson's product-moment correlation coefficient are equivalent.

Table 9.19 Example data for variables x and y with categories dummy-coded 0 and 1

	y		
x	0	1	Total
0	6	2	8
1	3	4	7
Total	9	6	15

Table 9.20 Cell frequencies, Y values, and exact hypergeometric point probability values for $M = 7$ possible arrangements of the observed data in Table 9.19

	Cell frequency					
Table	n_{11}	n_{12}	n_{21}	n_{22}	Yule's Y	Probability
1	2	6	7	0	−1.0000	0.5594×10^{-2}
2	3	5	6	1	−0.5195	0.7832×10^{-1}
3	4	4	5	2	−0.2251	0.2937
4	5	3	4	3	+0.0557	0.3916
5*	6	2	3	4	+0.3333	0.1958
6*	7	1	2	5	+0.6141	0.3357×10^{-1}
7*	8	0	1	6	+1.0000	0.1394×10^{-2}
Sum						1.0000

value of Yule's coefficient of colligation is

$$Y = \frac{\sqrt{(6)(4)} - \sqrt{(2)(3)}}{\sqrt{(6)(4)} + \sqrt{(2)(3)}} = \frac{2.4495}{7.3485} = +0.3333 \; .$$

For the frequency data given in Table 9.19, there are only

$$M = \min(a + b, a + c) - \max(0, a - d) + 1$$
$$= \min(8, 9) - \max(0, 6 - 4) + 1 = 8 - 2 + 1 = 7$$

possible, equally-likely arrangements in the reference set of all permutations of cell frequencies given the observed row and column marginal frequency distributions, $\{8, 7\}$ and $\{9, 6\}$, respectively, making an exact permutation analysis feasible. Since $M = 7$ is a very small number of arrangements, it will be illustrative to list the seven sets of cell frequencies, Yule's Y coefficients, and the associated hypergeometric point probability values in Table 9.20, where the rows with hypergeometric point probability values associated with Y values equal to or greater than the observed Y value are indicated with asterisks.

If the $M = 7$ possible arrangements in the reference set of all permutations of the frequency data given in Table 9.19 occur with equal chance, the exact probability value of Y under the null hypothesis is the sum of the hypergeometric point probability values associated with $Y = +0.3333$ or greater. Based on the hypergeometric probability distribution, the exact upper-tail probability value is

$$P = 0.1958 + 0.3357\times10^{-1} + 0.1394\times10^{-2} = 0.2308 \; .$$

In contrast to Yule's Y, for the frequency data given in Table 9.19, Yule's Q is

$$Q = \frac{ad - bc}{ad + bc} = \frac{(6)(4) - (2)(3)}{(6)(4) + (2)(3)} = \frac{18}{30} = +0.60 \, .$$

The relationships between Q and Y are given by

$$Q = \frac{2Y}{1 + Y^2} \quad \text{and} \quad Y = \frac{Q}{1 + \sqrt{1 - Q^2}} \, .$$

Thus, for the frequency data given in Table 9.19,

$$Q = \frac{2(0.3333)}{1 + 0.3333^2} = +0.60 \quad \text{and} \quad Y = \frac{0.60}{1 + \sqrt{1 - 0.60^2}} = +0.3333 \, .$$

9.7 The Odds Ratio

While useful by itself, the odds ratio has become an important component of medical research as well as more advanced statistical techniques.[13] The natural log (ln) of the odds ratio plays an important role in, for example, both logistic regression and log-linear analysis. Importantly, the odds ratio constitutes a measure of effect size unaffected by the proportional increases or decreases of the marginal frequency totals, e.g., doubling all the cell frequencies does not affect the value of the odds ratio [4, pp. 311–312].

In terms of the pairwise notation of Kendall, the odds ratio may be written as

$$\varphi = \frac{C}{D} \, ,$$

where C and D denote the number of concordant and discordant pairs, respectively.[14] More conventionally, given the notation of Table 9.15 on p. 533, the odds ratio is given by

$$\varphi = \frac{ad}{bc} \, .$$

To illustrate the calculation of the odds ratio, consider the frequency data given in Table 9.21 with $N = 18$ observations, where the observed value of the odds ratio is

$$\varphi = \frac{(7)(6)}{(2)(3)} = 7.00 \, ,$$

[13]The odds ratio is sometimes referred to as the "cross-product ratio."

[14]There appears to be no standardized symbol for indicating the odds ratio; in this section, φ is used to represent the odds ratio.

Table 9.21 Example data for variables x and y with categories dummy-coded 0 and 1

	y		
x	0	1	Total
0	7	2	9
1	3	6	9
Total	10	8	18

Table 9.22 Cell frequencies, odds ratios, and exact hypergeometric point probability values for $M = 7$ possible arrangements of the observed data in Table 9.21

	Cell frequency					
Table	n_{11}	n_{12}	n_{21}	n_{22}	Odds ratio	Probability
1	1	8	9	0	0.0000	0.2057×10^{-3}
2	2	7	8	1	0.0357	0.7404×10^{-2}
3	3	6	7	2	0.1429	0.6911×10^{-1}
4	4	5	6	3	0.4000	0.2419
5	5	4	5	4	1.0000	0.3628
6	6	3	4	5	2.5000	0.2410
7*	7	2	3	6	7.0000	0.6911×10^{-1}
8*	8	1	2	7	28.0000	0.7404×10^{-2}
9*	9	0	1	8	∞	0.2057×10^{-3}
Sum						1.0000

indicating that a subject classified as y_0 is 7 times as likely to be classified as x_0 as a subject classified as y_1. For the frequency data given in Table 9.21, there are only

$$M = \min(a+b, a+c) - \max(0, a-d) + 1$$
$$= \min(9, 10) - \max(0, 7-6) + 1 = 9 - 1 + 1 = 9$$

possible, equally-likely arrangements in the reference set of all permutations of cell frequencies given the observed row and column marginal frequency distributions, $\{9, 9\}$ and $\{10, 8\}$, respectively, making an exact permutation analysis feasible. Since $M = 9$ is a small number of arrangements, it will be illustrative to list the nine sets of cell frequencies, odds ratios, and the associated hypergeometric point probability values in Table 9.22, where the rows with hypergeometric point probability values associated with odds ratios equal to or greater than the observed odds ratio are indicated with asterisks.

If the $M = 9$ possible arrangements in the reference set of all permutations of the frequency data given in Table 9.21 occur with equal chance, the exact probability value of φ under the null hypothesis is the sum of the hypergeometric point probability values associated with $\varphi = 7.00$ or greater. Based on the hypergeometric probability distribution, the exact upper-tail probability value is

$$P = 0.6911\times 10^{-1} + 0.7404\times 10^{-2} + 0.2057\times 10^{-3} = 0.0767\ .$$

In contrast to the odds ratio, for the frequency data given in Table 9.21, Yule's Q is

$$Q = \frac{ad - bc}{ad + bc} = \frac{(7)(6) - (2)(3)}{(7)(6) + (2)(3)} = +0.75$$

and Yule's Y is

$$Y = \frac{\sqrt{ad} - \sqrt{bc}}{\sqrt{ad} + \sqrt{bc}} = \frac{\sqrt{(7)(6)} - \sqrt{(2)(3)}}{\sqrt{(7)(6)} + \sqrt{(2)(3)}} = +0.4514 \, .$$

The relationships between φ and Q are given by

$$\varphi = \frac{1 + Q}{1 - Q} \quad \text{and} \quad Q = \frac{\varphi - 1}{\varphi + 1} \, .$$

Thus, for the frequency data given in Table 9.21,

$$\varphi = \frac{1 + 0.75}{1 - 0.75} = 7.00 \quad \text{and} \quad Q = \frac{7.00 - 1}{7.00 + 1} = +0.75 \, .$$

The relationships between φ and Y are given by

$$\varphi = \frac{(Y + 1)^2}{(Y - 1)^2} \quad \text{and} \quad Y = \frac{\sqrt{\varphi} - 1}{\sqrt{\varphi} + 1} \, .$$

Thus, for the frequency data given in Table 9.21,

$$\varphi = \frac{(0.4514 + 1)^2}{(0.4514 - 1)^2} = 7.00 \quad \text{and} \quad Y = \frac{\sqrt{7.00} - 1}{\sqrt{7.00} + 1} = +0.4514 \, .$$

9.8 Goodman–Kruskal's t_a and t_b Measures

In 1954 Leo Goodman and William Kruskal published the first of four formative articles on measures of association for cross-classifications [23]. In this lead article Goodman and Kruskal introduced new asymmetric measures of association for two nominal-level variables that they called t_a for when variable a is the dependent variable and t_b for when variable b is the dependent variable. See Chap. 4, Sect. 4.3 for a more detailed description of Goodman and Kruskal's t_a and t_b measures of association.

A convenient calculation form for Goodman and Kruskal's t_a is given by

$$t_a = \frac{N \displaystyle\sum_{i=1}^{r} \sum_{j=1}^{c} \frac{n_{ij}^2}{n_{i.}} - \sum_{j=1}^{c} n_{.j}^2}{N^2 - \displaystyle\sum_{j=1}^{c} n_{.j}^2} , \tag{9.7}$$

where $n_{i.}$ denotes a marginal frequency total for the ith row, $i = 1, \ldots, r$, summed over all columns, $n_{.j}$ denotes a marginal frequency total for the jth column, $j = 1, \ldots, c$, summed over all rows, and n_{ij} denotes an observed cell frequency, $i = 1, \ldots, r$ and $j = 1, \ldots, c$. Thus,

$$n_{i.} = \sum_{j=1}^{c} n_{ij} , \quad n_{.j} = \sum_{i=1}^{r} n_{ij} , \quad \text{and} \quad N = \sum_{i=1}^{r} \sum_{j=1}^{c} n_{ij} .$$

As Goodman and Kruskal noted, it is clear that t_a takes values between 0 and 1; it is 0 if and only if a and b are independent, and 1 if and only if knowledge of variable b completely determines variable a [23, p. 760].

9.8.1 Example with Goodman and Kruskal's t_a

To illustrate the calculation of Goodman and Kruskal's t_a, consider the frequency data given in Table 9.23, where, following Eq. (9.7), the observed value of t_a is

$$t_a = \frac{N \displaystyle\sum_{i=1}^{r} \sum_{j=1}^{c} \frac{n_{ij}^2}{n_{i.}} - \sum_{j=1}^{c} n_{.j}^2}{N^2 - \displaystyle\sum_{j=1}^{c} n_{.j}^2}$$

$$= \frac{20 \left(\dfrac{8^2}{12} + \dfrac{4^2}{12} + \dfrac{2^2}{8} + \dfrac{6^2}{8} \right) - 10^2 - 10^2}{20^2 - 10^2 - 10^2} = 0.1667 ,$$

Table 9.23 Example data for variables a and b with categories dummy-coded 0 and 1

	a		
b	0	1	Total
0	8	4	12
1	2	6	8
Total	10	10	20

Table 9.24 Cell frequencies, t_a values, and exact hypergeometric point probability values for $M = 7$ possible arrangements of the observed data in Table 9.23

	Cell frequency					
Table	n_{11}	n_{12}	n_{21}	n_{22}	G–K t_a	Probability
1*	2	10	8	0	0.6667	0.3572×10^{-3}
2*	3	9	7	1	0.3750	0.9526×10^{-2}
3*	4	8	6	2	0.1667	0.7502×10^{-1}
4	5	7	5	3	0.0417	0.2401
5	6	6	4	4	0.0000	0.3500
6	7	5	3	5	0.0417	0.2401
7*	8	4	2	6	0.1667	0.7502×10^{-1}
8*	9	3	1	7	0.3750	0.9526×10^{-2}
9*	10	2	0	8	0.6667	0.3572×10^{-3}
Sum						1.0000

indicating an approximately 17% reduction in the number of prediction errors, given knowledge of the distribution of independent variable b over knowledge of the distribution of dependent variable a only.

For the frequency data given in Table 9.23, there are only

$$M = \min(a+b, a+c) - \max(0, a-d) + 1$$
$$= \min(12, 10) - \max(0, 8-6) + 1 = 10 - 2 + 1 = 9$$

possible, equally-likely arrangements in the reference set of all permutations of cell frequencies given the observed row and column marginal frequency distributions, $\{12, 8\}$ and $\{10, 10\}$, respectively, making an exact permutation analysis feasible. Since $M = 9$ is a very small number of arrangements, it will be illustrative to list the nine sets of cell frequencies, t_a values, and the associated hypergeometric point probability values in Table 9.24, where the rows with hypergeometric probability values associated with t_a values equal to or greater than the observed t_a value are indicated with asterisks.

If the $M = 9$ possible arrangements in the reference set of all permutations of the frequency data given in Table 9.23 occur with equal chance, the exact probability value of t_a under the null hypothesis is the sum of the hypergeometric point probability values associated with $t_a = 0.1667$ or greater. The hypergeometric point probability values associated with τ_b values equal to or greater than the observed τ_b value are indicated with asterisks in Table 9.24. Because the column marginals are evenly divided at $N/2 = 20/2$, i.e., $\{10, 10\}$, the discrete permutation distribution is symmetrical and the exact two-sided probability value is

$$P = 2\big(0.3572\times 10^{-3} + 0.9526\times 10^{-2} + 0.7502\times 10^{-1}\big) = 0.1698\ .$$

9.8.2 Example with Goodman and Kruskal's t_b

For 2×2 contingency tables, Goodman and Kruskal's t_a and t_b yield identical values. Thus, for the frequency data given in Table 9.23,

$$t_b = \frac{N \displaystyle\sum_{i=1}^{r} \sum_{j=1}^{c} \frac{n_{ij}^2}{n_{.j}} - \sum_{i=1}^{r} n_{i.}^2}{N^2 - \displaystyle\sum_{i=1}^{r} n_{i.}^2}$$

$$= \frac{20\left(\dfrac{8^2}{10} + \dfrac{4^2}{10} + \dfrac{2^2}{10} + \dfrac{6^2}{10}\right) - 12^2 - 8^2}{20^2 - 12^2 - 8^2} = 0.1667 ,$$

indicating an approximately 17% reduction in the number of prediction errors, given knowledge of the distribution of independent variable a over knowledge of the distribution of dependent variable b only.

If the

$$M = \min(a + b, a + c) - \max(0, a - d) + 1$$
$$= \min(12, 10) - \max(0, 8 - 6) + 1 = 10 - 2 + 1 = 9$$

possible, equally-likely arrangements in the reference set of all permutations of the frequency data given in Table 9.23 occur with equal chance, the exact probability value of t_b under the null hypothesis is the sum of the hypergeometric point probability values associated with $t_b = 0.1667$ or greater. Based on the hypergeometric probability distribution, the exact two-sided probability value is

$$P = 2\left(0.3572\times10^{-3} + 0.9526\times10^{-2} + 0.7502\times10^{-1}\right) = 0.1698 .$$

9.8.3 Goodman–Kruskal's t_a, t_b, and χ^2

Some interesting simplifications occur for Goodman and Kruskal's t_a and t_b test statistics, on the one hand, and χ^2, on the other hand, when $r = c = 2$, i.e., fourfold contingency tables,

$$t_a = t_b = \frac{\chi^2}{N} = \phi^2 = r_{xy}^2 .$$

For the frequency data given in Table 9.23, $t_a = t_b = 0.1667$ and $\chi^2 = 3.3333$. Thus,

$$t_a = t_b = \frac{\chi^2}{N} = \frac{3.3333}{20} = 0.1667 \; .$$

It is well known that χ^2/N is equal to Pearson's ϕ^2, which is equal to Pearson's r_{xy}^2 when the two categories of variables x and y are dummy-coded 0 and 1. Thus,

$$t_a = t_b = \frac{\chi^2}{N} = \phi^2 = r_{xy}^2 = 0.1667$$

for a 2×2 contingency table.

9.9 Somers' d_{yx} and d_{xy} Measures

In 1962 Robert Somers published a brief article titled "On the measurement of association" in *American Sociological Review*.[15] Somers proposed two new asymmetric measures of ordinal association that he labeled d_{yx}, with variable y the dependent variable, and d_{xy}, with variable x the dependent variable. See Chap. 5, Sect. 5.7 for a more detailed description of Somers' d_{yx} and d_{xy} measures of association.

Given the notation in Table 9.25, Somers' d_{yx} measure is given by

$$d_{yx} = \frac{C - D}{C + D + T_y} = \frac{S}{C + D + T_y} \; ,$$

where C denotes the number of concordant pairs, D denotes the number of discordant pairs, T_y denotes the number of pairs tied on variable y that are not tied on variable x, and S is Kendall's test statistic. Given the notation in Table 9.25,

$$C = ad \; , \quad D = bc \; , \quad \text{and} \quad T_y = ac + bd \; .$$

Table 9.25 Notation for variables x and y with categories dummy-coded 0 and 1

	y		
x	0	1	Total
0	a	b	$a+b$
1	c	d	$c+d$
Total	$a+c$	$b+d$	N

[15] In a number of articles and textbooks, Somers' last name is misspelled as "Sommers" [30, 38, p. 223]

9.9.1 Example with Somers' d_{yx}

To illustrate the calculation of Somers' d_{yx} measure of association, consider the frequency data given in Table 9.26 with $N = 30$ observations, where the observed value of Somers' d_{yx} is

$$d_{yx} = \frac{C - D}{C + D + T_y} = \frac{ad - bc}{ad + bc + ac + bd} = \frac{ad - bc}{(a + b)(c + d)}$$
$$= \frac{(12)(7) - (8)(3)}{(12 + 8)(3 + 7)} = +0.30 \; .$$

For the frequency data given in Table 9.26, there are only

$$M = \min(a + b, a + c) - \max(0, a - d) + 1$$
$$= \min(20, 15) - \max(0, 12 - 7) + 1 = 15 - 5 + 1 = 11$$

possible, equally-likely arrangements in the reference set of all permutations of cell frequencies given the observed row and column marginal frequency distributions, {20, 10} and {15, 15}, respectively, making an exact permutation analysis feasible. Since $M = 11$ is a small number of arrangements, it will be illustrative to list the 11 sets of cell frequencies, d_{yx} values, and the associated hypergeometric point probability values in Table 9.27, where the rows with hypergeometric point probability values associated with d_{yx} values equal to or greater than the observed d_{yx} value are indicated with asterisks.

If the $M = 11$ possible arrangements in the reference set of all permutations of the frequency data given in Table 9.26 occur with equal chance, the exact probability value of d_{yx} under the null hypothesis is the sum of the hypergeometric point probability values associated with $d_{yx} = +0.30$ or greater. Based on the hypergeometric probability distribution, the exact upper-tail probability value is

$$P = 0.9745 \times 10^{-1} + 0.2249 \times 10^{-1} + 0.2499 \times 10^{-2}$$
$$+ 0.9995 \times 10^{-4} = 0.1225 \; .$$

Table 9.26 Example data for variables x and y with categories dummy-coded 0 and 1

	y		
x	0	1	Total
0	12	8	20
1	3	7	10
Total	15	15	30

Table 9.27 Cell frequencies, d_{yx} values, and exact hypergeometric point probability values for $M = 11$ possible arrangements of the observed data in Table 9.26

	Cell frequency					
Table	n_{11}	n_{12}	n_{21}	n_{22}	d_{yx}	Probability
1	5	15	10	0	−0.75	0.9995×10^{-4}
2	6	14	9	1	−0.60	0.2499×10^{-2}
3	7	13	8	2	−0.45	0.2249×10^{-1}
4	8	12	7	3	−0.30	0.9745×10^{-1}
5	9	11	6	4	−0.15	0.2274
6	10	10	5	5	0.00	0.3001
7	11	9	4	6	+0.15	0.2274
8*	12	8	3	7	+0.30	0.9745×10^{-1}
9*	13	7	2	8	+0.45	0.2249×10^{-1}
10*	14	6	1	9	+0.60	0.2499×10^{-2}
11*	15	5	0	10	+0.75	0.9995×10^{-4}
Sum						1.0000

9.9.2 Example with Somers' d_{xy}

Somers' asymmetric measure of ordinal association with variable x considered to be the dependent variable is given by

$$d_{xy} = \frac{C - D}{C + D + T_x} = \frac{S}{C + D + T_x} ,$$

where C denotes the number of concordant pairs, D denotes the number of discordant pairs, T_x denotes the number of pairs tied on variable x that are not tied on variable y, and S is Kendall's test statistic. Given the notation in Table 9.25 on p. 544,

$$C = ad \; , \quad D = bc \; , \quad \text{and} \quad T_x = ab + cd \; .$$

To illustrate the calculation of Somers' d_{xy}, consider once again the frequency data given in Table 9.26, where the observed value of Somers' d_{xy} is

$$d_{xy} = \frac{C - D}{C + D + T_x} = \frac{ad - bc}{ad + bc + ab + cd} = \frac{ad - bc}{(a + c)(b + d)}$$
$$= \frac{(12)(7) - (8)(3)}{(12 + 3)(8 + 7)} = +0.2667 \; .$$

For the frequency data given in Table 9.26, there are only

$$M = \min(a+b, a+c) - \max(0, a-d) + 1$$
$$= \min(20, 15) - \max(0, 12-7) + 1 = 15 - 5 + 1 = 11$$

possible, equally-likely arrangements in the reference set of all permutations of cell frequencies given the observed row and column marginal frequency distributions, {20, 10} and {15, 15}, respectively, making an exact permutation analysis feasible. Since $M = 11$ is a small number of arrangements, it will be illustrative to list the 11 sets of cell frequencies, d_{xy} values, and the associated hypergeometric point probability values in Table 9.28, where the rows with hypergeometric point probability values associated with d_{xy} values equal to or greater than the observed d_{xy} value are indicated with asterisks.

If the $M = 11$ possible arrangements in the reference set of all permutations of cell frequencies in Table 9.26 occur with equal chance, the exact probability value of d_{xy} under the null hypothesis is the sum of the hypergeometric point probability values associated with $d_{xy} = +0.2667$ or greater. Based on the hypergeometric probability distribution, the exact upper-tail probability value is

$$P = 0.9745\times10^{-1} + 0.2249\times10^{-1} + 0.2499\times10^{-2} + 0.9995\times10^{-4} = 0.1225 .$$

Table 9.28 Cell frequencies, d_{xy} values, and exact hypergeometric point probability values for $M = 11$ possible arrangements of the observed data in Table 9.26

	Cell frequency					
Table	n_{11}	n_{12}	n_{21}	n_{22}	d_{xy}	Probability
1	5	15	10	0	−0.6667	0.9995×10^{-4}
2	6	14	9	1	−0.5333	0.2499×10^{-2}
3	7	13	8	2	−0.4000	0.2249×10^{-1}
4	8	12	7	3	−0.2667	0.9745×10^{-1}
5	9	11	6	4	−0.1333	0.2274
6	10	10	5	5	0.0000	0.3001
7	11	9	4	6	+0.1333	0.2274
8*	12	8	3	7	+0.2667	0.9745×10^{-1}
9*	13	7	2	8	+0.4000	0.2249×10^{-1}
10*	14	6	1	9	+0.5333	0.2499×10^{-2}
11*	15	5	0	10	+0.6667	0.9995×10^{-4}
Sum						1.0000

9.10 Percentage Differences

Simple percentage differences are commonly used by the mass media to contrast two groups in a simple-to-understand manner. However, percentage differences are more sophisticated than is immediately apparent. Consider the frequency data given in Table 9.29 and also consider Table 9.30 where the cell entries in Table 9.30 are expressed as proportions of the column marginal frequency totals. For the proportion data given in Table 9.30, the percentage difference for variable y is

$$D_y = |0.72 - 0.48| = |0.28 - 0.52| = 0.24 \ .$$

There are only

$$\begin{aligned} M &= \min(a+b, a+c) - \max(0, a-d) + 1 \\ &= \min(30, 25) - \max(0, 18-13) + 1 = 25 - 5 + 1 = 21 \end{aligned}$$

possible, equally-likely arrangements in the reference set of all permutations of cell frequencies in Table 9.29 given the observed row and column marginal frequency distributions, $\{30, 20\}$ and $\{25, 25\}$, respectively, making an exact permutation analysis feasible. Since $M = 21$ is a reasonably small number of arrangements, it will be illustrative to list the 21 sets of cell frequencies, the D_y values, and the associated hypergeometric point probability values in Table 9.31, where the rows with hypergeometric point probability values associated with D_y values equal to or greater than the observed D_y value are indicated with asterisks.

If the $M = 21$ possible arrangements in the reference set of all permutations of the frequency data given in Table 9.29 occur with equal chance, the exact probability value of D_y under the null hypothesis is the sum of the hypergeometric point probability values associated with $D_y = 0.24$ or greater. Because the column marginals are evenly divided at $N/2 = 50/2$, i.e., $\{25, 25\}$, the discrete permutation

Table 9.29 Example data for variables x and y with categories dummy-coded 0 and 1

	y		
x	0	1	Total
0	18	12	30
1	7	13	20
Total	25	25	50

Table 9.30 Example data from Table 9.29 with cell entries expressed as proportions of the column marginal frequency totals

	y	
x	0	1
0	0.72	0.48
1	0.28	0.52
Total	1.00	1.00

Table 9.31 Cell frequencies, D_y values, and exact hypergeometric point probability values for $M = 21$ possible arrangements of the observed data in Table 9.29

	Cell frequency					
Table	n_{11}	n_{12}	n_{21}	n_{22}	D_y	Probability
1*	5	25	20	0	0.80	0.1127×10^{-8}
2*	6	24	19	1	0.72	0.9394×10^{-7}
3*	7	23	18	2	0.64	0.3060×10^{-6}
4*	8	22	17	3	0.56	0.5278×10^{-4}
5*	9	21	16	4	0.48	0.5484×10^{-3}
6*	10	20	15	5	0.40	0.3685×10^{-2}
7*	11	19	14	6	0.32	0.1675×10^{-1}
8*	12	18	13	7	0.24	0.5304×10^{-1}
9	13	17	12	8	0.16	0.1193
10	14	16	11	9	0.08	0.1932
11	15	15	10	10	0.00	0.2267
12	16	14	9	11	0.08	0.1932
13	17	13	8	12	0.16	0.1193
14*	18	12	7	13	0.24	0.5304×10^{-1}
15*	19	11	6	14	0.32	0.1675×10^{-1}
16*	20	10	5	15	0.40	0.3685×10^{-2}
17*	21	9	4	16	0.48	0.5484×10^{-3}
18*	22	8	3	17	0.56	0.5278×10^{-4}
19*	23	7	2	18	0.64	0.3060×10^{-6}
20*	24	6	1	19	0.72	0.9394×10^{-7}
21*	25	5	0	20	0.80	0.1127×10^{-8}
Sum						1.0000

Table 9.32 Example data from Table 9.29 with cell entries expressed as proportions of the row marginal frequency totals

	y		
x	0	1	Total
0	0.60	0.40	1.00
1	0.35	0.65	1.00

distribution is symmetrical and, based on the hypergeometric probability distribution, the exact two-sided probability value is

$$P = 2\big(0.5304\times10^{-1} + 0.1675\times10^{-1} + 0.3685\times10^{-2} + 0.5484\times10^{-3} + 0.5278\times10^{-4} + 0.3060\times10^{-6} + 0.9394\times10^{-7} + 0.1127\times10^{-8}\big) = 2(0.0741) = 0.1482\ .$$

Percentage differences are asymmetric measures. For the proportions based on the row marginal frequency totals given in Table 9.32, the percentage difference for variable x is

$$D_x = |0.60 - 0.35| = |0.40 - 0.65| = 0.25\ .$$

There are only

$$M = \min(a+b, a+c) - \max(0, a-d) + 1$$
$$= \min(30, 25) - \max(0, 18-13) + 1 = 25 - 5 + 1 = 21$$

possible, equally-likely arrangements in the reference set of all permutations of cell frequencies in Table 9.29 given the observed row and column marginal frequency distributions, $\{30, 20\}$ and $\{25, 25\}$, respectively, making an exact permutation analysis feasible. Since $M = 21$ is a reasonably small number of arrangements, it will be illustrative to list the 21 sets of cell frequencies, the D_x values, and the associated hypergeometric point probability values in Table 9.33, where the rows with hypergeometric point probability values associated with D_x values equal to or greater than the observed D_x value are indicated with asterisks.

If the $M = 21$ possible arrangements of the frequency data given in Table 9.29 occur with equal chance, the exact probability value of D_x under the null hypothesis is the sum of the hypergeometric point probability values associated with $D_x =$ 0.25 or greater. Because the column marginals are evenly divided as $N/2 = 50/2$, i.e., $\{25, 25\}$, the discrete permutation distribution is symmetrical and, based on the

Table 9.33 Cell frequencies, D_x values, and exact hypergeometric point probability values for $M = 21$ possible arrangements of the observed data in Table 9.29

	Cell frequency					
Table	n_{11}	n_{12}	n_{21}	n_{22}	D_x	Probability
1∗	5	25	20	0	0.8333	0.1127×10^{-8}
2∗	6	24	19	1	0.7500	0.9394×10^{-7}
3∗	7	23	18	2	0.6667	0.3060×10^{-6}
4∗	8	22	17	3	0.5833	0.5278×10^{-4}
5∗	9	21	16	4	0.5000	0.5484×10^{-3}
6∗	10	20	15	5	0.4167	0.3685×10^{-2}
7∗	11	19	14	6	0.3333	0.1675×10^{-1}
8∗	12	18	13	7	0.2500	0.5304×10^{-1}
9	13	17	12	8	0.1667	0.1193
10	14	16	11	9	0.0833	0.1932
11	15	15	10	10	0.00	0.2267
12	16	14	9	11	0.0833	0.1932
13	17	13	8	12	0.1667	0.1193
14∗	18	12	7	13	0.2500	0.5304×10^{-1}
15∗	19	11	6	14	0.3333	0.1675×10^{-1}
16∗	20	10	5	15	0.4167	0.3685×10^{-2}
17∗	21	9	4	16	0.5000	0.5484×10^{-3}
18∗	22	8	3	17	0.5833	0.5278×10^{-4}
19∗	23	7	2	18	0.6667	0.3060×10^{-6}
20∗	24	6	1	19	0.7500	0.9394×10^{-7}
21∗	25	5	0	20	0.8333	0.1127×10^{-8}
Sum						1.0000

hypergeometric probability distribution, the exact two-sided probability value is

$$\begin{aligned}P &= 2\big(0.5304\times10^{-1} + 0.1675\times10^{-1} + 0.3685\times10^{-2} + 0.5484\times10^{-3} \\ &\quad + 0.5278\times10^{-4} + 0.3060\times10^{-6} + 0.9394\times10^{-7} + 0.1127\times10^{-8}\big) \\ &= 2(0.0741) = 0.1482\ .\end{aligned}$$

For comparison, given the frequency data given in Table 9.29, Somers' d_{xy} is

$$\begin{aligned}d_{xy} &= \frac{C - D}{C + D + T_x} = \frac{ad - bc}{ad + bc + ab + cd} = \frac{ad - bc}{(a + c)(b + d)} \\ &= \frac{(18)(13) - (12)(7)}{(18 + 7)(12 + 13)} = \frac{150}{625} = 0.24\end{aligned}$$

and Somers' d_{yx} is

$$\begin{aligned}d_{yx} &= \frac{C - D}{C + D + T_y} = \frac{ad - bc}{ad + bc + ac + bd} = \frac{ad - bc}{(a + b)(c + d)} \\ &= \frac{(18)(13) - (12)(7)}{(18 + 12)(7 + 13)} = \frac{150}{600} = 0.25\ ,\end{aligned}$$

demonstrating the equivalency between Somers' d_{xy} and d_{yx} and corresponding percentage differences, D_y and D_x, for 2×2 contingency tables [50].

It is easily demonstrated that, say, Somers' d_{yx} and the corresponding percentage difference are equivalent. Given the notation in Table 9.25 on p. 544, the percentage difference is

$$D_x = \frac{a}{a + b} - \frac{c}{c + d} = \frac{18}{30} - \frac{7}{20} = 0.25\ .$$

Now,

$$D_x = \frac{a}{a + b} - \frac{c}{c + d} = \frac{ad - bc}{(a + b)(c + d)} = \frac{ad - bc}{ad + bc + ac + bd}\ .$$

Then, substituting $C = ad$, $D = bc$, and $T_y = ac + bd$, yields

$$D_x = \frac{C - D}{C + D + T_y} = d_{yx}\ .$$

9.11 Kendall's τ_b Measure of Ordinal Association

In 1948 Maurice Kendall introduced a strongly monotonic measure of ordinal association given by

$$\tau_b = \frac{C - D}{\sqrt{(C + D + T_x)(C + D + T_y)}} ,$$

where C denotes the number of concordant pairs, D denotes the number of discordant pairs, T_x denotes the number of pairs tied on variable x but not tied on variable y, and T_y denotes the number of pairs tied on variable y but not tied on variable x [33, p. 35]. See Chap. 5, Sect. 5.4 for a more detailed description of Kendall's τ_b measure of association.

Given the notation in Table 9.34 for a 2×2 contingency table, the number of concordant pairs is $C = ad$, the number of discordant pairs is $D = bc$, the number of pairs tied on variable x is $T_x = ab+cd$, and the number of pairs tied on variable y is $T_y = ac + bd$. To illustrate the calculation of Kendall's τ_b for a 2×2 contingency table, consider the frequency data given in Table 9.35, where

$$C = ad = (16)(8) = 128 ,$$

$$D = bc = (4)(8) = 32 ,$$

$$T_x = ab + cd = (16)(4) + (8)(8) = 128 ,$$

$$T_y = ac + bd = (16)(8) + (4)(8) = 160 ,$$

and

$$\tau_b = \frac{C - D}{\sqrt{(C + D + T_x)(C + D + T_y)}}$$

$$= \frac{128 - 32}{\sqrt{(128 + 32 + 128)(128 + 32 + 160)}} = +0.3162 .$$

Table 9.34 Notation for variables x and y with categories dummy-coded 0 and 1

	y		
x	0	1	Total
0	a	b	$a+b$
1	c	d	$c+d$
Total	$a+c$	$b+d$	N

Table 9.35 Example data for variables x and y with categories dummy-coded 0 and 1

	y		
x	0	1	Total
0	16	4	20
1	8	8	16
Total	24	12	36

There are only

$$M = \min(a+b, a+c) - \max(0, a-d) + 1$$
$$= \min(20, 24) - \max(0, 16-8) + 1 = 20 - 8 + 1 = 13$$

possible, equally-likely arrangements in the reference set of all permutations of cell frequencies in Table 9.35 given the observed row and column marginal frequency distributions, {20, 16} and {24, 12}, respectively, making an exact permutation analysis feasible. Because $M = 13$ is a small number of arrangements, it will be illustrative to list the 13 sets of cell frequencies, τ_b values, and the associated hypergeometric point probability values in Table 9.36, where the rows with hypergeometric point probability values associated with τ_b values equal to or greater than the observed τ_b value are indicated with asterisks.

If the $M = 13$ possible arrangements in the reference set of all permutations of the frequency data in Table 9.35 occur with equal chance, the exact probability value of τ_b under the null hypothesis is the sum of the hypergeometric point probability values associated with $\tau_b = +0.3162$ or greater. Based on the hypergeometric probability distribution, the exact upper-tail probability value is

$$P = 0.4982\times10^{-1} + 0.1042\times10^{-1} + 0.1216\times10^{-2} + 0.6979\times10^{-4}$$
$$+ 0.1454\times10^{-5} = 0.0615\ .$$

Table 9.36 Cell frequencies, τ_b values, and exact hypergeometric point probability values for $M = 13$ possible arrangements of the observed data in Table 9.35

	Cell frequency					
Table	n_{11}	n_{12}	n_{21}	n_{22}	τ_b	Probability
1	8	12	16	0	−0.6325	0.1006×10^{-3}
2	9	11	15	1	−0.5139	0.2147×10^{-2}
3	10	10	14	2	−0.3953	0.1771×10^{-1}
4	11	9	13	3	−0.2767	0.7515×10^{-1}
5	12	8	12	4	−0.1581	0.1832
6	13	7	11	5	−0.0395	0.2705
7	14	6	10	6	+0.0791	0.2480
8	15	5	9	7	+0.1976	0.1417
9*	16	4	8	8	+0.3162	0.4982×10^{-1}
10*	17	3	7	9	+0.4348	0.1042×10^{-1}
11*	18	2	6	10	+0.5534	0.1216×10^{-2}
12*	19	1	5	11	+0.6720	0.6979×10^{-4}
13*	20	0	4	12	+0.7906	0.1454×10^{-5}
Sum						1.0000

For the frequency data given in Table 9.35, Somers' d_{xy} is

$$d_{xy} = \frac{C - D}{C + D + T_x} = \frac{ad - bc}{ad + bc + ab + cd} = \frac{ad - bc}{(a + c)(b + d)}$$
$$= \frac{(16)(8) - (4)(8)}{(16 + 8)(4 + 8)} = +0.3333 \,,$$

Somers' d_{yx} is

$$d_{yx} = \frac{C - D}{C + D + T_y} = \frac{ad - bc}{ad + bc + ac + bd} = \frac{ad - bc}{(a + b)(c + d)}$$
$$= \frac{(16)(8) - (4)(8)}{(16 + 4)(8 + 8)} = +0.30 \,,$$

and it is obvious that for 2×2 contingency tables, Kendall's τ_b measure of association is simply the geometric mean of Somers' two asymmetric measures, e.g.,

$$\tau_b = \sqrt{d_{xy} d_{yx}} = \sqrt{(0.3333)(0.30)} = \pm 0.3162 \,.$$

9.12 Kendall's τ_b and Pearson's r_{xy} Measures

It is readily apparent that Goodman and Kruskal's two asymmetric measures of ordinal association, t_a and t_b, are equal to each other for any 2×2 contingency table, and it is also well known that for a 2×2 contingency table both t_a and t_b are equal to χ^2/N, which, in turn, is equal to Pearson's ϕ^2 mean-squared contingency coefficient and Pearson's product-moment correlation coefficient r_{xy}^2 when two variables, x and y, are dummy-coded (0, 1) [41, pp. 75, 325]. Thus, for 2×2 contingency tables,

$$t_a = t_b = \frac{\chi^2}{N} = \phi^2 = r_{xy}^2 \quad \text{and} \quad \sqrt{t_a} = \sqrt{t_b} = \sqrt{\frac{\chi^2}{N}} = \pm\phi = \pm r_{xy} \,.$$

However, it is less well known that Kendall's τ_b measure of ordinal association is equivalent to Pearson's product-moment correlation coefficient, r_{xy}, for any 2×2 contingency table.

Table 9.37 Notation for the cross-classification of two categorical variables, X_i for $i = 1, \ldots, r$ and Y_j for $j = 1, \ldots, c$

	Y				
X	y_1	y_2	$\cdots$	y_c	Total
x_1	n_{11}	n_{12}	$\cdots$	n_{1c}	$n_{1.}$
x_2	n_{21}	n_{22}	$\cdots$	n_{2c}	$n_{2.}$
$\vdots$	$\vdots$	$\vdots$	$\ddots$	$\vdots$	$\vdots$
x_r	n_{r1}	n_{r2}	$\cdots$	n_{rc}	$n_{r.}$
Total	$n_{.1}$	$n_{.2}$	$\cdots$	$n_{.c}$	N

Kendall's τ_b measure of ordinal association is given by

$$\tau_b = \frac{C - D}{\sqrt{(C + D + T_x)(C + D + T_y)}} = \frac{S}{\sqrt{(C + D + T_x)(C + D + T_y)}} ,$$

where C denotes the number of concordant pairs, D denotes the number of discordant pairs, T_x denotes the number of pairs tied on variable x but not tied on variable y, and T_y denotes the number of pairs tied on variable y but not tied on variable x.

Consider an $r\times c$ contingency table such as depicted in Table 9.37, where categorical variables X and Y are cross-classified, n_{ij} denotes a cell frequency for $i = 1, \ldots, r$ and $j = 1, \ldots, c$, and N denotes the total of cell frequencies in the table. Denote by a dot $(\cdot)$ the partial sum of all rows or all columns, depending on the position of the $(\cdot)$ in the subscript list. If the $(\cdot)$ is in the first subscript position, the sum is over all rows, and if the $(\cdot)$ is in the second subscript position, the sum is over all columns. Thus, $n_{i.}$ denotes the marginal frequency total of the ith row, $i = 1, \ldots, r$, summed over all columns, and $n_{.j}$ denotes the marginal frequency total of the jth column, $j = 1, \ldots, c$, summed over all rows. It can easily be demonstrated that the following relationships hold:

$$C + D + T_x = \frac{1}{2}\left(N^2 - \sum_{j=1}^{c} n_{.j}^2\right) \tag{9.8}$$

and

$$C + D + T_y = \frac{1}{2}\left(N^2 - \sum_{i=1}^{r} n_{i.}^2\right) . \tag{9.9}$$

The importance of these relationships is that $C + D + T_x$ and $C + D + T_y$ are completely determined by the marginal frequency totals.[16]

[16]Equations (9.8) and (9.9) are not specific to 2×2 contingency tables and are applicable to any $r\times c$ contingency table.

Table 9.38 Notation for variables x and y, each with two categories

	y		
x	0	1	Total
0	a	b	$a+b$
1	c	d	$c+d$
Total	$a+c$	$b+d$	N

Now consider a 2×2 contingency table, such as given in Table 9.38. Then,

$$
\begin{aligned}
C &= ad\ ,\\
D &= bc\ ,\\
C+D+T_x &= \frac{1}{2}\Big[(a+b+c+d)^2-(a+c)^2-(b+d)^2\Big]\\
&= \frac{1}{2}\big(2ab+2ad+2bc+2cd\big)\\
&= ab+ad+bc+cd\\
&= (a+c)(b+d)\ ,
\end{aligned}
$$

$$
\begin{aligned}
C+D+T_y &= \frac{1}{2}\Big[(a+b+c+d)^2-(a+b)^2-(c+d)^2\Big]\\
&= \frac{1}{2}\big(2ac+2ad+2bc+2bd\big)\\
&= ac+ad+bc+bd\\
&= (a+b)(c+d)\ ,
\end{aligned}
$$

and

$$
\begin{aligned}
\tau_b &= \frac{C-D}{\sqrt{(C+D+T_x)(C+D+T_y)}}\\
&= \frac{ad-bc}{\sqrt{(a+c)(b+d)(a+b)(c+d)}} = \sqrt{\frac{\chi^2}{N}} = \phi = r_{xy}\ .
\end{aligned}
$$

Thus, if $t_a = t_b = r_{xy}^2$ and $\tau_b = r_{xy}$, then Goodman and Kruskal's t_a and t_b measures are equal to the square of Kendall's τ_b measure (τ_b^2) for any 2×2 contingency table.

9.12.1 Example

To illustrate the relationships between Pearson's χ^2, Pearson's ϕ^2, Pearson's r_{xy}^2, Goodman and Kruskal's t_a and t_b, and Kendall's τ_b test statistics, consider the 2×2 contingency table with $N = 10$ cases given in Table 9.39. For the frequency data given in Table 9.39, Pearson's chi-squared test statistic is given by

$$\chi^2 = \sum_{i=1}^{r} \sum_{j=1}^{c} \frac{(O_{ij} - E_{ij})^2}{E_{ij}} ,$$

where O_{ij} denotes the observed cell frequencies, $i, j = 1, 2$, E_{ij} denotes the expected cell values given by

$$E_{ij} = \frac{n_{i.}n_{.j}}{N} \qquad \text{for } i, j = 1, 2 ,$$

the expected values are

$$E_{11} = \frac{(4)(7)}{10} = 2.80 , \qquad E_{12} = \frac{(4)(3)}{10} = 1.20 ,$$

$$E_{21} = \frac{(6)(7)}{10} = 4.20 , \qquad E_{22} = \frac{(6)(3)}{10} = 1.80 ,$$

and Pearson's chi-squared test statistic is

$$\chi^2 = \sum_{i=1}^{r} \sum_{j=1}^{c} \frac{(O_{ij} - E_{ij})^2}{E_{ij}}$$

$$= \frac{(3-2.80)^2}{2.80} + \frac{(1-1.20)^2}{1.20} + \frac{(4-4.20)^2}{4.20} + \frac{(2-1.80)^2}{1.80} = 0.0794 .$$

Then, Pearson's mean-squared contingency coefficient is

$$\phi^2 = \frac{\chi^2}{N} = \frac{0.0794}{10} = 0.0079 .$$

Table 9.39 Example 2×2 contingency data for variables x and y with dummy (0, 1) coding

	y		
x	0	1	Total
0	3	1	4
1	4	2	6
Total	7	3	10

Table 9.40 Example dummy-coded values from the 2×2 contingency table in Table 9.39

	Variable	
Object	x	y
1	0	0
2	0	0
3	0	0
4	0	1
5	1	0
6	1	0
7	1	0
8	1	0
9	1	1
10	1	1

It is well known that Pearson's ϕ^2 is equivalent to Pearson's squared product-moment correlation coefficient when the categories of variables x and y are dummy-coded (0, 1). To illustrate the equivalency between Pearson's ϕ^2 and Pearson's r_{xy}^2, consider the 2×2 contingency table given in Table 9.39, where the row variable is denoted as x, the column variable is denoted as y, and the row and column categories are both coded (0, 1) . The frequency data given in Table 9.39 are recoded in Table 9.40, where Objects 1 through 3, coded (0, 0), represent the three objects in row 1 and column 1; Object 4, coded (0, 1), represents the single object in row 1 and column 2; Objects 5 through 8, coded (1, 0), represent the four objects in row 2 and column 1; and Objects 9 and 10, coded (1, 1), represent the two objects in row 2 and column 2 of Table 9.39.

For the binary-coded data listed in Table 9.40, $N = 10$,

$$\sum_{i=1}^{N} x_i = \sum_{i=1}^{N} x_i^2 = 6, \quad \sum_{i=1}^{N} y_i = \sum_{i=1}^{N} y_i^2 = 3, \quad \sum_{i=1}^{N} x_i y_i = +2 ,$$

and the squared Pearson product-moment correlation coefficient for variables x and y is

$$r_{xy}^2 = \frac{\left(N \sum_{i=1}^{N} x_i y_i - \sum_{i=1}^{N} x_i \sum_{i=1}^{N} y_i\right)^2}{\left[N \sum_{i=1}^{N} x_i^2 - \left(\sum_{i=1}^{N} x_i\right)^2\right]\left[N \sum_{i=1}^{N} y_i^2 - \left(\sum_{i=1}^{N} y_i\right)^2\right]}$$

$$= \frac{\left[(10)(+2) - (6)(3)\right]^2}{\left[(10)(6) - 6^2\right]\left[(10)(3) - 3^2\right]} = 0.0079 ,$$

which is identical to the value for Pearson's ϕ^2 contingency coefficient.

For the frequency data given in Table 9.39, Goodman and Kruskal's t_b is

$$t_b = \frac{N \displaystyle\sum_{j=1}^{c} \sum_{i=1}^{r} \frac{n_{ij}^2}{n_{.j}} - \sum_{i=1}^{r} n_{i.}^2}{N^2 - \displaystyle\sum_{i=1}^{r} n_{i.}^2}$$

$$= \frac{10\left(\dfrac{3^2}{7} + \dfrac{1^2}{7} + \dfrac{4^2}{3} + \dfrac{2^2}{3}\right) - 4^2 - 6^2}{10^2 - 4^2 - 6^2} = 0.0079 .$$

Similarly, Goodman and Kruskal's t_a is

$$t_a = \frac{N \displaystyle\sum_{i=1}^{r} \sum_{j=1}^{c} \frac{n_{ij}^2}{n_{i.}} - \sum_{j=1}^{c} n_{.j}^2}{N^2 - \displaystyle\sum_{j=1}^{c} n_{.j}^2}$$

$$= \frac{10\left(\dfrac{3^2}{4} + \dfrac{1^2}{4} + \dfrac{4^2}{6} + \dfrac{2^2}{6}\right) - 7^2 - 3^2}{10^2 - 7^2 - 3^2} = 0.0079 .$$

Now, consider Kendall's τ_b measure. For the cell frequency values given in Table 9.39,

$$\tau_b = \frac{C - D}{\sqrt{(C + D + T_x)(C + D + T_y)}} = \frac{(3)(2) - (1)(4)}{\sqrt{(7)(3)(4)(6)}} = 0.0891 , \qquad (9.10)$$

which is the square root of $\phi^2 = r_{xy}^2 = 0.0079$. Thus, $\phi^2 = r_{xy}^2 = t_a = t_b = \tau_b^2 = 0.0079$.

Finally, consider a conventional calculation formula for Pearson's product-moment correlation coefficient given by

$$r_{xy} = \frac{N \displaystyle\sum_{i=1}^{N} x_i y_i - \sum_{i=1}^{N} x_i \sum_{i=1}^{N} y_i}{\sqrt{\left[N \displaystyle\sum_{i=1}^{N} x_i^2 - \left(\sum_{i=1}^{N} x_i\right)^2\right]\left[N \displaystyle\sum_{i=1}^{N} y_i^2 - \left(\sum_{i=1}^{N} y_i\right)^2\right]}} . \qquad (9.11)$$

It is easily demonstrated that the numerator of Eq. (9.11),

$$N \sum_{i=1}^{N} x_i y_i - \sum_{i=1}^{N} x_i \sum_{i=1}^{N} y_i \; ,$$

is equal to $C - D$. Thus, for the binary-coded data listed in Table 9.40,

$$N = 10, \quad \sum_{i=1}^{N} x_i = \sum_{i=1}^{N} x_i^2 = 6, \quad \sum_{i=1}^{N} y_i = \sum_{i=1}^{N} y_i^2 = 3, \quad \sum_{i=1}^{N} x_i y_i = +2 \; ,$$

and

$$N \sum_{i=1}^{N} x_i y_i - \sum_{i=1}^{N} x_i \sum_{i=1}^{N} y_i = (10)(2) - (6)(3) = +2 \; .$$

For the frequency data given in Table 9.39,

$$C = ab = (3)(2) = 6 \; ,$$

$$D = cd = (1)(4) = 4 \; ,$$

$$T_x = ab + cd = (3)(1) + (4)(2) = 11 \; ,$$

$$T_y = ac + bd = (3)(4) + (1)(2) = 14 \; ,$$

and $C - D = 6 - 4 = +2$. Now, consider the factor on the left side of the denominator of Eq. (9.11),

$$N \sum_{i=1}^{N} x_i^2 - \left(\sum_{i=1}^{N} x_i \right)^2 \; ,$$

which is equal to $C + D + T_y$. Thus,

$$N \sum_{i=1}^{N} x_i^2 - \left(\sum_{i=1}^{N} x_i \right)^2 = (10)(6) - 6^2 = 60 - 36 = 24$$

and

$$C + D + T_y = 6 + 4 + 14 = 24 \; .$$

Similarly, consider the factor on the right side of the denominator of Eq. (9.11),

$$N \sum_{i=1}^{N} y_i^2 - \left(\sum_{i=1}^{N} y_i \right)^2 ,$$

which is equal to $C + D + T_x$. Thus,

$$N \sum_{i=1}^{N} y_i^2 - \left(\sum_{i=1}^{N} y_i \right)^2 = (10)(3) - 3^2 = 30 - 9 = 21$$

and

$$C + D + T_x = 6 + 4 + 11 = 21 .$$

9.12.2 An Alternative Proof

A more rigorous proof of the equality of Kendall's τ_b and Pearson's r_{xy} is offered in this section. Consider Tables 9.38, 9.39, and 9.40, replicated for convenience in Tables 9.41, 9.42, and 9.43, respectively. For the binary-coded data listed in Table 9.43,

$$N = 10, \quad \sum_{i=1}^{N} x_i = \sum_{i=1}^{N} x_i^2 = 6, \quad \sum_{i=1}^{N} y_i = \sum_{i=1}^{N} y_i^2 = 3, \quad \sum_{i=1}^{N} x_i y_i = +2 ,$$

Table 9.41 Notation for variables x and y with categories dummy-coded 0 and 1

	y		
x	0	1	Total
0	a	b	$a+b$
1	c	d	$c+d$
Total	$a+c$	$b+d$	N

Table 9.42 Example 2×2 contingency data for variables x and y with dummy (0, 1) coding

	y		
x	0	1	Total
0	3	1	4
1	4	2	6
Total	7	3	10

Table 9.43 Example dummy-coded values from the 2×2 contingency table in Table 9.42

	Variable	
Object	x	y
1	0	0
2	0	0
3	0	0
4	0	1
5	1	0
6	1	0
7	1	0
8	1	0
9	1	1
10	1	1

and the Pearson product-moment correlation coefficient for variables x and y is

$$r_{xy} = \frac{N\sum_{i=1}^{N} x_i y_i - \sum_{i=1}^{N} x_i \sum_{i=1}^{N} y_i}{\sqrt{\left[N\sum_{i=1}^{N} x_i^2 - \left(\sum_{i=1}^{N} x_i\right)^2\right]\left[N\sum_{i=1}^{N} y_i^2 - \left(\sum_{i=1}^{N} y_i\right)^2\right]}}$$

$$= \frac{(10)(+2) - (6)(3)}{\sqrt{[(10)(6) - 6^2][(10)(3) - 3^2]}} = +0.0891 \,. \qquad (9.12)$$

From Tables 9.41 and 9.42,

$$N = a + b + c + d = 3 + 1 + 4 + 2 = 10 \,,$$

$$\sum_{i=1}^{N} x_i = \sum_{i=1}^{N} x_i^2 = (0)(a+b) + (1)(c+d) = c + d = 4 + 2 = 6 \,,$$

$$\sum_{i=1}^{N} y_i = \sum_{i=1}^{N} y_i^2 = (0)(a+c) + (1)(b+d) = b + d = 1 + 2 = 3 \,,$$

$$\sum_{i=1}^{N} x_i y_i = (0)(0)(a) + (0)(1)(b) + (1)(0)(c) + (1)(1)(d) = d = +2 \,,$$

$$N\sum_{i=1}^{N} x_i y_i - \sum_{i=1}^{N} x_i \sum_{i=1}^{N} y_i$$
$$= (a+b+c+d)(d) - (c+d)(b+d)$$
$$= ad + bd + cd + d^2 - bc - cd - bd - d^2$$
$$= ad - bc = C - D \ ,$$

$$N\sum_{i=1}^{N} x^2 - \left(\sum_{i=1}^{N} x_i\right)^2$$
$$= (a+b+c+d)(c+d) - c^2 - 2cd - d^2$$
$$= ac + ad + bc + bd + c^2 + cd + cd + d^2 - c^2 - 2cd - d^2$$
$$= (a+b)(c+d) = C + D + T_y \ ,$$

and

$$N\sum_{i=1}^{N} y^2 - \left(\sum_{i=1}^{N} y_i\right)^2$$
$$= (a+b+c+d)(b+d) - b^2 - 2bd - d^2$$
$$= ab + ad + b^2 + bd + cb + cd + bd + d^2 - b^2 - 2bd - d^2$$
$$= (a+c)(b+d) = C + D + T_x \ .$$

Then, substituting into Eq. (9.12),

$$r_{xy} = \frac{N\sum_{i=1}^{N} x_i y_i - \sum_{i=1}^{N} x_i \sum_{i=1}^{N} y_i}{\sqrt{\left[N\sum_{i=1}^{N} x_i^2 - \left(\sum_{i=1}^{N} x_i\right)^2\right]\left[N\sum_{i=1}^{N} y_i^2 - \left(\sum_{i=1}^{N} y_i\right)^2\right]}}$$
$$= \frac{C - D}{\sqrt{(C + D + T_y)(C + D + T_x)}} = \tau_b \ .$$

9.13 Pearson's Correlation Coefficient

Pearson's product-moment correlation coefficient can be adapted for 2×2 contingency tables when the two variables are dummy-coded (0, 1), as in Table 9.35 on p. 552, replicated in Table 9.44 for convenience. See Chap. 7, Sect. 7.1 for a more detailed description of Pearson's product-moment correlation coefficient. Table 9.45 displays the $N = 36$ dummy-coded frequencies, where Objects 1 through 16, coded $(0, 0)$, represent the sixteen objects in row 1 and column 1 of Table 9.44; Objects 17 through 20, coded (0, 1), represent the four objects in row 1 and column 2; Objects 21 through 28, coded $(1, 0)$, represent the eight objects in row 2 and column 1; and Objects 29 through 36, coded $(1, 1)$, represent the eight objects in row 2 and column 2. For the dummy-coded frequencies listed in Table 9.45, $N = 36$,

$$\sum_{i=1}^{N} x_i = \sum_{i=1}^{N} x_i^2 = 16\,, \quad \sum_{i=1}^{N} y_i = \sum_{1=1}^{N} y_i^2 = 12\,, \quad \sum_{i=1}^{N} x_i y_i = +8\,,$$

Table 9.44 Example data for variables x and y with categories dummy-coded 0 and 1

	y		
x	0	1	Total
0	16	4	20
1	8	8	16
Total	24	12	36

Table 9.45 Example dummy-coded values from the 2×2 contingency table in Table 9.44

	Variable	
Object	x	y
1	0	0
⋮	⋮	⋮
16	0	0
17	0	1
⋮	⋮	⋮
20	0	1
21	1	0
⋮	⋮	⋮
28	1	0
29	1	1
⋮	⋮	⋮
36	1	1

and Pearson's product-moment correlation coefficient is

$$r_{xy} = \frac{N\sum_{i=1}^{N} x_i y_i - \sum_{i=1}^{N} x_i \sum_{i=1}^{N} y_i}{\sqrt{\left[N\sum_{i=1}^{N} x_i^2 - \left(\sum_{i=1}^{N} x_i\right)^2\right]\left[N\sum_{i=1}^{N} y_i^2 - \left(\sum_{i=1}^{N} y_i\right)^2\right]}}$$

$$= \frac{(36)(+8) - (16)(12)}{\sqrt{[(36)(16) - 16^2][(36)(12) - 12^2]}} = +0.3162\ .$$

It is well known that r_{xy} is equal to Pearson's ϕ coefficient for 2×2 contingency tables; thus,

$$\phi = \sqrt{\frac{\chi^2}{N}} = \sqrt{\frac{3.60}{36}} = \sqrt{0.1000} = \pm 0.3162\ .$$

Also, Pearson's r_{xy} is equivalent to Kendall's τ_b for 2×2 contingency tables, as shown in Sect. 9.12.2. Thus,

$$\tau_b = \frac{C - D}{\sqrt{(C + D + T_x)(C + D + T_y)}}$$

$$= \frac{128 - 32}{\sqrt{(128 + 32 + 128)(128 + 32 + 160)}} = +0.3162\ .$$

There are only

$$M = \min(a + b, a + c) - \max(0, a - d) + 1$$

$$= \min(20, 24) - \max(0, 20 - 12) + 1 = 20 - 8 + 1 = 13$$

possible, equally-likely arrangements in the reference set of all permutations of the cell frequencies in Table 9.44 given the observed row and column marginal frequency distributions, {20, 16} and {24, 12}, respectively, making an exact permutation analysis feasible. Because $M = 13$ is a small number of arrangements, it will be illustrative to list the 13 sets of cell frequencies, r_{xy} values, and the associated hypergeometric point probability values in Table 9.46, where the rows with hypergeometric point probability values associated with r_{xy} values equal to or greater than the observed value of $r_{xy} = +0.3162$ are indicated with asterisks.

If the $M = 13$ possible arrangements of the frequency data given in Table 9.44 occur with equal chance, the exact probability value of r_{xy} under the null hypothesis is the sum of the hypergeometric point probability values associated with $r_{xy} = +0.3162$ or greater. Based on the hypergeometric probability distribution, the exact

Table 9.46 Cell frequencies, r_{xy} values, and exact hypergeometric point probability values for $M = 13$ possible arrangements of the observed data in Table 9.44

	Cell frequency					
Table	n_{11}	n_{12}	n_{21}	n_{22}	r_{xy}	Probability
1	8	12	16	0	−0.6325	0.1006×10^{-3}
2	9	11	15	1	−0.5139	0.2147×10^{-2}
3	10	10	14	2	−0.3953	0.1771×10^{-1}
4	11	9	13	3	−0.2767	0.7515×10^{-1}
5	12	8	12	4	−0.1581	0.1832
6	13	7	11	5	−0.0395	0.2705
7	14	6	10	6	+0.0791	0.2480
8	15	5	9	7	+0.1976	0.1417
9*	16	4	8	8	+0.3162	0.4982×10^{-1}
10*	17	3	7	9	+0.4348	0.1042×10^{-1}
11*	18	2	6	10	+0.5534	0.1216×10^{-2}
12*	19	1	5	11	+0.6720	0.6979×10^{-4}
13*	20	0	4	12	+0.7906	0.1454×10^{-5}
Sum						1.0000

upper-tail probability value is

$$P = 0.4982\times10^{-1} + 0.1042\times10^{-1} + 0.1216\times10^{-2} + 0.6979\times10^{-4} + 0.1454\times10^{-5} = 0.0615\,.$$

9.14 Unstandardized Regression Coefficients

Consider once again the binary-coded data listed in Table 9.45. Given $N = 36$,

$$\sum_{i=1}^{N} x_i = \sum_{i=1}^{N} x_i^2 = 16\,, \quad \sum_{i=1}^{N} y_i = \sum_{1=1}^{N} y_i^2 = 12\,, \quad \text{and} \quad \sum_{i=1}^{N} x_i y_i = +8\,,$$

the unstandardized regression equation for variable y, conditioned on variable x, yields

$$b_{yx} = \frac{N\sum_{i=1}^{N} x_i y_i - \sum_{i=1}^{N} x_i \sum_{i=1}^{N} y_i}{N\sum_{i=1}^{N} x_i^2 - \left(\sum_{i=1}^{N} x_i\right)^2} = \frac{(36)(+8) - (16)(12)}{(36)(16) - 16^2} = +0.30$$

and the unstandardized regression equation for variable x, conditioned on variable y, yields

$$b_{xy} = \frac{N\sum_{i=1}^{N} x_i y_i - \sum_{i=1}^{N} x_i \sum_{i=1}^{N} y_i}{N\sum_{i=1}^{N} y_i^2 - \left(\sum_{i=1}^{N} y_i\right)^2} = \frac{(36)(+8) - (16)(12)}{(36)(12) - 12^2} = +0.3333 .$$

The unstandardized slopes are illustrated in Fig. 9.3 where, when variable y is considered to be the dependent variable, the intercept is $a_{yx} = +0.20$ and the slope is $b_{yx} = +0.30$, and when variable x is considered to be the dependent variable, the intercept is $a_{xy} = +0.3333$ and the slope is $b_{xy} = +0.3333$.

It may be of some interest to note that when the two regression lines are drawn on the same graph, assuming that the two variables, x and y, have been standardized as in Fig. 9.3, there is a direct relationship between Pearson's product-moment correlation coefficient, r_{xy}, and the acute angle, θ, expressed in degrees, between the two regression lines. Specifically,

$$\theta = 90° - 2\tan^{-1}\sqrt{b_{yx}b_{xy}} \quad \text{and} \quad r_{xy} = \tan\left(\frac{90° - \theta}{2}\right) .$$

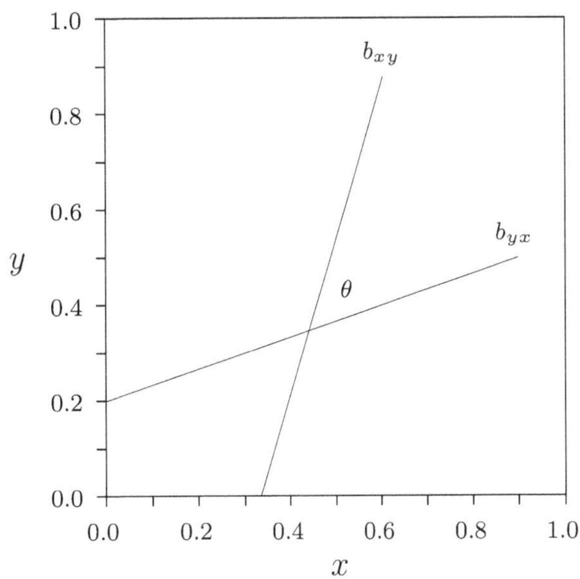

Fig. 9.3 Graphic depicting the two regression lines for the data listed in Table 9.45

Table 9.47 Example data for variables x and y with categories dummy-coded 0 and 1

	y		
x	0	1	Total
0	16	4	20
1	8	8	16
Total	24	12	36

If the scatter of points is circular, $r_{xy} = 0$ and $\theta = 90°$, so that the two regression lines are orthogonal to each other, and if $r_{xy} = +1$, then $\theta = 0°$ and the two regression lines are superimposed on each other.

Thus, for the data given in Table 9.45,

$$\theta = 90° - 2\tan^{-1}\sqrt{b_{yx}b_{xy}} = 90° - 2\tan^{-1}\sqrt{(+0.30)(+0.3333)} = 54.9032°$$

and

$$r_{xy} = \tan\left(\frac{90° - \theta}{2}\right) = \tan\left(\frac{90° - 54.9032°}{2}\right) = +0.3162\ .$$

Now consider the frequency data given in Table 9.35 on p. 552, replicated in Table 9.47 for convenience, where the percentage differences are

$$D_x = \frac{16}{20} - \frac{8}{16} = 0.30 \quad \text{and} \quad D_y = \frac{16}{24} - \frac{4}{12} = 0.3333\ ,$$

and Somers' two asymmetric measures are

$$d_{yx} = \frac{(16)(8) - (4)(8)}{(20)(16)} = 0.30 \quad \text{and} \quad d_{xy} = \frac{(16)(8) - (4)(8)}{(24)(12)} = 0.3333\ .$$

Note that the percentage differences, the unstandardized regression coefficients, and Somers' two asymmetric measures are all equivalent for 2×2 contingency tables; thus, for 2×2 contingency tables,

$$D_x = b_{yx} = d_{yx} = 0.30 \quad \text{and} \quad D_y = b_{xy} = d_{xy} = 0.3333\ .$$

It is not widely recognized that, given a 2×2 contingency table, a percentage difference is really just the slope of a regression line [3], and that Somers' d_{yx} and d_{xy} measures thereby reduce to simple percentage differences.[17]

[17] Somers observed that d_{yx} and d_{xy} were equivalent to the corresponding percentage differences in 2×2 contingency tables [50, p. 805].

On the other hand, it is well known that the Pearson product-moment correlation coefficient is simply the geometric mean of the slopes of the two regression lines, i.e.,

$$r_{xy} = \sqrt{b_{yx}b_{xy}} = \sqrt{(0.30)(0.3333)} = \pm 0.3162\ .$$

Therefore, for a 2×2 contingency table, r_{xy} is also the geometric mean of Somers' two asymmetric coefficients of association, i.e.,

$$r_{xy} = \sqrt{d_{yx}d_{xy}} = \sqrt{(0.30)(0.3333)} = \pm 0.3162\ ,$$

as well as the geometric mean of the two percentage differences, i.e.,

$$r_{xy} = \sqrt{D_x D_y} = \sqrt{(0.30)(0.3333)} = \pm 0.3162\ .$$

9.15 Pearson's ϕ^2 and Cohen's κ Measures

Given a 2×2 contingency table and following the notation in Table 9.41 on p. 561, replicated in Table 9.48 for convenience, where $N = a + b + c + d$, Pearson's mean-squared contingency coefficient may be defined as

$$\phi^2 = \frac{(ad - bc)^2}{(a + b)(c + d)(a + c)(b + d)}\ .$$

Kraemer [36] suggested that Cohen's unweighted measure of inter-rater agreement may be defined more generally as

$$\kappa_k = \frac{ad - bc}{(a + b)(c + d)(k) + (a + c)(b + d)(k - 1)}\ ,$$

where $k = 0$ yields an index of specificity, i.e., the proportion of objects without the desired attribute that are correctly identified by the test; $k = 1$ yields an index of sensitivity, i.e., the proportion of objects with the desired attribute that are correctly identified by the test; and $k = 1/2$ yields Cohen's kappa measure [51].

Table 9.48 Notation for variables x and y with categories dummy-coded 0 and 1

	y		
x	0	1	Total
0	a	b	$a + b$
1	c	d	$c + d$
Total	$a + c$	$b + d$	N

If $k = 0$

$$\kappa_0 = \frac{ad - bc}{(a+b)(c+d)(0) + (a+c)(b+d)(1-0)} = \frac{ad - bc}{(a+c)(b+d)}$$

and if $k = 1$

$$\kappa_1 = \frac{ad - bc}{(a+b)(c+d)(1) + (a+c)(b+d)(1-1)} = \frac{ad - bc}{(a+b)(c+d)} .$$

Then it can be demonstrated that

$$\phi^2 = \kappa_0\kappa_1 \quad \text{and} \quad \phi = \sqrt{\kappa_0\kappa_1} ,$$

establishing the relationship between Cohen's unweighted kappa measure and Pearson's mean-squared contingency coefficient [36, 51].

9.15.1 Example

To illustrate the relationships between κ_k, ϕ^2, and other measures, consider the example frequency data given in Table 9.49 with $N = 20$ objects cross-classified into four categories. For the frequency data given in Table 9.49,

$$\phi^2 = \frac{(ad - bc)^2}{(a+b)(c+d)(a+c)(b+d)} = \frac{[(8)(6) - (4)(2)]^2}{(12)(8)(10)(10)} = 0.1667 ,$$

$$\kappa_0 = \frac{ad - bc}{(a+c)(b+d)} = \frac{(8)(6) - (4)(2)}{(10)(10)} = 0.40 ,$$

$$\kappa_1 = \frac{ad - bc}{(a+b)(c+d)} = \frac{(8)(6) - (4)(2)}{(12)(8)} = 0.4167 ,$$

$$\phi^2 = \kappa_0\kappa_1 = (0.40)(0.4167) = 0.1667 ,$$

Table 9.49 Notation for variables x and y with categories dummy-coded 0 and 1

	y		
x	0	1	Total
0	8	4	12
1	2	6	8
Total	10	10	20

and

$$\phi = \sqrt{\kappa_0 \kappa_1} = \sqrt{(0.40)(0.4167)} = 0.4082 \; .$$

Since, for any 2×2 contingency table, $\phi^2 = r_{xy}^2$, then

$$r_{xy}^2 = \kappa_0 \kappa_1 \quad \text{and} \quad r_{xy} = \sqrt{\kappa_0 \kappa_1} \; .$$

Also, for any 2×2 contingency table,

$$\phi^2 = \frac{\chi^2}{N} \quad \text{and} \quad N\phi^2 = \chi^2 \; ,$$

then

$$\chi^2 = N\phi^2 = N\kappa_0\kappa_1 = (20)(0.40)(0.4167) = 3.3333$$

and

$$r_{xy}^2 = \phi^2 = \kappa_0\kappa_1 = \frac{\chi^2}{N} = \frac{3.3333}{20} = 0.1667 \; .$$

Finally, it can be demonstrated that for any 2×2 contingency table, Kraemer's $\kappa_0\kappa_1$, Pearson's ϕ^2, Tschuprov's T^2, Cramér's V^2, Pearson's r_{xy}^2, the unstandardized regression coefficients b_{yx} and b_{xy}, the square of Kendall's τ_b measure, Goodman and Kruskal's t_x and t_y coefficients, Somers' d_{yx} and d_{xy} asymmetric measures, and percentage differences D_x and D_y are all inter-related. Thus, for the frequency data given in Table 9.49, Kraemer's $\kappa_0\kappa_1$ is

$$\kappa_0\kappa_1 = \left[\frac{ad - bc}{(a+c)(b+d)}\right]\left[\frac{ad - bc}{(a+b)(c+d)}\right]$$
$$= \left[\frac{(8)(6) - (4)(2)}{(10)(10)}\right]\left[\frac{(8)(6) - (4)(2)}{(12)(8)}\right] = 0.1667 \; ,$$

Pearson's chi-squared statistic is

$$\chi^2 = \frac{N(ad - bc)^2}{(a+b)(c+d)(a+c)(b+d)} = \frac{20[(8)(6) - (4)(2)]^2}{(12)(8)(10)(10)} = 3.3333 \; ,$$

Pearson's mean-squared contingency coefficient is

$$\phi^2 = \frac{\chi^2}{N} = \frac{3.3333}{20} = 0.1667 \; ,$$

Tschuprov's T^2 is

$$T^2 = \frac{\chi^2}{N\sqrt{(r-1)(c-1)}} = \frac{3.3333}{20\sqrt{(2-1)(2-1)}} = 0.1667 ,$$

Cramér's V^2 is

$$V^2 = \frac{\chi^2}{N \min(r-1, c-1)} = \frac{3.3333}{20 \min(2-1, 2-1)} = 0.1667 ,$$

and Pearson's squared product-moment correlation coefficient is

$$r_{xy}^2 = \frac{(ad-bc)^2}{(a+b)(c+d)(a+c)(b+d)} = \frac{[(8)(6)-(4)(2)]^2}{(12)(8)(10)(10)} = 0.1667 .$$

The unstandardized regression coefficients, b_{xy} and b_{yx}, are equivalent to κ_0 and κ_1, respectively; thus,

$$b_{xy} = \frac{ad-bc}{(a+c)(b+d)} = \frac{(8)(6)-(4)(2)}{(10)(10)} = 0.40$$

and

$$b_{yx} = \frac{ad-bc}{(a+b)(c+d)} = \frac{(8)(6)-(4)(2)}{(12)(8)} = 0.4167 .$$

Define the number of concordant pairs as $C = ad$, the number of discordant pairs as $D = bc$, the number of pairs tied on variable x as $T_x = ab + cd$, and the number of pairs tied on variable y as $T_y = ac + bd$. Then the square of Kendall's τ_b measure of ordinal association is identical to Kraemer's $\kappa_0\kappa_1$; thus,

$$\tau_b^2 = \frac{(C-D)^2}{(C+D+T_x)(C+D+Y_y)}$$

$$= \frac{(ad-bc)^2}{(ad+bc+ac+bd)(ad+bc+ab+cd)}$$

$$= \frac{[(8)(6)-(4)(2)]^2}{[(8)(6)+(4)(2)+(8)(2)+(4)(6)][(8)(6)+(4)(2)+(8)(4)+(2)(6)]}$$

$$= 0.1667 .$$

Goodman and Kruskal's asymmetric measures, t_x and t_y, are also equivalent to Kraemer's $\kappa_0\kappa_1$; thus,

$$t_x = \frac{N\left(\dfrac{a^2+c^2}{a+c} + \dfrac{b^2+d^2}{b+d}\right) - (a+b)^2 - (c+d)^2}{N^2 - (a+b)^2 - (c+d)^2}$$

$$= \frac{20\left(\dfrac{8^2+2^2}{10} + \dfrac{4^2+6^2}{10}\right) - 12^2 - 8^2}{20^2 - 12^2 - 8^2} = 0.1667\ ,$$

and

$$t_y = \frac{N\left(\dfrac{a^2+b^2}{a+b} + \dfrac{c^2+d^2}{c+d}\right) - (a+c)^2 - (b+d)^2}{N^2 - (a+c)^2 - (b+d)^2}$$

$$= \frac{20\left(\dfrac{8^2+4^2}{12} + \dfrac{2^2+6^2}{8}\right) - 10^2 - 10^2}{20^2 - 10^2 - 10^2} = 0.1667\ .$$

Somers' asymmetric d_{xy} and d_{yx} measures of ordinal association are equivalent to κ_0 and κ_1, respectively; thus,

$$d_{xy} = \frac{C-D}{C+D+T_x} = \frac{ad-bc}{ad+bc+(a)(b)+(c)(d}$$

$$= \frac{(8)(6)-(4)(2)}{(8)(6)+(4)(2)+(8)(4)+(2)(6)} = 0.40$$

and

$$d_{yx} = \frac{C-D}{C+D+T_y} = \frac{ad-bc}{ad+bc+ac+bd}$$

$$= \frac{(8)(6)-(4)(2)}{(8)(6)+(4)(2)+(8)(2)+(4)(6)} = 0.4167\ .$$

Finally, the simple percentage differences D_y and D_x are also equivalent to κ_0 and κ_1, respectively; thus,

$$D_y = \frac{a}{a+c} - \frac{b}{b+d} = \frac{ad-bc}{(a+c)(b+d)} = \frac{(8)(6)-(4)(2)}{(10)(10)} = 0.40$$

and

$$D_x = \frac{a}{a+b} - \frac{c}{c+d} = \frac{ad-bc}{(a+b)(c+d)} = \frac{(8)(6)-(4)(2)}{(12)(8)} = 0.4167\ .$$

9.16 Coda

Chapter 9 examined measures of association for 2×2 contingency tables. Included in Chap. 9 were permutation statistical methods applied to Pearson's ϕ coefficient of contingency, Pearson's tetrachoric correlation coefficient, Yule's Q and Yule's Y measures of nominal association, Leik and Gove's d_N^c measure of nominal association, the odds ratio, Goodman and Kruskal's t_a and t_b asymmetric measures of nominal association, Somers' d_{yx} and d_{xy} measures of ordinal association, simple percentage differences, and Kendall's τ_b measure of ordinal association.

Chapter 10 continues the discussion of 2×2 contingency tables with consideration of symmetrical 2×2 contingency tables, where each marginal frequency total is equal to $N/2$. Included in Chap. 10 are permutation statistical methods applied to Pearson's ϕ^2, Tschuprov's T^2, Cramér's V^2, Pearson's product-moment correlation coefficient, Leik and Gove's d_N^c measure, Goodman and Kruskal's t_a and t_b asymmetric measures, Kendall's τ_b and Stuart's τ_c measures, Somers' d_{yx} and d_{xy} asymmetric measures, simple percentage differences, Yule's Y measure of nominal association, and Cohen's unweighted and weighted κ measures of inter-rater agreement.

Also included in Chap. 10 are extensions to multiple 2×2 contingency tables and 2×2×2 contingency tables, including the Mantel–Haenszel test for combined 2×2 contingency tables, Cohen's kappa measure of inter-rater agreement, McNemar's and Cochran's Q tests, Fisher's exact test for 2×2×2 and 2×2×2×2 contingency tables, and tests for interactions in 2×2×2 and 2×2×2×2 contingency tables.

References

1. Bergmann, R., Ludbrook, J., Spooren, W.P.J.M.: Different outcomes of the Wilcoxon–Mann–Whitney test from different statistics packages. Am. Stat. **54**, 72–77 (2000)
2. Berry, K.J., Martin, T.W., Olson, K.F.: A note on fourfold point correlation. Educ. Psychol. Meas. **34**, 53–56 (1974)
3. Blalock, H.M.: A double standard in measuring degree of association. Am. Sociol. Rev. **28**, 988–989 (1963)
4. Blalock, H.M.: Social Statistics, 2nd edn. McGraw–Hill, New York (1979)
5. Bonett, D.G., Price, R.M.: Inferential methods for the tetrachoric correlation coefficient. Psych. Rep. **30**, 213–225 (2005)
6. Brown, M.B.: Algorithm AS-116: The tetrachoric correlation and its asymptotic standard error. Appl. Stat. **26**, 343–351 (1977)
7. Camp, B.H.: Karl Pearson and mathematical statistics. J. Am. Stat. Assoc. **28**, 395–401 (1933)
8. Castellan, N.J.: On the estimation of the tetrachoric correlation coefficient. Psychometrika **31**, 67–73 (1966)
9. Cohen, J.: A coefficient of agreement for nominal scales. Educ. Psychol. Meas. **20**, 37–46 (1960)
10. Costner, H.L.: Criteria for measures of association. Am. Sociol. Rev. **30**, 341–353 (1965)
11. Cramér, H.: Mathematical Methods of Statistics. Princeton University Press, Princeton, NJ (1946)

12. Cureton, E.E.: Note on $\phi/\phi_{\max}$. Psychometrika **24**, 89–91 (1959)
13. Duggan, T.J., Dean, C.W.: Common misinterpretations of significance levels in sociological journals. Am. Sociol. **3**, 45–46 (1968)
14. Eden, T., Yates, F.: On the validity of Fisher's z test when applied to an actual example of non-normal data. J. Agric. Sci. **23**, 6–17 (1933)
15. Edwards, A.W.F.: The measure of association in a 2×2 table. J. R. Stat. Soc. A Gen. **126**, 109–114 (1963)
16. Ekström, J.: The phi-coefficient, the tetrachoric correlation coefficient, and the Pearson–Yule debate. Department of Statistics, University of California at Los Angeles (2011). http://escholarship.org/uc/item/7qp4604r (25 Oct 2011) Accessed 7 Mar 2016
17. Everitt, P.F.: Tables of the tetrachoric functions for fourfold correlation tables. Biometrika **7**, 437–451 (1910)
18. Ferguson, G.A.: Statistical Analysis in Psychology and Education, 5th edn. McGraw–Hill, New York (1981)
19. Fisher, R.A.: Statistical Methods for Research Workers. Oliver and Boyd, Edinburgh (1925)
20. Fleiss, J.L.: Statistical Methods for Rates and Proportions, 2nd edn. Wiley, New York (1981)
21. Francis, R.G.: The Rhetoric of Science: A Methodological Discussion of the Two-by-Two Table. University of Minnesota Press, Minneapolis, MN (1961)
22. Geary, R.C.: Some properties of correlation and regression in a limited universe. Metron **7**, 83–119 (1927)
23. Goodman, L.A., Kruskal, W.H.: Measures of association for cross classifications. J. Am. Stat. Assoc. **49**, 732–764 (1954)
24. Greer, T., Dunlap, W.P., Beatty, G.O.: A Monte Carlo evaluation of the tetrachoric correlation coefficient. Educ. Psychol. Meas. **63**, 931–950 (2003)
25. Guilford, J.P.: Fundamental Statistics in Psychology and Education. McGraw–Hill, New York (1950)
26. Guilford, J.P., Lyons, T.C.: On determining the reliability and significance of a tetrachoric coefficient of correlation. Psychometrika **7**, 243–249 (1942)
27. Hooker, R.H.: Discussion on Mr. Yule's paper. J. R. Stat. Soc. **75**, 646–647 (1912)
28. Hutchinson, T.P.: Kappa muddles together two sources of disagreement: Tetrachoric correlation is preferable. Res. Nurs. Health **16**, 313–315 (1993)
29. Kang, T.S.: Linking form of hypothesis to type of statistic: An application of Goodman's Z. Am. Soc. Rev. **37**, 357–365 (1972)
30. Kang, T.S.: Ordinal measures of association. Sociol. Quart. **14**, 235–248 (1973)
31. Kendall, M.G.: George Udny Yule C.B.E, F.R.S. J. R. Stat. Soc. A Gen. **115**, 156–161 (1952)
32. Kendall, M.G.: Studies in the history of probability and statistics: XI. Daniel Bernoulli on maximum likelihood. Biometrika **48**, 1–18 (1961)
33. Kendall, M.G.: Rank Correlation Methods, 3rd edn. Griffin, London (1962)
34. Kendall, M.G., Stuart, A.: The Advanced Theory of Statistics, Vol. 2. Hafner, New York (1961)
35. Kim, J.-O.: Predictive measures of ordinal association. Am. J. Soc. **76**, 891–907 (1971)
36. Kraemer, H.C., Kazdin, A.E., Offord, D.R., Kessler, R.C., Jensen, P.S., Kupfer, D.J.: Measuring the potency of risk factors for clinical or policy significance. Psychol. Methods **4**, 257–271 (1999)
37. Leik, R.K., Gove, W.R.: The conception and measurement of asymmetric monotonic relationships in sociology. Am. J. Sociol. **74**, 696–709 (1969)
38. Loether, H.J., McTavish, D.G.: Descriptive and Inferential Statistics: An Introduction, 4th edn. Allyn and Bacon, Boston (1993)
39. Long, M.A., Berry, K.J., Mielke, P.W.: Tetrachoric correlation: A permutation alternative. Educ. Psychol. Meas. **69**, 429–437 (2009)
40. McNemar, Q.: Psychological Statistics. Wiley, New York (1962)
41. Mielke, P.W., Berry, K.J.: Permutation Methods: A Distance Function Approach, 2nd edn. Springer–Verlag, New York (2007)
42. Nunnally, J.C.: Psychometric Theory, 2nd edn. McGraw–Hill, New York (1978)

43. Pearson, K.: On the criterion that a given system of deviations from the probable in the case of a correlated system of variables is such that it can be reasonably supposed to have arisen from random sampling. Philos. Mag. 5 **50**, 157–175 (1900)
44. Pearson, K.: On the probable error of a coefficient of correlation as found from a fourfold table. Biometrika **9**, 22–27 (1913)
45. Pearson, K., Heron, D.: On theories of association. Biometrika **9**, 159–315 (1913)
46. Pitman, E.J.G.: Significance tests which may be applied to samples from any populations. Suppl. J. R. Stat. Soc. **4**, 119–130 (1937)
47. Pitman, E.J.G.: Significance tests which may be applied to samples from any populations: II. The correlation coefficient test. Suppl. J. R. Stat. Soc. **4**, 225–232 (1937)
48. Pitman, E.J.G.: Significance tests which may be applied to samples from any populations: III. The analysis of variance test. Biometrika **29**, 322–335 (1938)
49. Senn, S.: Tea for three: Of infusions and inferences and milk in first. Significance **9**, 30–33 (Dec 2012)
50. Somers, R.H.: A new asymmetric measure of association for ordinal variables. Am. Sociol. Rev. **27**, 799–811 (1962)
51. Streiner, D.L.: Diagnosing tests: Using and misusing diagnostic and screening tests. J. Person. Assess. **81**, 209–219 (2003)
52. Uebersax, J.S.: The tetrachoric and polychoric correlation coefficients (2006). http://ourworld.compuserve.com/homepage/jsuebersax/tetra.htm Assessed 20 Dec 2007
53. Yule, G.U.: On the methods of measuring association between two attributes. J. R. Stat. Soc. **75**, 579–652 (1912). [Originally a paper read before the Royal Statistical Society on 23 April 1912]
54. Yule, G.U.: Prof. Karl Pearson, F.R.S. Nature **137**, 856–857 (1936)
55. Yule, G.U., Filon, L.N.G.: Karl Pearson. 1857–1936. Obit. Notices Fellows Roy. Soc. **2**, 73–110 (1936)

Tschuprov's measure of nominal association is

$$T^2 = \frac{\chi^2}{N\sqrt{(r-1)(c-1)}} = \frac{1.3333}{12\sqrt{(2-1)(2-1)}} = 0.1111$$

and $T = \sqrt{T^2} = \sqrt{0.1111} = 0.3333$. Also, Cramér's measure of nominal association is

$$V^2 = \frac{\chi^2}{N\big[\min(r-1, c-1)\big]} = \frac{1.3333}{12\big[\min(2-1, 2-1)\big]} = 0.1111$$

and $V = \sqrt{V^2} = \sqrt{0.1111} = 0.3333$. Thus, Pearson's ϕ, Tschuprov's T, and Cramér's V are equivalent for a symmetrical 2×2 contingency table.

10.1.2 Pearson's r_{xy} Correlation Coefficient

Next, consider Pearson's product-moment correlation coefficient given by

$$r_{xy} = \frac{N\sum_{i=1}^{N} x_i y_i - \sum_{i=1}^{N} x_i \sum_{i=1}^{N} y_i}{\sqrt{\left[N\sum_{i=1}^{N} x_i^2 - \left(\sum_{i=1}^{N} x_i\right)^2\right]\left[N\sum_{i=1}^{N} y_i^2 - \left(\sum_{i=1}^{N} y_i\right)^2\right]}} .$$

The binary-coded (0, 1) data listed in Table 10.3 were obtained from the frequency data given in Table 10.2, where Objects 1 through 4, coded (0, 0), represent the four

Table 10.3 Example dummy-coded (0, 1) values from the 2×2 contingency table in Table 10.2

	Variable	
Object	x	y
1	0	0
2	0	0
3	0	0
4	0	0
5	0	1
6	0	1
7	1	0
8	1	0
9	1	1
10	1	1
11	1	1
12	1	1

objects in row 1 and column 1 of Table 10.2; Objects 5 and 6, coded (0, 1), represent the two objects in row 1 and column 2; Objects 7 and 8, coded (1, 0), represent the two objects in row 2 and column 1; and Objects 9 through 12, coded (1, 1), represent the four objects in row 2 and column 2 of Table 10.2.

For the binary-coded data listed in Table 10.3,

$$N = 12\,, \quad \sum_{i=1}^{N} x_i = \sum_{i=1}^{N} x_i^2 = \sum_{i=1}^{N} y_i = \sum_{i=1}^{N} y_i^2 = 6\,, \quad \sum_{i=1}^{N} x_i y_i = +4\,,$$

Pearson's product-moment correlation coefficient is

$$r_{xy} = \frac{N\sum_{i=1}^{N} x_i y_i - \sum_{i=1}^{N} x_i \sum_{i=1}^{N} y_i}{\sqrt{\left[N\sum_{i=1}^{N} x_i^2 - \left(\sum_{i=1}^{N} x_i\right)^2\right]\left[N\sum_{i=1}^{N} y_i^2 - \left(\sum_{i=1}^{N} y_i\right)^2\right]}}$$

$$= \frac{(12)(+4) - (6)(6)}{\sqrt{[(12)(6) - 6^2][(12)(6) - 6^2]}} = +0.3333\,,$$

and $r_{xy}^2 = (+0.3333)^2 = 0.1111$.

10.1.3 Regression Coefficients

For the binary-coded data listed in Table 10.3, the slope (unstandardized regression coefficient) of the regression line with variable y the dependent variable is

$$b_{yx} = \frac{N\sum_{i=1}^{N} x_i y_i - \sum_{i=1}^{N} x_i \sum_{i=1}^{N} y_i}{N\sum_{i=1}^{r} x_i^2 - \left(\sum_{i=1}^{r} x_i\right)^2} = \frac{(12)(+4) - (6)(6)}{(12)(6) - 6^2} = +0.3333$$

and the standardized regression coefficient with variable x the dependent variable is

$$\hat{\beta}_{yx} = b_{yx}\left(\frac{s_x}{s_y}\right) = +0.3333\left(\frac{0.5222}{0.5222}\right) = +0.3333\,.$$

Also the unstandardized regression coefficient with variable x the dependent variable is

$$b_{xy} = \frac{N\sum_{i=1}^{N} x_i y_i - \sum_{i=1}^{N} x_i \sum_{i=1}^{N} y_i}{N\sum_{i=1}^{r} y_i^2 - \left(\sum_{i=1}^{r} y_i\right)^2} = \frac{(12)(+4) - (6)(6)}{(12)(6) - 6^2} = +0.3333$$

and the standardized regression coefficient with variable y the dependent variable is

$$\hat{\beta}_{xy} = b_{xy}\left(\frac{s_x}{s_y}\right) = +0.3333\left(\frac{0.5222}{0.5222}\right) = +0.3333\ .$$

Thus it is demonstrated that $\phi = T = V = r_{xy} = b_{yx} = b_{xy} = \hat{\beta}_{yx} = \hat{\beta}_{xy}$ for a symmetrical 2×2 contingency table.

10.1.4 Leik and Gove's d_N^c Statistic

Leik and Gove's d_N^c test statistic for two nominal-level variables is described in detail in Chap. 4, Sect. 4.9. As noted by Leik and Gove, for symmetrical 2×2 contingency tables, d_N^c is equivalent to the traditional chi-squared-based measures such as Pearson's ϕ^2, Tschuprov's T^2, and Cramér's V^2 [15, p. 291]. Test statistic d_N^c is based on three $r\times c$ contingency tables: one $r\times c$ contingency table containing the observed cell frequency values, a second $r\times c$ contingency table containing the expected cell frequency values, and a third $r\times c$ contingency table containing the maximized cell frequency values. Here, the observed values of concordant pairs, C; discordant pairs, D; pairs tied on variable x, T_x; pairs tied on variable y, T_y; and pairs tied on both variables x and y, T_{xy}, are indicated without primes, the expected values of concordant pairs, C; discordant pairs, D; pairs tied on variable x, T_x; pairs tied on variable y, T_y; and pairs tied on both variables x and y, T_{xy}, are indicated with a single prime ($'$), and the maximized values of concordant pairs, C; discordant pairs, D; pairs tied on variable x, T_x; pairs tied on variable y, T_y; and pairs tied on both variables x and y, T_{xy}, are indicated with double primes ($''$).

Consider d_N^c for a symmetrical 2×2 contingency table, where

$$d_N^c = \frac{T_y' - T_y}{T_y' - T_y''} = \frac{T_x' - T_x}{t_x' - T_x''} = \frac{T_{xy}' - T_{xy}}{T_{xy}' - T_{xy}''} = \frac{(C' + D') - (C + D)}{(C' + D') - (C'' + D'')}\ .$$

Table 10.4 Observed values for a 2×2 contingency table with categories dummy-coded 0 and 1

	y		
x	0	1	Total
0	4	2	6
1	2	4	6
Total	6	6	12

For the observed data given in Table 10.2 on p. 578, replicated in Table 10.4 for convenience, the observed values of C, D, T_x, T_y, and T_{xy} are

$$\begin{aligned}
C &= ad = (4)(4) = 16\,,\\
D &= bc = (2)(2) = 4\,,\\
T_x &= ab + cd = (4)(2) + (2)(4) = 16\,,\\
T_y &= ac + bd = (4)(2) + (2)(4) = 16\,,\\
T_{xy} &= \frac{1}{2}\big[(a)(a-1) + (b)(b-1) + (c)(c-1) + (d)(d-1)\big]\\
&= \frac{1}{2}\big[(4)(3) + (2)(1) + (2)(1) + (4)(3)\big] = 14\,,
\end{aligned}$$

and

$$\begin{aligned}
C + D + T_x + T_y + T_{xy} &= 16 + 4 + 16 + 16 + 14\\
&= \frac{N(N-1)}{2} = \frac{12(12-1)}{2} = 66\,.
\end{aligned}$$

Next, consider the expected values for the observed data in Table 10.4, given in Table 10.5, where

$$E_{11} = E_{12} = E_{21} = E_{22} = \frac{(6)(6)}{12} = 3\,.$$

Table 10.5 Expected values for the 2×2 contingency table data in Table 10.4

	y		
x	0	1	Total
0	3	3	6
1	3	3	6
Total	6	6	12

For the expected cell values given in Table 10.5,

$$C' = ad = (3)(3) = 9 ,$$

$$D' = bc = (3)(3) = 9 ,$$

$$T_x' = ab + cd = (3)(3) + (3)(3) = 18 ,$$

$$T_y' = ac + bd = (3)(3) + (3)(3) = 18 ,$$

$$T_{xy}' = \frac{1}{2}\big[(a)(a-1) + (b)(b-1) + (c)(c-1) + (d)(d-1)\big]$$

$$= \frac{1}{2}\big[(3)(2) + (3)(2) + (3)(2) + (3)(2)\big] = 12 ,$$

and

$$C' + D' + T_x' + T_y' + T_{xy}' = 9 + 9 + 18 + 18 + 12$$

$$= \frac{N(N-1)}{2} = \frac{12(12-1)}{2} = 66 .$$

Finally, consider the maximized cell frequencies for the data in Table 10.4, given in Table 10.6. For the maximized values given in Table 10.6,

$$C'' = ad = (6)(6) = 36 ,$$

$$D'' = bc = (0)(0) = 0 ,$$

$$T_x'' = ab + cd = (6)(0) + (0)(6) = 0 ,$$

$$T_y'' = ac + bd = (6)(0) + (0)(6) = 0 ,$$

$$T_{xy}'' = \frac{1}{2}\big[(a)(a-1) + (b)(b-1) + (c)(c-1) + (d)(d-1)\big]$$

$$= \frac{1}{2}\big[(6)(5) + (6)(5)\big] = 30 ,$$

Table 10.6 Maximized values for the 2×2 contingency table data in Table 10.4

	y		
x	0	1	Total
0	6	0	6
1	0	6	6
Total	6	6	12

and

$$C'' + D'' + T_x'' + T_y'' + T_{xy}'' = 36 + 0 + 0 + 0 + 30$$
$$= \frac{N(N-1)}{2} = \frac{12(12-1)}{2} = 66 \; .$$

Then, Leik and Gove's d_N^c measure is

$$d_N^c = \frac{T_y' - T_y}{T_y' - T_y''} = \frac{18-16}{18-0} = 0.1111 \; ,$$

or

$$d_N^c = \frac{T_x' - T_x}{T_x' - T_x''} = \frac{18-16}{18-0} = 0.1111 \; ,$$

or

$$d_N^c = \frac{T_{xy}' - T_{xy}}{T_{xy}' - T_{xy}''} = \frac{12-14}{12-30} = 0.1111 \; ,$$

or

$$d_N^c = \frac{(C' + D') - (C + D)}{(C' + D') - (C'' + D'')} = \frac{(9+9) - (16+4)}{(9+9) - (36-0)} = 0.1111 \; .$$

Thus it is demonstrated that $\phi^2 = T^2 = V^2 = r_{xy}^2 = d_N^c$ for a symmetrical 2×2 contingency table.

10.1.5 Goodman and Kruskal's t_a and t_b Statistics

Goodman and Kruskal's t_a and t_b measures of nominal association are discussed in Chap. 4, Sect. 4.3. Consider the notation for a 2×2 contingency table given in Table 10.7. For the frequency data given in Table 10.4 on p. 582, Goodman and Kruskal's asymmetric measure of association with variable a the dependent

Table 10.7 Notation for a 2×2 contingency data for variables a and b with dummy (0, 1) coding

	a		
b	0	1	Total
0	n_{11}	n_{12}	$n_{1.}$
1	n_{21}	n_{22}	$n_{2.}$
Total	$n_{.1}$	$n_{.2}$	N

variable is

$$t_a = \frac{N \sum_{j=1}^{c} \sum_{i=1}^{r} \frac{n_{ij}^2}{n_{.j}} - \sum_{i=1}^{r} n_{i.}^2}{N^2 - \sum_{i=1}^{r} n_{i.}^2}$$

$$= \frac{12 \left(\frac{4^2 + 2^2 + 2^2 + 4^2}{6} \right) - 6^2 - 6^2}{12^2 - 6^2 - 6^2} = 0.1111$$

and Goodman and Kruskal's asymmetric measure with variable b the dependent variable is

$$t_b = \frac{N \sum_{i=1}^{r} \sum_{j=1}^{c} \frac{n_{ij}^2}{n_{i.}} - \sum_{j=1}^{c} n_{.j}^2}{N^2 - \sum_{j=1}^{c} n_{.j}^2}$$

$$= \frac{12 \left(\frac{4^2 + 2^2 + 2^2 + 4^2}{6} \right) - 6^2 - 6^2}{12^2 - 6^2 - 6^2} = 0.1111 .$$

10.1.6 Kendall's τ_b Statistic

Kendall's τ_b measure of ordinal association is detailed in Chap. 5, Sect. 5.4. For the frequency data given in Table 10.4 on p. 582, the number of concordant pairs is

$$C = ad = (4)(4) = 16 ,$$

the number of discordant pairs is

$$D = bc = (2)(2) = 4 ,$$

the number of pairs tied on variable x but not tied on variable y is

$$T_x = ab + cd = (4)(2) + (2)(4) = 16 ,$$

and the number of pairs tied on variable y but not tied on variable x is

$$T_y = ac + bd = (4)(2) + (2)(4) = 16 .$$

Then, Kendall's τ_b measure is

$$\tau_b = \frac{C - D}{\sqrt{(C + D + T_x)(C + D + T_y)}}$$

$$= \frac{16 - 4}{\sqrt{(16 + 4 + 16)(16 + 4 + 16)}} = +0.3333 .$$

Alternatively, following the notation given in Table 10.1,

$$\tau_b = \frac{ad - bc}{\sqrt{(a + b)(c + d)(a + c)(b + d)}} = \frac{(4)(4) - (2)(2)}{\sqrt{(6)(6)(6)(6)}} = +0.3333 .$$

10.1.7 Stuart's τ_c Statistic

Stuart's τ_c measure of ordinal association is discussed in Chap. 5, Sect. 5.5 and is given by

$$\tau_c = \frac{2mS}{N^2(m - 1)} ,$$

where m is the minimum number of rows or columns. For the frequency data given in Table 10.4 on p. 582, $m = \min(r, c) = \min(2, 2) = 2$, the number of concordant pairs is

$$C = ad = (4)(4) = 16 ,$$

the number of discordant pairs is

$$D = bc = (2)(2) = 4 ,$$

Kendall's S is

$$S = C - D = 16 - 4 = +12 ,$$

and Stuart's τ_c measure is

$$\tau_c = \frac{2mS}{N^2(m - 1)} = \frac{2(2)(+12)}{12^2(2 - 1)} = +0.3333 .$$

10.1.8 Somers' d_{yx} and d_{xy} Statistics

Somers' d_{yx} and d_{xy} asymmetric measures of ordinal association are discussed in Chap. 5, Sect. 5.7. For the frequency data given in Table 10.4 on p. 582, Somers' asymmetric measure of association with variable y the dependent variable is

$$d_{yx} = \frac{C - D}{C + D + T_y} = \frac{16 - 4}{16 + 4 + 16} = +0.3333$$

and Somers' asymmetric measure with variable x the dependent variable is

$$d_{xy} = \frac{C - D}{C + D + T_x} = \frac{16 - 4}{16 + 4 + 16} = +0.3333 \; .$$

Alternatively,

$$d_{yx} = \frac{ad - bc}{(a + c)(b + d)} = \frac{(4)(4) - (2)(2)}{(6)(6)} = +0.3333$$

and

$$d_{xy} = \frac{ad - bc}{(a + b)(c + d)} = \frac{(4)(4) - (2)(2)}{(6)(6)} = +0.3333 \; .$$

10.1.9 Percentage Differences

Percentage differences are discussed in Chap. 9, Sect. 9.10. For the frequency data given in Table 10.4 on p. 582, the percentage difference for variable x is

$$D_x = \left| \frac{a}{a + b} - \frac{c}{c + d} \right| = \left| \frac{4}{6} - \frac{2}{6} \right| = |0.6667 - 0.3333| = 0.3333$$

and the percentage difference for variable y is

$$D_y = \left| \frac{a}{a + c} - \frac{b}{b + d} \right| = \left| \frac{4}{6} - \frac{2}{6} \right| = |0.6667 - 0.3333| = 0.3333 \; .$$

10.1.10 Yule's Y Statistic

Yule's Y measure of nominal association is discussed in Chap. 9, Sect. 9.6. For the frequency data given in Table 10.4 on p. 582, Yule's coefficient of colligation is

$$Y = \frac{\sqrt{ad} - \sqrt{bc}}{\sqrt{ad} + \sqrt{bc}} = \frac{\sqrt{(4)(4)} - \sqrt{(2)(2)}}{\sqrt{(4)(4)} + \sqrt{(2)(2)}} = +0.3333 \, .$$

10.1.11 Cohen's κ Statistic

Cohen's unweighted kappa measure of inter-rater agreement is discussed in Chap. 4, Sect. 4.5, and Cohen's linear and quadratic weighted kappa measures of inter-rater agreement are discussed in Chap. 6, Sect. 6.5. For the frequency data given in Table 10.4 on p. 582, let O_{ii} for $i = 1, 2$ denote the observed cell frequencies on the principal diagonal and E_{ii} for $i = 1, 2$ denote the expected cell frequencies on the principal diagonal. Then, Cohen's unweighted chance-corrected coefficient of inter-rater agreement is

$$\kappa = \frac{\displaystyle\sum_{i=1}^{r} O_{ii} - \sum_{i=1}^{r} E_{ii}}{\displaystyle N - \sum_{i=1}^{r} E_{ii}} = \frac{(4+4) - (3+3)}{12 - (3+3)} = +0.3333 \, .$$

Cohen's weighted kappa measure of inter-rater agreement for $b = 2$ judges and c categories is given by

$$\kappa_w = 1 - \frac{\displaystyle N \sum_{i=1}^{c} \sum_{j=1}^{c} w_{ij} n_{ij}}{\displaystyle \sum_{i=1}^{c} \sum_{j=1}^{c} w_{ij} R_i C_j} \, , \qquad (10.1)$$

where n_{ij} denotes the observed cell frequencies, w_{ij} denotes the cell weights, R_i and C_j denote the observed row and column marginal frequency totals for $i, j = 1, \ldots, c$, and

$$N = \sum_{i=1}^{c} \sum_{j=1}^{c} n_{ij}$$

denotes the table frequency total. For Cohen's unweighted kappa measure of inter-rater agreement, the cell disagreement "weights" are given by

$$w_{ij} = \begin{cases} 0 & \text{if } i = j \,, \\ 1 & \text{otherwise} \,, \end{cases}$$

and for Cohen's weighted kappa measure of inter-rater agreement the cell disagreement weights are given by

$$w_{ij} = \begin{cases} 0 & \text{if } i = j \,, \\ |i - j| & \text{otherwise} \,, \end{cases}$$

for linear weighting, and

$$w_{ij} = \begin{cases} 0 & \text{if } i = j \,, \\ (i - j)^2 & \text{otherwise} \,, \end{cases}$$

for quadratic weighting. For the frequency data given in Table 10.4 on p. 582, Cohen's linear-weighted kappa measure of inter-rater agreement is $\kappa_w = +0.3333$ and Cohen's quadratic-weighted kappa measure of inter-rater agreement is $\kappa_w = +0.3333$.

10.2 Inter-relationships Among the Measures

The inter-relationships among the various measures for a symmetrical 2×2 contingency table can be summarized as follows. The Pearson product-moment correlation coefficient, r_{xy}; the unstandardized slopes of the two regression lines, b_{yx} and b_{xy}; Yule's coefficient of colligation, Y; Pearson's mean-square contingency coefficient, ϕ; Tschuprov's T measure; Cramér's V measure; Kendall's τ_b measure; Stuart's τ_c measure; Somers' d_{yx} and d_{xy} asymmetric measures; the two percentage differences, D_x and D_y; and Cohen's κ unweighted and weighted measures of chance-corrected inter-rater agreement are all equivalent measures, i.e.,

$$r_{xy} = b_{yx} = b_{xy} = Y = \phi = T = V = \tau_b = \tau_c = d_{yx} = d_{xy}$$
$$= D_x = D_y = \kappa = \kappa_w \,.$$

Also, Pearson's squared product-moment correlation coefficient, r_{xy}^2; Pearson's mean-squared contingency coefficient, ϕ^2; Tschuprov's T^2 measure; Cramér's V^2 measure; Leik and Gove's d_N^c measure; and Goodman and Kruskal's t_b and t_a

measures of association are all equivalent measures, i.e.,

$$r_{xy}^2 = \phi^2 = T^2 = V^2 = d_N^c = t_b = t_a \ .$$

10.2.1 Notational Inconsistencies

Measures of association for 2×2 contingency tables in particular, and $r \times c$ contingency tables in general, can be very confusing. First, some measures are denoted by uppercase Latin letters, e.g., Yule's Q and Y, Tschuprov's T^2, and Cramér's V^2; some measures are denoted by lowercase Latin letters, e.g., Somers' d_{yx} and d_{xy}, Leik and Gove's d_N^c, and Goodman and Kruskal's t_a and t_b; and some measures are denoted by lowercase Greek letters, e.g., Pearson's ϕ, Kendall's τ_b, and Cohen's κ. While it would be preferable to reserve Greek letters for population parameters that are being estimated by sample statistics and Latin letters for sample statistics, once symbols are in common use it is difficult to standardize usage.[1] Second, certain measures of association appear as squared, whereas others do not. In particular, for the 2×2 case, the non-squared symbols t_b and t_a for Goodman and Kruskal's asymmetric measures of nominal association are equivalent to Pearson's symmetric measures ϕ^2 and r_{xy}^2. Third, some measures norm between 0 and 1 for 2×2 contingency tables, e.g., Goodman and Kruskal's t_a and t_b; others norm between -1 and $+1$, e.g., Kendall's τ_b and Cramér's V; and still others norm between 0 and ∞, e.g., the odds ratio. Finally, some measures identify the two variables as x and y, e.g., Somers' d_{yx} and d_{xy}, while others identify the two variables as a and b, e.g., Kendall's τ_a and τ_b.

10.3 Extended Fourfold Contingency Tables

In some cases, measures of association have been introduced to analyze fourfold tables that have either been extended to analyze a series of 2×2 contingency tables or redesigned to consider multidimensional contingency tables with two categories in each dimension. In this section a small number of such measures are considered, including the Mantel–Haenszel test, McNemar's Q test, Cochran's Q test, Cohen's chance-corrected measure of inter-rater agreement, Fisher's exact probability test for 2×2×2 contingency tables, and tests for interactions in 2×2×2 and 2×2×2×2 contingency tables

[1] It was not too many years ago that while μ_x and σ_x^2 denoted the population mean and variance, respectively, $\hat{\mu}_x$ and $\hat{\sigma}_x^2$ denoted the unbiased sample-estimated population mean and variance. The *American Psychological Association* presently recommends using M for the sample mean instead of the conventional $\bar{x}$.

Table 10.8 General layout of a 3-way contingency table with $r = 2$ rows, $c = 2$ columns, and S strata

Stratum		Column 1	Column 2	Total	Stratum total	Table total
1	Row 1	n_{111}	n_{121}	$n_{1.1}$		
	Row 2	n_{211}	n_{221}	$n_{2.1}$		
	Total	$n_{.11}$	$n_{.21}$		$n_{..1}$	
2	Row 1	n_{112}	n_{122}	$n_{1.2}$		
	Row 2	n_{212}	n_{222}	$n_{2.2}$		
	Total	$n_{.12}$	$n_{.22}$		$n_{..2}$	
⋮	⋮	⋮	⋮	⋮	⋮	
S	Row 1	n_{11S}	n_{12S}	$n_{1.S}$		
	Row 2	n_{21S}	n_{22S}	$n_{2.S}$		
	Total	$n_{.1S}$	$n_{.2S}$		$n_{..S}$	
Row 1 Total		$n_{11.}$	$n_{12.}$	$n_{1..}$		
Row 2 Total		$n_{21.}$	$n_{22.}$	$n_{2..}$		
Column Total		$n_{.1.}$	$n_{.2.}$			
Table Total						$n_{...}$

10.4 The Mantel–Haenszel Test

The Mantel–Haenszel test, developed by Nathan Mantel and William Haenszel in 1959, is a test of significance for S combined $2{\times}2$ contingency tables.[2] Suppose that a treatment is compared with a control in each of S strata, where the outcome is binary: success or failure. Of interest is whether or not the treatment increases the probability of success.

Let n_{ijk} denote the cell frequency for $i, j = 1, 2$ discrete categories and $k = 1, \ldots, S$ discrete strata for a $2{\times}2{\times}S$ contingency table. Table 10.8 illustrates a three-way contingency table with $r = 2$ rows, $c = 2$ columns, and S strata. Denote by a dot $(\cdot)$ the partial sum of all rows, all columns, or all strata, depending on the position of the $(\cdot)$ in the subscript list. If the $(\cdot)$ is in the first subscript position, the sum is over all rows; if the $(\cdot)$ is in the second subscript position, the sum is over all columns; and if the $(\cdot)$ is in the third subscript position, the sum is over all strata. Thus, $n_{i..}$ denotes the marginal frequency total of the ith row, $i = 1, 2$, summed over all columns and strata; $n_{.j.}$ denotes the marginal frequency total of the jth column, $j = 1, 2$, summed over all rows and strata; $n_{..k}$ denotes the marginal frequency total of the kth stratum, $k = 1, \ldots, S$, summed over all rows and columns; and $n_{...}$ denotes the table frequency total. The Mantel–Haenszel statistical model, under the null hypothesis, states that the S $2{\times}2$ contingency tables are independent and the marginal frequency totals for each of the $2{\times}2$ contingency tables are fixed [17].

[2] The test is often called the Cochran–Mantel–Haenszel test as William Cochran presented essentially the same test in an earlier paper [5].

Then, the probability for the n_{11k} frequency of each of the 2×2 contingency tables under the null hypothesis is the hypergeometric point probability value given by

$$p\left(n_{11k}|n_{1.k}, n_{.1k}, n_{..k}\right) = \binom{n_{.1k}}{n_{11k}}\binom{n_{.2k}}{n_{12k}}\binom{n_{..k}}{n_{1.k}}^{-1}$$
$$= \frac{n_{1.k}!\, n_{2.k}!\, n_{.1k}!\, n_{.2k}!}{n_{..k}!\, n_{11k}!\, n_{12k}!\, n_{21k}!\, n_{22k}!}\,, \qquad (10.2)$$

where $n_{..k} = n_{11k} + n_{12k} + n_{21k} + n_{22k}$, $n_{2.k} = n_{..k} - n_{1.k}$, $n_{.2k} = n_{..k} - n_{.1k}$, and $k = 1, \ldots, S$.

The test statistic of interest is given by

$$T = \sum_{k=1}^{S} n_{11k}\,,$$

where the summation is over only one cell since for any 2×2 contingency table with fixed marginal frequency totals the entry in any one cell determines the entries in the remaining three cells.

Under the null hypothesis (H_0) of the model in Eq. (10.2), the mean and variance of test statistic T are given by

$$\mathrm{E}\left[T|H_0\right] = \sum_{k=1}^{S} \frac{n_{1.k}\, n_{.1k}}{n_{..k}}$$

and

$$\mathrm{VAR}\left(T|H_0\right) = \sum_{k=1}^{S} \frac{n_{1.k}\, n_{2.k}\, n_{.1k}\, n_{.2k}}{(n_{..k})^2(n_{..k} - 1)}\,,$$

respectively. The Mantel–Haenszel test statistic, corrected for continuity, is given by

$$M = \frac{\left(\left|T - \mathrm{E}[T|H_0]\right| - \frac{1}{2}\right)^2}{\mathrm{VAR}(T|H_0)}\,.$$

The Mantel–Haenszel test statistic, M, is approximately distributed as Pearson's chi-squared with one degree of freedom as $N \to \infty$.[3]

[3]The symbol M for the Mantel–Haenszel test should not be confused with the symbol M for the number of possible, equally-likely arrangements of the observed data under the Fisher–Pitman permutation model.

10.4.1 Example Analysis

Consider the example data set given in Table 10.9 with $r = 2$ rows, $c = 2$ columns, $S = 3$ strata, and $n_{...} = 74$ total observations. For the data listed in Table 10.9, the observed value of test statistic T is

$$T_o = \sum_{k=1}^{S} n_{11k} = 2 + 2 + 4 = 8.00 ,$$

the expected value of T under the null hypothesis is

$$\mathrm{E}[T|H_0] = \sum_{k=1}^{S} \frac{n_{1.k}\, n_{.1k}}{n_{..k}} = \frac{(3)(7)}{32} + \frac{(4)(4)}{24} + \frac{(5)(5)}{18} = 2.7118 ,$$

the variance of T is

$$\begin{aligned} \mathrm{VAR}\,(T|H_0) &= \sum_{k=1}^{S} \frac{n_{1.k}\, n_{2.k}\, n_{.1k}\, n_{.2k}}{(n_{..k})^2(n_{..k}-1)} \\ &= \frac{(3)(29)(7)(25)}{(32)^2(32-1)} + \frac{(4)(20)(4)(20)}{(24)^2(24-1)} + \frac{(5)(13)(5)(13)}{(18)^2(18-1)} = 1.7272 , \end{aligned}$$

Table 10.9 General layout of a 3-way contingency table with $r = 2$ rows, $c = 2$ columns, and $S = 3$ strata

Stratum		Column 1	Column 2	Total	Stratum total	Table total
1	Row 1	2	1	3		
	Row 2	5	24	29		
	Total	7	25		32	
2	Row 1	2	2	4		
	Row 2	2	18	20		
	Total	4	20		24	
3	Row 1	4	1	5		
	Row 2	1	12	13		
	Total	5	13		18	
Row 1 Total		8	4	12		
Row 2 Total		8	54	62		
Column Total		16	58			
Table Total						74

and the observed Mantel–Haenszel test statistic is

$$M_{\rm o} = \frac{\left(\left|T_{\rm o} - {\rm E}[T|H_0]\right| - \frac{1}{2}\right)^2}{{\rm VAR}(T|H_0)} = \frac{\left(\left|8.00 - 2.7118\right| - \frac{1}{2}\right)^2}{1.7272} = 13.2742\ . \tag{10.3}$$

Mantel and Haenszel's M test statistic is approximately distributed as Pearson's chi-squared with one degree of freedom. For the observed value of $M_{\rm o} = 13.2742$ the approximate chi-squared probability value is $P = 0.2691\times10^{-3}$.

In Eq. (10.3), ${\rm E}[T|H_0]$, ${\rm VAR}(T|H_0)$, and the correction factor, are all invariant under permutation, leaving only variable T. Thus, for the data listed in Table 10.9 the approximate Monte Carlo resampling probability value based on $L = 1{,}000{,}000$ random arrangements of the observed data under the null hypothesis is

$$P(M \geq M_{\rm o}|H_0) = \frac{\text{number of } M \text{ values } \geq M_{\rm o}}{L}$$
$$= P(T \geq T_{\rm o}|H_0) = \frac{\text{number of } T \text{ values } \geq T_{\rm o}}{L} = \frac{2{,}555}{1{,}000{,}000}$$
$$= 0.2555\times10^{-2}\ .$$

10.4.2 Measures of Effect Size

Two types of measures of effect size have been proposed to represent the strength of a treatment effect [32]. One type, designated the d-family, is based on one or more measures of the differences between groups or levels of an independent variable. Representative of the d-family is Cohen's d, which calculates the effect size by the number of standard deviations separating the means of the groups or levels [8]. The second type of measure of effect size, designated the r-family, represents some sort of correlation between the independent variables. Measures in the r-family are typically measures of correlation or association, the most prominent being Pearson's squared product-moment correlation coefficient. Since the Mantel–Haenszel test is based on a $2\times2\times S$ contingency table, the d-family is not applicable.

The r-family measures of effect size contains two types of measures: putative maximum-corrected and chance-corrected. Maximum-corrected measures of effect size standardize the observed test statistic value by the maximum possible value of the test statistic. Maximum-corrected measures of effect size are bounded between 0 and 1 and are interpretable as the proportion of the maximum possible value of the test statistic. On the other hand, chance-corrected measures of effect size standardize the observed test statistic value by the expected value of the test statistic. Chance-corrected measures of effect size can attain a maximum value of $+1$, but may be less than 0 when the test statistic value is less than expected by chance and are interpretable as the proportion above, or below, what is expected by chance. In 2010 Berry, Johnston, and Mielke developed two measures of effect size for the Mantel–Haenszel test statistic: a maximum-corrected and a chance-corrected measure of effect size [2].

Maximum-Corrected Measure of Effect Size

Let M_o and T_o denote the observed values of M and T, respectively. Then, the maximum-corrected measure of effect size is given by M_o divided by the maximum possible value of M. The maximum value of T for an observed $2{\times}2{\times}S$ contingency table is given by

$$T_{\max} = \sum_{k=1}^{S} \min(n_{1.k}, n_{.1k}) ,$$

where $\min(n_{1.k}, n_{.1k})$ is the maximum value of n_{11k} in the kth of S $2{\times}2$ contingency tables. Thus, the maximum value of M is given by

$$M_{\max} = \frac{\left(\left|T_{\max} - \mathrm{E}[T|H_0]\right| - \frac{1}{2}\right)^2}{\mathrm{VAR}(T|H_0)}$$

and the maximum-corrected measure of effect size for M is given by the observed value of M divided by the maximum value of M, i.e.,

$$\mathrm{ES}_{\mathrm{M}} = \frac{M_o}{M_{\max}} .$$

For the frequency data given in Table 10.2 on p. 578, the maximum value of T is

$$T_{\max} = \sum_{k=1}^{S} \min(n_{1.k}, n_{.1k}) = 3 + 4 + 5 = 12.00 ,$$

the maximum value of M is

$$M_{\max} = \frac{\left(\left|T_{\max} - \mathrm{E}[T|H_0]\right| - \frac{1}{2}\right)^2}{\mathrm{VAR}(T|H_0)} = \frac{\left(\left|12.00 - 2.7118\right| - \frac{1}{2}\right)^2}{1.7272} = 44.7162 ,$$

and the maximum-corrected measure of effect size is

$$\mathrm{ES}_{\mathrm{M}} = \frac{M_o}{M_{\max}} = \frac{13.2742}{44.7162} = 0.2969 ,$$

indicating that $M_o = 13.2742$ accounts for approximately 30% of the maximum value of M, given the observed row, column, and stratum marginal frequency distributions, {12, 62}, {16, 58}, and {32, 24, 18}, respectively.

Chance-Corrected Measure of Effect Size

A chance-corrected measure of effect size for the Mantel–Haenszel test may be given by statistic M, standardized by the expected value of M. Thus, the chance-corrected measure is given by

$$\mathrm{ES_C} = \frac{M - \mathrm{E}[M|H_0]}{M_{\max} - \mathrm{E}[M|H_0]} = 1 - \frac{M_{\max} - M}{M_{\max} - 1} ,$$

where $\mathrm{E}[M] = 1$ since the mean of a chi-squared distribution is equal to the degrees of freedom and M is approximately distributed as chi-squared with one degree of freedom. For the frequency data given in Table 10.2, the chance-corrected measure of effect size is

$$\mathrm{ES_C} = 1 - \frac{44.7162 - 13.2742}{44.7162 - 1} = +0.2808 ,$$

indicating that $M_o = 13.2742$ accounts for approximately 28% above what is expected by chance. In general, chance-corrected measures of effect size, such as $\mathrm{ES_C}$, tend to slightly smaller values than maximum-corrected measures, such as $\mathrm{ES_M}$, for the same set of data [2, pp. 398–399].

10.5 Cohen's Kappa Measure

In 1960 Jacob Cohen introduced statistic kappa, an unweighted, chance-corrected measure of inter-rater agreement between two judges for a set of c disjoint, unordered categories [6]. In 1968 Cohen expanded kappa to include weighting for measuring the agreement between two judges for a set of c disjoint, ordered categories [7]. Unweighted kappa is discussed more completely in Chap. 4, Sect. 4.5, and weighted kappa is discussed in detail in Chap. 6, Sect. 6.5. Whereas unweighted kappa for categorical data did not distinguish among magnitudes of disagreement, weighted kappa for ordinal-level data incorporated the magnitude of each disagreement and provided partial credit for disagreements when agreement was not complete [16]. Weighted kappa is easily extended to interval-level data [3]. The usual approach is to assign weights to each disagreement pair with larger weights indicating greater disagreement. In the cases of both, unweighted and weighted kappa, kappa is equal to +1 when perfect agreement between the two judges occurs, 0 when agreement is equal to that expected under independence, and negative when agreement is less than expected by chance. Unweighted kappa and weighted kappa are conventionally designated as κ and κ_w, respectively. Two forms of weighting are popular for weighted kappa: linear weighting, in which category disagreement weights progress outward linearly from the agreement diagonal, and quadratic weighting, in which category disagreement weights progress outward geometrically from the agreement diagonal. In keeping with the theme of this chapter—fourfold contingency tables—κ and κ_w are extended to multiple judges with $c = 2$ categories.

Consider first $b = 2$ judges and $c = 2$ categories. A generalized calculation formula that applies to both unweighted and weighted kappa for $b = 2$ judges and c categories is given by

$$\kappa = 1 - \frac{N \displaystyle\sum_{i=1}^{c} \sum_{j=1}^{c} w_{ij} n_{ij}}{\displaystyle\sum_{i=1}^{c} \sum_{j=1}^{c} w_{ij} R_i C_j}\,, \tag{10.4}$$

where n_{ij} denotes the observed cell frequencies, w_{ij} denotes the cell weights, R_i and C_j denote the observed row and column marginal frequency totals for $i, j = 1, \ldots, c$, and

$$N = \sum_{i=1}^{c} \sum_{j=1}^{c} n_{ij}$$

denotes the table frequency total.

Given a $c \times c$ agreement table with N objects cross-classified by the ratings of two independent judges into c disjoint categories, an exact permutation test generates all M possible, equally-likely arrangements of the N objects in the c^2 cells, while preserving the total number of objects in each category, i.e., the marginal frequency distributions. For each arrangement of cell frequencies with fixed marginal frequency distributions, the kappa statistic, κ, and the exact point probability, $p(n_{ij}|n_{i.}, n_{.j}, N)$, are calculated, where

$$p(n_{ij}|R_i, C_j, N) = \frac{\left(\displaystyle\prod_{i=1}^{c} R_i!\right)\left(\displaystyle\prod_{j=1}^{c} C_j!\right)}{N! \displaystyle\prod_{i=1}^{c} \prod_{j=1}^{c} n_{ij}!}$$

is the conventional hypergeometric probability of a $c \times c$ contingency table.

Let κ_o denote the value of the observed weighted kappa statistic and M denote the total number of distinct cell frequency arrangements of the N objects in the $c \times c$ agreement table, given fixed marginal frequency totals. Then the exact probability value of κ_o under the null hypothesis is given by

$$P(\kappa_o | H_0) = \sum_{k=1}^{M} \Psi(\kappa_k)\, p(n_{ij} | R_i, C_j, N) ,$$

where

$$\Psi(\kappa_k) = \begin{cases} 1 & \text{if } \kappa_k \geq \kappa_o , \\ 0 & \text{otherwise} . \end{cases}$$

When M is very large, exact permutation analyses quickly become impractical and Monte Carlo resampling procedures become necessary. Let L denote a random sample of all M possible values of κ. Then, under the null hypothesis the resampling approximate probability value for the observed value of κ, κ_o is given by

$$P(\kappa_o) = \frac{1}{L} \sum_{l=1}^{L} \Psi_l(\kappa) ,$$

where

$$\Psi_l(\kappa) = \begin{cases} 1 & \text{if } \kappa \geq \kappa_o , \\ 0 & \text{otherwise} . \end{cases}$$

To calculate Cohen's unweighted kappa with Eq. (10.4) on p. 597, the cell disagreement "weights" are given by

$$w_{ij} = \begin{cases} 0 & \text{if } i = j , \\ 1 & \text{otherwise} . \end{cases}$$

To calculate Cohen's weighted kappa with linear weighting, the cell disagreement weights are given by

$$w_{ij} = \begin{cases} 0 & \text{if } i = j , \\ |i - j| & \text{otherwise} . \end{cases}$$

To calculate Cohen's weighted kappa with quadratic weighting, the cell disagreement weights are given by

$$w_{ij} = \begin{cases} 0 & \text{if } i = j \ , \\ (i-j)^2 & \text{otherwise} \ . \end{cases}$$

Thus, as demonstrated, for $b = 2$ judges and $c = 2$ categories, the cell disagreement weights are the same for unweighted kappa (κ) and weighted kappa (κ_w) with either linear or quadratic weighting.

10.5.1 Example 1

To illustrate the application of Cohen's unweighted kappa with $b = 2$ judges and $c = 2$ categories, consider the frequency data given in Table 10.10, where $b = 2$ independent judges have each assigned $N = 123$ observations to $c = 2$ disjoint, unordered categories labeled Pro and Con. Assign the number 1 to the categories labeled "Pro" and the number 2 to the categories labeled "Con." Then following Eq. (10.4) on p. 597,

$$\kappa = 1 - \frac{N \displaystyle\sum_{i=1}^{c} \sum_{j=1}^{c} w_{ij} n_{ij}}{\displaystyle\sum_{i=1}^{c} \sum_{j=1}^{c} w_{ij} R_i C_j}$$

$$= 1 - \frac{123\big[(0)(42) + (1)(23) + (1)(18) + (0)(40)\big]}{(0)(65)(60) + (1)(65)(63) + (1)(58)(60) + (0)(58)(63)}$$

$$= +0.3343 \ ,$$

indicating approximately 33% agreement between the two judges above that expected by chance.

For the frequency data given in Table 10.10, there are only

$$M = \min(a+b, a+c) - \max(0, a-d) + 1$$

$$= \min(65, 60) - \max(0, 42-40) + 1 = 60 - 2 + 1 = 59$$

Table 10.10 Example 2×2 contingency table for $b = 2$ independent judges and $c = 2$ disjoint categories

	Judge 2		
Judge 1	Pro	Con	Total
Pro	42	23	65
Con	18	40	58
Total	60	63	123

possible, equally-likely arrangements in the reference set of all permutations of the cell frequencies in Table 10.10 given the observed row and column marginal frequency distributions, {65, 58} and {60, 63}, respectively, making an exact permutation analysis possible. If the $M = 59$ possible arrangements of the frequency data given in Table 10.10 occur with equal chance, the exact probability value of κ under the null hypothesis is the sum of the hypergeometric point probability values associated with $\kappa = +0.3343$ or greater.

Table 10.11 lists the n_{11} cell frequency values, unweighted kappa values, and associated hypergeometric probability values for the frequency data given in Table 10.10, where the n_{11} cell values associated with κ values equal to or greater

Table 10.11 Listing of the $M = 59$ possible arrangements of cell frequencies, unweighted kappa values, and associated hypergeometric probability values for the data given in Table 10.10

n_{11}	Kappa	Probability	n_{11}	Kappa	Probability
2	−0.9648	0.2825×10^{-32}	32	$+0.9505\times10^{-2}$	0.1425
3	−0.9328	0.3441×10^{-29}	33	$+0.4198\times10^{-1}$	0.1287
4	−0.8998	0.1520×10^{-26}	34	$+0.7446\times10^{-1}$	0.1022
5	−0.8673	0.3462×10^{-24}	35	+0.1069	0.7033×10^{-1}
6	−0.8349	0.4760×10^{-22}	36	+0.1394	0.4370×10^{-1}
7	−0.8024	0.4333×10^{-20}	37	+0.1719	0.2349×10^{-1}
8	−0.7699	0.2775×10^{-18}	38	+0.2044	0.1106×10^{-1}
9	−0.7374	0.1305×10^{-16}	39	+0.2368	0.4552×10^{-2}
10	−0.7049	0.4660×10^{-15}	40	+0.2693	0.1635×10^{-2}
11	−0.6725	0.1295×10^{-13}	41	+0.3018	0.5113×10^{-3}
12	−0.6400	0.2855×10^{-12}	42*	+0.3343	0.1388×10^{-3}
13	−0.6075	0.5078×10^{-11}	43*	+0.3667	0.3259×10^{-4}
14	−0.5750	0.7388×10^{-10}	44*	+0.3992	0.6595×10^{-5}
15	−0.5426	0.8888×10^{-9}	45*	+0.4317	0.1145×10^{-5}
16	−0.5101	0.8928×10^{-7}	46*	+0.4642	0.1697×10^{-6}
17	−0.4776	0.7548×10^{-7}	47*	+0.4966	0.2135×10^{-7}
18	−0.4451	0.5410×10^{-6}	48*	+0.5291	0.2262×10^{-8}
19	−0.4127	0.3306×10^{-5}	49*	+0.5616	0.2004×10^{-9}
20	−0.3802	0.1732×10^{-4}	50*	+0.5941	0.1470×10^{-10}
21	−0.3477	0.7814×10^{-4}	51*	+0.6265	0.8822×10^{-12}
22	−0.3152	0.3047×10^{-3}	52*	+0.6590	0.4275×10^{-13}
23	−0.2828	0.1031×10^{-2}	53*	+0.6915	0.1645×10^{-14}
24	−0.2503	0.3034×10^{-2}	54*	+0.7240	0.4921×10^{-16}
25	−0.2178	0.7788×10^{-2}	55*	+0.7564	0.1114×10^{-17}
26	−0.1853	0.1747×10^{-1}	56*	+0.7889	0.1842×10^{-19}
27	−0.1529	0.3433×10^{-1}	57*	+0.8214	0.2115×10^{-21}
28	−0.1204	0.5913×10^{-1}	58*	+0.8539	0.1563×10^{-23}
29	-0.8792×10^{-1}	0.8941×10^{-1}	59*	+0.8863	0.6507×10^{-26}
30	-0.5545×10^{-1}	0.1188	60*	+0.9188	0.1122×10^{-28}
31	-0.2297×10^{-1}	0.1387			

than the observed value of $\kappa = +0.3343$ are indicated with asterisks. Because there is only one degree of freedom, it is sufficient to list the cell frequency values for only one cell, n_{11}. For the frequency data given in Table 10.10, the exact upper-tail hypergeometric probability value of the observed κ value is

$$P = 0.1388\times10^{-3} + 0.3259\times10^{-4} + \cdots + 0.6507\times10^{-26} + 0.1122\times10^{-28} = 0.1793\times10^{-3}.$$

10.5.2 Example 2

Although weighted and unweighted kappa were originally formulated to compare only two judges, both κ and κ_w can be generalized to accommodate multiple judges [25]. However, with multiple judges an exact permutation analysis becomes impractical except for very small sample sizes; therefore, a Monte Carlo resampling permutation analysis is preferred when analyzing agreement data from multiple judges. The analysis for b multiple judges may be conceptualized as a b-way contingency table with $c = 2$ categories on each axis. Figure 10.1 illustrates a $2\times2\times2$ contingency table with $b = 3$ judges and $c = 2$ disjoint, unordered categories labeled Pro and Con.

To illustrate the application of Cohen's kappa with multiple judges and $c = 2$ disjoint categories, consider the frequency data given in Table 10.12, where $b = 3$ judges have independently assigned $N = 254$ observations to $c = 2$ categories labeled Pro and Con. A generalized calculation formula that applies to

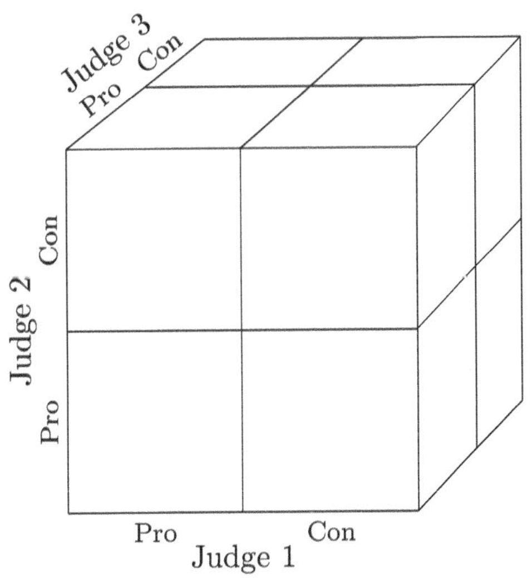

Fig. 10.1 Graphic depiction of a $2\times2\times2$ contingency table with $b = 3$ independent judges and $c = 2$ disjoint categories

Table 10.12 Example 2×2×2 contingency table for $b = 3$ independent judges and $c = 2$ disjoint categories

		Judge 3	
Judge 1	Judge 2	Pro	Con
Pro	Pro	42	23
	Con	18	40
Con	Pro	41	29
	Con	33	28

both unweighted and weighted kappa for $b = 3$ judges and c categories is given by

$$\kappa = 1 - \frac{N^2 \sum_{i=1}^{c} \sum_{j=1}^{c} \sum_{k=1}^{c} w_{ijk} n_{ijk}}{\sum_{i=1}^{c} \sum_{j=1}^{c} \sum_{k=1}^{c} w_{ijk} R_i C_j S_k} , \tag{10.5}$$

where n_{ijk} denotes the observed cell frequencies, w_{ijk} denotes the cell weights, R_i, C_j, and S_k denote the observed row, column, and slice marginal frequency totals for $i, j, k = 1, \ldots, c$, and

$$N = \sum_{i=1}^{c} \sum_{j=1}^{c} \sum_{k=1}^{c} n_{ijk}$$

denotes the table frequency total.

Given a $c{\times}c{\times}c$ agreement table with N objects cross-classified by $b = 3$ independent judges, an exact permutation test involves generating all possible, equally-likely arrangements of the N objects to the c^3 cells, while preserving the observed row, column, and slice marginal frequency distributions, $\{123, 131\}$, $\{135, 119\}$, and $\{134, 120\}$, respectively. For each arrangement of cell frequencies, the kappa statistic, κ, and the exact hypergeometric point probability value under the null hypothesis, $p(n_{ijk}|R_i, C_j, S_k, N)$, are calculated, where

$$p(n_{ijk}|R_i, C_j, S_k, N) = \frac{\left(\prod_{i=1}^{c} R_i!\right)\left(\prod_{j=1}^{c} C_j!\right)\left(\prod_{k=1}^{c} S_k!\right)}{(N!)^2 \prod_{i=1}^{c} \prod_{j=1}^{c} \prod_{k=1}^{c} n_{ijk}!}$$

[20].

If κ_o denotes the value of the observed kappa test statistic, the exact probability value of κ_o under the null hypothesis is given by

$$P(\kappa_o|H_0) = \sum_{l=1}^{M} \Psi_l\left(n_{ijk}|R_i, C_j, S_k, N\right) ,$$

where

$$\Psi_l\left(n_{ijk}|R_i, C_j, S_k, N\right) = \begin{cases} p(n_{ijk}|R_i, C_j, S_k, N) & \text{if } \kappa \geq \kappa_o , \\ 0 & \text{otherwise} , \end{cases}$$

and M denotes the total number of possible, equally-likely arrangements in the reference set of all permutations of cell frequencies in Table 10.12 given the observed marginal frequency distributions. When M is very large, as is typical with multi-way contingency tables, exact tests are impractical and Monte Carlo resampling becomes necessary, where a random sample, L, of the M possible arrangements of cell frequencies provides for a comparison of κ test statistics calculated on the L random tables with the κ test statistic calculated on the observed table.

Unweighted Kappa

Unweighted kappa and weighted kappa, with either linear or quadratic weighting, yield the same result when analyzing agreement data for $b = 2$ judges and $c = 2$ categories. For $b > 2$ judges and $c = 2$ categories, unweighted kappa and weighted kappa usually yield different results, but weighted kappa with linear weighting and weighted kappa with quadratic weighting yield the same result. For the frequency data given in Table 10.12, assign the number 1 to the categories labeled "Pro" and the number 2 to the categories labeled "Con." Then the cell disagreement "weights" for unweighted kappa are given by

$$w_{ijk} = \begin{cases} 0 & \text{if } i = j = k , \\ 1 & \text{otherwise} . \end{cases}$$

Following Eq. (10.5) on p. 602, Cohen's unweighted kappa coefficient is $\kappa = +0.1862$, indicating approximately 19% agreement among the $b = 3$ judges above that expected by chance. If κ_o denotes the observed value of κ, the approximate Monte Carlo resampling probability value based on $L = 1{,}000{,}000$ random arrangements of the cell frequencies, given the observed row, column, and slice marginal frequency distributions, {123, 131}, {135, 119}, and {134, 120}, respectively, is

$$P(\kappa \geq \kappa_o | H_0) = \frac{\text{number of } \kappa \text{ values } \geq \kappa_o}{L} = \frac{2{,}250}{1{,}000{,}000} = 0.0023 \, .$$

Weighted Kappa

For the frequency data given in Table 10.12, assign the number 1 to the categories labeled "Pro" and the number 2 to the categories labeled "Con." Then the linear cell disagreement weights are given by

$$w_{ijk} = |i - j| + |i - k| + |j - k|$$

and the quadratic cell disagreement weights are given by

$$w_{ijk} = (i - j)^2 + (i - k)^2 + (j - k)^2$$

for $i, j, k = 1, \ldots, c$. Table 10.13 lists the eight cell indices and the associated linear and quadratic weights for a 2×2×2 agreement table, demonstrating that with $c = 2$ categories, the linear and quadratic weights are identical.

Following Eq. (10.5) on p. 602, Cohen's weighted kappa with linear weighting is $\kappa_w = +0.0342$, indicating approximately 3% agreement among the $b = 3$ judges above that expected by chance. If κ_o denotes the observed value of κ_w, the approximate Monte Carlo resampling probability value based on $L = 1{,}000{,}000$ random arrangements of the cell frequencies, given the observed row, column, and slice marginal frequency distributions, {123, 131}, {135, 119}, and {134, 120}, respectively, is

$$P(\kappa_w \geq \kappa_o | H_0) = \frac{\text{number of } \kappa_w \text{ values } \geq \kappa_o}{L} = \frac{190{,}610}{1{,}000{,}000} = 0.1906 \, .$$

Table 10.13 Cells, linear weights, and quadratic weights for $b = 3$ independent judges and $c = 2$ disjoint categories

	Weight	
Cell	Linear	Quadratic
111	0	0
112	2	2
121	2	2
122	2	2
211	2	2
212	2	2
221	2	2
222	0	0

Because with $c = 2$ categories the linear and quadratic weights are the same, the results are identical with quadratic weighting, i.e., $\kappa_w = +0.0342$ and $P = 0.1906$.

10.5.3 Example 3

For this third example of Cohen's chance-corrected measure of inter-rater agreement, consider $b = 4$ judges who independently assign $N = 76$ observations to $c = 2$ disjoint, unordered categories labeled Pro and Con. The frequency data are given in Table 10.14.

A generalized calculation formula that applies to both unweighted and weighted kappa for $b = 4$ judges and c categories is given by

$$\kappa = 1 - \frac{N^3 \displaystyle\sum_{i=1}^{c} \sum_{j=1}^{c} \sum_{k=1}^{c} \sum_{l=1}^{c} w_{ijkl} n_{ijkl}}{\displaystyle\sum_{i=1}^{c} \sum_{j=1}^{c} \sum_{k=1}^{c} \sum_{l=1}^{c} w_{ijkl} R_i C_j S_k L_l}, \tag{10.6}$$

where n_{ijkl} denotes the observed cell frequencies, w_{ijkl} denotes the cell weights, R_i, C_j, S_k, and L_l denote the observed row, column, slice, and level marginal frequency totals for $i, j, k, l = 1, \ldots, c$, and

$$N = \sum_{i=1}^{c} \sum_{j=1}^{c} \sum_{k=1}^{c} \sum_{l=1}^{c} n_{ijkl}$$

denotes the table frequency total.

Given a $c \times c \times c \times c$ agreement table with N objects cross-classified by $b = 4$ independent judges, an exact permutation test involves generating all possible, equally-likely arrangements of the N objects to the c^4 cells, while preserving the

Table 10.14 Example $2 \times 2 \times 2 \times 2$ contingency table for $b = 4$ independent judges and $c = 2$ disjoint categories

			Judge 4	
Judge 1	Judge 2	Judge 3	Pro	Con
Pro	Pro	Pro	5	2
		Con	4	1
	Con	Pro	7	3
		Con	9	2
Con	Pro	Pro	8	4
		Con	1	9
	Con	Pro	7	3
		Con	3	8

observed row, column, slice, and level marginal frequency distributions, $\{33, 43\}$, $\{34, 42\}$, $\{39, 37\}$, and $\{44, 32\}$, respectively. For each arrangement of cell frequencies, the kappa statistic, κ, and the exact hypergeometric point probability value under the null hypothesis, $p(n_{ijkl}|R_i, C_j, S_k, L_l, N)$, are calculated, where

$$p(n_{ijkl}|R_i, C_j, S_k, L_l, N) = \frac{\left(\prod_{i=1}^{c} R_i!\right)\left(\prod_{j=1}^{c} C_j!\right)\left(\prod_{k=1}^{c} S_k!\right)\left(\prod_{l=1}^{c} L_l!\right)}{(N!)^3 \prod_{i=1}^{c}\prod_{j=1}^{c}\prod_{k=1}^{c}\prod_{l=1}^{c} n_{ijkl}!}$$

[20].

If κ_o denotes the value of the observed kappa test statistic, the exact probability value of κ_o under the null hypothesis is given by

$$P(\kappa_o|H_0) = \sum_{l=1}^{M} \Psi_l\left(n_{ijkl}|R_i, C_j, S_k, L_l, N\right) ,$$

where

$$\Psi_l\left(n_{ijkl}|R_i, C_j, S_k, L_l, N\right) = \begin{cases} p(n_{ijkl}|R_i, C_j, S_k, L_l, N) & \text{if } \kappa \geq \kappa_o , \\ 0 & \text{otherwise} , \end{cases}$$

and M denotes the total number of possible, equally-likely arrangements in the reference set of all permutations of cell frequencies in Table 10.14 given the row, column, slice, and level observed marginal frequency distributions, $\{33, 43\}$, $\{34, 42\}$, $\{39, 37\}$, and $\{44, 32\}$, respectively. When M is very large, as is typical with multi-way contingency tables, exact tests are impractical and Monte Carlo resampling becomes necessary, where a random sample, L, of the M possible arrangements of cell frequencies provides for a comparison of κ test statistics calculated on the L random tables with the κ test statistic calculated on the observed table.

Unweighted Kappa

For the frequency data given in Table 10.14, assign the number 1 to the categories labeled "Pro" and the number 2 to the categories labeled "Con." Then the cell disagreement "weights" for unweighted kappa are given by

$$w_{ijkl} = \begin{cases} 0 & \text{if } i = j = k = l , \\ 1 & \text{otherwise} . \end{cases}$$

Following Eq. (10.6) on p. 605, Cohen's unweighted kappa coefficient is $\kappa = +0.0561$, indicating approximately 6% agreement among the $b = 4$ judges above that expected by chance. If κ_o denotes the observed value of κ, the approximate Monte Carlo resampling probability value based on $L = 1{,}000{,}000$ random arrangements of the cell frequencies, given the observed marginal frequency distributions, is

$$P(\kappa \geq \kappa_o | H_0) = \frac{\text{number of } \kappa \text{ values } \geq \kappa_o}{L} = \frac{9{,}475}{1{,}000{,}000} = 0.0095 .$$

Weighted Kappa

For the frequency data given in Table 10.14, assign the number 1 to the categories labeled "Pro" and the number 2 to the categories labeled "Con." Then the linear cell disagreement weights are given by

$$w_{ijkl} = |i - j| + |i - k| + |i - l| + |j - k| + |j - l| + |k - l|$$

and the quadratic cell disagreement weights are given by

$$w_{ijkl} = (i - j)^2 + (i - k)^2 + (i - l)^2 + (j - k)^2 + (j - l)^2 + (k - l)^2$$

for $i, j, k, l = 1, \ldots, c$.

Table 10.15 lists the 16 cell indices and the associated linear and quadratic weights for a 2×2×2×2 agreement table. Note that for $c = 2$ categories, the linear and quadratic weights are identical.

Table 10.15 Cells, linear weights, and quadratic weights for $b = 4$ independent judges and $c = 2$ disjoint categories

	Weight	
Cell	Linear	Quadratic
1111	0	0
1112	3	3
1121	3	3
1122	4	4
1211	3	3
1212	4	4
1221	4	4
1222	3	3
2111	3	3
2112	4	4
2121	4	4
2122	3	3
2211	4	4
2212	3	3
2221	3	3
2222	0	0

Following Eq. (10.6) on p. 605, Cohen's weighted kappa with linear weighting is $\kappa_w = +0.0654$, indicating approximately 7% agreement among the $b = 4$ judges above that expected by chance. If κ_o denotes the observed value of κ_w, the approximate Monte Carlo resampling probability value based on $L = 1{,}000{,}000$ random arrangements of the cell frequencies, given the observed row, column, slice, and level marginal frequency distributions, {33, 43}, {34, 42}, {39, 37}, and {44, 32}, respectively, is

$$P(\kappa_w \geq \kappa_o | H_0) = \frac{\text{number of } \kappa_w \text{ values } \geq \kappa_o}{L} = \frac{3{,}967}{1{,}000{,}000} = 0.0040 \, .$$

Because, with $c = 2$ categories, the linear and quadratic weights are the same, the results are identical to those obtained with quadratic weighting, i.e., $\kappa_w = +0.0654$ and $P = 0.0040$.

10.6 McNemar's and Cochran's *Q* Tests for Change

In 1947 Quinn McNemar proposed a test for change over $k = 2$ time periods [18]. In 1950 William Cochran developed a test for change for $k \geq 2$ time periods [4]. For $k = 2$, Cochran's Q test for related proportions is identical to McNemar's Q test for related proportions. The McNemar and Cochran Q tests are described in detail in Chap. 4, Sects. 4.6 and 4.7, respectively.

10.6.1 McNemar's Q Test for Change

Represent a 2×2 contingency table as in Table 10.16. Then, McNemar's test for change is given by

$$Q = \frac{(B - C)^2}{B + C} \, ,$$

where B and C represent the two cells of change, i.e., Pro to Con and Con to Pro.

Table 10.16 Notation for a 2×2 cross-classification for McNemar's test for change

	Time 2		
Time 1	Pro	Con	Total
Pro	A	B	$A + B$
Con	C	D	$C + D$
Total	$A + C$	$B + D$	N

Illustration

To illustrate the calculation of probability values for McNemar's Q test for change, consider the frequency data given in Table 10.17, where $N = 9$ subjects have been recorded as either Pro or Con on a specified issue at Time 1 and again on the same issue at Time 2. For the frequency data given in Table 10.17, the observed value of McNemar's Q test statistic is

$$Q = \frac{(B - C)^2}{B + C} = \frac{(5 - 1)^2}{5 + 1} = 2.6667 \; .$$

The exact probability value of an observed value of Q, under the null hypothesis, is given by the sum of the hypergeometric point probability values associated with the Q values equal to or greater than the observed value of Q. For the frequency data given in Table 10.17, there are only

$$\begin{aligned} M &= \min(A + B, A + C) - \max(0, A - D) + 1 \\ &= \min(7, 3) - \max(0, 2 - 1) + 1 = 3 - 1 + 1 = 3 \end{aligned}$$

possible, equally-likely arrangements in the reference set of all permutations of cell frequencies given the two cell frequencies of change, 5 and 1, and only two Q values are equal to or greater than the observed value of $Q = 2.6667$. The exact upper-tail probability of the observed Q value is $P = 0.9167$, i.e., the sum of the hypergeometric point probability values associated with values of $Q = 2.6667$ or greater.

More specifically, Table 10.18 displays the complete reference set of three possible 2×2 contingency tables given the row and column marginal frequency distributions, {7, 2} and {3, 6}, respectively. For Table A in Table 10.18, $Q = 2.0000$ and the associated hypergeometric point probability value is $p = 0.0833$. For

Table 10.17 Example frequency data for McNemar's test for change with $N = 9$ subjects

	Time 2		
Time 1	Pro	Con	Total
Pro	2	5	7
Con	1	1	2
Total	3	6	9

Table 10.18 Three possible cell arrangements given the marginal frequency distributions {7, 2} and {3, 6}, Q values, and hypergeometric point probability values

Table	Frequency		Q	Probability
A	1	6		
	2	0	2.0000	0.0833
B	2	5		
	1	1	2.6667	0.5000
C	3	4		
	0	2	4.0000	0.4167

Table B in Table 10.18, the observed table, $Q = 2.6667$ and the associated hypergeometric point probability value is $p = 0.5000$. And for Table C in Table 10.18, $Q = 4.0000$ and the associated hypergeometric point probability value is $p = 0.4167$. Thus, the cumulative hypergeometric probability value for $Q = 2.6667$ is the sum of the hypergeometric point probability values associated with values of $Q = 2.6667$ or greater; in this case, the probability values associated with $Q = 2.6667$ and $Q = 4.0000$, i.e., $P = 0.5000 + 0.4167 = 0.9167$.

McNemar's Q test statistic is approximately distributed as chi-squared with 1 degree of freedom. While no responsible researcher would knowingly fit a chi-squared distribution function to only three possible outcomes, small samples, such as in Table 10.17, sometimes occur inadvertently. Suppose a researcher is employed by a national food service provider and begins with a reasonable, but small sample of subjects. As the research analysis proceeds, an interest develops in a subset of subjects composed of only women, breast-feeding their first child, and residing on a Native American reservation. Such unplanned small samples are relatively common and are not suitable for a conventional analysis. The chi-squared value for the observed data in Table 10.17 is $\chi^2 = 0.3214$ and the probability value is $P = 0.5708$, which, as expected, is far removed from the exact probability value of $P = 0.9167$.

Example

A more realistic example illustrating McNemar's Q test for change is given in Table 10.19, where $N = 70$ subjects were recorded as either Pro or Con on a specified issue at Time 1 and again on the same issue at Time 2. At Time 1, 40 of the 70 subjects were in favor of the issue and 30 subjects were opposed. At Time 2, 50 subjects were in favor and 20 were opposed. Of those subjects that changed, seven changed from Pro to Con and 17 changed from Con to Pro. For the frequency data given in Table 10.19, McNemar's test statistic is

$$Q = \frac{(B - C)^2}{B + C} = \frac{(7 - 17)^2}{7 + 17} = \frac{100}{24} = 4.1667\,.$$

Table 10.19 Example frequency data for McNemar's test for change with $N = 70$ subjects

	Time 2		
Time 1	Pro	Con	Total
Pro	33	7	40
Con	17	13	30
Total	50	20	70

For the frequency data given in Table 10.19, there are only

$$M = \min(A + B, A + C) - \max(0, A - D) + 1$$
$$= \min(40, 50) - \max(0, 33 - 13) + 1 = 40 - 20 + 1 = 21$$

possible, equally-likely arrangements in the reference set of all permutations of cell frequencies given the observed row and column marginal frequency distributions, {40, 30} and {50, 20}, respectively, making an exact permutation analysis possible. Since $M = 21$ is a reasonably small number of arrangements, it will be illustrative to list the 21 sets of cell frequencies, McNemar's Q values, and the associated hypergeometric point probability values in Table 10.20, where the rows with hypergeometric probability values associated with Q values equal to or greater than the observed value of $Q = 4.1667$ are indicated with asterisks.

If the $M = 21$ possible arrangements of the frequency data given in Table 10.19 occur with equal chance, the exact probability of Q under the null hypothesis is the sum of the hypergeometric point probability values associated with $Q = 4.1667$ or greater. For the frequency data given in Table 10.19, the exact upper-tail probability

Table 10.20 Cell frequencies, McNemar's Q values, and exact hypergeometric point probability values for $M = 21$ possible arrangements of the observed data in Table 10.19

	Cell frequencies					
Table	n_{11}	n_{12}	n_{21}	n_{22}	Q	Probability
1	20	20	30	0	2.0000	0.8515×10^{-6}
2	21	19	29	1	2.0833	0.2433×10^{-4}
3	22	18	28	2	2.1739	0.3047×10^{-3}
4	23	17	27	3	2.2727	0.2225×10^{-2}
5	24	16	26	4	2.3809	0.1064×10^{-1}
6	25	15	25	5	2.5000	0.3541×10^{-1}
7	26	14	24	6	2.6316	0.8512×10^{-1}
8	27	13	23	7	2.7778	0.1513
9	28	12	22	8	2.9412	0.2020
10	29	11	21	9	3.1250	0.2043
11	30	10	20	10	3.3333	0.1573
12	31	9	19	11	3.5714	0.9227×10^{-1}
13	32	8	18	12	3.8462	0.4019×10^{-1}
14*	33	7	17	13	4.1667	0.1379×10^{-1}
15*	34	6	16	14	4.5455	0.3448×10^{-2}
16*	35	5	15	15	5.0000	0.6305×10^{-3}
17*	36	4	14	16	5.5556	0.8210×10^{-4}
18*	37	3	13	17	6.2500	0.7309×10^{-5}
19*	38	2	12	18	7.1429	0.4167×10^{-6}
20*	39	1	11	19	8.3333	0.1350×10^{-7}
21*	40	0	10	20	10.0000	0.1856×10^{-9}
Sum						1.0000

of the observed value of Q value is

$$P = 0.1379\times10^{-1} + 0.3448\times10^{-2} + 0.6305\times10^{-3} + 0.8210\times10^{-4} + 0.7309\times10^{-5} + 0.4167\times10^{-6} + 0.1350\times10^{-7} + 0.1856\times10^{-9} = 0.0180\,.$$

For comparison, the value of chi-squared for the frequency data given in Table 10.19 is $\chi^2 = 5.6058$ and with 1 degree of freedom, the probability value is $P = 0.0179$, which compares favorably with the exact probability value of $P = 0.0180$.

10.6.2 Cochran's Q Test for Change

Cochran's Q test for $k \geq 2$ treatments can be considered an extension of McNemar's Q test for $k = 2$ treatments or time periods. Cochran's Q test is described more completely in Chap. 4, Sect. 4.7.

Cochran's Q test for the analysis of k treatment conditions (columns) and N subjects (rows) is given by

$$Q = \frac{(k-1)\left(k\sum_{j=1}^{k} C_j^2 - A^2\right)}{kA - B}\,, \tag{10.7}$$

where

$$C_j = \sum_{i=1}^{N} x_{ij}$$

is the number of 1s in the jth of k columns,

$$R_i = \sum_{j=1}^{k} x_{ij}$$

is the number of 1s in the ith of N rows,

$$A = \sum_{i=1}^{N} R_i\,, \quad B = \sum_{i=1}^{N} R_i^2\,,$$

and x_{ij} denotes the cell entry of either 0 or 1 associated with the ith of N rows and the jth of k columns. The null hypothesis stipulates that each of the

$$M = \prod_{i=1}^{N} \binom{k}{R_i}$$

distinguishable arrangements of 1s and 0s within each of the N rows occurs with equal probability, given that the values of $R_1, \ldots, R_N$ are fixed [21].

Example

To illustrate Cochran's Q test for change, consider the binary data listed in Table 10.21 consisting of the responses (1 or 0) for $N = 9$ subjects evaluated over $k = 3$ time periods, where a 1 indicates success on a prescribed task and a 0 indicates failure. For the binary data listed in Table 10.21,

$$\sum_{j=1}^{k} C_j^2 = 1^2 + 8^2 + 5^2 = 90 ,$$

$$A = \sum_{i=1}^{N} R_i = 2 + 2 + 2 + 2 + 1 + 1 + 1 + 1 + 2 = 14 ,$$

$$B = \sum_{i=1}^{N} R_i^2 = 2^2 + 2^2 + 2^2 + 2^2 + 1^1 + 1^2 + 1^2 + 1^2 + 2^2 = 24 ,$$

Table 10.21 Successes (1) and failures (0) of $N = 9$ subjects on a series of $k = 3$ time periods

	Time			
Subject	1	2	3	R_i
1	0	1	1	2
2	0	1	1	2
3	0	1	1	2
4	0	1	1	2
5	0	1	0	1
6	0	1	0	1
7	1	0	0	1
8	0	1	0	1
9	0	1	1	2
C_j	1	8	5	14

and, following Eq. (10.7) on p. 612, the observed value of Cochran's Q is

$$Q = \frac{(k-1)\left(k\sum_{j=1}^{k} C_j^2 - A^2\right)}{kA - B} = \frac{(3-1)[(3)(90) - 14^2]}{(3)(14) - 24} = 8.2222\,.$$

For the binary data listed in Table 10.21, there are only

$$M = \prod_{i=1}^{N} \binom{k}{R_i} = \binom{3}{1}^4 \binom{3}{2}^5 = (3^4)(3^5) = 19{,}683$$

possible, equally-likely arrangements in the reference set of all permutations of the observed binary data, making an exact permutation analysis feasible. Based on $M = 19{,}683$ arrangements of the observed data, there are 312 Q values equal to or greater than the observed value of $Q = 8.2222$. If Q_o denotes the observed value of Q, the exact upper-tail probability value of the observed data is

$$P\big(Q \geq Q_o | H_0\big) = \frac{\text{number of } Q \text{ values } \geq Q_o}{M} = \frac{312}{19{,}683} = 0.0159\,.$$

For comparison, under the null hypothesis Cochran's Q is approximately distributed as chi-squared with $k-1$ degrees of freedom. The approximate probability of $Q = 8.2222$ with $k-1 = 3-1 = 2$ degrees of freedom is $P = 0.0164$.

10.7 Fisher's Exact Probability Test

Fisher's exact probability test was independently developed by R.A. Fisher, Joseph Irwin, and Frank Yates in the early 1930s [11, 14, 34]. Characteristically, Fisher's exact test is applied to 2×2 contingency tables, but can be generalized and extended to more complex contingency tables. The eponymous exact test for 2×2 tables and several extensions are detailed in Chap. 4, Sects. 4.11 and 4.12. In this chapter on fourfold contingency tables, only 2×2 and 2×2×2 contingency tables are considered.

10.7.1 Analysis of 2×2 Contingency Tables

Consider a 2×2 contingency table containing N cases, where x_o denotes the observed frequency of any cell and r and c represent the row and column marginal frequency totals, respectively, corresponding to x_o. Table 10.22 illustrates the notation for a 2×2 contingency table.

Table 10.22 Example notation for a 2×2 contingency table

	A_1	A_2	Total
B_1	x	$r-x$	r
B_2	$c-x$	$N-r-c+x$	$N-r$
Total	c	$N-c$	N

Table 10.23 Example 2×2 contingency table for Fisher's exact test

	A_1	A_2	Total
B_1	13	2	15
B_2	7	8	15
Total	20	10	30

Given the notation in Table 10.22, Fisher's exact test for 2×2 contingency tables is given by

$$P = \sum_{x=a}^{b} p(x|r, c, N) ,$$

where $a = \max(0, r + c - N)$, $b = \min(r, c)$, and the hypergeometric point probability value is given by

$$p(x|r, c, N) = \binom{c}{x}\binom{N-c}{r-x}\binom{N}{r}^{-1} = \frac{r!\,(N-r)!\,c!\,(N-c)!}{N!\,x!\,(r-x)!\,(N-r-c-x)!} .$$

To illustrate Fisher's exact probability test for a multi-way contingency table, consider the 2×2 contingency table given in Table 10.23 where $x_o = 13$, $r = 15$, $c = 20$, and $N = 30$.

For the frequency data given in Table 10.23, there are only

$$\begin{aligned} M &= \min(r, c) - \max(0, r + c - N) + 1 \\ &= \min(15, 20) - \max(0, 15 + 20 - 30) + 1 = 15 - 5 + 1 = 11 \end{aligned}$$

possible, equally-likely arrangements in the reference set of all permutations of cell frequencies given the observed row and column marginal frequency distributions, {15, 15} and {20, 10}, respectively, making an exact permutation analysis possible. Table 10.24 lists the $M = 11$ possible values of x and associated hypergeometric point probability values to nine decimal places.

The exact probability value is obtained by summing all the hypergeometric point probability values equal to or less than the hypergeometric point probability value of the observed table, indicated with asterisks in Table 10.24. Thus,

$$P = 0.022488756 + 0.002498751 + 0.000099950 = 0.025087457$$

Table 10.24 Probability values for $M = 11$ possible arrangements of cell frequencies in Table 10.23, given the marginal frequency distributions {15, 15} and {20, 10}

x	$p(x\|r, c, N)$
5	0.000099950
6	0.002498751
7	0.022488756
8	0.097451274
9	0.227386307
10	0.300149925
11	0.227386307
12	0.097451274
13*	0.022488756
14*	0.002498751
15*	0.000099950
Total	1.000000000

for the upper tail of the distribution, i.e., the sum of the hypergeometric point probability values associated with $x = 13$, 14, and 15. Since the probability distribution is symmetric in this case, the exact hypergeometric probability value is twice the probability of the upper tail, i.e., $P = 2(0.0251) = 0.0502$.

10.7.2 Analysis of 2×2×2 Contingency Tables

Analyses of multi-way contingency tables are more complex than simple two-way tables; see Chap. 4, Sect. 4.12. For a two-way contingency table the degrees of freedom are given by $df = (r-1)(c-1)$, where r denotes the number of rows and c denotes the number of columns. Thus, in the case of a 2×2 contingency table the degrees of freedom are $(2-1)(2-1) = 1$ and only one cell frequency need be permuted over its range. In the 2×2 example above, the chosen cell (A_1B_1) was designated as x in Table 10.22.

For multi-way contingency tables the degrees of freedom are given by

$$df = \prod_{i=1}^{r} c_i - \sum_{i=1}^{r} (c_i - 1) - 1 ,$$

where r denotes the number of dimensions and c_i denotes the number of categories in each dimension, $i = 1, \ldots, r$ [24, p. 309]. Thus, for a 2×2×2 contingency table with $c = 2$ disjoint categories in each of $r = 3$ dimensions,

$$df = 2^3 - 3(2-1) - 1 = 4 .$$

Consider a 2×2×2 contingency table where n_{ijk} denotes the cell frequency of the ith row, jth column, and kth slice for $i, j, k = 1, 2$. Let $A = n_{1..}$, $B = n_{.1.}$,

$C = n_{..1}$, and $N = n_{...}$ denote the observed marginal frequency totals of the first row, first column, first slice, and entire table, respectively, such that $1 \leq A \leq B \leq C \leq N/2$. Also, let $w = n_{111}$, $x = n_{112}$, $y = n_{121}$, and $z = n_{211}$ denote four cell frequencies of the 2×2×2 contingency table. Then, the probability for any specified w, x, y, and z is given by

$$p(w, x, y, z|A, B, C, N) = \big[A!\,(N-A)!\;B!\,(N-B)!\;C!\,(N-C)!\big] \times \big[(N!)^2\;w!\;x!\;y!\;z!\;(A-w-x-y)!\;(B-w-x-z)!\;(C-w-y-z)!\;(N-A-B-C+2w+x+y+z)!\big]^{-1}$$

[26].

The bounds for w, x, y, and z are

$$0 \leq w \leq M_w\ ,$$

$$0 \leq x \leq M_x\ ,$$

$$0 \leq y \leq M_y\ ,$$

and

$$L_x \leq z \leq M_z\ ,$$

respectively, where $M_w = A$, $M_x = A - w$, $M_y = A - w - x$, $M_z = \min(B - w - x, C - w - y)$, and $L_z = \max(0, A + B + C - N - 2w - x - y)$. If w_o, x_o, y_o, and z_o denote the values of w, x, y, and z in the observed contingency table, then Fisher's exact probability value for a 2×2×2 contingency table is given by

$$P = \sum_{w=0}^{M_w} \sum_{x=0}^{M_x} \sum_{y=0}^{M_y} \sum_{z=L_z}^{M_z} p(w, x, y, z|A, B, C, N)\psi(w, x, y, z)\ ,$$

where

$$\psi(w, x, y, x) = \begin{cases} 1 & \text{if } p(w, x, y, z) \leq p(w_o, x_o, y_o, z_o)\ , \\ 0 & \text{otherwise}\ . \end{cases}$$

To illustrate Fisher's exact probability test, consider the 2×2×2 contingency table given in Table 10.25 where $N = 75$ and the observed values of w, x, y, and z are $w_o = 13$, $x_o = 8$, $y_o = 4$, and $z_o = 18$. For the frequency data given in Table 10.25 there are $M = 77{,}910$ possible arrangements in the reference set of all permutations of cell frequencies given the observed row, column, and

Table 10.25 Example 2×2×2 contingency table for Fisher's exact test

		Judge 3	
Judge 1	Judge 2	Pro	Con
Pro	Pro	13	8
	Con	4	11
Con	Pro	18	5
	Con	9	7

slice marginal distributions, {44, 31}, {44, 31}, and {44, 31}, respectively, making an exact permutation analysis feasible. Fisher's exact probability is the sum of the hypergeometric point probability values equal to or less than the probability value associated with the observed contingency table; in this case, there are 2,991 tables with probability values equal to or less than the probability value of the observed table, i.e., $p = 0.1743 \times 10^{-4}$, yielding $P = 0.0384$.

10.8 Contingency Table Interactions

It is occasionally necessary to test the independence among multiple classification variables, each of which consists of two mutually exclusive classes, e.g., a 2×2×2 or 2^3 contingency table. In this section exact permutation procedures are described for analyzing interactions in 2×2×2 and 2×2×2×2 contingency tables.

10.8.1 Analysis of 2×2×2 Contingency Tables

Mielke, Berry, and Zelterman provided a procedure for determining the exact global probability value obtained from an examination of all possible arrangements of the eight cell frequencies of a 2×2×2 contingency table, conditioned on the observed marginal frequency totals [26]. An alternative approach that is not as computationally intensive and, quite possibly, more fruitful is to examine the first- and second-order interactions of a 2×2×2 table when the observed marginal frequency totals are considered to be fixed [22]. This approach was first proposed by Bartlett [1] and has been discussed by Darroch [9, 10], Haber [12, 13], Odoroff [27], Plackett [29], Pomar [30], Simpson [33], and Zachs and Solomon [35]. In this section an algorithm is described that computes the exact probability values of the three first-order (two-variable) interactions and the single second-order (three-variable) interaction.

The logic on which the algorithm is based was apparently first developed by Lambert Adolphe Jacques Quetelet to calculate binomial probability values in 1846 [31]. Beginning with a small arbitrary initial value, a simple recursion procedure generates relative frequency values for all possible 2×2×2 contingency tables, given the observed marginal frequency totals. The desired exact probability value is obtained by summing the relative frequency values equal to or less than the observed relative frequency value and dividing the resultant sum by the unrestricted relative frequency total.

Consider a sample of N independent observations arranged in a 2×2×2 contingency table. Let n_{ijk} denote the observed cell frequency of the ith row, jth column, and kth slice, and let p_{ijk} denote the corresponding cell probability for $i, j, k = 1, 2$. Also let $n_{.jk}$, $n_{i.k}$, $n_{ij.}$, $n_{1..}$, $n_{.j.}$, $n_{..k}$, and $n_{...}$ indicate the observed marginal frequency totals of the 2×2×2 contingency table, and let the corresponding marginals over p_{ijk} be indicated by $p_{.jk}$, $p_{i.k}$, $p_{ij.}$, $p_{1..}$, $p_{.j.}$, $p_{..k}$, and $p_{...}$, respectively, for $i, j, k = 1, 2$. Because the categories are mutually exclusive and exhaustive, $n_{...} = N$ and $p_{...} = 1$.

Let r denote the number of dimensions and c_i denote the number of categories in each dimension, $i = 1, \ldots, r$. Then for a 2×2×2 contingency table there are

$$\prod_{i=1}^{r} c_i - \sum_{i=1}^{r} (c_i - 1) - 1$$
$$= (2)(2)(2) - [(2-1) + (2-1) + (2-1)] - 1 = 8 - 3 - 1 = 4$$

degrees of freedom and, consequently, four interaction terms to be considered: three first-order and one second-order. Following Bartlett, the null hypotheses for the three first-order interactions are

$$H_0\colon p_{.11}p_{.22} = p_{.12}p_{.21} \ ,$$

$$H_0\colon p_{1.1}p_{2.2} = p_{1.2}p_{2.1} \ ,$$

and

$$H_0\colon p_{11.}p_{22.} = p_{12.}p_{21.}$$

[1]. The null hypothesis for the second-order interaction is

$$H_0\colon p_{111}p_{122}p_{212}p_{221} = p_{112}p_{121}p_{211}p_{222}$$

[1, 13, 28].

For simplicity, set $x = n_{111}$, $a = n_{.11}$, $b = n_{1.1}$, $c = n_{11.}$, $A = n_{1..}$, $B = n_{.1.}$, $C = n_{..1}$, and $N = n_{...}$. The point probability of x is given by

$$P(x|a, b, c, A, B, C, N) = \left[A!\,(N-A)!\,B!\,(N-B)!\,C!\,(N-C)!\right]$$
$$\times \left[(N!)^2\,x!\,(a-x)!\,(b-x)!\,(c-x)!\,(A-b-c+x)!\right.$$
$$\left.(B-a-c+x)!\,(C-a-b+x)!\,(N-A-B-C+a+b+c-x)!\right]^{-1} .$$

If $H(k)$, given a, b, c, A, B, C, and N, is a recursively defined positive function, then solving the recursive relation $H(k+1) = H(k) \times g(k)$ yields

$$g(k) = \frac{(a-k)(b-k)(c-k)(N-A-B-C+a+b+c-k)}{(k+1)(A-b-c+k+1)(B-a-c+k+1)(C-a-b+k+1)} ,$$

which may be used to enumerate the distribution of $P(k|a, b, c, A, B, C, N)$, $v \leq k \leq w$, where

$$v = \max(0, b+c-A, a+c-B, a+b-C) ,$$

$$w = \min(a, b, c, N-A-B-C+a+b+c) ,$$

and where $H(v)$ is initially set to some small value, such as 10^{-20}. The total over the completely enumerated distribution may be found by

$$T = \sum_{k=v}^{w} H(k) .$$

The exact second-order interaction probability value is found by

$$P = \sum_{k=v}^{w} \frac{H(k) I_k}{T} ,$$

where

$$I_k = \begin{cases} 1 & \text{if } H(k) \leq H(x), \\ 0 & \text{otherwise} . \end{cases}$$

A 2×2×2 Contingency Table Example

Table 10.26 depicts a 2×2×2 contingency table based on $N = 76$ responses to a question (Yes, No) classified by gender (Female, Male), in two elementary school grades (First, Fourth).

Table 10.26 Cross-classification of yes/no responses, categorized by gender and elementary school grade

	Gender			
	Female		Male	
Grade	Yes	No	Yes	No
First	10	4	2	16
Fourth	6	11	15	12

Table 10.27 provides the cell frequencies for Grade by Gender, conditioned on Response. The first-order interaction probability value associated with the cell frequencies in Table 10.27 is

$$P(a|a+b,a+c,N) = \binom{a+c}{a}\binom{b+d}{b}\binom{N}{a+b}^{-1}$$

$$= \binom{31}{14}\binom{45}{18}\binom{76}{32}^{-1} = \frac{32!\;44!\;31!\;45!}{76!\;14!\;18!\;17!\;27!} = 0.8134\;.$$

Table 10.28 provides the cell frequencies for Gender by Response, conditioned on Grade. The first-order interaction probability value associated with the cell frequencies in Table 10.28 is

$$P(a|a+b,a+c,N) = \binom{a+c}{a}\binom{b+d}{b}\binom{N}{a+b}^{-1}$$

$$= \binom{33}{16}\binom{43}{15}\binom{76}{31}^{-1} = \frac{31!\;45!\;33!\;43!}{76!\;16!\;15!\;17!\;28!} = 0.2496\;.$$

Table 10.29 provides the cell frequencies for Grade by Response, conditioned on Gender The first-order interaction probability value associated with the cell

Table 10.27 Grade by Gender, conditioned on Response

	Gender		
Grade	Female	Male	Total
First	14	18	32
Fourth	17	27	44
Total	31	45	76

Table 10.28 Gender by Response, conditioned on Grade

	Response		
Gender	Yes	No	Total
Female	16	15	31
Male	17	28	45
Total	33	43	76

Table 10.29 Grade by Response, conditioned on Gender

	Response		
Grade	Yes	No	Total
First	12	20	32
Fourth	21	23	44
Total	33	43	76

frequencies in Table 10.29 is

$$P(a|a+b, a+c, N) = \binom{a+c}{a}\binom{b+d}{b}\binom{N}{a+b}^{-1}$$

$$= \binom{33}{12}\binom{43}{20}\binom{76}{32}^{-1} = \frac{32!\ 44!\ 33!\ 43!}{76!\ 12!\ 20!\ 21!\ 23!} = 0.4830\ .$$

The second-order interaction probability value for the frequency data given in Table 10.29 is $P = 0.9036\times10^{-3}$ and the global probability of a table this extreme or more extreme than the observed table in Table 10.29 is $P = 0.4453\times10^{-2}$ [26].

10.8.2 Analysis of 2×2×2×2 Contingency Tables

Utilizing the recursion procedure presented in the previous example, it is possible to analyze a 2×2×2×2 or 2^4 contingency table [23]. The conditional probability value of a 2×2×2×2 contingency table is a special case of the conditional probability of an r-way contingency table as defined in Mielke and Berry [20]. Zelterman, Chan, and Mielke [36] provided an algorithm for the exact global probability value obtained from an examination of all possible arrangements of the 16 cell frequencies of a 2×2×2×2 contingency table, conditioned on the observed marginal frequency totals. An alternative approach is to examine the first-, second-, and third-order interactions in a 2×2×2×2 table when the observed marginal frequency totals are considered to be fixed.

Let r denote the number of dimensions and c_i denote the number of categories in each dimension, $i = 1, \ldots, r$, then for a 2×2×2×2 contingency table there are

$$\prod_{i=1}^{r} c_i - \sum_{i=1}^{r}(c_i - 1) - 1$$

$$= (2)(2)(2)(2) - [(2-1) + (2-1) + (2-1) + (2-1)] - 1$$

$$= 16 - 4 - 1 = 11$$

degrees of freedom and, consequently, 11 interaction terms to be considered: six first-order and four second-order, and one third-order. In this section, a procedure is described for computing the exact probability values of the six first-order (two-variable) interactions, the four second-order (three-variable) interactions, and the single third-order (four-variable) interactions for a 2×2×2×2 contingency table.

Following Mielke [19], let $p_{i_1i_2i_3i_4}$ denote the probability of cell $i_1i_2i_3i_4$ in a 2×2×2×2 contingency table, where the index $i_j = 1$ or 2 for $j = 1, 2, 3, 4$. The six null hypotheses of no first-order interactions for a 2×2×2×2 contingency table are

$$H_0\colon p_{1100}p_{2200} = p_{1200}p_{2100} \ ,$$

$$H_0\colon p_{1010}p_{2020} = p_{1020}p_{2010} \ ,$$

$$H_0\colon p_{1001}p_{2002} = p_{1002}p_{2001} \ ,$$

$$H_0\colon p_{0110}p_{0220} = p_{0120}p_{0210} \ ,$$

$$H_0\colon p_{0101}p_{0202} = p_{0102}p_{0201} \ ,$$

and

$$H_0\colon p_{0011}p_{0022} = p_{0012}p_{0021} \ ,$$

where the usual summation convention is employed. Thus, p_{0101} is the sum over indices i_1 and i_3. The four null hypotheses of no second-order interaction for a 2×2×2×2 contingency table are

$$H_0\colon p_{1110}p_{2210}p_{1220}p_{2120} = p_{1120}p_{2220}p_{1210}p_{2110} \ ,$$

$$H_0\colon p_{1101}p_{2201}p_{1202}p_{2102} = p_{1102}p_{2202}p_{1201}p_{2101} \ ,$$

$$H_0\colon p_{1011}p_{2021}p_{1022}p_{2012} = p_{1012}p_{2022}p_{1021}p_{2011} \ ,$$

and

$$H_0\colon p_{0111}p_{0221}p_{0122}p_{0212} = p_{0112}p_{0222}p_{0121}p_{0211} \ .$$

The null hypothesis of no third-order interaction for a 2×2×2×2 contingency table is given by

$$H_0\colon p_{1111}p_{2211}p_{1221}p_{2121}p_{1122}p_{2222}p_{1212}p_{2112} = p_{1112}p_{2212}p_{1222}p_{2122}p_{1121}p_{2221}p_{1211}p_{2111} \ .$$

Table 10.30 contains data from a 2×2×2×2 contingency table based on $N = 1{,}356$ responses classified on four dichotomous variables: A, B, C, and D. The first-, second-, and third-order interaction exact probability values associated with the data listed in Table 10.30 are given in Table 10.31.

Table 10.30 Example data for a 2×2×2×2 contingency table

Variable				
A	B	C	D	Frequency
1	1	1	1	187
1	1	1	2	15
1	1	2	1	42
1	1	2	2	40
1	2	1	1	256
1	2	1	2	42
1	2	2	1	34
1	2	2	2	62
2	1	1	1	177
2	1	1	2	14
2	1	2	1	30
2	1	2	2	63
2	2	1	1	194
2	2	1	2	27
2	2	2	1	52
2	2	2	2	121
N				1,356

Table 10.31 Interactions and associated exact hypergeometric probability values for the data listed in Table 10.30

Interaction	Probability
A×B	0.3822×10^{-9}
A×C	0.4891×10^{-3}
A×D	0.8690×10^{-4}
B×C	0.2181
B×D	0.5475×10^{-5}
C×D	1.0000
A×B×C	0.4491
A×B×D	0.2792×10^{-1}
A×C×D	0.7999
B×C×D	0.4021×10^{-2}
A×B×C×D	0.6517×10^{-1}

10.9 Coda

Chapter 10 applied exact and Monte Carlo permutation statistical methods to measures of association for symmetrical 2×2 contingency tables. Included in Chap. 10 were discussions of Pearson's ϕ, Tschuprov's T^2, and Cramér's V^2 coefficients of contingency, Pearson's product-moment correlation coefficient, Leik and Gove's d_N^c measure, Goodman and Kruskal's t_a and t_b asymmetric measures of nominal association, Kendall's τ_b and Stuart's τ_c measures of ordinal association, Somers' d_{yx} and d_{xy} asymmetric measures of ordinal association, Yule's Y measure of nominal association, simple percentage differences, and Cohen's unweighted and weighted κ measures of inter-rater agreement.

Chapter 10 concluded with an examination of extensions to multiple 2×2 contingency tables and 2×2×2 contingency tables, including the Mantel–Haenszel test for combined 2×2 contingency tables, Cohen's chance-corrected measure of inter-rater agreement, McNemar's and Cochran's Q tests for change, Fisher's exact test for 2×2×2 and 2×2×2×2 contingency tables, and tests for interactions in 2×2×2 and 2×2×2×2 contingency tables.

References

1. Bartlett, M.S.: Contingency table interactions. Suppl. J. R. Stat. Soc. **2**, 248–252 (1935)
2. Berry, K.J., Johnston, J.E., Mielke, P.W.: Maximum-corrected and chance-corrected measures of effect size for the Mantel–Haenszel test. Psychol. Rep. **107**, 393–401 (2010)
3. Berry, K.J., Mielke, P.W.: A generalization of Cohen's kappa agreement measure to interval measurement and multiple raters. Educ. Psychol. Meas. **48**, 921–933 (1988)
4. Cochran, W.G.: The comparison of percentages in matched samples. Biometrika **37**, 256–266 (1950)
5. Cochran, W.G.: Some methods for strengthening the common χ^2 test. Biometrics **10**, 417–452 (1954)
6. Cohen, J.: A coefficient of agreement for nominal scales. Educ. Psychol. Meas. **20**, 37–46 (1960)
7. Cohen, J.: Weighted kappa: Nominal scale agreement with provision for scaled disagreement or partial credit. Psychol. Bull. **70**, 213–220 (1968)
8. Cohen, J.: Statistical Power Analysis for the Behavioral Sciences, 2nd edn. Erlbaum, Hillsdale, NJ (1988)
9. Darroch, J.N.: Interactions in multi-factor contingency tables. J. R. Stat. Soc. B Meth. **24**, 251–263 (1962)
10. Darroch, J.N.: Multiplicative and additive interaction in contingency tables. Biometrika **61**, 207–214 (1974)
11. Fisher, R.A.: The logic of inductive inference (with discussion). J. R. Stat. Soc. **98**, 39–82 (1935)
12. Haber, M.: Sample sizes for the exact test of "no interaction" in 2×2×2 tables. Biometrics **39**, 493–498 (1983)
13. Haber, M.: A comparison of tests for the hypothesis of no three-factor interaction in 2×2×2 contingency tables. J. Stat. Comp. Sim. **20**, 205–215 (1984)
14. Irwin, J.O.: Tests of significance for differences between percentages based on small numbers. Metron **12**, 83–94 (1935)
15. Leik, R.K., Gove, W.R.: Integrated approach to measuring association. In: Costner, H.L. (ed.) Sociological Methodology, pp. 279–301. Jossey Bass, San Francisco, CA (1971)
16. Maclure, M., Willett, W.C.: Misinterpretation and misuse of the kappa statistic. Am. J. Epidemiol. **126**, 161–169 (1987)
17. Mantel, N., Haenszel, W.: Statistical aspects of the analysis of data from retrospective studies of disease. J. Natl. Cancer I **22**, 719–748 (1959)
18. McNemar, Q.: Note on the sampling error of the differences between correlated proportions and percentages. Psychometrika **12**, 153–157 (1947)
19. Mielke, P.W.: Some exact and nonasymptotic analyses of discrete goodness-of-fit and r-way contingency tables. In: Johnson, N.L., Balakrishnan, N. (eds.) Advances in the Theory and Practice of Statistics: A Volume in Honor of Samuel Kotz, pp. 179–192. Wiley, New York (1997)
20. Mielke, P.W., Berry, K.J.: Cumulant methods for analyzing independence of r-way contingency tables and goodness-of-fit frequency data. Biometrika **75**, 790–793 (1988)

21. Mielke, P.W., Berry, K.J.: Nonasymptotic inferences based on Cochran's Q test. Percept. Motor Skill **81**, 319–322 (1995)
22. Mielke, P.W., Berry, K.J.: Exact probabilities for first-order and second-order interactions in $2 \times 2 \times 2$ contingency tables. Educ. Psychol. Meas. **56**, 843–847 (1996)
23. Mielke, P.W., Berry, K.J.: Exact probabilities for first-order, second-order, and third-order interactions in $2{\times}2{\times}2{\times}2$ contingency tables. Percept. Motor Skill **86**, 760–762 (1998)
24. Mielke, P.W., Berry, K.J.: Permutation Methods: A Distance Function Approach, 2nd edn. Springer–Verlag, New York (2007)
25. Mielke, P.W., Berry, K.J., Johnston, J.E.: Resampling probability values for weighted kappa with multiple raters. Psychol. Rep. **102**, 606–613 (2008)
26. Mielke, P.W., Berry, K.J., Zelterman, D.: Fisher's exact test of mutual independence for $2{\times}2{\times}2$ cross-classification tables. Educ. Psychol. Meas. **54**, 110–114 (1994)
27. Odoroff, C.L.: A comparison of minimum logit chi-square estimation and maximum likelihood estimation in $2{\times}2{\times}2$ and $3{\times}2{\times}2$ contingency tables: Tests for interaction. J. Am. Stat. Assoc. **65**, 1617–1631 (1970)
28. O'Neill, M.E.: A comparison of the additive and multiplicative definitions of second-order interaction in $2{\times}2{\times}2$ contingency tables. J. Stat. Comp. Sim. **15**, 33–50 (1982)
29. Plackett, R.L.: A note on interactions in contingency tables. J. R. Stat. Soc. B Meth. **24**, 162–166 (1962)
30. Pomar, M.I.: Demystifying loglinear analysis: Four ways to assess interaction in a $2{\times}2{\times}2$ table. Sociol. Persp. **27**, 111–135 (1984)
31. Quetelet, L.A.J.: Lettres à S. A. R. le Duc Régnant de Saxe–Cobourg et Gotha, sur la Théorie des Probabilitiés Appliquée aux Sciences Morales et Politiques. Hayez, Bruxelles (1846). [English translation, *Letters Addressed to H.R.H. the Grand Duke of Saxe Coburg and Gotha on the Theory of Probabilities as Applied to the Moral and Political Sciences*, by O.G. Downes and published by Charles & Edwin Layton, London, 1849]
32. Rosenthal, R.: Parametric measures of effect size. In: Cooper, H., Hedges, L.V. (eds.) The Handbook of Research Synthesis, pp. 231–234. Russell Sage, New York (1994)
33. Simpson, E.H.: The interpretation of interaction in contingency tables. J. R. Stat. Soc. B Meth. **13**, 238–241 (1951)
34. Yates, F.: Contingency tables involving small numbers and the χ^2 test. Suppl. J. R. Stat. Soc. **1**, 217–235 (1934)
35. Zachs, S., Solomon, H.: On testing and estimating the interaction between treatments and environmental conditions in binomial experiments: The case of two stations. Commun. Stat. Theor. M **5**, 197–223 (1976)
36. Zelterman, D., Chan, I.S., Mielke, P.W.: Exact tests of significance in higher dimensional tables. Am. Stat. **49**, 357–361 (1995)

Epilogue

The purpose of *The Measurement of Association: A Permutation Approach* is twofold. First, to introduce exact and Monte Carlo resampling permutation statistical methods for obtaining probability values for a variety of measures of association, and second, to complement the authors' previous work on *Permutation Statistical Methods: An Integrated Approach*, which provided a synthesis of a number of tests and measures under a common model given by the generalized Minkowski distance function [2]. While *Permutation Statistical Methods* concentrated on statistical tests of differences, such as two-sample t tests and various analysis of variance designs, *The Measurement of Association* concentrates on statistical measures of relationships, including association, agreement, and correlation.

In particular, two models of statistical inference are described and compared: the conventional population model and the lesser-known permutation model. The population model assumes random sampling from one or more fully specified populations. Under the population model, the level of statistical significance that results from applying a statistical test to the results of an experiment or survey corresponds to the frequency with which the null hypothesis would be rejected in repeated random sampling from a specified population or populations. Because repeated sampling of the specified population(s) is usually impractical, it is assumed that the sampling distribution of test statistics generated under repeated random sampling conforms to an approximating theoretical distribution, such as the normal distribution. The size of a statistical test is the probability under the null hypothesis that repeated outcomes based on random samples of the same size are equal to or more extreme than the observed outcome.

In contrast, the permutation model does not assume random sampling, but is completely data-dependent, relying entirely on the observed data. Thus, a test statistic is computed for the observed data and the observations are then permuted over all possible arrangements of the observed data and the selected test statistic is computed for each arrangement. The proportion of arrangements with test statistic values equal to or more extreme than the observed test statistic yields the exact

K. J. Berry et al., *The Measurement of Association*,
https://doi.org/10.1007/978-3-319-98926-6

probability of the observed test statistic value. When the number of possible arrangements of the observed data is very large, exact permutation methods are impractical and Monte Carlo resampling permutation methods become necessary. Resampling methods generate a random sample of all possible arrangements of the observed data and the resampling probability is the proportion of arrangements with test statistic values equal to or more extreme than the observed test statistic.

Throughout the book, emphasis is on permutation statistical methods, both exact and Monte Carlo resampling methods. Permutation statistical methods have a long history with beginnings in the 1920s and 1930s stemming from the early works of R.A. Fisher, T. Eden and F. Yates, and E.J.G. Pitman [1]. Permutation methods possess several advantages over conventional statistical methods.

1. Permutation statistical methods are entirely data dependent, in that all of the information required for analysis is contained within the observed data set.
2. Permutation statistical methods do not depend on the assumptions associated with traditional parametric tests, such as normality and homogeneity of variance.
3. Permutation statistical methods provide exact probability values based on the discrete permutation distribution of equally-likely test statistic values, rather than an approximate probability value based on a theoretical distribution, such as a normal, chi-squared, t, or F distribution.
4. Although permutation statistical methods are suitable when a random sample is obtained from a specified population, permutation methods are also appropriate for nonrandom samples, such as are common in everyday research.
5. Permutation statistical methods are appropriate for analyzing entire populations, as permutation methods are not predicated on repeated random sampling from a specified population.
6. Permutation statistical methods can be defined for nearly any selected test statistic. Thus, researchers have the option of using a wide variety of statistics, including the majority of conventional statistics utilized in classical statistical approaches.
7. Permutation statistical methods are ideal for small data sets, when hypothetical distribution functions may provide very poor fits.
8. Appropriate permutation statistical methods are highly resistant to extreme values, such as are common in demographic data, e.g., age at first marriage, income, and so on. Consequently, the need for any data transformation is mitigated in the permutation context and in general is not recommended, e.g., square root, logarithmic, arc cosine, and other transformations, including the conversion of raw scores to ranks.
9. Permutation statistical methods provide data-dependent statistical inferences only to the actual experiment or survey that has been analyzed, and are not dependent on knowledge of a super population. On the other hand, if random sampling from a specified population has been accomplished, then permutation tests can provide inferences to the population.

The Measurement of Association is organized around the three traditional levels of measurement, which have typically defined existing measures of association:

nominal (categorical), ordinal (ranked), and interval level measurements. Chapter 1 introduced measures of association, correlation, and agreement. Chapter 2 provided an overview of permutation statistical methods, including exact, Monte Carlo resampling, and moment-approximation permutation methods. Chapter 3 focused on exact and Monte Carlo resampling permutation statistical methods for measures of association designed for two nominal-level (categorical) variables that are based on chi-squared, e.g., Pearson's ϕ^2, Tschuprov's T^2, and Cramér's V^2.

Chapter 4 supplemented Chap. 3 with discussions of exact and Monte Carlo permutation statistical methods for measures of association designed for two nominal-level variables that are not based on chi-squared, e.g., Goodman and Kruskal's λ_a, λ_b, t_a, and t_b measures and Fisher's exact probability test. Chapter 5 presented exact and Monte Carlo permutation statistical methods for measures of association designed for two ordinal-level (ranked) variables that are based on pairwise comparisons of differences, e.g., Kendall's τ_a and τ_b measures and Goodman and Kruskal's γ measure. Chapter 6 supplemented Chap. 5 with discussions of exact and Monte Carlo permutation statistical methods for measures of association designed for two ordinal-level variables that are not based on pairwise comparisons of differences, e.g., Spearman's rank-order correlation coefficient and Bross's ridit analysis.

Chapter 7 focused on exact and Monte Carlo permutation statistical methods for measures of association designed for two interval-level variables, e.g., ordinary least squares (OLS) and least absolute deviation (LAD) correlation and Pearson's intraclass correlation. Chapter 8 examined exact and Monte Carlo permutation statistical methods for measures of association for two variables that are measured at different levels of measurement: nominal-ordinal, nominal-interval, and ordinal-interval, e.g., Freeman's θ, Cureton's rank-biserial correlation coefficient, and Jaspen's multiserial correlation coefficient.

Chapter 9 was confined to exact and Monte Carlo permutation statistical methods for measures of association applied to 2×2 contingency tables, where levels of measurement are less relevant, e.g., Yule's Q and Y measures, Pearson's tetrachoric correlation coefficient, and simple percentage differences, D_x and D_y. Chapter 10 supplemented Chap. 9 with discussions of exact and Monte Carlo permutation statistical methods for measures of association applied to symmetrical 2×2 contingency tables, e.g., Pearson's ϕ coefficient of contingency, Yule's Y measure of nominal association, Goodman and Kruskal's t_a and t_b asymmetric measures of nominal association, Somers' d_{yx} and d_{xy} measures of ordinal association, percentage differences, and Kendall's τ_b measure of ordinal association. Also included in Chap. 10 were extensions to multiple 2×2 contingency tables, including the Mantel–Haenszel test for combined 2×2 contingency tables, Cohen's unweighted and weighted kappa measures of chance-corrected inter-rater agreement, McNemar's and Cochran's Q tests for change, Fisher's exact test for 2×2×2 and 2×2×2×2 contingency tables, and tests for interactions in 2×2×2 and 2×2×2×2 contingency tables.

In this manner, permutation statistical methods, both exact and Monte Carlo resampling, were applied to a wide variety of measures of association at the usual three levels of measurement. The result is a new approach to existing measures that is entirely data-dependent, does not depend on the usual assumptions of normality and homogeneity, is ideal for small samples, and is appropriate for both random and nonrandom samples.

References

1. Berry, K.J., Johnston, J.E., Mielke, P.W.: A Chronicle of Permutation Statistical Methods: 1920–2000 and Beyond. Springer–Verlag, Cham, CH (2014)
2. Berry, K.J., Mielke, P.W., Johnston, J.E.: Permutation Statistical Methods: An Integrated Approach. Springer–Verlag, Cham, CH (2016)

Author Index

An "n" following a page number indicates an entry contained within a footnote on that page, an *italic* number indicates an entry in a table or figure heading, and a page number in Roman type indicates a textural reference.

K. J. Berry et al., *The Measurement of Association*,
https://doi.org/10.1007/978-3-319-98926-6

L

M

Subject Index

A **bold** page number indicates an important or comprehensive entry on that page and a page number in Roman type indicates a textural reference.

K. J. Berry et al., *The Measurement of Association*,
https://doi.org/10.1007/978-3-319-98926-6

R

S

CPSIA information can be obtained
at www.ICGtesting.com
Printed in the USA
LVHW011920121118
596823LV00007B/28/P